CRC SERIES IN NUTRITION AND FOOD

Editor-in-Chief

Miloslav Rechcigl, Jr.

Handbook of Nutritive Value for Processed Food
Volume I: Food for Human Use
Volume II: Animal Feedstuffs

Handbook of Nutritional Requirements in a Functional Context
Volume I: Development and Conditions of Physiologic Stress
Volume II: Hematopoiesis, Metabolic Function, and Resistance to Physical Stress

Handbook of Agricultural Productivity
Volume I: Plant Productivity
Volume II: Animal Productivity

CRC Handbook of Agricultural Productivity

Volume II
Animal Productivity

Miloslav Rechcigl, Jr., Editor

Nutrition Advisor and Director
Interregional Research Staff
Agency for International Development
U.S. Department of State
Bethesda, Maryland

CRC Series in Nutrition and Food
Editor-in-Chief
Miloslav Rechcigl, Jr.

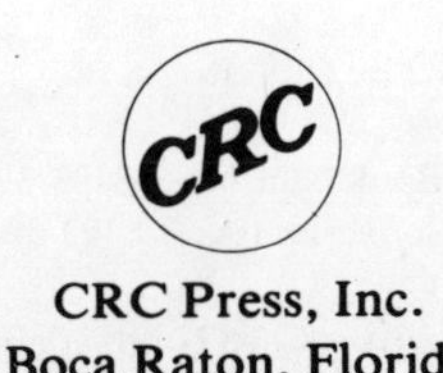

CRC Press, Inc.
Boca Raton, Florida

Library of Congress Cataloging in Publication Data

Main entry under title:

Handbook of agricultural productivity.

(CRC series in nutrition and food)
Bibliography: p.
Includes index.
CONTENTS: v. 1. Plant productivity.—v. 2. Animal productivity.
1. Agricultural productivity. 2. Agriculture.
I. Rechcigl, Miloslav. II. Series.
S494.5.P75H36 631.5 80-15628
ISBN 0-8493-3960-X (set)
ISBN 0-8493-3961-8 (v. 1)
ISBN 0-8493-3963-4 (v. 2)

Direct all inquiries to CRC Press, Inc., 2000 N.W. 24th Street, Boca Raton, Florida 33431.

International Standard Book Number 0-8493-3961-8 (Volume I)
International Standard Book Number 0-8493-3963-4 (Volume II)

Library of Congress Card Number 80-15628
Printed in the United States

PREFACE
CRC SERIES IN NUTRITION AND FOOD

Nutrition means different things to different people, and no other field of endeavor crosses the boundaries of so many different disciplines and abounds with such diverse dimensions. The growth of the field of nutrition, particularly in the last 2 decades, has been phenomenal, the nutritional data being scattered literally in thousands and thousands of not always accessible periodicals and monographs, many of which, furthermore, are not normally identified with nutrition.

To remedy this situation, we have undertaken an ambitious and monumental task of assembling in one publication all the critical data relevant in the field of nutrition.

The *CRC Series in Nutrition and Food* is intended to serve as a ready reference source of current information on experimental and applied human, animal, microbial, and plant nutrition presented in concise tabular, graphical, or narrative form and indexed for ease of use. It is hoped that this projected open-ended multivolume compendium will become for the nutritionist what the *CRC Handbook of Chemistry and Physics* has become for the chemist and physicist.

Apart from supplying specific data, the comprehensive, interdisciplinary, and comparative nature of the *CRC Series in Nutrition and Food* will provide the user with an easy overview of the state of the art, pinpointing the gaps in nutritional knowledge and providing a basis for further research. In addition, the series will enable the researcher to analyze the data in various living systems for commonality or basic differences. On the other hand, an applied scientist or technician will be afforded the opportunity of evaluating a given problem and its solutions from the broadest possible point of view, including the aspects of agronomy, crop science, animal husbandry, aquaculture and fisheries, veterinary medicine, clinical medicine, pathology, parasitology, toxicology, pharmacology, therapeutics, dietetics, food science and technology, physiology, zoology, botany, biochemistry, developmental and cell biology, microbiology, sanitation, pest control, economics, marketing, sociology, anthropology, natural resources, ecology, environmental science, population, law politics, nutritional and food methodology, and others.

To make more facile use of the series, the publication has been organized into separate handbooks of one or more volumes each. In this manner the particular sections of the series can be continuously updated by publishing additional volumes of new data as they become available.

The Editor wishes to thank the numerous contributors many of whom have undertaken their assignment in pioneering spirit, and the Advisory Board members for their continuous counsel and cooperation. Last but not least, he wishes to express his sincere appreciation to the members of the CRC editorial and production staffs, particularly President Bernard J. Starkoff, Earl Starkoff, Sandy Pearlman, Pamela Woodcock, Lisa Levine Eggenberger, John Hunter, and Amy G. Skallerup for their encouragement and support.

We invite comments and criticism regarding format and selection of subject matter, as well as specific suggestions for new data which might be included in subsequent editions. We should also appreciate it if the readers would bring to the attention of the Editor any errors or omissions that might appear in the publication.

Miloslav Rechcigl, Jr.
Editor-in-Chief

PREFACE

HANDBOOK OF AGRICULTURAL PRODUCTIVITY

The greatest challenge of our time is to produce sufficient food to keep pace with the rapidly growing population. In the opinion of experts, during the next 25 years there will be a need for as much food as was produced in the entire history of mankind to date. Of the various measures available, improvement in agricultural productivity is judged as the ultimate means of augmenting food production and supplies.

In this Handbook, an international team of experts consider the most important factors affecting production of both crops and livestock. This Handbook is intended as a scientific guide to practitioners and students, as well as to researchers, who should find here stimulating ideas for further exploration.

THE EDITOR

Miloslav Rechcigl, Jr. is a Nutrition Advisor and Chief of Research and Methodology Division in the Agency for International Development.

He has a B.S. in Biochemistry (1954), a Master of Nutritional Science degree (1955), and a Ph.D. in nutrition, biochemistry, and physiology (1958), all from Cornell University. He was formerly a Research Biochemist in the National Cancer Institute, National Institutes of Health and subsequently served as Special Assistant for Nutrition and Health in the Health Services and Mental Health Administration, U.S. Department of Health, Education and Welfare.

Dr. Rechcigl is a member of some 30 scientific and professional societies, including being a Fellow of the American Association for the Advancement of Science, Fellow of the Washington Academy of Sciences, Fellow of the American Institute of Chemists, and Fellow of the International College of Applied Nutrition. He holds membership in the Cosmos Club, the Honorary Society of Phi Kappa Pi, and the Society of Sigma Xi, and is recipient of numerous honors, including an honorary membership certificate from the International Social Science Honor Society Delta Tau Kappa. In 1969, he was a delegate to the White House Conference on Food, Nutrition, and Health and in 1975 a delegate to the ARPAC Conference on Research to Meet U.S. and World Food Needs. He served as President of the District of Columbia Institute of Chemists and Councillor of the American Institute of Chemists, and currently is a delegate to the Washington Academy of Sciences and a member of the Program Committee of the American Institute of Nutrition.

His bibliography extends over 100 publications including contributions to books, articles in periodicals, and monographs in the fields of nutrition, biochemistry, physiology, pathology, enzymology, molecular biology, agriculture, and international development. Most recently he authored and edited *Nutrition and the World Food Problem* (S. Karger, Basel, 1979), *World Food Problem: a Selective Bibliography of Reviews* (CRC Press, 1975), and *Man, Food and Nutrition: Strategies and Technological Measures for Alleviating the World Food Problem* (CRC Press, 1973) following his earlier pioneering treatise on *Enzyme Synthesis and Degradation in Mammalian Systems* (S. Karger, Basel, 1971), and that on *Microbodies and Related Particles, Morphology, Biochemistry and Physiology* (Academic Press, New York, 1969). Dr. Rechcigl also has initiated a new series on *Comparative Animal Nutrition* and was Associated Editor of *Nutrition Reports International.*

ADVISORY BOARD MEMBERS

ADVISORY BOARD MEMBERS (Continued)

CONTRIBUTORS

M. W. Adams, Ph.D.
Professor of Crop Sciences
Department of Crop and Soil Sciences
Michigan State University
East Lansing, Michigan

Rodney J. Arkley, Ph. D
Soil Morphologist and Lecturer
Department of Plant and Soil Biology
University of California
Berkeley, California

Billy J. Barfield, Ph.D.
Professor of Agricultural Engineering
Department of Agricultural Engineering
University of Kentucky
Lexington, Kentucky

Keith C. Barrons, Ph.D.
Agricultural Consultant
Holmes Beach, Florida

A. Bondi, Ph.D.
Professor of Animal Nutrition and Biochemistry (Emeritus)
Faculty of Agriculture
Hebrew University of Jerusalem
Rehovot, Israel

Eileen Brennan, Ph.D.
Professor of Plant Pathology
Plant Pathology Department
Rutgens University
New Brunswick, New Jersey

M. J. Burridge, Ph.D.
Associate Professor of Epidemiology
College of Veterinary Medicine
University of Florida
Gainesville, Florida

Theodore C. Byerly, Ph.D.
Consultant, Winrock International Livestock Research and Training Center and
Adjunct Professor
University of Maryland
College Park, Maryland

David L. Carter, Ph.D.
Supervisory Soil Scientist
Snake River Conservation Research Center
Kimberly, Idaho

G. I. Christison, Ph.D.
Associate Professor
Department of Animal and Poultry Science
University of Saskatchewan
Saskatoon, Canada

Walter Couto, Ph.D.
Senior Soil Scientist
Tropical Pasture Program
Centro Internacional de Agricultura Tropical
Planaltina, Brazil

Robert J. Collier, Ph.D.
Assistant Professor
Dairy Science Department
University of Florida
Gainesville, Florida

S. H. Crowdy, Ph.D.
Professor
Department of Biology
The University
Southampton, England

S. E. Curtis, Ph.D.
Professor of Animal Science
College of Agriculture
University of Illinois
Urbana, Illinois

R. H. Daines, Ph.D.
Adjunct Professor
Department of Botany and Range Science
Brigham Young University
Provo, Utah

J. B. Derbyshire, Ph.D.
Chairman, Department of Veterinary Microbiology and Immunology
Ontario Veterinary College
University of Guelph
Ontario, Canada

V. Alejandro Deregibus, Ph.D.
Agronomic Engineer
Department of Ecology
Faculty of Agronomy
University of Buenos Aires
Argentina

J. G. Drummond, Ph.D.
Research Microbiologist
Life Sciences Research Division
IIT Research Institute
Chicago, Illinois

C. F. Eagles, Ph.D.
Principal Scientific Officer
Welsh Plant Breeding Station
University College of Wales
Plas Gogerddan near Aberystwyth
England

R. H. Ellis, Ph.D.
Research Fellow
Department of Agriculture and Horticulture
University of Reading
Reading, England

G. LeRoy Hahn
Agricultural Engineer and Technical Advisor for Livestock Environment Research
Roman L. Hruska U.S. Meat Animal Research Center
Science and Education Administration
U.S. Department of Agriculture
Clay Center, Nebraska

A. E. Hall, Ph.D.
Associate Professor of Plant Physiology
Department of Botany and Plant Sciences
University of California
Riverside, California

R. W. F. Hardy, Ph.D.
Director-Life Sciences
Central Research and Development Department
E. I. du Pont de Nemours & Co.
Experimental Station
Wilmington, Delaware

Henry Hellmers, Ph.D
Professor of Botany and Forestry
Department of Botany
Duke University
Durham, North Carolina

Rodney E. Henderson
Research Associate
Agronomy Department
Louisiana State University
Baton Rouge, Louisiana

Donald A. Jameson, Ph.D.
Professor of Range Science
Department of Range Science
Colorado State University
Fort Collins, Colorado

Harold D. Johnson, Ph.D.
Project Leader, Environmental Physiology
Dairy Science Department
University of Missouri-Columbia
Columbia, Missouri

Paul J. Kramer, Ph.D.
James B. Duke Professor of Botany, Emeritus
Department of Botany
Duke University
Durham, North Carolina

Ida Leone
Professor in Plant Pathology
Cook College, Rutgers University
New Brunswick, New Jersey

J. J. Lynch, Ph.D.
Principal Research Scientist
Division of Animal Production
Commonwealth Scientific Industrial Research Organization
Armidale, Australia

James D. McQuigg, Ph.D
McQuigg Consultants, Inc.
Columbia, Missouri

Henry Olivier, C.M.G., Ph.D.
Senior Partner-Consulting Engineer
Henry Olivier and Associates
Johannesburg
South Africa

R. A. Olson, Ph.D.
Professor of Agronomy
University of Nebraska-Lincoln
Lincoln, Nebraska

William H. Patrick, Jr., Ph.D.
Boyd Professor
Marine Sciences Department
Louisiana State University
Baton Rouge, Louisiana

Robert K. Ringer, Ph.D.
Professor of Physiology and Animal Science
Department of Animal Science
College of Agriculture and Natural Resources
Michigan State University
East Lansing, Michigan

E. H. Roberts, Ph.D.
Professor of Crop Production
Department of Agriculture and Horticulture
University of Reading
Reading, England

H. E. Smalley, D. V. M.
Consultant in Veterinary Toxicology
College Station, Texas

Arthur H. Smith
Department of Animal Physiology
University of California, Davis
Davis, California

B. C. Stenning, Esq.
Lecturer in Environmental Control
National College of Agricultural Engineering
Silsoe, Bedford
England

Donald R. Sumner, Ph.D.
Associate Professor of Plant Pathology
Department of Plant Pathology
University of Georgia
Coastal Plain Experimental Station
Tifton, Georgia

Howard M. Taylor, Ph.D.
Supervisory Soil Scientist
Soil and Water Conservation Research Unit
Agricultural Research, Science and Education Administration
U.S. Department of Agriculture
Ames, Iowa

Edward E. Terrell, Ph.D.
Botanist
Plant Taxonomy Laboratory
Plant Genetics and Germplasm Institute
Science and Educational Administration
U.S. Department of Agriculture
Beltsville, Maryland

William W. Thatcher, Ph.D.
Professor (Physiology)
Institute of Food and Agricultural Sciences
Dairy Science Department
University of Florida
Gainesville, Florida

Glover B. Triplett, Jr., Ph.D.
Professor of Agronomy
Ohio Agricultural Research and Development Center
Wooster, Ohio

M. J. Trlica
Associate Professor of Range Science
Range Science Department
Colorado State University
Fort Collins, Colorado

J. D. Turton, D.T.V.M.
Director, Commonwealth Bureau of Animal Breeding and Genetics
Edinburgh, Scotland

D. H. Wallace, Ph.D.
Professor
Department of Plant Breeding and Biometry and of Vegetable Crops
Cornell University
Ithaca, New York

C. M. Williams, Ph.D.
Professor and Head
Department of Animal and Poultry Science
University of Saskatchewan
Saskatoon, Canada

Ian J. Warrington
Scientist
Department of Scientific and Industrial Research
Palmerston North
New Zealand

David Wilson, Ph.D.
Senior Principal Scientific Officer
Welsh Plant Breeding Station
University College of Wales
Plas Gogerddan near Aberystwyth
England

R. W. Willey, Ph.D.
Principal Agronomist
International Crop Research Institute for the Semi-Arid Tropics
Patancheru P.O.
India

Mary Hotze Witt, Ph.D.
Associate Professor of Horticulture
Department of Horticulture and Landscape Architecture
University of Kentucky
Lexington, Kentucky

Richard W. Zobel, Ph.D.
Research Geneticist, USDA-SEA and Professor
Departments of Plant Breeding and of Agronomy
Cornell University
Ithaca, New York

DEDICATION

To my inspiring teachers at Cornell University—Harold H. Williams, John K. Loosli, the late Richard H. Barnes, the late Clive M. McCay, and the late Leonard A. Maynard. And to my supportive and beloved family—Eva, Jack, and Karen.

TABLE OF CONTENTS

Volume I

TABLE OF CONTENTS

Volume II

Physical Factors

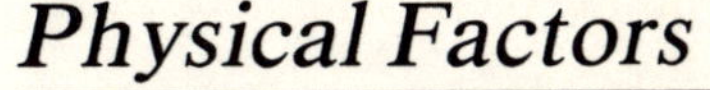

CLIMATE AND ANIMAL PRODUCTIVITY*

H. D. Johnson and G. L. Hahn

INTRODUCTION

Climate, in the general context, includes physical factors such as temperature, humidity, wind, radiation, rainfall, and altitude; chemical factors such as air composition; and indirect factors such as quantity and quality of feed and water, disease, parasites, soil, and fertility. Animal management, shelter provisions, and the many factors associated with modern animal industry alter climatic influences of a temperate, arctic, or tropical environment.

All species of the plant and animal kingdom have an optimal environmental zone or set of conditions in which they function most productively and, usually, most efficiently. In this chapter, information on the environment is limited to primary climatic factors such as temperature, humidity, air velocity, radiation (when available and the effects these factors have on productivity of domestic animals. Data on domestic animals of major agricultural importance (cattle, sheep, poultry, and swine) are presented. Factors of productivity such as milk production, egg production, growth, reproduction, and associated physiological functions such as feed intake, body temperature, and heat balance are briefly categorized. Lactation of mammals and egg production of birds are productive functions that are dependent upon an optimal climate and environment for optimum growth, and time required for sexual maturity. The processes of lactation and ovulation are regulated by the neuroendocrine system, which in turn is strongly influenced directly and indirectly by climatic environmental factors. Reproduction and growth of birds and mammals are similarly influenced. Efficiency of all these productive functions is dependent upon availability and utilization of indirect factors of the environment such as quantity and quality of feed and water. The response to altered heat balance that operates to maintain homeothermy affects all of these as well as other animal functions described.

The climatic temperature for optimal productivity is summarized in Table 1; current recommended practices in the production of cattle, swine, and poultry are summarized in Table 2.[2]

Figure 1 is a generalized illustration of the productivity of pigs, laying hens, and dairy cows at temperatures ranging from 4.4 to 37.8°C.[3] Other environmental factors such as humidity, air flow, radiation, level of feeding, and breed and age differences modify these general curves. More specific information is presented in subsequent sections on growth, and egg and milk production.

Zones of thermoneutrality are similar to zones of optimal productivity for the various species and breeds and, of course, may vary due to many factors such as age, level of feed intake, physical activity, and acclimation. Data included in the section on heat production and heat loss substantiate the thermoneutral zone designations.

REPRODUCTION

Cattle

Seasonal variation in fertility occurs in both dairy and beef cattle. In the cool northern latitudes, fertility in the female is usually lowest during the winter months. In warm humid areas, however, cow fertility is lowest during late summer and fall. Semen quality and fertility in the male are depressed during the summer in most locations. Expo-

* Tables follow text, beginning on page 21.

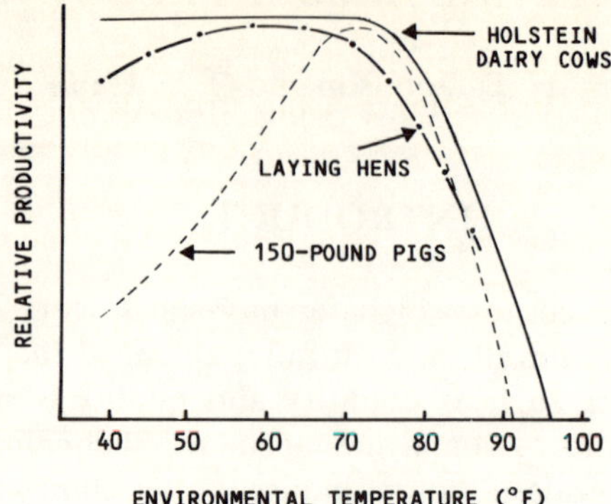

FIGURE 1. Influence of environmental temperature on growth rate of pigs and milk- and egg-production trends of farm animals (40, 50, 60, 70, 80, 90, 100°F = 4.4, 10, 15.6, 21.1, 26.7, 32.2, and 37.8°C, respectively.) (From Bond, T. E. and Kelly, C. F., in *Environment of Animals,* U.S. Department of Agriculture, Washington, D.C., 1960, 231. With permission.)

sure of bulls to high temperature impairs spermatogenesis, and several weeks are required for semen quality to return to normal.

Female

In the female, heat stress of sufficient duration and intensity delays puberty, causes anestrus, depresses estrual activity, lowers conception rates, induces abortions, and increases perinatal mortality. Cows are most susceptible to the depressing effects of heat stress on fertility near the time of breeding; a negative relationship exists between body temperature at insemination and subsequent conception rates. There are significant differences among breeds in their ability to adapt to heat stress, and the degree of adaptability determines the physiologic response to such stress. Increased blood progestins and lowered luteinizing hormone (LH) and cortisol found in heat-stressed cows arouse speculation that an altered hormonal status may be a contributing factor in reduced fertility.[4,5] Recent research on other species indicates that high temperatures can also have a direct detrimental effect on developing spermatozoa and embryos.[6]

Puberty in Shorthorn and Brahman heifers is delayed when animals are reared at 27°C compared to those reared at 10°C, but Santa Gertrudis heifers are unaffected.[7] Length of the estrous cycle in heifers is longer under hot climatic conditions, but duration and intensity of estrus is decreased.[8,9] There is a higher incidence of clinical anestrus among heifers in hot climate-controlled chambers.[8]

In U.S. Department of Agriculture studies, five experiments were undertaken to determine the long-term effects of thermal stress (32°C) on reproductive performance in heifers of several beef breeds.[10] When winter-conditioned heifers were exposed to high temperature, they became anestrous, with inactive ovaries, but later became acclimatized and reestablished their estrous cycles by the 16th week. In one trial, the heifers were bred after becoming acclimatized and five of six conceived and produced normal calves. Only one of six summer-conditioned heifers became anestrous when subjected to 32°C, but when exposed to 38°C, five of the six became anestrous.

Cows with high body temperature at time of insemination have lower conception rates than cows with normal body temperature.[11-14] To more precisely determine the critical period of this phenomenon, 25 Hereford heifers were exposed to 32°C for 72 hr immediately after breeding.[15] None of these heifers conceived, compared to 12 of 25 heifers that conceived after exposure to 21°C. After removal of the heifers from the hot chamber, 72 hr postbreeding plasma progesterone content, as measured by competitive protein-binding procedures, was significantly higher in those animals exposed to the higher temperature (0.55 ng at 21°C, 0.97 ng at 32°C).[16] The physiological importance of increased progesterone content on fertility remains to be determined.

Considerable research has been conducted in Arizona on the effects of heat stress on fertility in dairy cows.[17,18] Heat stress beginning 10 days after breeding during the cool weather months did not decrease fertility; the first 4 to 6 days following breeding was determined to be the most critical period. Attempts were made to improve fertility during hot summer months by moving cows in estrus to a refrigerated building for 4 to 6 days. However, this practice only slightly improved reproductive performance, which suggests that other physiological factors in addition to increased body temperature during estrus caused lowered conception rates. The adrenal glands of heat-stressed cows had significantly higher progesterone content than those of control cows. In another study, cows maintained under evaporatively cooled shades during summer months had significantly higher reproductive performance and lower blood progesterone content than cows with conventional shades.

High temperatures can also have detrimental effects on pregnant cows during late gestation. A 27-hr exposure at 38°C caused two Holstein-Friesian cows, 4½ to 6 months pregnant, to abort 2 days later.[19] Calves born in the summer in South Africa from cows of British breeds were 20% lighter in weight than calves born in the winter.[20] This seasonal difference in calf size was not noted in well-adapted breeds.

The numerical data presented on conception rates of well-managed Holstein cattle fed adequately for a good level of milk production are those of Ingraham et al.[21] Conception rates for the herd, which was near Culiacan on the west coast of Mexico, were evaluated with respect to the average temperature-humidity index (THI)* of the 2 days prior to breeding, the day of breeding, and the day following breeding. Average daily THI for 3 years ranged from 62 to 86. Average daily ambient temperature and relative humidity (RH) for indices 76 and 82 were 26.5°C, 68% RH, and 29.7°C, 75% RH, respectively. Conception rates for 191 cows serviced on days with an average index under 66 was 67%, as compared to 21% for 818 cows serviced on days averaging above 76. The average temperature-humidity index of the second day prior to breeding had the most influence on conception rates, with these rates declining from 55 to 10% as the average index of the second day prior to breeding increased from 70 to 84 (correlation coefficient of 0.995). In the range of THI values between 68 and 82, conception rates averaged 10.4% lower (31.9%), if the average THI of the 2 days prior to breeding was higher than on the day of breeding, compared to the conception rates when the index of

$$\mathrm{THI} = t_{db} + 0.36 \times t_{dp} + 41.2$$

the 2 days prior to breeding was higher than on the day of breeding. This observation indicates that temperature and humidity of individual days prior to breeding influenced breeding efficiency. Conception rates throughout the year are shown in Table 3.[21]

Conception rates are considerably higher in Florida, which has a milder climate than the Mexican region. Relationship to temperature is shown in Figure 2, with a maximum conception rate at approximately 18°C.[22]

Dairy cattle in Arizona demonstrate extremely low fertility during the summer, es-

* Temperature-humidity index (THI) is a derived statistic computed from the relation where $+_{db}$ = dry-bulb temperature, °C and t_{dp} = dew point temperature, °C.

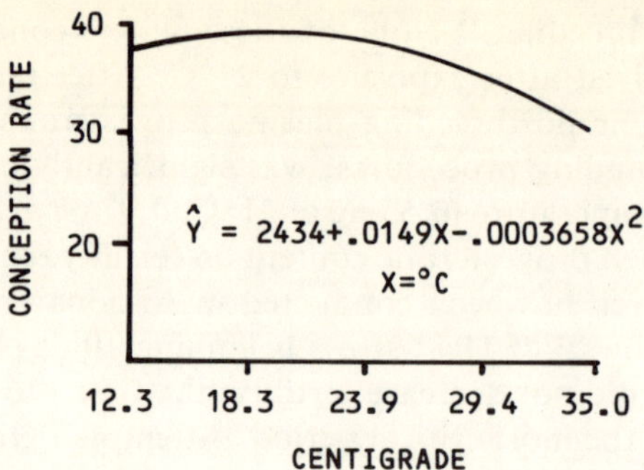

FIGURE 2. Relationship of maximum ambient temperature on conception rate in cattle the day after insemination. (From Guazduskas, F. C., Wilcox, C. J., and Thatcher, W. W., *J. Dairy Sci.*, 58(1), 88, 1975. With permission.)

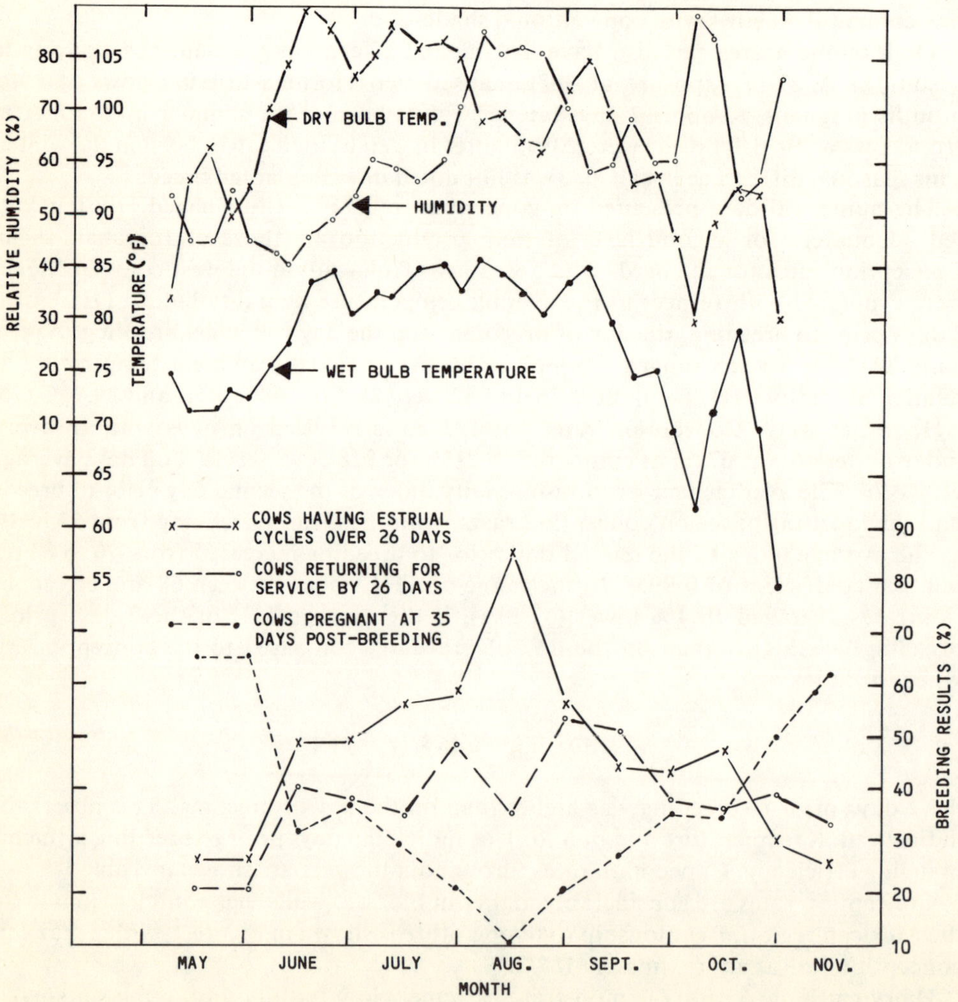

FIGURE 3. Relationship of environmental temperature and humidity on reproductive efficiency in Holstein cattle during an Arizona summer. Metric equivalents are 70°F (21.1°C), 80° (26.7°C), 90°F (32.2°C), and 100°F (32.8°C). (From Stott, G. H. and Williams, R. J., *J. Dairy Sci.*, 45, 1369, 1962. With permission.)

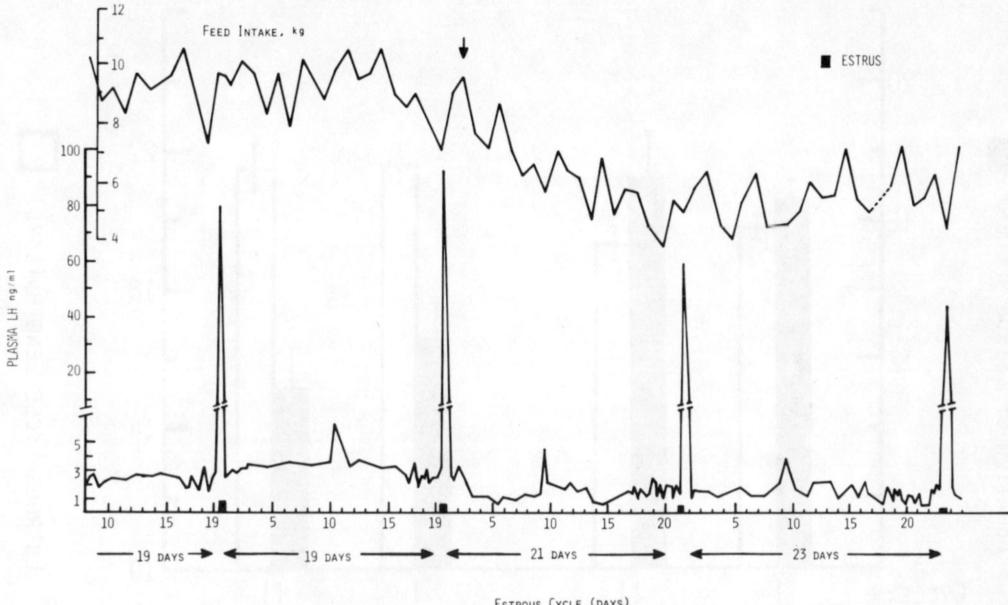

FIGURE 4. Plasma LH of a single animal measured through consecutive estrous cycles at two temperature conditions. Figure shows the relation between onset of estrus, LH peak, and feed consumed by the animal. (Arrow designates the change in chamber temperature conditions from 18.2 to 33.5°C.) (From Madan, M. L. and Johnson, H. D., *J. Dairy Sci.*, 56(11), 1420, 1973. With permission.)

pecially in August, when the relative humidity becomes higher. This is verified by the data in Figure 3, which show that conception rates of well-managed dairies can be as low as 10% during summer heat.[23] Table 4 illustrates the influence of shelter evaporative cooling on conception of cattle in Arizona.[24]

Missouri laboratory data (Figure 4) show that animals exposed to 33.5°C as compared to 18.2°C had a lower LH hormone peak of 61 ± 5 vs. 85 ng/mℓ near the onset of estrus; the surge persisted 8 to 16 hr.[25] Basal LH which was approximately 2.43 ng/mℓ for all heifers, rose significantly during the luteal phase of the cycle on day 10 to 3.5 ± 0.27 ng/mℓ and declined thereafter. Under high temperature conditions of 33.5°C and a body temperature that remained elevated by 1 to 1.5°C, base line as well as peak LH was lower at 1.25 ± 0.48 ng/mℓ (day 1 postestrus) and 44.5 ± 4.3 ng/mℓ, respectively.

The mean average duration of estrus of 16.8 hr at 18.2°C differed from 11.9 hr at 33.5°C (Figure 5).[26] Mean length of the estrous cycle was 19.5 days at 18°C and 21.6 days at 33.5°C, with some cycles lasting as long as 23 days under the hot conditions.

Male

Exposure to high environmental temperature lowers fertility in the male bovine.[27,28] Heat-impaired fertility is accompanied by alterations in semen volume, sperm motility, and sperm morphology, reflecting deleterious changes in spermatogenesis.[29,30] The effects of elevated environmental temperature on spermatogenesis in the bull are well documented and appear to be similar to effects observed in males of other mammalian species.[31-33]

In an attempt to determine the role of heat stress in the decline of fertility during warmer seasons of the year, detailed studies have been conducted in climate-controlled chambers in which climatic variables can be precisely controlled.

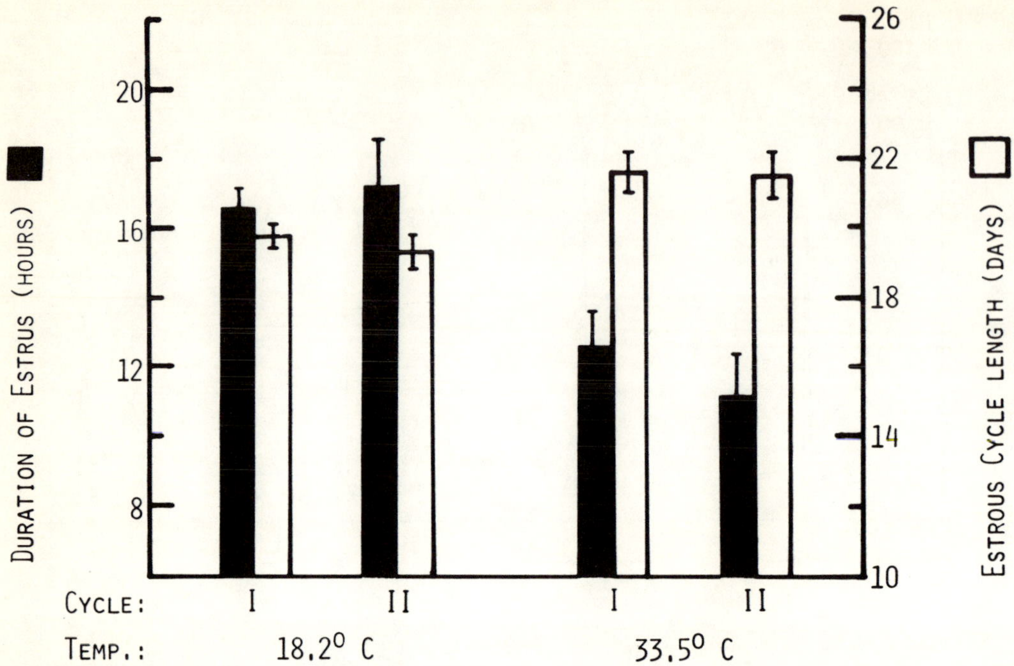

FIGURE 5. Effects of environmental temperature of 18.2 and 33.5°C on the duration of estrus and estrous cycling of Guernsey heifers. (From Johnson, H. D., in *Progress in Biometeorology*, Tromp, S. W., Ed., Swets & Zeitlinger, Amsterdam, 1972, 43. With permission.)

In a study on the effects of heat stress on puberty, ten Jersey bull calves were placed in a chamber heated to 35 to 36°C for 8 hr daily from 26 weeks of age until puberty.[34] An additional eight bull calves sired by the same bull were maintained at ambient temperatures. The high temperature retarded puberty and lowered semen quality, but did not alter libido.

Exposure of Guernsey bulls to 29°C impaired spermatogenesis.[34] When temperatures of 32 to 38°C were used, spermatogenesis was adversely affected within 2 weeks; it took 6 to 8 weeks before semen quality returned to normal. Environmental temperature was varied each day in another study in order to better simulate summer conditions.[35] A 7-day exposure to cycled hot climatic conditions (28 to 40°C) had deleterious effects upon semen quality. Red Sindhi crossbred bulls were less affected than Holstein-Friesian and Brown Swiss bulls, and recovery of semen quality was more rapid in crossbred than in purebred bulls.

Four experiments were conducted in climate-controlled chambers to determine the length of exposure to heat stress (40°C) that is required to impair spermatogenesis in both *Bos indicus* (Afrikaner) and *Bos taurus* (Friesian) breeds.[36] Semen quality was not as severely affected in the *B. indicus* breed as in the *B. taurus* breed. Furthermore, exposure for a period as short as 12 hr adversely affected spermatogenesis. It was concluded that short-term heat stress may be an important factor in bovine fertility under practical conditions.

Artificial insulation of the scrotum for periods as short as 24 to 72 hr depressed semen quality in Hereford bulls, which indicated that the normal thermoregulatory mechanisms of the testes were inhibited.[37] An increase in primary abnormalities was observed in five bulls after placing the scrotum in a water bath maintained at 43°C for varying intervals.[38] Spermatozoa in the cauda epididymides were more resistant to heat than those in the caput epididymides.[39]

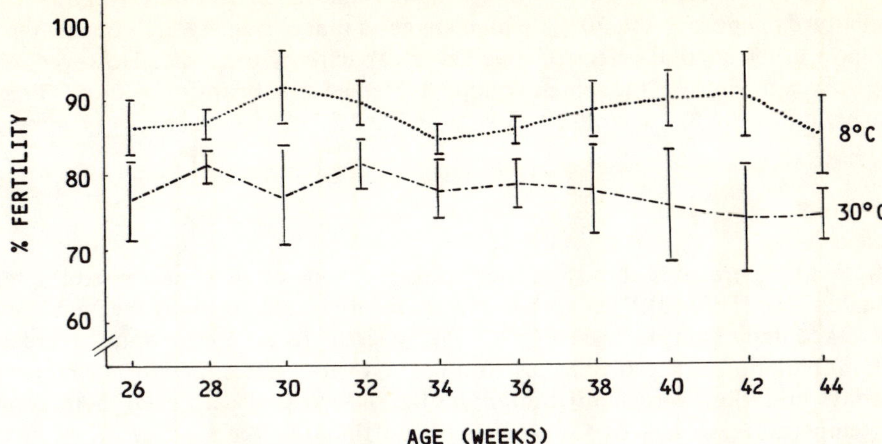

FIGURE 6. Percentage of fertility of eggs from hens exposed to different environmental temperatures and mated to males held at 19°C. (From Houston, T. M., *Poult. Sci.*, 54(4), 1180, 1975. With permission.)

Similar results have also been observed using laboratory animals. Heat stress can directly affect spermatozoa and developing embryos.[40,41] Incubation of rabbit spermatozoa for 3 hr at 40°C compared to 38°C did not alter their fertilizing capacity, but increased embryonic death in those inseminated with the heat-stressed sperm.[42] When one-celled rabbit embryos were cultured for 6 hr at 40°C, they had lower survival rates after transfer than did embryos cultured at 38°C.[43,44] Chance of survival was greatly improved, however, if heat stress was delayed until later cell stages.[6]

To better understand the mechanisms of decreased fertility in cattle, plasma testosterone was measured in Hereford bulls subjected to climatic stress. These bulls were placed in a temperature- and humidity-controlled chamber and exposed to 21°C, 50% relative humidity (RH) for 7 weeks (control period), and subsequently to 35.5°C, 50% RH for 7 weeks (heat period). Rectal temperature and respiration rates rose, and testosterone (Table 5) declined rapidly during the first 2 days of heat treatment.[45] Testosterone plasma concentration fell to 43% of control levels during subsequent weeks, as shown in Table 6.[45] Spermatogenesis, evaluated by semen characteristics and histological examination of testes at the termination of the experiment, was impaired by heat.

Fowl

Female

The fertility of female chickens is also affected by high environmental temperatures. Fertility was significantly lower in hens kept at 30°C than in similar groups held at an environment of 8°C. The fertility of eggs of hens maintained at 8 or 30°C is shown in Figure 6.[46]

Male

In studies made to determine the influence of environmental temperature on the fertility of domestic fowl, it was found that a cold environmental temperature depressed testes growth and delayed spermatogenesis in maturing cockerels. There was also a highly significant difference in the fertility of mature males kept at different environmental temperatures; males housed at 19°C had higher fertility than those kept at either 30 or 8°C.

Table 7 shows a highly significant difference in the fertility of males held at different environmental temperatures ($p < 0.01$).[46] This difference occurred between birds held at 19°C and those held at 8 and 30°C. No significant differences in fertility were found between birds kept at 8 and 30°C, which suggests that extremely high or low temperatures have a detrimental effect on fertilizing capacity of the male. However, only in the hot environment was the semen volume depressed significantly ($p<0.05$). The mean semen volumes for 8, 19, and 30°C were 0.75, 0.77, and 0.64 mℓ, respectively, per ejaculate.

Swine

Female

Ambient temperatures above the thermoneutral zone of 26°C decreased the fertility of female swine (Table 8).[47] As ambient temperature increased, daily feed consumption and average daily gain decreased ($p<0.05$), whereas rectal temperatures increased ($p < 0.05$). Ovulation rate (corpora lutea) and the overall percentage of swine pregnant at 25 days gestation were significantly ($p<0.05$) decreased with each increase in ambient temperature; degree of failure was proportional to the severity of the stress. A higher THI (as defined earlier) reduces the number of piglets born alive from Large White and Landrace pigs.[48]

Male

In a recent extensive study, Wettemann et al. collected semen twice weekly from boars to determine sperm output and quality.[49] Semen volume and gel weight per ejaculum were not altered during elevated ambient temperature; however, sperm motility and the percentage of normal cells with nonaged acrosomes decreased, and the percentage of abnormal cells and cells with aged acrosomes increased by the second week of treatment. Sperm output was reduced in stressed boars during the second through sixth week of treatment. Only 28.6% of 77 gilts bred with semen from stressed boars conceived, compared to 41.2% of 88 gilts bred with control semen. At day 30 ± 3 of pregnancy, embryonic survival was 71.2 ± 3.7% in gilts bred with semen from control boars and 48.5 ± 5.2% for gilts bred with semen from stressed boars.

Sheep

Female

It has been established that reproductive performance of ewes during the breeding period is adversely affected by constant high ambient temperatures of 32 to 35°C[50-53] and favorably affected by constant lower ambient temperatures of 16 to 21°C.[50,54,55]

The female as well as the male reacts to hot humid environmental conditions with increased body temperature, increased respiratory rate, decreased feed consumption, and lethargy in proportion to the severity of the thermal environment imposed. In addition, these environments exact a penalty in reproductive performance, which also appears to be in proportion to the severity of the thermal environment and duration of the exposure. Environmental heat reduces the percentage of ova fertilized and increases the number of abnormal ova (Table 9).[52] Environmental heat-exposure time in relation to time of breeding is an important factor in fertility of ewes.[52] Fertilization rate in ewes exposed to elevated air temperature (32.2°C) on the 12th day of the cycle before breeding was significantly lower ($p<0.01$) than the rate for control ewes. During two breeding seasons, 92.6% of ova from control ewes was cleaved, compared to 51.9% from ewes in the hot room. Heat treatment resulted in an increase in the percentage of abnormal ova; only 3.7% of ova from control ewes examined 3 days after breeding was classified as morphologically abnormal, compared to 44.2% from ewes in the hot room. Embryo loss, estimated as the percent of fertilized ova that died, was significantly higher in ewes exposed to the heat before breeding. For control ewes during two breeding seasons, the estimated embryo loss was 4.0%, compared to an estimated loss of 91.7% for ewes exposed to the heat before breeding. When ewes were not exposed to the heated room until 8 days postbreeding, the estimated embryo loss (15.4%) was not significantly different from control ewes. Out of 20 ewes, 17 lambed when bred and exposed to the heat 8 days later, but only 1 out of 20 ewes lambed when exposed to the heat before breeding. Fertilization rate and survival of the early embryo in ewes appear to be more susceptible to heat damage than is the 8-day-old embryo.

Rectal temperatures and pulse rates of the ewes in the hot room were significantly increased ($p < 0.01$) over those for control ewes. Hot-room sheared ewes had lower average rectal temperatures and pulse rates than the unsheared ewes. The adverse effects of heat on fertilization rate, percentage of abnormal ova, and embryo loss were less severe when ewes were sheared before being exposed to the elevated temperature.

Male

Effects of heat on ram fertility are similar to those on other domestic males, but perhaps even more drastic reductions in fertility occur. Semen from rams kept in thermoneutral conditions was superior to semen of rams held in hot environments. These effects are summarized in Table 10.[56] Even local heating of the scrotal contents of rams to approximately 40°C for 1½ to 2 hr causes a sharp increase in the proportion of morphologically abnormal spermatozoa in the ejaculate 14 to 16 days later.[57] This period of delay approximates to the epididymal passage time for ram spermatozoa[58,59] and has been cited as evidence that spermatozoa undergoing epididymal passage at the time of heating are resistant to damage.[57,60]

Turkeys

Female

Constant environmental temperatures have a pronounced effect on breeder turkeys. High temperature seems to increase the percentage of birds molting and subsequently stop laying eggs. In one study (Table 11), the average percentage of birds molting was 45.7, 44.4, and 76.6% in the 12.8, 21.1 and 29.4°C temperature environments, respectively.[61] The fact that molting birds generally reduce egg production indicates that high temperature may have played a significant role in reducing egg production at high temperatures.

Male

At present, no published data are available concerning the effects of climate on fertility of male turkeys.

MILK PRODUCTION

Major climatic factors that affect milk quantity and quality are temperature, humidity, radiation, wind velocity, barometric pressure, and rainfall. An adverse biometeorological factor can influence milk production by alteration of the animal's behavioral activity and thermal, water, and energy balance; such functions are interrelated and involve the neuroendocrine system.[62] These biometeorological factors also influence milk production indirectly by altering the quantity and quality of feed and water intake and also may determine whether specific disease or parasites survive and are transmitted. In the tropics, the meteorological factors (high temperature, relative humidity, and thermal radiation) and such indirect factors such as inadequate nutrition and parasites severely limit milk production. Environmental pollution of air, water, and soil by animals themselves or by industry in more urban areas provide chemical modification of the environment, which may influence production. However, the emphasis in this summary is on major, direct meteorological factors.

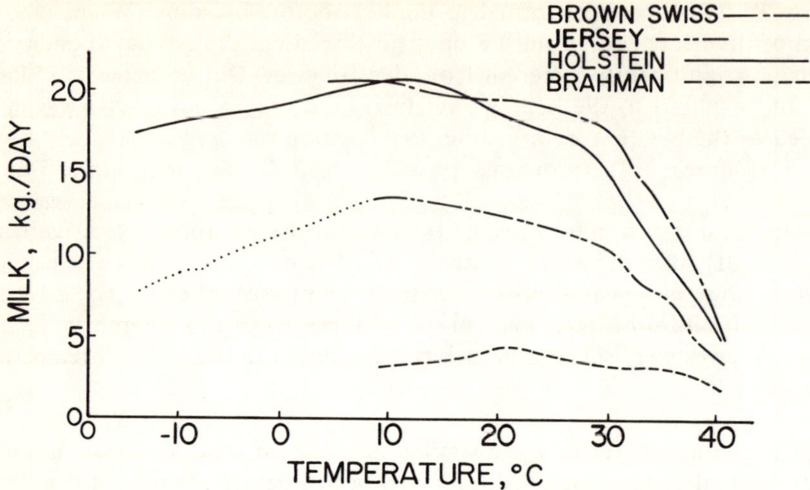

FIGURE 7. Breed differences in the effect of environmental temperature on milk yield of cattle in controlled-temperature laboratory at relative humidity of 40 to 60%.

Table 12 illustrates breed differences in response to climate by the lower milk production of a Criollo (Zebu type) cattle and the results of crossbreeding with *B. taurus* (Holstein), which increases lactation in a tropical environment.[62] Another major advantage is the greater reproductive efficiency of the Criollo-Friesian crosses. Some dairy breeds or species can acclimate quite readily to varied biometeorological or climatic environments, resulting in less impairment of the lactation functions. Highly productive *B. taurus* cattle are commonly crossbred with the more heat-tolerant and disease-resistant *B. indicus* cattle to increase production as well as retain heat and disease tolerance under tropical management conditions.

Recent reviews and reports of the meteorological effects on milk yield are those of Bianca[63] and Johnson.[60,64] Generally, the yield and composition of milk are much the same within the temperature range of 10 to 20°C. From 20 to 27°C, yield decreases slowly and fat percentage is reduced; but beyond 27°C, decline in yield is much more marked, whereas fat percentage increases and the content of nonfat solids is usually decreased. Data of Moody et al.[65] reemphasize the effects of temperature on milk composition and the fatty acid composition of the milk changes, as shown in Table 13.[65]

Figure 7 describes the milk production of temperate-evolved Holstein, Brown Swiss, Jersey, and tropically evolved Brahman cows.[66,66a] Milk production plotted as a function of dry bulb temperature (approximately 50% relative humidity) indicates a maximum between 4 and 21°C; it generally declines above and below this comfort zone. More specifically, at high environmental temperatures, yield declined for Holstein animals at approximately 21°C, Brown Swiss and Jersey at about 24 to 27°C, and Brahman at approximately 32°C. The most pronounced decline in lactation was shown by the Holstein animals.

The cold influences on lactation also lower milk production as shown by milk yield and composition data from mature Holstein-Freisian cows managed under low fluctuating environmental temperatures at the University of Saskatchewan.[67] As temperature decreased below −3.9°C, daily yield of milk decreased significantly. Milk yield was unaffected by degree hours per day at mean temperatures greater than −3.9°C (600 degree hr/day); on days colder than 600 degree hr/day, the effect of temperature on milk yield was curvilinear. Rate of decline in milk yield (kg) was four times greater on days when daily minimum ambient air temperature (DMAAT) was below −12.2°C

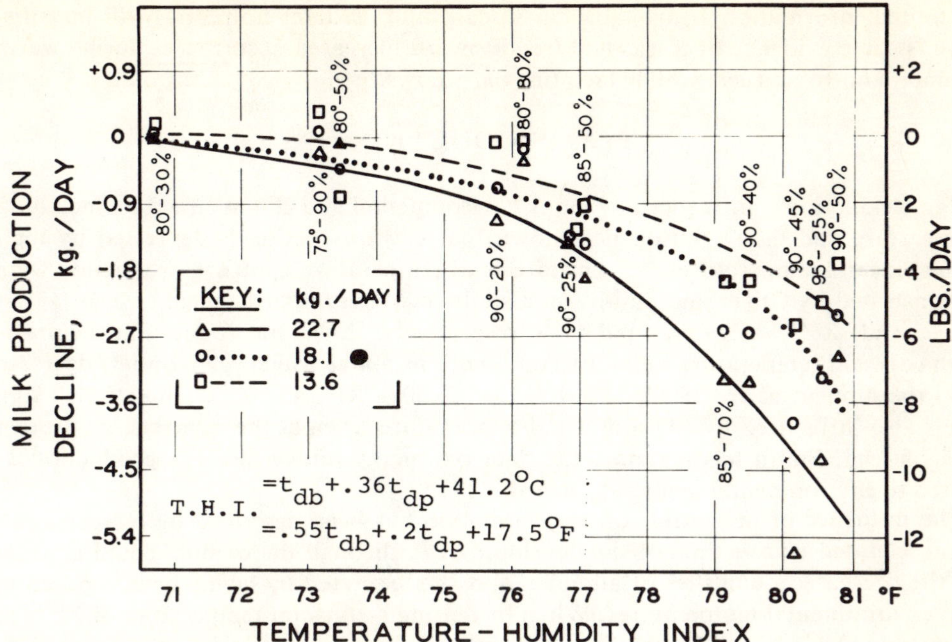

FIGURE 8. Declines in milk production from base 18°C values (switchback design) at various THI conditions. (From Johnson, H. D., in *Progress in Biometeorology*, Tromp, S. W., Ed., Swets & Zeitlinger, Amsterdam, 1972, 43. With permission.)

than on days when DMAAT was above −12.2°C. Although DMAAT had a significant effect on milk total-solids percentage and a highly significant negative effect on crude protein yield, the effect of degree hr/day on these two factors was not significant. DMAAT and degree hr/day had no significant effect on crude protein percentage, butterfat and solids-not-fat yield and percentage, or fat-corrected milk and total-solids yield. Table 14 illustrates the relative effects of temperature on milk production, feed intake, and the conversion of feed to milk by these four breeds.[68,69]

Milk yields are affected by humidities at temperatures above 27°C.[70] These relationships were quantified by establishing milk production decline as a function of the THI (previously discussed).[71] Figure 8 illustrates the effects of various temperature-humidity conditions on animals producing approximately 23, 18, and 14 kg/day.[26]

These values were based on declines in production from base (18°C) values. A switchback procedure was used for the various temperature-humidity conditions, thus eliminating the persistency effects on lactation.

Critical temperatures have been calculated for maintenance of 10- and 20-kg milk levels at −4 and −10°C, respectively.[72]

Data from Table 15 demonstrate that increased wind speed is advantageous at air temperatures between 27 and 35°C, although velocities above 5 mi/hr had no additional benefits.[26] Increased wind speed has the practical result of shifting the comfort zone to higher temperatures. Air velocities of 5 and 9 mi/hr proved beneficial in recovering milk production at an air temperature of 35°C that was otherwise lost when the velocity was only 0.4 mi/hr.[73]

When the air is hot, radiation augments the decline in milk production; exposure to 180 Btu/ft^2/hr did not affect milk production at 8°C, but did cause a decline at 21°C and above.[74] The data of Table 16 verify that, at 27°C, the decline in milk production by Holstein or Jersey was sharpest when radiation was greatest.

Limited information is available on disease and climate; however, with mastitis, there is some evidence of a seasonal trend toward increased occurrences during warm summer months and early fall in lactating dairy cows.[75]

EGG PRODUCTION

Egg production is influenced by many environmental and climatic factors, including temperature and light. Wilson has shown that egg production is depressed by high environmental temperatures.[76,77] The effects of temperature upon egg production were demonstrated by Oliver and Smith[78] in a study in which the percentage of eggs laid at 21, 32, and 38°C was 79, 72, and 41%, respectively. Payne has found that the maximum constant temperature-humidity combinations above which egg numbers decrease from thermoneutral are 28°C, 75% RH; 31°C, 50% RH; and 33°C, 30% RH.[79] Egg size is also influenced by environmental temperature, even at the same energy protein level of feed. Smith has reviewed the data on energy intake and egg production as related to environmental temperature (Table 17).[80]

The influence of heat stress on egg formation has been described by Nordstrom.[81] An accelerated transit time of the developing egg through the oviduct could account for the decreased quantities of albumen and shell secreted by laying hens exposed to high environmental temperatures. When increasing a constant temperature of 21°C to a constant 32 ± 1°C for 3 weeks, the time interval between successive eggs was significantly greater (p <0.01) at 32°C (27.7 hr) than at 21°C (25.6 hr). Egg weight, shell weight (percentage of egg weight), and laying rate were all decreased at the higher temperature. Thus, the developing egg appears to spend a slightly longer period of time (about 2 hr) in the shell gland at 32°C than at 21°C.

Table 18 shows the effects of environmental temperature on mortality, egg production, feed consumption, and body weight of Leghorn pullets from 150 to 435 days of age.[82]

GROWTH*

Man's interest in the growth of domestic animals results from his need for a high-quality protein for human consumption (with the exception of female poultry and dairy cattle, which are maintained to produce eggs and milk). Growth of domestic animals is influenced by climatic factors, as are other productive functions. Extremely cold (especially if animals are unprotected) and hot climates lessen growth rates and efficiency of gains. Climatic factors of temperature, humidity, wind, and radiation should be considered in all growth trials. However, many times they are not measured, and the effects are usually attributed to random variation.

Cattle

Recent data from Canada (Table 19) summarize the effects of cold upon beef cattle productivity.[83] Feedlot cattle in western Canada are exposed to more severe cold conditions than those experienced by intensively managed livestock in other parts of the world. Average daily gain is greater in summer at an average temperature of 17°C than during the colder seasons of the year. These data, which were taken from performance records for the university feedlot and collected monthly over a period of 7 years on a total of 1970 finishing steers, showed that during December, January, and February (mean monthly temperature, −17°C; wind velocity, 15 km/hr; precipitation, 2.2 cm/month), productivity was markedly depressed. Average daily gain fell to 1.03

* Growth data for sheep were not available at this time.

from 1.47 kg/day, feed per gain rose to 9.8 from 6.6, and energy per unit of gain rose to 23.3 from 16.7 Mcal ME/kg gain, when compared to values for the balance of the year (March to November). These differences were not due to seasonal variations in weight or maturity. Opportunity, therefore, exists to improve livestock productivity through additional environmental protection. Williams demonstrated that shelter from wind and adequate bedding both markedly improved the performance of feedlot steers.[84] Evidence from other areas in Canada also indicated that winter performance improves when cattle are provided with shelter.[85,86]

The effects of higher temperatures on cattle growth are described in Table 20.[87,88] In this study, six breeds were raised under constant laboratory conditions at 10 or 27°C; with the exception of Brahman cattle, gains were greater at 10°C. Table 21 shows similar results for Hereford × Angus steers.[89]

Swine

Weight gain of young pigs was maximal at 15°C in this study, with lower values above and below this temperature (Table 22).[90] Pigs of various ages and weights were grown at various cold and hot temperatures; again, the maximal gains were in the thermoneutral range of 15 to 20°C (Table 23).[91]

Chickens

Data demonstrate that for a constant temperature maximal growth rate occurred near 20°C, but that feed conversion was highest at 34°C (Table 24).[92]

Turkeys

Optimal environmental temperature for growth gain of turkeys is in the range of 15 to 21°C (Table 25). Feed conversion and fat digestive values also suggest that this environmental temperature range is optimal.

FEED INTAKE

It is well established that low environmental temperatures stimulate appetites and increase metabolic rates and that higher environmental temperatures lessen the desire of all domestic animals to eat. The temperature zone between these extremes provides the most efficient energy conversion. Quality and composition of rations may alter the productive response to adverse climates. In some instances, rectal temperature and water intake data are included with feed data because they also vary with climate and feed level.

Cattle

Table 26 summarizes feed and water data for various breeds of cattle at different environmental temperatures. Results of an intensive study on the effects of temperature-humidity on feed intake of Holstein cattle under controlled laboratory conditions are shown in Table 27 and Figure 9.[70]

Swine

Tables 28[98] and 29[99] describe water and feed consumption for pigs at different temperatures. Water intake expressed per unit body weight or as a function of feed level increased above 20°C; feed intake was markely lower at temperatures above 20°C.

Sheep

High temperatures and ration variations on feed intake, water consumption, and urine output values are summarized in Table 30.[100] Feed intake was decreased; water

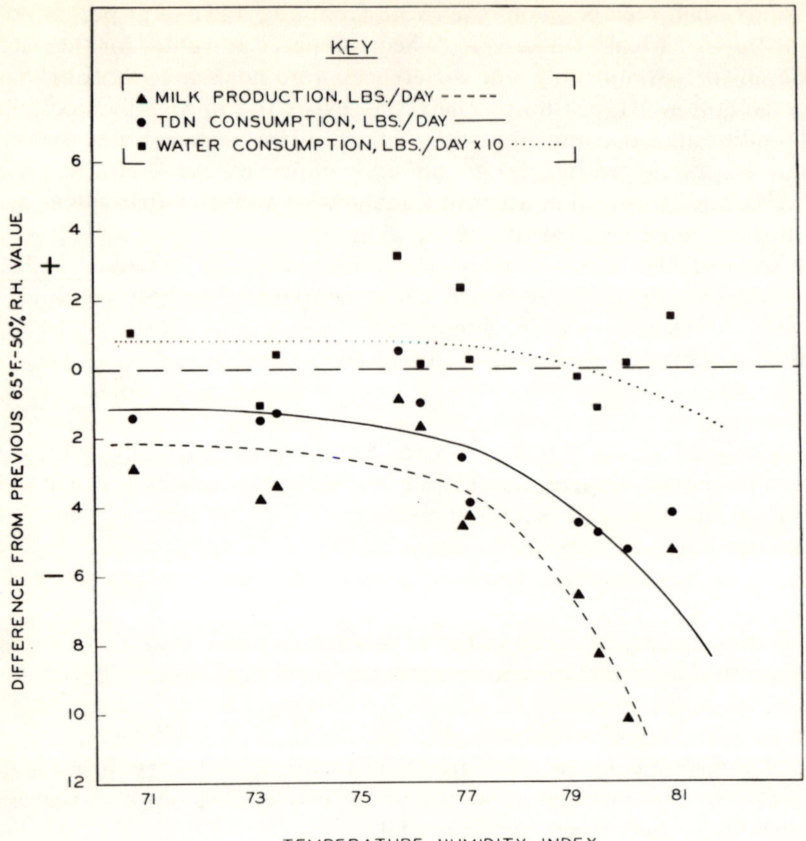

FIGURE 9. Expression of milk production, TDN consumption, and water consumption at various temperature-humidity conditions vs. THI index. (77 THI may be approximately 90°F [32.2°C], 25% RH or 85°F [29.4°C], 50% RH, etc. Each data point is the difference from previous 65°F (18.3°C) based on a 12-cow average.) (From Johnson, H. D., Ragsdale, A. C., Berry, I. L., and Shanklin, M. D., *Mo. Agric. Exp. Stn. Res. Bull.*, 846, 1, 1963. With permission.)

intake was increased; and, urine volume increased at the high temperature of 32°C and 88% relative humidity.

Turkeys and Chickens

Table 31 summarizes available data concerning the effects of temperature on feed and water intake and rectal temperature of turkeys. Turkeys appear to be quite sensitive to the higher environmental temperatures. This table (and Tables 32 and 33)[104] also includes additional data on chickens, swine, and rabbits.

HEAT PRODUCTION AND LOSS

As described earlier, low environmental temperatures increase appetites, calorie intake, and metabolic rates; higher fiber ratios for ruminants and higher caloric intake for nonruminants reduce the need for animals to withdraw fat stores. Vasoconstriction and insulation of skin and hair aid in conserving body heat to meet heat maintenance requirements.

Higher temperatures decrease appetite, lower metabolic rate and cause increased efforts by the animal to lose body heat through an evaporative process in an attempt to maintain.

Thus, domestic animals utilize heat-producing and heat-loss processes to adjust to variations in climate, level of feeding, and physical activity. Animals attempt to maintain their heat balance within the limits of physical, chemical, and behavioral responses, so that increases or decreases in body temperature do not alter efficiency of reproduction, lactation, egg production, or growth functions. Efficiencies may be altered in tropical or arctic climates or during seasonal extremes in temperate climates.

Available values for metabolism or heat production and loss are shown in Tables 34 to 42:

1. Table 34 describes total heat production for several dairy and beef breeds at various environmental temperatures. In most instances (with the exception of the Brown Swiss) total heat production is reduced at the higher environmental temperature of 26°C.
2. Table 35 is a comparison of lactating and nonlactating cattle, breed differences, and lactation effects on heat production.[108]
3. Table 36 also compares the heat production of lactating and nonlactating Holstein cattle and describes the relationship of heat loss and heat production in the Jersey breed.
4. Table 37 presents levels of swine heat production as determined by partitional calorimetry at environmental temperatures ranging from 5 to 30°C.[112]
5. Table 38 shows effects of fasting on swine maintained in outdoor seasonal conditions at average temperatures of 13 and 23°C.
6. Table 39 partitions heat loss for sheep maintained at 12 to 38°C and compares shorn to unshorn sheep. Also, heat production data are available for closely clipped sheep held at similar temperatures.
7. Table 40 presents partitional calorimetry data on turkeys, both male and female, at temperatures of 10 to 35°C.
8. Table 41 shows heat production values for fasting chickens at 5, 20, and 34°C and cyclic conditions.
9. Table 42 cites heat production data on rabbits for temperatures of 9 and 28°C.[109]

LIVESTOCK PRODUCTION ECONOMICS

An assessment of the impact of climatic effects on livestock productivity is required in order to determine any resulting penalties (economic or otherwise). Shelters and other environmental modification practices for livestock are usually considered in view of potential economic returns and energy availability. An optimum environment for maximum animal productivity or efficiency, or both, is not necessarily the optimum for investment and energy inputs.

Hahn has reviewed the rationale for selection and application of environmental modification practices to livestock production systems.[1] The primary orientation of that review is toward reduction of economic penalties resulting from heat stress, which causes a greater decline in livestock production than does cold stress, provided that nutritional requirements of the animals are met. Teter and DeShazer have evaluated the nutrient requirements of meat animals that are affected by temperatures below thermoneutral.[119]

Economic penalties incurred from livestock production in adverse climates are dependent upon many factors, including species, breed, location, and level of production. Established quantitative relationships that permit evaluation of penalties to pro-

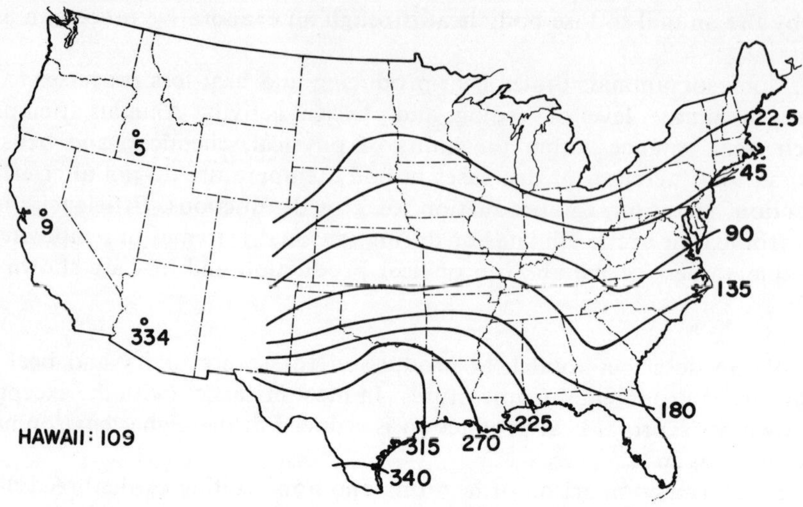

FIGURE 10. Expected summer-season (June 1 to September 30) milk-production losses (kilogram per cow per season) for cows with a normal production level of 22.5 kg/day. (Solar radiation shades, hot-weather rations, and adequate water are assumed available; if not provided, production losses would be larger.) (From Hahn, G. L. and Osburn, D. D. *Trans. ASAE,* 12, 448, 1969. With permission.)

duction and efficiency resulting from adverse climates are few; most livestock environmental research has been comparative in nature (e.g., shade vs. no shade) at a given location, which does not provide a generally applicable relationship for prediction of performance in other locations. For lactating dairy cattle and finishing swine, rates of change in performance have been developed in terms of indices combining the effects of air temperature and humidity. These relationships can then be used with climatological data for specific locations to predict animal performance.[120]

For summer weather (June through September) in natural environments throughout the U.S., Figure 10 presents expected production losses for dairy cows with a production potential of 22.5 kg/day, and Figure 11 shows the percentage of normal growth expected for swine in the finishing phase of production.[127,128] Feed-intake declines for dairy cows, which occur as a result of summer weather (June through September), are indicated in Figure 12. Predicted values for milk production of dairy cows have been reasonably validated.[121] Dairy cow performance in natural and modified environments permits evaluation of the feasibility of environmental modification practices.[122]

Compensatory growth ability is a factor that must be considered for growing animals exposed to adverse climates. A series of studies with *ad libitum* -fed beef cattle, swine, and broilers in the finishing stage before marketing have indicated that moderate heat stress does not reduce attainable market weight or quality of the animals, providing they have a 1- or preferably 2-week recovery period at lower temperatures after a prolonged period of hot weather.[123,124] When adequate managerial flexibility exists to take advantage of compensatory growth, the impact of hot weather on finishing hogs may be less than that shown in Figure 11.

Variability of livestock production due to differences between years can be an important factor in making decisions relative to stability of production as well as to selection of environmental modification practices. Figure 13 illustrates this year-to-year variability for dairy cows during hot weather in Columbia, Mo.,[125] and Figure 14 shows an overview of milk production variability at selected U.S. locations.[126]

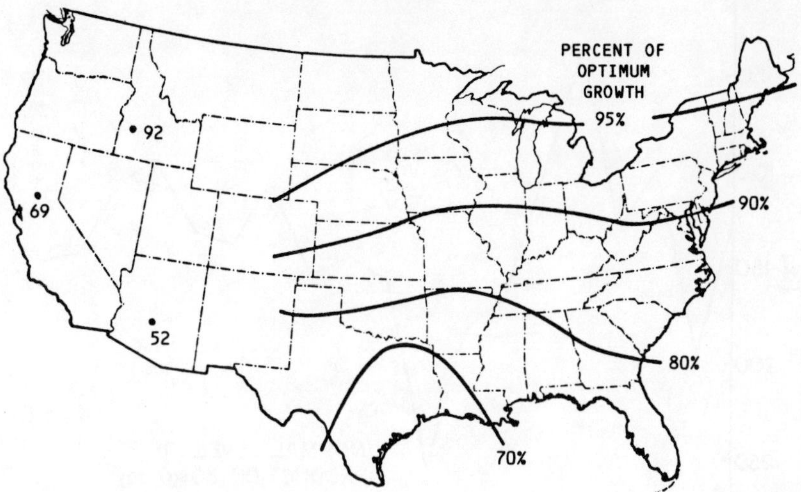

FIGURE 11. Expected production losses as percentages of optimum growth rates for shade 70-kg finishing hogs subjected to natural summer weather (June 1 to September 30). (From Morrison, S. R., Hahn, G. L., and Bond, T. E., Predicting Summer Production Losses for Swine, Production Res. Rep. 118, U.S. Department of Agriculture, Washington, D.C., 1970. With permission.)

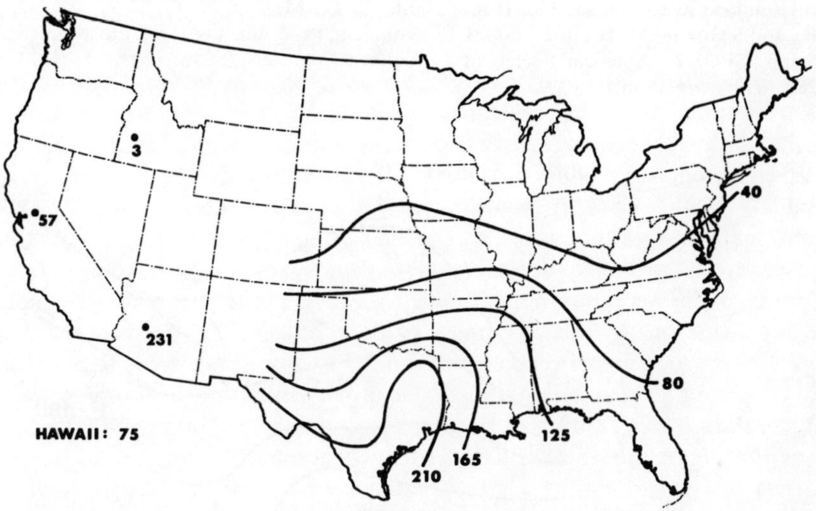

FIGURE 12. Expected decrease in hay consumption (kilogram per cow) for 122-day summer period from June 1 through September 30. (From Hahn, G. L. and Osburn, D. D., *Trans. ASAE,* 12, 448, 1969. With permission.)

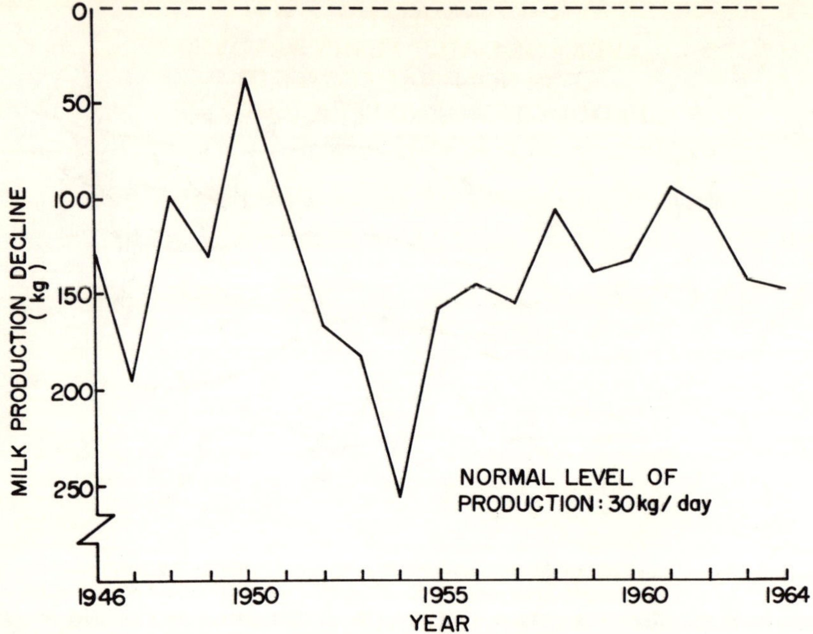

FIGURE 13. Year-to-year variability in predicted summertime production decline for cows with a normal production level of 30 kg/day exposed to the naturally varying environment at Columbia, Mo. (From Hahn, G. L., Meador, N. F., Thompson, G. B., and Shanklin, M. D., in *Livestock Environment*, Proc. Int. Livestock Environment Symp., SPO1-74, American Society of Agricultural Engineers, St. Joseph, Mich., 1974, 288. With permission.)

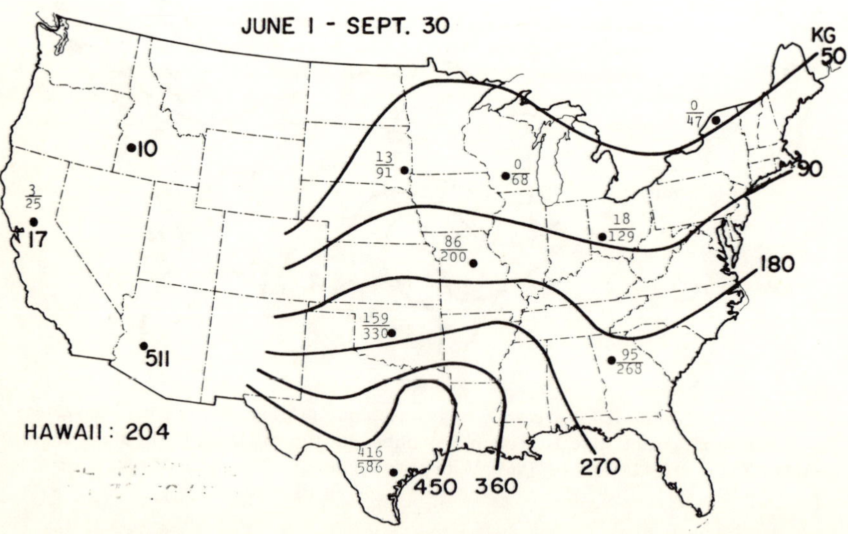

FIGURE 14. Expected milk production losses for dairy cows with a normal production level of 32 kg/day during the June 1 to September 30 summer season. (Values by selected stations, e.g., 86/200, represent the 10th and 90th percentile production losses for that station, indicating the variability in production due to climate fluctuations.) (From Hahn, G. L. and Nienaber, J. A., Summer Weather Variability and Livestock Production, ASAE Paper No. 76-1033, American Society of Agricultural Engineers, St. Joseph, Mich., 1976.

Table 1
AVERAGE DAILY TEMPERATURES FOR NOMINAL LOSSES IN PRODUCTION AND EFFICIENCY OF LIVESTOCK

Animal	Acceptable temperature range[a]
Dairy cattle —	
lactating or within 2 weeks of breeding	4—24°C
Calves	10—26°C
Beef cattle	4—26°C
Sheep	4—24°C
Hogs	
Weaning to market weight	10—24°C[b]
Farrowing sows	10—16°C
Poultry	
Growing (over 10 days old)	13—27°C[b]
Laying hens	7—21°C

[a] Acceptable average daily temperatures for long-term exposure (concurrent relative humidity less than 75%). The range should be shifted downward at least 3°C for high radiant heat loads (greater than 1 cal/cm^2/min). Nutrition, management, housing, and other factors can also alter the acceptable range.

[b] Optimum temperature shifts downward within this range as weights increase.

From Hahn, G. L., in *Progress in Animal Biometeorology,* Johnson, H. D., Ed., Swets & Zeitlinger, Amsterdam, 1976, 496. With permission.

Table 2
TEMPERATURE, HUMIDITY, VENTILATION RATE, AND SPACE REQUIREMENTS FOR CATTLE, SWINE, AND POULTRY

	Cattle	Swine	Poultry
Animal	**Stall barns**	**Farrowing houses**	**Broiler houses**
Temperature range	1.7—23.9°C	10—23.9°C (with small areas warmed for pigs to 26.7°C by means of brooders or heat lamps; cold drafts and temperature extremes must be avoided)	15.6—18.3°C[a] 29.4—32.2°C, (reducing 5°/week until room temperature is reached)[b]
Relative humidity	55—75%	Up to 75% maximum	50—80%
Ventilation rate	50—200 cfm per cow (the lower rate for poorly insulated shelters in extremely cold weather)	10—50 cfm per sow (the low rate for winter and with newborn pigs; the high rate when outdoor temperatures are above 1.7°C and the pigs are ready for weaning)	0.5—1 cfm/lb of live weight in winter; 2 cfm/lb of live weight in summer
Space	—	—	0.6—1.0 ft² per bird (7—9 in² per chick under brooder)
	Milking barns	**Nursery houses**	**Laying houses[c]**
Temperature range	10—23.9°C (for operator comfort)	10—23.9°C	7.2—29.4°C
Relative humidity	55—75%	75% maximum in winter; no established limit in summer	—
Ventilation rate	50—200 cfm per cow (the lower rate for poorly insulated shelters in extremely cold weather)	6—9 cfm per pig below 1.7°C outdoor temperature; above 1.7°C 13—50 cfm per pig (the low rate is for 45.5-kg pigs and moderate temperatures; the high rate is for 113.6-kg pigs and hot weather)	1—3 cfm per bird in winter and 4—6 cfm per bird in summer
Space	—	—	On litter, 3—4 ft² per hen (may be reduced for small breeds); on litter with utility pit, 1—2.5 ft² per hen; on slats, 1—2 ft² per hen

			Laying houses, birds in cages
Temperature range	—	—	7.2—29.4°C
Relative humidity	—	—	50—80%
Ventilation rate	—	—	5—6 cfm per hen (with provisions for opening windows or side walls in summer)
Space	—	—	1—2 ft^2 per hen

[a] Room temperature.
[b] Temperature under brooder hover.
[c] With birds on litter and slatted floors.

From ASHRAE Guide & Data Book, Applications Volume, MacPhee, C. W., Ed., American Society of Heating, Refrigeration, and Air-conditioning Engineers, New York, 1971, 203. Reprinted with permission from the 1971 Applications Volume, ASHRAE Handbook and Product Directory.

Table 3
SEASONAL EFFECTS ON CONCEPTION RATE OF HOLSTEIN CATTLE IN SUBTROPICAL ZONE[21]

	Temperature and humidity		Conception rate	
Month	Maximum temperature (°C)	Humidity (% RH)	First service only	All breedings
Fall	32.8	73.2	35.2	36.7
Winter	28.7	67.8	70.2	59.0
Spring	33.5	58.5	45.9	44.0
Summer	35.0	76.7	17.4	16.8

Table 4
INFLUENCE OF SHELTER COOLING ON CONCEPTION RATES OF HOLSTEIN COWS IN ARIZONA

Breeding results	July		August		September		Total	
	Control	Cooled	Control	Cooled	Control	Cooled	Control	Cooled
Number bred	27	30	66	60	102	99	195	189
Percentage pregnant	15	33	9	25	16	33	14[a]	31[b]

[a] Breedings per pregnancy for control cows = 7.3.
[b] Breedings per pregnancy for cooled cows = 3.1.

From Stott, G. H., Wiersma, F., and Woods, J. M., *J. Am. Vet. Med. Assoc.*, 161(11), 1339, 1972. With permission.

Table 5
PLASMA TESTOSTERONE CONCENTRATION OF HEREFORD BULLS DURING THE INITIAL 7 DAYS OF EXPOSURE TO 35.5°C, 50% RH

Day of exposure[a]						
1	2	3	4	5	6	7
2.80±0.58	1.69±0.14	2.77±0.64	1.96±0.30	2.39±0.40	1.47±0.36	1.62±0.28

Note: Plasma testosterone concentration is in ng/mℓ.

[a] Each value represents the mean ± SE of eight bulls.

From Rynes, W. E. and Ewing, L. L., *Endocrinology*, 92(2), 509, 1973. With permission.

Table 6
PLASMA TESTOSTERONE CONCENTRATION OF HEREFORD BULLS DURING CONFINEMENT IN ENVIRONMENTAL ROOM

Temperature (°C)	RH (%)	Week of exposure 1	2	3	4	5	6	7	Av.
21.0	50	3.10[a]±0.60	3.52±0.53	2.57±0.42	3.18±0.41	3.99±0.45	3.48±0.59	3.39±0.56	3.32±0.23
35.5	50	1.62±0.28	1.40±0.21	2.22±0.34	2.76±0.47	1.98±0.45	2.27±0.45	2.74±0.62	2.20±0.21

Note: Plasma testosterone concentration is in ng/mℓ.

[a] Each value represents the mean ± SE of eight bulls.

From Rhynes, W. E. and Ewing, L. L., *Endocrinology*, 92(2), 509, 1973. With permission.

Table 7
EFFECTS OF ENVIRONMENTAL TEMPERATURE UPON SPERMATOGENESIS OF MATURING FOWL

	Age in weeks		Number of birds per temperature		Spermatogenesis per age group (%)				
	Trial 1	Trial 2	Trial 1	Trial 2	Trial 1		Trial 2		
					8°	30°	8°	19°	30°
	—	10	—	10	—	—	0.0	0.0	0.0
	11	11	8	10	0.0	0.0	0.0	20.0	0.0
	13	12	8	10	0.0	37.5	0.0	20.0	10.0
	15	13	8	10	25.0	100.0	40.0	60.0	50.0
	17	14	8	10	50.0	100.0	40.0	70.0	90.0
	19	15	8	10	87.5	100.0	50.0	80.0	80.0
Average					32.5	67.5[a]	23.0	42.0[a]	35.0[a]

[a] Means significantly higher ($p<0.5$) than that of the groups from 8°C.

From Houston, T. M., *Poult. Sci.*, 54(4), 1180, 1975. With permission.

Table 8
A SUMMARY OF OBSERVATIONS ON SWINE OBTAINED IN THE CONTROLLED TEMPERATURE ROOMS AND OBSERVATIONS AT SLAUGHTER 25 DAYS AFTER BREEDING

	Dry-bulb temperature (°C)		
	26.7°	30.0°	33.3°
Average daily feed intake (kg)	2.11	2.03	1.86
Average daily gain (kg)	0.47	0.46	0.35
Average rectal temperature (°C)	38.4	39.3	39.9
Breeding and reproductive performance			
Number returning to estrus after breeding	2	8	8
Number failing to come into estrus in rooms	0	2	7
Number not pregnant at slaughter (did not return to heat after breeding)	5	2	3
Number pregnant (25 days)	67	67	62
Average number corpora lutea (25 days)	14.2	13.6	13.1
Average number live embyros (25 days)	10.3	9.7	9.8
Percent pregnant (at 25 days)	90.5	84.8	77.5

Note: Summary is adjusted for differences in age and initial weight.

From Teague, H. S., Roller, W. L., and Grifo, A. P., Jr., *J. Anim. Sci.*, 27(2), 408, 1968. With permission.

Table 9
DEGREE OF THERMAL STRESS AND REPRODUCTIVE RESPONSES IN EWES

		Hot-room ewes (32.2°C, 60% RH)	
	Control[a]	Sheared	Unsheared
Rectal temperature (°C)	39.1±0.04	40.1±0.12	40.6±0.13
Ova fertilized (%)	92.6	64.0	40.7
Abnormal ova (%)	3.7	32.0	55.6

[a] Control = natural environment in October in Kentucky.

From Dutt, R. H., Ellington, E. F., and Carlton, W. W., *J. Anim. Sci.*, 18, 1308, 1959. With permission.

Table 10
EFFECT OF ENVIRONMENTAL TEMPERATURE ON SEMEN QUALITY OF RAMS

	Treatment			
Semen quality (av)	Cooled (20.6°C)	Number of observations	Heated (26.7°C)	Number of observations
Semen volume (mℓ)	0.92	11	1.20	8[a]
Motility[b]	3.5	14[c]	1.8	12
Live sperm (%)	67	14[a]	35	12
Normal sperm (%)	73	14[a]	43	12
Sperm concentration	3.48	14[c]	1.43	12

Note: Semen data of the last two collection periods.

[a] $p = 0.05$.
[b] Concentration expressed in millions per mm^3.
[c] $p = 0.01$.

From Brooks, J. R. and Ross, C. V., *Mo. Agric. Exp. Stn. Res. Bull.*, 801, 1, 1962. With permission.

Table 11
EGG PRODUCTION OF TURKEYS AND FERTILITY OF EGGS AT VARIOUS ENVIRONMENTAL TEMPERATURES[61]

Temperature (°C)	Feed per bird (kg)		Egg production per bird		Settable egg production (%)		Egg weight (g)	Shell thickness (mm)	Fertile eggs (%)	Hatchable fertile eggs (%)
	0—12 weeks	0—24 weeks	12 weeks	24 weeks	12 weeks	24 weeks				
12.8	19.07	37.79	43.9	75.2	83.4	81.1	86.6	34.4	74.8	62.6
21.1	17.36	33.38	42.6	72.0	87.8	84.3	86.0	33.8	74.3	63.6
29.4	15.04	28.76	31.4	43.5	86.7	85.1	83.0	33.4	79.4	58.2

Table 12
LACTATION AND REPRODUCTION EFFICIENCY OF TROPICALLY EVOLVED CRIOLLO AND HOLSTEIN CATTLE AND VARIED CROSSES

Breed	Lactation		Reproduction	
	Yield (kg/day)	Days	Percent pregnant by 100 days after calving	Services per conception
U.S. Fresian (F)	11	305	55	3.0
U.S. Brown Swiss	11	305	67	2.6
Criollo (CCC) (Conteño ConCuernos)	5	180	65	1.7
½ F and ½ CCC	10	300	81	1.9
¾ F and ¼ CCC	10	298		

Adapted from Pearson, L. and Devaccaro, L. P., *World Anim. Rev.*, 12, 8, 1974.

Table 13
MILK YIELD, FAT, AND FATTY ACID COMPOSITION OF HOLSTEIN CATTLE AT THERMONEUTRAL (15 to 24°C) AND HOT (32°C) TEMPERATURES[65]

Temperature (°C)	Milk yield per day (kg)	Milk fat (%)	$C_{12:0}$ (%)	$C_{14:0}$ (%)	$C_{14:1-15:0}$ (%)	$C_{15:1}$ (%)	$C_{16:0}$ (%)	$C_{16:1}$ (%)	$C_{18:0}$ (%)	$C_{18:1}$ (%)	$C_{18:2}$ (%)
15—24[a]	18.4	3.4	2.56	8.63	1.31	0.95	26.38	2.24	10.10	35.49	2.51
32[a]	12.8	2.8	2.19	8.27	1.08	0.91	29.14	2.04	11.75	32.65	2.05
Cool vs. hot	$p < 0.01$	$p < 0.01$	$p < 0.05$		$p < 0.05$		$p < 0.01$		$p < 0.01$	$p < 0.01$	$p < 0.01$

[a] 60% RH.

Table 14A
EFFECTS OF −13°C AS COMPARED TO 10°C ON MILK PRODUCTION, TDN INTAKE, AND THE RATIO OF CONVERSION[a]

	Milk (kg/day)		TDN (kg/day)		Ration of conversion (feed/milk)	
Breed	**10°C**	**−13°C**	**10°C**	**−13°C**	**10°C**	**−13°C**
Holstein	15	14	10.4	11.2	0.70	0.80
Brown Swiss						
Jersey	7.6	3.5	5.9	7.4	0.78	2.1
Brahman			4.5	6.2		

Table 14B
EFFECTS OF 38°C AS COMPARED TO 10°C ON MILK PRODUCTION, TDN INTAKE, AND RATIO OF CONVERSION

	Milk (kg/day)		TDN (kg/day)		Ratio of conversion (feed/milk)	
	10°C	**38°C**	**10°C**	**38°C**	**10°C**	**38°C**
Holstein	18.6	4.9	12.1	2.6	0.65	0.53
Brown Swiss	20.4	9.5	12.2	2.5	0.60	0.26
Jersey	13.5	5.1	8.8	2.8	0.65	0.55
Brahman	3.6	3.2	5.2	3.3	1.44	1.03

Note: $\frac{\text{Feed kg/day}}{\text{Milk kg/day}}$ = kilograms of feed (TDN) required to produce 1 kg milk.

[a] Data from References 68 and 69.

Adapted from Johnson, H. D., in *Progress in Biometeorology,* Tromp, S. W., Ed., Swets & Zeitlinger, Amsterdam, 1972, 43. With permission.

Table 15
EFFECT OF WIND ON MILK PRODUCTION AT FOUR TEMPERATURES

Wind mi/hr (km/hr)	Milk production (% normal)											
	−8°C			10°C			27°C			35°C		
	Holstein	Jersey	Brown Swiss	Holstein	Jersey	Brown Swiss	Holstein	Jersey	Brown Swiss	Holstein	Jersey	Brown Swiss
0.4 (0.64)	76	36	72	100	100	100	85	100	100	63	74	83
5.0 (8.05)	85	39	74	100	100	100	95	100	100	79	94	90
9.0 (14.48)	84	35	75	100	100	100	95	100	100	79	94	90

Note: RH range is 60 to 70% at all four temperatures.

From Johnson, H. D., in *Progress in Biometeorology*, Tromp, S. W., Ed, Swets & Zeitlinger, Amsterdam, 1972, 43. With permission.

Table 16
EFFECT OF RADIATION ON MILK PRODUCTION AT THREE AIR TEMPERATURES

Level of radiation (cal/cm² −min)	Milk production (% normal)					
	8°C		21°C		27°C	
	Holstein	Jersey	Holstein	Jersey	Holstein	Jersey
Variable	100	100	99	99	84	94
5 (0.02)	100	100	100	100	93	99
40 (0.19)	100	100	100	99	92	94
90 (0.42)	100	100	93	95	77	93
130 (0.60)	100	100	90	97	69	87
180 (0.84)	100	100	88	95	57	79

From Johnson, H. D., in *Progress in Biometeorology*, Tromp, S. W., Ed., Swets & Zeitlinger, Amsterdam, 1972, 43. With permission.

Table 17
EGG PRODUCTION AS AFFECTED BY ENVIRONMENTAL TEMPERATURE, ENERGY INTAKE, AND HEAT PRODUCTION BY WHITE LEGHORN LAYING PULLETS

Temperature °C	Temperature °F	Estimated daily energy intake per kilogram metabolic body weight (kcal)		Estimated daily heat production per kilogram metabolic body weight (kcal)	Difference, i.e., energy available for egg production per day per kilogram metabolic body weight (kcal)	Energy available for egg production converted to 1.489 kg metabolic body weight (1.7 kg body weight) (kcal)	Possible production of 57 g eggs by 1.7 kg pullet (assuming 90 kcal per egg) (%)
26.5	80	195.2	(290.7)[a]	145.4	49.8	74.2	82
29.5	85	190.1	(283.1)[a]	142.2	47.9	71.3	79
32.0	90	173.8	(258.8)[a]	131.8	42.0	62.6	70
35.0	95	146.3	(217.8)[a]	114.1	32.2	48.0	53
38.0	100	107.6[b]	(160.2)[a]	89.2[b]	18.4	27.5	31

[a] Estimated metabolizable energy intake of a laying pullet weighing 1.7 kg.

[b] Extrapolated figures; heat production at 38°C is probably higher than indicated in this table.

From Smith, A. J., *Anim. Health Prod.*, 5, 259, 1973. With permission.

Table 18
EFFECT OF ENVIRONMENTAL TEMPERATURE ON MORTALITY, EGG PRODUCTION, FEED CONSUMPTION, AND BODY WEIGHT ON SINGLE-COMB WHITE LEGHORN PULLETS FROM 150 TO 435 DAYS OF AGE[82]

	Temperature		
	Constant		Cycling
	32.2°C	12.8°C	12.8 to 32.2°C
Mortality (%)	17	3	2
Average egg production of survivors	140	179	190
Average egg production per pullet housed	129	177	188
Feed consumption per pullet per day (kg)	0.09	0.13	0.11
Feed per dozen eggs (kg)	2.36	2.45	2.00
Average body weight (kg)	1.77	2.00	2.00

Table 19
SUMMARY OF STEER PERFORMANCE BY SEASONS AND MEAN SEASONAL CLIMATIC CONDITIONS

Month	Air temperature (°C)	Days per month below −23°C	Dew point (°C)	Wind chill (kcal/m^2/hr)	Wind velocity (km/hr)	Precipitation (cm/month)	Average weight (kg)	Average daily gain (kg)	Actual/predicted gain[a]	Daily feed (kg)	Feed/gain[b]	Daily kcal ME/kg body weight
December to February	−17	11	−15	1302	15	2.2	419	1.03	0.99	8.95	9.8	56.7
March to May	2	1	− 3	837	16	1.8	390	1.33	1.18	9.18	7.2	59.7
June to August	17	0	11	420	17	7.0	372	1.51	1.51	7.97	5.6	54.3
September to November	3	1	1	767	15	3.2	431	1.57	1.30	10.68	6.9	60.1

[a] Calculated on the basis of net energy intake (National Research Council, 1970).
[b] Feed per gain values are the average of results for individual pens and were not calculated from the overall means of feed and gain.

From Christison, G. I. and Milligan, J. D., in *Livestock Environment,* American Society of Agricultural Engineers, St. Joseph, Mich., 1974, 296. With permission.

Table 20
WEIGHT GAIN COMPARISONS OF CATTLE AT TWO ENVIRONMENTAL TEMPERATURES

Species	Air temperature (°C)	Weight at 4 months (kg)	Weight at 12 months (kg)	Total gain for 8-month period (kg)	Difference in gain from 10°C values (kg)	Ref.
Santa Gertrudis	10	126.1	342.9	216.8		87
	27	128.4	313.0	184.6	−32.2	87
Brahman	10	112.9	285.8	172.8		87
	27	116.6	297.6	181.0	+ 8.2	87
Shorthorn	10	93.0	298.5	201.9		87
	27	73.9	209.1	135.2	−66.7	87
Holstein	10	103.5	333.3	203.3		88
	27	95.3	302.7	207.4	−22.9	88
Brown Swiss	10	74.2	303.3	229.1		88
	27	89.0	310.2	221.2	− 7.9	88
Jersey	10	65.5	210.0	144.5		88
	27	56.7	197.3	140.6	−3.9	88

Table 21
TEMPERATURE EFFECTS ON WEIGHT GAIN, FEED CONSUMPTION, AND FEED EFFICIENCY OF STEERS

Species	Air temperature (°C)	Rectal temperature (°C)	Weight gain (kg/day)	Feed consumption (kg/day)	Efficiency feed/gain (kg)	Remarks
Hereford × Angus steers[a]	32.6	39.4	1.16	7.56	6.54	Outside continuously, seasonal heat in Imperial Valley, Calif.
	23.9	39.1	1.29	8.46	6.77	Inside continuously, cooled 24 hr/day

[a] Average of four animals per treatment for 3 years.

Table 22
FEED CONSUMPTION OF 8-WEEK-OLD PIGS

Air temperature (°C)	Body weight (kg)	Food consumption (kg/week)	Weight gain (kg/week)
10	29.9	11.15	4.03
15	33.4	12.84	5.39
20	37.5	12.17	5.10
25	38.4	12.77	4.72
30	29.2	9.11	4.56

Note: Data represent average values for feed consumption.

From Fuller, M. F., *Br. J. Nutr.*, 19, 531, 1965. With permission.

Table 23
EFFECT OF AMBIENT AIR TEMPERATURE AND MEAN LIVEWEIGHT ON RATE OF GAIN IN SWINE

Average Daily Gain per Pig (kg)

Mean liveweight (kg)	Air temperature (°C)							
	4.4	10.0	15.6	21.1	26.7	32.2	37.8	43.3
45.36		0.62	0.72	0.91	0.89	0.64	0.18	−0.60
68.04	0.58	0.67	0.79	0.98	0.83	0.52	−0.09	−1.18
90.72	0.54	0.71	0.87	1.01	0.76	0.40	−0.35	
113.40	0.50	0.76	0.94	0.97	0.68	0.28	−0.62	
136.40	0.46	0.80	1.02	0.93	0.62	0.16	−0.88	
158.76	0.43	0.85	1.09	0.90	0.55	0.05	−1.15	

Adapted from Heitman, H., Jr., Kelly, C. F., and Bond, T. E., *J. Anim. Sci.*, 17, 62, 1958. With permission.

Table 24
GROWTH AND FEED CONVERSION FOR CHICKENS

Species	Air temperature (°C)	Body weight (kg)	Growth rate (g/day)	Conversion g/g gain	Ref.
Chickens	5	1.49	17.9	5.1	92
	5—20 (cyclic)	1.50	19.3	3.9	92
	20	1.44	17.2	4.3	92
	20—34 (cyclic)	1.20	15.0	3.5	92
	34	1.09	13.4	3.1	92
Chickens (broilers)	7	1.61		2.50	117
	13	1.60		2.39	117
	18	1.64		2.26	117
	24	1.57		2.20	117

Table 25
AVERAGE VALUES FOR WEIGHT GAIN AND FAT DEPOSITION OF MALE TURKEYS FROM 12 TO 24 WEEKS OF AGE[93]

	Temperature (°C)			
	10	15.6	21.1	26.7
Fat deposition (%)	7.0	7.9	7.1	4.5
Average gain (kg/week)	3.86	4.35	4.31	3.76
Feed conversion (kg/kg gain)	3.40	3.08	2.95	2.99

Table 26
FEED AND WATER CONSUMPTION AND RECTAL TEMPERATURE

Species	Air temperature (°C)	Rectal temperature (°C)	Body weight (kg)	Feed (kg/day)	TDN (kg/day)	Water ℓ/day	Remarks	Ref.
Holstein	18	38.7	513.0	21.0	—	94.2	Lactating, 2-week exposure	94
	29	39.6	504.1	18.1	—	88.2	9-week exposure	94
	18	38.5	589.0	12.1	—	52.1	Dry cows, 2-week exposure	94
	29	38.7	600.0	11.6	—	53.7	9-week exposure	94
	−15	—	616.7	—	10.85	—	Lactating	119
	18.3	—	619.1	—	10.19	—	Lactating	119
	34.7	—	604.8	—	8.33	—	Lactating	119
Brown Swiss (heifers)	2	38.7	—	2.1	4.97	25.7	Fixed feed concentrate; hay *ad libitum;* 5—9 day exposure	95
	10	38.6	—	—	4.60	26.9		
	21	38.7	399.2	—	4.29	31.4		
	27	38.7	—	—	4.29	41.3		
	32	39.7	—	—	3.53	66.2		
	35	39.6	417.3	—	3.69	72.7		
Holstein (heifers)	2	38.7	—	—	5.96	23.9		
	10	38.6	—	—	5.63	23.9		
	21	38.7	426.4	—	5.21	27.3		
	27	38.9	—	—	5.12	31.8		
	32	39.9	—	—	3.55	55.3		
	35	40.1	435.5	—	3.30	67.4		

Jersey	2	38.6	—	—	3.51	19.0		
(heifers)	10	38.5	—	—	3.37	19.4		
	21	38.6	263.1	—	3.07	28.1		
	27	38.6	—	—	2.94	35.0		
	32	39.2	—	—	1.89	60.6		
	35	39.4	272.2	—	1.80	61.7		
	−15	—	395.5	—	7.72	—	Lactating	119
	18.3	—	405.5	—	7.09	—	Lactating	119
	34.7	—	402.3	—	5.86	—	Lactating	119
Brahman	10	38.8	329.8	6.9	3.33	16.7	8-month av.	88, 96
	27	39.0	347.0	6.6	3.51	29.2		87, 88, 96
Santa Gertrudis	10	29.0	405.5	7.9	3.97	23.5		87, 88, 96
	27	39.2	365.1	6.7	3.46	31.0		87, 88, 96
Shorthorn	10	39.0	351.5	7.4	3.82	23.5		87, 88, 96
	27	40.2	261.3	9.4	2.95	57.5		87, 88, 96
Scottish Highland	9[a]	38.6	352.0	7.6	—		High roughage	97
	18[a]	38.7	378.9	6.9	—	38.0		97
	31[a]	39.8	392.4	4.1	—	55.0	Low concentrate feed	97
Zebu	9[a]	29.0	353.7	6.4	—	—		97
	18[a]	38.9	372.3	6.0	—	22.0		97
	31[a]	38.9	379.8	5.2	—	36.0		97

[a] Four-week exposure.

Table 27
TEMPERATURE AND HUMIDITY EFFECTS ON HAY, TDN, AND WATER CONSUMPTION

Environmental conditions				Hay			TDN			Water		
Dry bulb (°C)	Relative humidity (%)	Vapor pressure (mmHg)	Dew point (°C)	Mean difference	SEM	Level of significance[a]	Mean difference	SEM	Level of significance	Mean difference (ℓ/day)	SEM	Level of significance
23.9	90	20.0	22.1	+0.07[b]	0.60	n.s.	−0.47[b]	0.38	n.s.	− 1.59[b]	2.23	n.s.
26.7	30	8.0	7.6	−2.37	1.20	0.10	−1.40	0.83	n.s.	+ 4.92	2.61	0.10
26.7	50	13.0	15.3	−2.48	0.89	0.02	−1.30	0.51	0.05	+ 1.89	3.29	n.s.
26.7	80	21.0	22.9	−1.95	0.45	0.01	−1.00	0.27	0.01	− 0.38	1.97	n.s.
29.4	50	15.5	17.9	−4.65	1.40	0.01	−3.10	0.80	0.01	+ 0.79	4.20	n.s.
29.4	70	21.5	23.3	−5.83	1.38	0.01	−4.13	0.94	0.01	− 1.14	5.45	n.s.
32.2	20	7.0	6.4	+1.72	0.95	0.10	+0.50	0.60	n.s.	+14.76	3.07	0.01
32.2	25	9.0	9.7	−3.65	1.44	0.05	−2.58	0.89	0.02	+10.60	3.97	0.05
32.2	40	14.5	16.8	−9.98	1.40	0.01	−5.90	0.72	0.01	− 5.30	3.71	n.s.
32.2	50	18.0	20.4	−7.81	1.09	0.01	−4.20	0.58	0.01	+ 6.81	7.19	n.s.
35.0	25	10.0	11.9	−8.17	1.30	0.01	−5.30	0.80	0.01	+ 1.32[c]	3.52	n.s.

Note: Based on average differences for 12 cows at 65° F, 50% RH as compared to treatments.

[a] Significance determined by student's *t* test; n.s. = not significant.
[b] Cow 844 omitted due to acute mastitis (23.9°C, 90% RH).
[c] Eleven cows (35°C, 25% RH).

Adapted from Johnson, H. D., Ragsdale, A. C., Berry, I. L., and Shanklin, M. D., *Mo. Agric. Exp. Stn. Res. Bull.*, 846, 1, 1963. With permission.

Table 28
RECTAL TEMPERATURE AND WATER INTAKES AT VARIOUS ENVIRONMENTAL TEMPERATURES

Species	Air temperature (°C)	Rectal temperature (°C)	Body weight (kg)	Water uptake		Remarks
				ℓ/kg/Body wt	ℓ/kg/Feed	
Swine	7	39.1	25.8	0.136	2.88	Average value for 3 animals
	12	39.4	37.6	0.122	2.76	Average value for 5 animals
	20	39.6	34.8	0.123	2.74	
	30	39.8	35.1	0.181	4.28	

From Close, W. H., Mount, L. E., and Stuart, I. B., *Anim. Prod.*, 13, 285, 1971. With permission.

Table 29
FEED CONSUMPTION OF LANDRACE SWINE

Air temperature (°C)	Feed consumption (per $kg^{0.72}$/week)	Remarks
10	1.10	Castrated males
15	1.08	
20	0.99	
25	0.97	
30	0.85	

From Fuller, M. F., *Br. J. Nutr.*, 19, 531, 1965. With permission.

Table 30
EFFECT OF AMBIENT TEMPERATURE AND FEEDING REGIMES ON DAILY FEED INTAKE, WATER CONSUMPTION, AND URINE OUTPUT IN SHEEP

Ration Roughage level (%) Trial	1 25			2 50			3 75			4 75 + Fat			Mean		
	1	2	3	1	2	3	1	2	3	1	2	3	1	2	3
Ambient Temperature	Normal	High	Normal	Normal	High	Normal	Normal	High	Normal	Normal	High	Normal	Normal	High	Normal
Feed intake (g/day)	758[a]	652[b]	662[b]	804[a]	518[b]	626[c]	879[a]	447[b]	686[b]	624[a]	484[b]	540[b]	766[a]	525[b]	629[b]
Water consumption (ℓ/day)	2.34[a]	3.66[b]	2.48[a]	1.54[a]	2.50[b]	2.20[c]	2.05[a]	3.18[b]	2.64[a]	2.17[a]	3.01[b]	2.10[a]	2.03[a]	3.08[b]	2.35[a]
Urine volume (mℓ/day)	712[a]	1175[b]	806[a]	404[a]	643[b]	453[c]	674[a]	950[b]	684[a]	483[a]	832[b]	558[a]	568[a]	900[b]	625[a]

Note: Rations 1, 2, and 3 contained barley hay in the levels of 25.50 and 75%, respectively. The fourth ration contained 75% hay and no barley grain; instead 6% tallow was incorporated to make it isocaloric to ration 1. Ambient temperature: normal, 22°C and 65% RH; high, 32°C and 88% RH.

[a,b,c] Means having different superscripts in the same row under the same ration are significantly different ($p < 0.05$).

From Bhattacharya, A. N. and Hussain, F., *J. Anim. Sci.*, 38(4), 877, 1974. With permission.

Table 31
FEED AND WATER CONSUMPTION AND RECTAL TEMPERATURE

Species	Air temperature (°C)	Rectal temperature (°C)	Body weight (kg)	Feed (kg/day)	Water (ℓ/day)	Remarks	Ref.
Turkeys	10	39.9	14.81	0.46	0.35	Adult males, 28-day exposure	101
	21	40.2	13.23	0.37	0.61	Adult males, 28-day exposure	101
	32	40.9	12.47	0.32	1.03	Adult males, 28-day exposure	101
	38	41.7	11.91	0.24	1.26	Adult males, 28-day exposure	101
Chickens							
Laying hens	22	—		0.11	—	250-kcal/day diet	102
	30	—		0.11	—	250-kcal/day diet	102
Roosters	22	—		0.06	—	250-kcal/day diet	102
	30	—		0.05	—	250-kcal/day diet	102
Broilers[a]							
Rabbits	9	38.3	4.37	0.15	0.20	250-kcal/day diet	103
	28	38.8	3.65	0.09	0.23	250-kcal/day diet	103
Swine	7	39.1	25.8	—	—	250-kcal/day diet	98
	12	39.4	37.6	—	—	250-kcal/day diet	98
	20	39.6	34.8	—	—	250-kcal/day diet	98
	30	39.8	35.1	—	—	250-kcal/day diet	98

[a] Data in Table 32.

Table 32
TEMPERATURE AND HUMIDITY EFFECTS ON FEED AND WATER CONVERSION OF GROWING BROILERS

	21.1°C				26.7°C		35.0°C	
	48% RH	58% RH	70% RH	90% RH	40% RH	93% RH	30% RH	90% RH
kg H_2O/kg gain (3—10 weeks of age)[a]	4.60	4.29	3.85	3.57	4.64	4.30	11.2	11.0
kg H_2O/kg feed (3—10 weeks of age)[a]	1.91	1.78	1.75	1.62	2.20	1.90	5.2	4.2

[a] Five to ten weeks at 26.7 and 35.0°C.

From Winn, P. N. and Godfrey, E. F., *Int. J. Biometeorol.*, 11(1), 39, 1967. With permission.

Table 33
WATER CONSUMPTION OF CHICKS 4 TO 10 WEEKS OF AGE AT TWO ENVIRONMENTAL TEMPERATURES

	Water consumption (ℓ/day/1000 birds)	
Age in weeks	7.2°C, 63%RH	35.0°C, 32%RH
4	55.0	140.0
5	90.0	180.0
10	200.0	340.0

From Winn, P. N. and Godfrey, E. F., *Int. J. Biometeorol.*, 11(1), 39, 1967. With permission.

Table 34
HEAT PRODUCTION

Species	Sex	Age (months)	Body weight (kg)	Acclimation indoors (°C)	Temperature (°C)	Duration	Consumption O_2		Remarks	Ref.
							ℓ/kg/hr	kJ/kg/hr[a]		
Brahman	F	15.6	341	10	18	1 Month	0.140	2.76	Fasting	105
		16.0	364	26.6	18	1 Month	0.154	3.03	Fasting	105
		16.1	350	10	10	14 Months	0.229	4.61	Resting	105
		16.6	375	26.6	26.6	14 Months	0.224	4.51	Resting	105
Angus	M	30	525	15—20	3.8	4 Days	0.211	4.24	Steers	106
		30	527	15—20	14.8	4 Days	0.198	3.98	Resting	106
		30	519	15—20	24.8	4 Days	0.201	4.04	Resting	106
		30	528	15—20	35.2	4 Days	0.207	4.16	Resting	106
Brown Swiss	F	11	300	10	10	10 Months	0.33	6.64	Resting	107
		10.8	300	26.7	26.7	10 Months	0.34	6.84	Resting	107
Holstein	F	10.6	325	10	10	10 Months	0.35	7.04	Resting	107
		11.1	300	26.7	26.7	10 Months	0.34	6.84	Resting	107
Jersey	F	10.6	200	10	10	10 Months	0.395	7.94	Resting	107
		11.3	200	26.7	26.7	10 Months	0.355	7.14	Resting	107
Shorthorn	F	16.4	375	10	10	14 Months	0.258	5.19	Resting	105
		16.4	301	26.6	18	1 Month	0.209	4.12	Fasting	105
		16.4	300	26.6	26.6	14 Months	0.283	5.69	Resting	105
		16.6	380	10	18	1 Month	0.164	3.23	Fasting	105
Santa Gertrudis	F	15.3	425	10	10	14 Months	0.249	5.01	Resting	105
		15.5	416	10	18	1 Month	0.162	3.19	Fasting	105
		16.0	385	26.6	18	1 Month	0.147	2.89	Fasting	105
		16.0	375	26.6	26.6	14 Months	0.229	4.61	Resting	105

Note: Total heat production is reduced at the higher environmental temperature of 26°C, with the exception of the Brown Swiss.

[a] Conversion: ℓO_2/kg/hr × TE (4.8 normal, 4.7 fasting) × 4.19 = kJ/kg/hr.

Table 35
HEAT-PRODUCTION VALUES FOR SELECTED CATTLE UNDER NORMAL CONDITIONS[108]

Species	Rectal temperature (°C)	Body weight (kg)	Heat production (kJ/hr)	Remarks
Brahman				
Lactating	38.1	331	2053	Resting
Dry	38.4	431	2095	Resting
Jersey				
Lactating	38.1	376	2597	Resting
Holstein				
Lactating	38.2	553	3561	Resting
Brown Swiss				
Lactating	38.0	608	3771	Resting
Dry	38.6	190	1466	Resting

Note: Normal conditions = average values for each breed between 4.4 and 15.6°C environmental temperature, the apparent comfort zone for these cows.

Table 36
HEAT PRODUCTION AND HEAT LOSS

Species	Temperature (°C)	Body weight (kg)	Evaporative		Nonevaporative total (kJ/m²/hr)	Heat production (kJ/hr)	Remarks	Ref.
			Respiratory kJ/m²/hr	Cutaneous kJ/m²/hr				
Holstein	10	—	—	—	—	4692	Control fed	109
Lactating								
	20	—	—	—	—	4609	Control fed	109
	30	—	—	—	—	4064	Control fed	109
	40	—	—	—	—	3561	Control fed	109
Nonlactating	10	—	—	—	—	3561	Resting	109
	20	—	—	—	—	3393	Resting	109
	30	—	—	—	—	2681	Resting	109
	40	—	—	—	—	220	Resting	109
Jersey	−10	385.7	41.9	67.0	599	3268	Resting	110, 111
	0	380.3	50.3	83.8	586	3310	Resting	110, 111
	10	389.0	62.9	92.2	481	2974	Resting	110, 111
	20	410.0	75.4	188.6	335	2933	Resting	110, 111
	30	420.3	100.6	318.4	125	2723	Resting	110, 111
	35	402.3	134.1	293.3	62	2304	Resting	110, 111

Table 37
RELATION BETWEEN METABOLIC RATE AND AMBIENT TEMPERATURE FOR NEWBORN AND 90-KG PIGS[112]

Swine	Temperature (°C)	Metabolic rate: kcal/m², or hr	Metabolic rate: kJ/m², or hr
Newborn	5	—	—
90 kg	5	78	326
Newborn	10	139	582
90 kg	10	69	289
Newborn	15	134	561
90 kg	15	60	251
Newborn	20	120	502
90 kg	20	50	209
Newborn	25	104	435
90 kg	25	50	209
Newborn	30	79	331
90 kg	30	50	209

Table 38
HEAT PRODUCTION AND METABOLISM: SWINE

Age (months)	Body weight (kg)	Acclimation	Temperature (°C)	Duration	O_2 consumption: ℓ/kg/hr	O_2 consumption: kJ/kg/hr[a]	Remarks	Ref.
43	98.0	Outdoors, seasonal	13.4	4—5 days	0.240	4.83	Fasting	113
46	139.0	Outdoors, seasonal	13.4	4—5 days	0.179	3.60	Fasting	113
48	169.0	Outdoors, seasonal	23.7	4—5 days	0.110	2.21	Fasting	113
	22.7	—	10.0	—	—	17.74	Resting	129
	90.7	—	10.0	—	—	8.30	Resting	129
	181.0	—	10. 0	—	—	6.62	Resting	129
	22.7	—	22.0	—	—	15.41	Resting	129
	90.7	—	22.0	—	—	7.01	Resting	129
	181.0	—	22.0	—	—	5.15	Resting	129
	22.7	—	32.0	—	—	15.64	Resting	129
	90.7	—	32.0	—	—	6.43	Resting	129
	181.0	—	32.0	—	—	4.63	Resting	129

[a] Conversion: ℓO_2/kg/hr × 4.7 (TE) × 4.19 = kJ/kg/hr.

Table 39
HEAT PRODUCTION AND HEAT LOSS

Species	Temperature (°C)	Evaporative Total (kJ/kg·hr)	Evaporative Respiratory (kJ/kg·hr)	Evaporative Cutaneous (kJ/kg·hr)	Nonevaporative total heat loss (kJ/kg·hr)	Heat production (kJ/m²/hr)	Remarks	Ref.
Sheep	12	1.5	0.9	0.6	5.4	—	3—8 cm, wool	114
	20	1.9	1.4	0.6	5.4	—	5—8 cm, wool	114
	30	3.3	2.8	0.5	5.4	—	3—8 cm, wool	114
	38	5.1	3.9	1.2	5.5	—	Shorn sheep	114
Sheep (closely clipped)	10	—	—	—	—	—	600 g feed	115
		—	—	—	—	480	1200 g feed	115
		—	—	—	—	515	1800 g feed	115
	20	—	—	—	—	349	600 g feed	115
		—	—	—	—	345	1200 g feed	115
		—	—	—	—	366	1800 g feed	115
	30	—	—	—	—	223	600 g feed	115
		—	—	—	—	272	1200 g feed	115
		—	—	—	—	296	1800 g feed	115
	40	—	—	—	—	201	600 g feed	115
		—	—	—	—	270	1200 g feed	115
		—	—	—	—	349	1800 g feed	115

Table 40
HEAT PRODUCTION IN TURKEYS

Sex	Temperature (°C)	Body weight (kg)	Evaporative total (kJ/hr)	Heat loss (kJ/hr)	Remarks	Ref.
M	10.0	17.2	14.5	136.2	Total	116
F	10.0	9.9	5.3	83.8	Total	116
M	20.0	16.8	25.7	118.9	Total	116
F	20.0	9.6	15.3	73.3	Total	116
M	30.0	16.8	44.5	91.7	Total	116
F	30.0	9.1	21.8	49.8	Total	116
M	35.0	15.9	57.1	80.7	Total	116
F	35.0	8.7	24.1	43.8	Total	116
M	29.4	0.11	—	3.49	Age 7 days	130
M	35.0	0.11	—	4.36	Age 6 days	130
M	40.6	0.13	—	9.07	Age 8 days	130
M	23.9	0.57	—	4.36	Age 27 days	130
M	26.7	0.63	—	6.63	Age 28 days	130
M	32.2	0.74	—	10.47	Age 29 days	130

Table 41
HEAT PRODUCTION IN CHICKENS

Species	Temperature (°C)	Body weight (kg)	Heat production (kJ/hr)	Total vaporization (kJ/hr)	Remarks	Ref.
Chickens	5	1.49	18.5	—	25 Day temperature exposure, 24-hr fast	92
	5—20 (cyclic)	1.50	19.1	—		92
	20	1.44	16.3	—		92
	20—34 (cyclic)	1.20	16.0	—		92
	34	1.09	11.5	—		92
Broilers	19.4	1.13	35.51	6.89	Resting	131
	19.4	2.04	41.50	7.16	Resting	131
	25.0	0.36	15.69	3.48	Resting	131
	25.0	0.72	24.25	5.43	Resting	131
	28.9	0.045	2.88	0.37	Resting	131
	28.9	0.13	6.52	1.65	Resting	131

Table 42
HEAT PRODUCTION VALUES FOR RABBITS[109]

Temperature (°C)	Body weight (kg)	Heat production (kJ/hr)
9	4.37	88.0
28	3.65	71.2

REFERENCES

1. **Hahn, G. L.**, Shelter engineering for cattle and other domestic animals, in *Progress in Animal Biometeorology,* Johnson, H. D., Ed., Swets & Zeitlinger, Amsterdam, 1976, 496—503.
2. *ASHRAE Guide & Data Book,* Applications Volume, MacPhee, C. W., Ed., American Society of Heating, Refrigeration and Air-conditioning Engineers, New York, 1971, 203—222.
3. **Bond, T. E. and Kelly, C. F.**, in *Environment of Animals,* U.S. Department of Agriculture, Washington, D.C., 1960, 231—242.
4. **Johnson, H. D., Lippincott, A. C., and Vanjonack, W. J.**, *Trans. Mo. Acad. Sci.,* 3, 6, 1975.
5. **Abilay, T. A. and Johnson, H. D.**, *J. Dairy Sci.,* 56(5), 642, 1973.
6. **Vincent, C. K.**, *J. Am. Vet. Med. Assoc.,* 161(11), 1333—1338, 1972.
7. **Dale, H. E., Ragsdale, A. C., and Cheng, C. S.**, *J. Anim. Sci.,* 18, 1363—1366, 1959.
8. **Gangwar, P. D., Branton, C., and Evans, D. L.**, *J. Dairy Sci.,* 48, 222—227, 1965.
9. **Hall, J. G., Branton, C., and Stone, E. J.**, *J. Dairy Sci.,* 42, 1086—1094, 1959.
10. **Vincent, C. K.**, *J. Am. Med. Assoc.,* 161(11), 1333—1338, 1972.
11. **Fallon, G. R.**, *J. Reprod. Fertil.,* 3, 116—123, 1962.
12. **Long, C. R., Nipper, W. A., and Vincent, C. K.**, *La. Agric.,* 12, 12—13, 1969.
13. **Ulberg, L. C. and Burfening, P. J.**, *J. Anim. Sci.,* 26, 571—577, 1967.
14. **Vincent, C. K. and Nipper, W. A.**, *La. Cattleman,* 70, 6—7, 1970.
15. **Dunlap, S. E. and Vincent, C. K.**, *J. Anim. Sci.,* 32, 1216—1218, 1971.
16. **Mercier, E. and Salisbury, G. W.**, *Cornell Vet.,* 36, 301—311, 1946.
17. **Wiersma, F. and Stott, G. H.**, *Trans. ASAE,* 9, 309—313, 1966.
18. **Wiersma, F. and Stott, G. H.**, *Trans. ASAE,* 12, 130—132, 1969.
19. **Ragsdale, A. C., Brody, S., Thompson, H. J., and Worstell, D. M.**, *Mo. Agric. Exp. Stn. Res. Bull.,* 425, 1—27, 1948.
20. **Bonsma, J. C.**, *J. Agric. Sci.,* 39, 204—221, 1949.
21. **Ingraham, R. H., Gillette, D. D., and Wagner, W. D.**, *J. Dairy Sci.,* 57(4), 476—482, 1974.
22. **Gwazduskas, F. C., Wilcox, C. J., and Thatcher, W. W.**, *J. Dairy Sci.,* 58(1), 88—92, 1975.
23. **Stott, G. H. and Williams, R. J.**, *J. Dairy Sci.,* 45, 1369—1375, 1962.
24. **Stott, G. H., Wiersma, F., and Woods, J. M.**, *J. Am. Vet. Med. Assoc.,* 161(11), 1339—1344, 1972.
25. **Madan, M. L. and Johnson, H. D.**, *J. Dairy Sci.,* 56(11), 1420—1423, 1973.
26. **Johnson, H. D.**, in *Progress in Biometeorology,* Tromp, S. W., Ed., Swets & Zeitlinger, Amsterdam, 1972, 43—51.
27. **Erb, R. E., Wilbur, J. W., and Hilton, J. H.**, *J. Dairy Sci.,* 23, 549, 1940.
28. **Kelly, J. W. and Hurst, V.**, *J. Am. Vet. Med. Assoc.,* 143, 40—43, 1963.
29. **Casady, R. B., Myers, R. M., and Legates, J. C.**, *J. Dairy Sci.,* 36, 14—23, 1953.
30. **Skinner, J. D. and Louw, G. N.**, *J. Appl. Physiol.,* 21, 1784—1790, 1966.
31. **Chowdhury, A. K. and Steinberger, E.**, *Am. J. Anat.,* 115, 509, 1964.
32. **Moule, G. R. and Waites, G. M. H.**, *J. Reprod. Fertil.,* 5, 433, 1963.
33. **Rhynes, W. E. and Ewing, L. L.**, *Endocrinology,* 92(2), 509—512, 1973.
34. **Casady, R. B., Myers, R. M., and Legates, J. E.**, *J. Dairy Sci.,* 36, 14—23, 1953.
35. **Johnston, J. E., Naelapaa, H., and Frye, J. B., Jr.**, *J. Anim. Sci.,* 22, 432—436, 1963.
36. **Skinner, J. D. and Louw, G. N.**, *J. Appl. Physiol.,* 21, 1784—1790, 1966.
37. **Austin, J. W., Hupp, E. W., and Murphree, R. L.**, *J. Anim. Sci.,* 20, 307—310, 1961.
38. **El-Azab, E. A.**, *Anim. Breed. Abstr.,* 36, 340, 1968.
39. **Waites, G. M. H. and Setchell, B. P.**, *Some physiological aspects of the function of the testis,* in *The Gonads,* McKerns, K. W., Ed., Appleton-Century-Crofts, New York, 1969, 649—714.
40. **Ulberg, L. C.**, Effect of macro- and micro-environment on the biology of mammalian reproduction, in *Ground Level Climatology,* Shaw, R. H., Ed., American Association for the Advancement of Science, Washington, D.C., 1967, 265—276.
41. **Ulberg, L. C. and Burfening, P. J.**, *J. Anim. Sci.,* 26, 571— 577, 1967.
42. **Burfening, P. J. and Ulberg, L. C.**, *J. Reprod. Fertil.,* 15, 87—92, 1968.
43. **Alliston, C. W., Howarth, B., and Ulberg, L. C.**, *J. Reprod. Fertil.,* 9, 337—341, 1965.
44. **Burfening, P. J., Alliston, C. W., and Ulberg, L. C.**, *J. Exp. Zool.,* 170, 55—59, 1969.
45. **Rhynes, W. E. and Ewing, L. L.**, *Endocrinology,* 92(2), 509—512, 1973.
46. **Houston, T. M.**, *Poult. Sci.,* 54(4), 1180—1184, 1975.
47. **Teague, H. S., Roller, W. L., and Grifo, A. P., Jr.**, J. Anim. Sci., *27(2), 408—411, 1968.*
48. **Steinbach, J.**, Proc. 6th Int. Congr. Animal Reproduction Artificial Insemination, Paris, 1968, 325—327.
49. **Wettemann, R. P., Wells, M. E., Omtvedt, I. T., Pope, C. E., and Turman, E. J.**, *J. Anim. Sci.,* 42(3), 664—669, 1976.
50. **Alliston, C. W., Egli, G. E., and Ulberg, L. C.**, *J. Appl. Physiol.,* 16(2), 89, 1957.

51. Alliston, C. W. and Ulberg, L. C., *J. Anim. Sci.*, 20, 608, 1961.
52. Dutt, R. H., Ellington, E. F., and Carlton, W. W., *J. Anim. Sci.*, 18, 1308—1318, 1959.
53. Dutt, R. H., *J. Anim. Sci.*, 22, 713, 1963.
54. Wilson, R. L., Godley, W. C., and Hurst, V., *J. Anim. Sci.*, 20, 693, 1961.
55. Godley, W. C., Wilson, R. L., and Hurst, V., *J. Anim. Sci.*, 25, 212, 1966.
56. Brooks, J. R. and Ross, C. V., *Mo. Agric. Exp. Stn. Res. Bull.*, 801, 1—20, 1962.
57. Braden, A. W. H. and Mattner, P. E., *Aust. J. Agric. Res.*, 21, 509—518, 1970.
58. Dawson, R. M. C., *Biochem. J.*, 68, 512, 1958.
59. Amir, D. and Ortavant, R., *Ann. Biol. Anim. Biochim. Biophys.*, 8, 195, 1968.
60. Johnson, H. D., *Meteorol. Monogr.*, 6(28), 109—122, 1965.
61. Thomason, D. M., Leighton, A. T., Jr., and Mason, J. P., Jr., *Poult. Sci.*, 51(4), 1438—1449, 1972.
62. Pearson, L. and Devaccaro, L. P., *World Anim. Rev.*, 12, 8—13, 1974.
63. Bianca, W., *J. Dairy Sci.*, 32, 291—345, 1965.
64. Johnson, H. D., *Int. J. Biometeorol.*, 9(2), 103—116, 1965.
65. Moody, C. G., Van Soest, P. J., McDowell, R. E., and Ford, G. S., *J. Dairy Sci.*, 54(10), 1457—1460, 1971.
66. Ragsdale, A. C., Thompson, H. J., Worstell, D. M., and Brody, S., *Mo. Agric. Exp. Stn. Res. Bull.*, 471, 1—24, 1950.
66a. Ragsdale, A. C., Thompson, H. J., Worstell, D. M., and Brody, S., *Mo. Agric. Exp. Stn. Res. Bull.*, 521, 1—23, 1950.
67. MacDonald, M. A. and Bell, J. M., *Can. J. Anim. Sci.*, 38, 160—170, 1958.
68. Ragsdale, A. C., Thompson, H. J., Worstell, D. M., and Brody, S., *Mo. Agric. Exp. Stn. Res. Bull.*, 460, 1—28, 1950.
69. Ragsdale, A. C., Thompson, H. J., Worstell, D. M., and Brody, S., *Mo. Agric. Exp. Stn. Res. Bull.*, 471, 1—24, 1951.
70. Johnson, H. D., Ragsdale, A. C., Berry, I. L., and Shanklin, M. D., *Mo. Agric. Exp. Stn. Res. Bull.*, 846, 1—22, 1963.
71. Johnson, H. D., Ragsdale, A. C., Berry, I. L., and Shanklin, M. D., *Mo. Agric. Exp. Stn. Res. Bull.*, 791, 1—22, 1962.
72. Hamada, T., *J. Dairy Sci.*, 54(11), 1704—1705, 1971.
73. Brody, S., Ragsdale, A. C., Thompson, H. J., and Worstell, D. M., *Mo. Agric. Exp. Stn. Res. Bull.*, 545, 1—20, 1954.
74. Brody, S., Ragsdale, A. C., Thompson, H. J., and Worstell, D. M., *Mo. Agric. Exp. Stn. Res. Bull.*, 556, 1—20, 1954.
75. Paape, M. J., Schultze, W. D., Miller, R. H., and Smith, J. W., *J. Dairy Sci.*, 56(1), 84—91, 1973.
76. Wilson, W. O., *Poult. Sci.*, 28, 581—592, 1949.
77. Wilson, W. O., McNally, E. H., and Ota, H., *Poult. Sci.*, 36, 1254—1261, 1957.
78. Smith, A. J. and Oliver, J., *Rhod. J. Agric. Res.*, 10, 43—60, 1972.
79. Payne, C. G., The influence of environmental temperature on egg production; a review, in *Environmental Control in Poultry Production,* Carter, T. C., Ed., Oliver & Boyd, London, 1967, 40—54.
80. Smith, A. J., *Anim. Health Prod.*, 5, 259—271, 1973.
81. Nordstrom, J. O., *Poult. Sci.*, 52(5), 1687—1690, 1973.
82. Mueller, W. J., *Poult. Sci.*, 40, 1562—1572, 1961.
83. Christison, G. I. and Milligan, J. D., A seven year study of winter performance of feedlot steers in western Canada, in *Livestock Environment,* American Society of Agricultural Engineers St. Joseph, Mich., 1974, 296—300.
84. Williams, C. M., in *Stockman's Day Report,* 14, University of Sasketchewan, Saskatoon, 1969, 21—26.
85. Webster, A. J. F., Chlumecky, J., and Young, B. A., *Can. J. Anim. Sci.*, 50, 89—100, 1970.
86. Hidiroglou, M. and Lessard, J. R., *Can. J. Anim. Sci.*, 51, 111—120, 1971.
87. Johnson, H. D., Ragsdale, A. C., and Yeck, R. G., *Mo. Agric. Exp. Stn. Res. Bull.*, 683, 1—31, 1958.
88. Johnson, H. D. and Ragsdale, A. C., *Mo. Agric. Exp. Stn. Res. Bull.*, 705, 1—31, 1959.
89. Mendel, V. E., Morrison, S. R., Bond, T. E., and Lofgreen, G. P., *J. Anim. Sci.*, 33(4), 850—854, 1971.
90. Fuller, M. F., *Br. J. Nutr.*, 19, 531—546, 1965.
91. Heitman, H., Jr., Kelly, C. F., and Bond, T. E., *J. Anim. Sci.*, 17, 62—67, 1958.
92. Swain, S. and Farrell, D. J., *Poult. Sci.*, 54(2), 513—520, 1975.
93. Hellickson, M. A., Butchbaker, A. F., Witz, R. L., and Bryant, R. L., *Trans. ASAE,* 10(6), 793—795, 1967.
94. Johnson, H. D., Hahn, L., Kibler, H. H., Shanklin, M. D., and Edmondson, J. E., *Mo. Agric. Exp. Stn. Res. Bull.*, 916, 1—32, 1967.

95. Johnson, H. D. and Yeck, R. G., *Mo. Agric. Exp. Stn. Res. Bull.*, 865, 1—37, 1964.
96. Ragsdale, A. C., Cheng, C. S., and Johnson, H. D., *Mo. Agric. Exp. Stn. Res. Bull.*, 642, 1—31, 1957.
97. Olbrich, S. E., Martz, F. A., and Hilderbrand, E. S., *J. Anim. Sci.*, 37(2), 574—580, 1973.
98. Close, W. H., Mount, L. E., and Start, I. B., *Anim. Prod.*, 13, 285—294, 1971.
99. Fuller, M. F., *Br. J. Nutr.*, 19, 531—546, 1965.
100. Bhattacharya, A. N. and Hussain, F., *J. Anim. Sci.*, 38(4), 877—886, 1974.
101. Parker, J. T., Boone, M. A., and Knechtges, J. F., *Poult. Sci.*, 51(2), 659—664, 1972.
102. Ahmad, M. M., Mather, F. B., and Gleaves, E. W., *Poult. Sci.*, 53(3), 927—935, 1974.
103. Johnson, H. D., Ragsdale, A. C., and Cheng, C. S., *Mo. Agric. Exp. Stn. Res. Bull.*, 646, 1—52, 1957.
104. Winn, P. N. and Godfrey, E. F., *Int. J. Biometeorol.*, 11(1), 39—50, 1967.
105. Kibler, H. H., *Mo. Agric. Exp. Stn. Res. Bull.*, 643, 1—32, 1957.
106. Blaxter, K. L. and Wainman, F. W., *J. Agric. Sci.*, 56, 81—90, 1961.
107. Kibler, H. H., *Mo. Agric. Exp. Stn. Res. Bull.*, 743, 1—38, 1960.
108. Worstell, D. M. and Brody, S., *Mo. Agric. Exp. Stn. Res. Bull.*, 515, 1—42, 1953.
109. Johnson, H. D., Ragsdale, A. C., and Cheng, C. S., *Mo. Agric. Exp. Stn. Res. Bull.*, 646, 1—52, 1957.
110. Kibler, H. H. and Brody, S., *Mo. Agric. Exp. Stn. Res. Bull.*, 450, 1—28, 1949.
111. Kibler, H. H. and Brody, S., *Mo. Agric. Exp. Stn. Res. Bull.*, 461, 1—19, 1950.
112. Mount, L. E., Effects of heat and cold on energy metabolism of the pig in *Progress in Animal Biometeorology, The Effect of Weather and Climate on Animals,* Johnson, H. D., Ed., Swets & Zeitlinger, Amsterdam, 1976, 227—238.
113. Capstick, J. W. and Wood, T. B., *J. Agric. Sci.*, 12, 257, 1922.
114. Johnson, K. G., Evaporative temperature regulation in sheep, in *Progress in Animal Biometeorology, The Effect of Weather and Climate on Animals,* Johnson, H. D., Ed., Swets & Zeitlinger, Amsterdam, 1976, 140—147.
115. Knox, K. L., Effects of heat on energy metabolism of sheep, in *Progress in Animal Biometeorology, The Effect of Weather and Climate on Animals,* Johnson, H. D., Ed., Swets & Zeitlinger, Amsterdam, 1976, 189—194.
116. Malhotra, R. K., Partitional Heat Losses of Mature Broad-Breasted Bronze Turkeys, Ph.D. thesis, University of Missouri, Columbia, 1967.
117. Deaton, James W., Proc. of 5th Annu. Southern Regional Avian Environmental Physiology and Bioengineering Study Group, Mobile, Ala., 1969, 102—107.
118. Ragsdale, A. C., Worstell, D. M., Thompson, H. J., and Brody, S., *Mo. Agric. Exp. Stn. Res. Bull.*, 449, 1—23, 1949.
119. Teter, N. C. and Deshazer, J. A., *Proc. Int. Symp. Feed Composition, Animal Nutrient Requirements, and Computer Formulation,* Fonnesbeck, P. V., Harris, L. E., and Kararl, L. C., Eds., Utah Agricultural Experimental Station, Logan, Utah, 1976, 497—501.
120. Hahn, G. L. and McQuigg, J. D., *Agric. Meteorol.*, 7, 131—141, 1970.
121. Hahn, G. L., *J. Dairy Sci.*, 52, 800—802, 1969.
122. Hahn, G. L., Osburn, D. D., and McQuigg, J. D., in *Proc. Natl. Dairy Housing Conf.*, SPO1-73, American Society of Agricultural Engineers, St. Joseph, Mich., 1973, 131—141.
123. Hahn, G. L., in *Livestock Environment,* Proc. Int. Livestock Environment Symp., SPO1-74, American Society of Agricultural Engineers, St. Joseph, Mich., 1974, 232—236.
124. Hahn, G. L., Meador, N. F., Stevens, D. G., Shanklin, M. D., and Johnson, H. D., Compensatory Growth in Livestock Subjected to Heat Stress, ASAE Paper No. 75-4008, American Society of Agricultural Engineers, St. Joseph, Mich., 1975.
125. Hahn, G. L., Meador, N. F., Thompson, G. B., and Shanklin, M. D., in *Livestock Environment,* Proc. Int. Livestock Environment Symp. SPO1-74, American Society of Agricultural Engineers, St. Joseph, Mich., 1974, 288—295.
126. Hahn, G. L., and Nienaber, J. A., Summer Weather Variability and Livestock Production, ASAE Paper No. 76-1033, American Society of Agricultural Engineers, St. Joseph, Mich., 1976.
127. Morrison, S. R., Hahn, G. L., and Bond, T. E., *Predicting Summer Production Losses for Swine,* Production Res. Rep. 118, U.S. Department of Agriculture, Washington, D.C., 1970, 1—14.
128. Hahn, G. L. and Osburn, D. D., *Trans. ASAE,* 12, 448—451, 1969.
129. Bond, T. E., Kelly, C. E., and Heitman, H., *Trans. ASAE,* 2(1), 1—4, 1959.
130. DeShazer, J. A., Olson, L. L., and Mathur, F. B., *Poult. Sci.*, 53(6), 2047—2054, 1974.
131. Longhouse, A. D., Hajime, O., Emerson, R. E., and Heishman, J. D., *Trans. ASAE,* 11, 694—700, 1968.

PHOTOPERIODISM AND PRODUCTIVITY OF DOMESTICATED ANIMALS

Robert K. Ringer

CIRCADIAN AND CIRCENNIAL RHYTHM

Biological observations over time have made scientists acutely aware of periodic functions in many animals. These observations suggest the intervention of some agencies that tend to adjust these periodic functions, which vary in frequency from cycles per minute to that of about one cycle/year. These cycles, of which there are many, are continually present within an animal.

Of importance in a discussion of photoperiodic influence on animal productivity are two such biological rhythms: (1) circadian rhythms, with a frequency of more than 20- but less than 28-hr and (2) circa-annual or circennian rhythms, with a period of about 1 year.

Circadian rhythms are inherited.[1] Within limits, these endogenous biological clocks can be changed by external stimuli such as the dark-light photoperiod. If the stimuli are out of phase with the animal's endogenous biological clock, a shift in the animal's cycle must occur in order for the two cycles to become in phase. A shift may be a delay or an advance. An example of this endogenous biological clock synchronization with photoperiodic control and its relationship to animal productivity will be discussed later.

SYNCHRONIZATION OF BIOLOGICAL RHYTHMS

Light, by virtue of its daily and seasonal variations, is one of the principal synchronizing agents or cues for many species. It furnishes a reliable clock for diurnal rhythms and a calendar by which the animal schedules reproductive functions, metabolic adjustments, molts, and migrations that are compatible with other environmental alterations. These latter adjustments have been of adaptive significance and, in the case of reproduction, ensure that the young are born at the most propitious time for survival.

Marshall[2] was the first to emphasize the dependence of the breeding season in many species on environmental or "exteroreceptive" factors. He suggested that such factors exert their influence by nervous and reflex stimulation of the secretion of gonadotrophic hormones, primarily follicle-stimulating hormone (FSH), from the anterior pituitary. He also pointed out that internal sexual rhythms are usually adjusted to external seasonal changes, and, in general, a species indigenous to one hemisphere adjusts its breeding season to the new calendar when moved across the equator, so that within 1 or 2 years, the time of the new breeding season coincides with the previous period of sexual response.

No all-encompassing generalization can be made about the role light plays in controlling animal functions. In some species, it has a major controlling influence on reproduction; at the other extreme, research has failed to show any essentiality. In addition, many animals such as birds and mink breed in response to "long-day" breeding seasons (increased photoperiod) in the spring, while goats and sheep show reproductive behavior in response to "short-day" light periods (decreased photoperiod) of autumn. The most important factor controlling this seasonal reproduction is the direction of change of the photoperiod rather than its absolute length. However, some animals kept under conditions of continual light or constant total darkness do show cyclic changes in reproductive behavior. At the equator, where no annual variation in the photoperiod occurs, seasonal reproductive cycles are still observed, indicating that stimuli other than photoperiod enter into the sexual rhythm of many animals.

Other stimuli that are known to influence or synchronize reproductive cycles include:

1. Auditory stimuli: Two examples are (a) vocalization of birds (associated with precopulatory behavior), which stimulates egg laying in budgerigars[3] and (b) "chuckling" by the male mink, which contributes to early breeding of the female and is used by fur ranchers for stimulating reproduction.
2. Visual stimuli: Examples include (a) isolation of female pigeons, resulting in failure to produce eggs; the introduction of a mirror or the placing of a male within sight results in egg laying[4] and (b) stimulated sexual response of bulls exposed to a visual stimuli.[5]
3. Olfactory stimuli: Exemplified by (a) the introduction of a ram, which stimulates the initiation of estrus in sheep and synchronizes the estrus cycle of ewes that are not cycling but does not synchronize cycling ewes[6] and (b) the blocking of pregnancy in mice exposed to the odor of a strange male.
4. Rainfall: In areas of low precipitation, reproductive activity of some birds follows heavy rains.[7,8]

MODE OF ACTION OF PHOTOPERIODIC CONTROL

Photoperiodic and environmental light control have enabled us to regulate special functions in husbandry practices. Examples in poultry husbandry are the control of the onset of egg laying in chickens, manipulation of the light regime following onset of egg production for maximizing egg production, the alternating light-dark sequence in broilers, often used to increase growth, utilization of feed, and the diminution of light intensity for prevention of cannibalism.

Light periodicity influences animal function through two modes of interaction:

1. Annual cycling, responsive to the gradual variation in the duration of the photoperiod and scotoperiod; the direction of the change is photostimulatory or photoinhibitory to a particular system.
2. Endogenous diurnal cycling (circadian rhythm), synchronized by the dark-light sequence provided by the environment.

The physiological pathways of mediation of these two actions of light are totally different.[9,10] The annual cycle, as exemplified by the breeding cycle in many animals, is mediated via retinal and/or extraretinal (encephalic) receptors and the neuroendocrine system (hypothalamus, median eminence, and adenohypophysis) (see Figure 1). In the case of the circadian cycle, recent research indicates that it is probably the pineal organ that transforms nervous information concerning alternation of light and dark sequences into biochemical information that goes to the brain and endocrine system.[11-13]

To examine light as it influences reproduction, one must consider its physiological pathway of action. Light energy induces within the hypothalamus the production of the releasing hormones for FSH, luteinizing hormone (LH), and either the inhibiting hormone for prolactin (in mammals) or the releasing hormone for prolactin (in birds). The neurohormones, via the portal vessels of the hypothalamus and median eminence, in turn affect the release of gonadotrophins by the adenohypophysis. That the pineal may be involved in the entrainment of the annual cycle of reproduction cannot be discounted. Findings in hamsters, in which the pineal gland is strongly antigonadal,

(a)

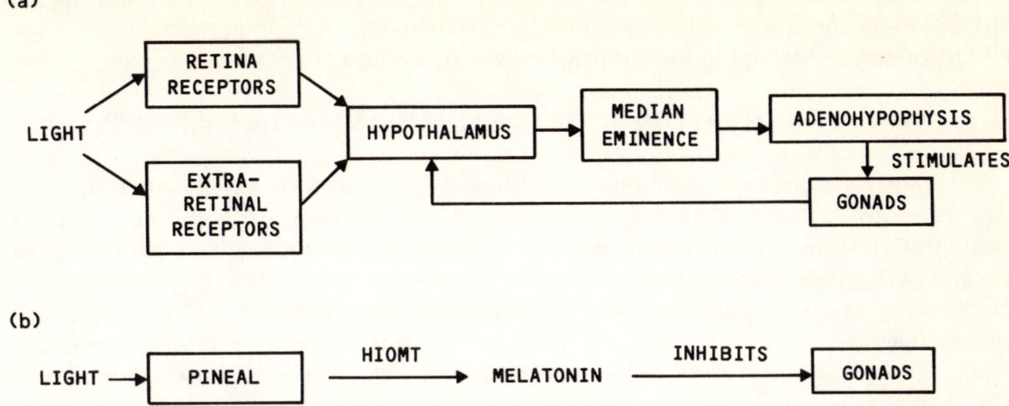

(b)

FIGURE 1. Two pathways whereby light mediates its action upon the gonads. Pathway (a) is that which is responsible for the annual reproductive cycle in many birds and some mammals and (b) influences certain mammals but has not been clearly demonstrated to influence avian species.

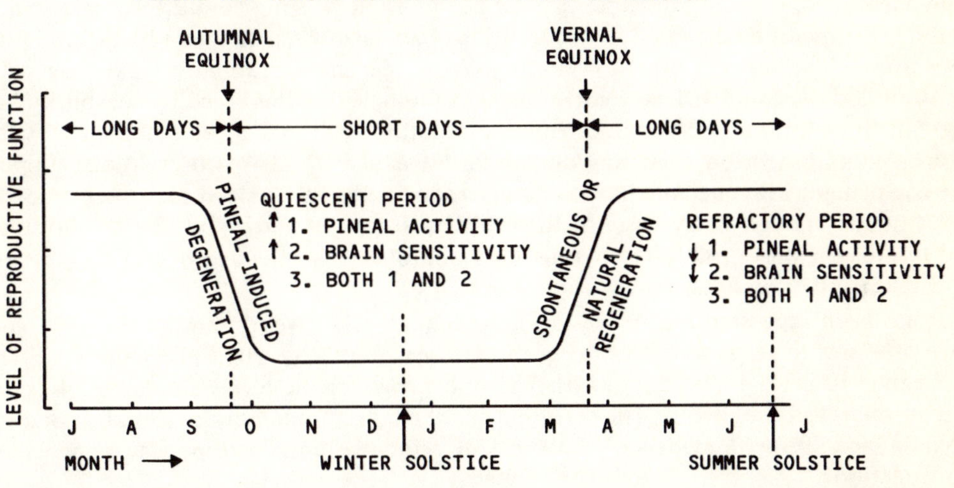

FIGURE 2. Possible relations between the pineal gland, the photoperiod, and seasonal reproductive events in the hamster. During the short day period (winter months), the pineal gland is maximally stimulated and the sexual organs regress. There is possibly an increased sensitivity of the brain to the pineal substances as well. During the summer (long days), the pineal is inhibited and the gonads are reproductively capable. During the summer, the reproductive system may be refractory to the influence of the pineal gland. (Reproduced, with permission, from Comparative physiology: pineal gland, by Russel J. Reiter, in *Annual Review of Physiology,* Vol. 35, © 1973 by Annual Reviews, Inc. All rights reserved.)

suggest that this gland (Figure 2) is the critical determinant between seasonal reproductive fluctuations and changing photoperiodic conditions.[14] During the "long-day" season, the pituitary-gonadal axis may be refractory to the influence of the pineal gland (Figure 1).

The pathway by which light influences feeding activity and thus growth probably involves the pineal. It is not via the production of growth hormone or its releasing hormone. That there is no direct growth stimulation by light can be demonstrated in chicks, in which the growth reponse to light disappears when groups are pair-fed. Growth is a response to the eating-activity pattern of the endogenous circadian clock.

Efficient livestock production of certain animals has been achieved by imposing artificial conditions to control environmental variables. The following is a brief coverage of one such variable, light, and its influence on life cycles of domesticated animals.

LONG-DAY PHOTOPERIODIC STIMULATION IN MAMMALS

No known functions in mammals are obligately controlled by day length under natural conditions; however, photoperiodism appears to be involved in the more precise timing of functions that occur because of endogenous periodicities, which are not as precise as the daily photoperiod.[15]

Domesticated mammals have been divided into three divisions based upon their reproductive response to photoperiodic influence:[16] (1) those that reproduce during seasons of long daylight, (2) those that reproduce during seasons of short daylight, and (3) those that domestication has caused to become insensitive to photoperiodic stimulation.

Stimulation of reproductive activity in ferrets, mink, martens, badgers, raccoons, cats, hamsters, voles, rabbits, and horses occurs in response to increasing photoperiods.

In horses, the onset of the breeding season of the mare occurs in the spring and coincides with increasing daylight as well as favorable grazing conditions and warmer ambient temperatures; these latter conditions have also been suggested as stimulating to mares. However, exposure of mares out of season to gradually increasing daily photoperiods (using artificial light) advances the onset of the breeding season.[17-20] In the fall, most mares become anestrous, a condition believed to be controlled by the decreasing photoperiod occurring during that season.[21, 22] These observations support the use of light as a cue for the breeding season in horses. A fixed photoperiod of 16 or 24 hr also induces early onset of the breeding season in mares, but a 9-hr photoperiod retards the onset (table 1).[21] Long daily photoperiods extended over a long period during the fall delay anestrus.

It has been suggested that mares do not become refractive to photoperiods.[22] Exposure of mares to 16 hr of light during the fall season of anestrus caused estrous cycles to begin within 45 to 60 days, with LH and progesterone levels similar to those of estrous mares in the spring. The stallion, like the mare, undergoes seasonal changes in gonadal activity, with evidence of decreasing semen volume in response to decreasing photoperiods.[23]

The ferret was one of the first animals in which light stimulation of estrus was reported,[24] and it has been studied intensively since then. In ferrets, normally annual breeders, exposure throughout the year to long-day photoperiods (14L:10D) for 2 months followed by exposure to short-day photoperiods (6L:18D) for 2 months results in an estrous cycle each 4-month period.[25] Photostimulatory conditions produce estrous in ferrets between 30 and 40 days after exposure. The threshold of intensity necessary for photostimulation in the ferret is about 4.5 lx (0.42 fc).[25] Under continual light, ferrets come into estrus at any time during the year.

Mink and marten are two species that have delayed implantation, but they differ widely with regard to length of the delay. Mink have short while marten have long delayed implantation, with reproduction occurring in the spring season of increasing photoperiod for both species. Enders and Pearson reported that marten subjected to gradually increasing lighting during their long delayed implantation showed induced early implantation, as evidenced by the birth of young in December.[26] Artificially increasing the photoperiod stimulated both the follicular and luteal development in these species,[27] thus accelerating the beginning and completion of the estrous period and the length of pregnancy.[28-30]

Table 1
EFFECT OF DAILY PHOTOPERIOD ON OVULATION OF MARES

Group[a]	Total no. of mares	No. of mares that ovulated by June 13, 1974	Mean interval to first postanestrous ovulation (days± SE)[b]
Control	8	8	192.1(a) ± 3.3
L24:D0	8	7	>156.1(b) ± 12.2
L16:D8	9	9	107.1(c) ± 11.1
L9:D15	9	4	>200.3(a) ± 5.8

[a] Treatments began on Nov. 13, 1973. Daily photoperiods were control — natural daylength; L:D — fixed hours light and dark.

[b] Means with different-letters within parentheses are significantly different

From Kooistra, L. H. and Ginther, O. J., *Am. J. Vet. Res.*, 36, 1415, 1975. With permission.

Artificial prolongation of the photoperiod (2.5 hr) during gestation in mink leads to an increase in fertility (reduced embryonic mortality) and a shortening of the gestation period.[31] These changes depend upon the interval between the last mating of the females and the beginning of the additional photoperiod; the shorter the interval the more efficient is the additional illumination. Based upon observations of vaginal smears, female mink that produce a normal litter of young in the spring can be stimulated by 3 months of photoperiod restriction, short-day, followed by 3 months of photostimulation, long-day, so that estrus is produced 6 months from the breeding season in the spring.[32] Males under this light regime fail to produce sperm. Thus, in order to induce gonadal stimulation, it is apparently necessary that the animals not be subjected to photostimulation until after completion of the winter furring cycle, which occurs during the photoperiodic restriction. This is a form of photorefractiveness. These are but a few examples of how increasing photoperiods induce reproduction in mammals.

SHORT-DAY PHOTOPERIODIC SYNCHRONIZATION OR STIMULATION IN MAMMALS

Light plays a major role in the annual periodicity of sexual activities in sheep[34,35] and goats.[36,37] In sheep from tropical areas, light plays a minor role in reproductive cycling. In species of the Northern Hemisphere, reproductive activity is generally at a maximum during the autumn, when the daily photoperiod begins to decrease.[38] Anestrus extends approximately from February until July or August, at which time some sheep show the first signs of cyclic behavior, and by September, all sheep are in estrus and ovulate.

The hypophyseal LH and FSH contents are higher in sheep under short photoperiods than in those under long photoperiods.[39,40] More important than the hypophyseal content is the fact that the circulating-blood levels of LH in sheep increase under short-day photoperiods and decrease under long-day photoperiods.[40] The absolute value of daylight length is not as important as is the direction of the light variation, the increasing photoperiod being nonstimulatory or less stimulatory than the decreasing photoperiod.

The number of spermatozoa per collection in rams reaches a maximum during the autumn and a minimum in late spring.[41] Rams subjected to an experimental photoperiodic "year" shortened to 6 months will reach a maximum spermatogenic activity twice during a 12-month period. This maximum activity occurs when the daily photoperiod is decreasing.[42] Thus, the male gonads repond as do those of the female.

The use of artificial light to reduce the interval between lambing and remating is of interest in certain intensive systems of lamb production.[43-45] Exposure of sheep to continual light for 3 years results in breeding seasons at the normal time of the year.[46] As Nalbandov[38] has pointed out, there may be factors other than light that play a significant role in the regulation of the breeding season of sheep, because the onset of the season from year to year is not as regular as is the time at which daylength decreases or increases. However, Hunter and Van Aarde[47] found that the level of nutrition did not influence the interval to estrus post partum, but photoperiod did alter the interval (Figure 3).

Hence, in sheep, there is ample evidence that a decreasing rather than an increasing photoperiod plays a predominant role in sexual activity regulation. Studies of goats are not as numerous, but those conducted follow closely those of sheep.

MAMMALIAN SPECIES WITH NO REPRODUCTIVE RESPONSE TO CHANGING PHOTOPERIODS

Husnain and Quddus[48] reported that in cows, generally considered nonresponsive to photoperiodic control, 285 of 425 onsets of heat occurred in October to March, while 140 occurred from April to September, suggesting that photoperiodicity plays a role in the onset of heat.

Seasonal variations in serum prolactin concentrations were reported in cows and bulls,[49,50] with highest concentrations in the summer months and lowest concentrations in the winter months. Decreasing the daily photoperiod from 16 to 8 hr reduced serum prolactin (from 48 to 10 ng/mℓ) and, conversely, increasing the photoperiod from 8 to 16 hr increased prolactin fourfold (from 25 to 100 ng/mℓ).[51] Thus, photoperiodic changes may account for part of the seasonal changes in serum prolactin of cattle.

Exposure of swine to either 9 or 24 hr of light per day did not influence ovulation rate.[52] Additional illumination before mating had no influence on the number of ovulations, but when given throughout gestation, light enhanced the function of the corpora lutea, as evidenced by larger weight and activity.[53] Continual light prolonged the estrous cycle in these animals.

PHOTOPERIODICITY AND AVIAN REPRODUCTION

The avian species is by far the most widely studied. Photoperiodic control of reproductive activity has received more extensive experimentation in avian species than in any other classification of animals. Many reviews have been written that detail both circadian rhythms and circa-annual rhythms in domestic and wildlife species.[9,10,54-58] Studies of wildlife species have examined the effect of the photoperiod on testicular recrudescence, fat deposition, migration, and molting, as well as the physiological parameters controlling these changes. In domestic species, the female has received more attention recently because of the economical factors involved in egg production. The interplay between the dark-light sequence and ovulation rate, delaying the onset of reproduction and egg size, and the influence of color and intensity of light have been areas of study. Avian species have been classified by Farner into three groups according to their pattern of reproductive response to various natural photoperiods. These include (1) species that are obligately dependent upon long-day photoperiods for control of the annual reproductive period, (2) species with endogenous circa-annual reproductive activity but in which environmental information plays a less significant role,

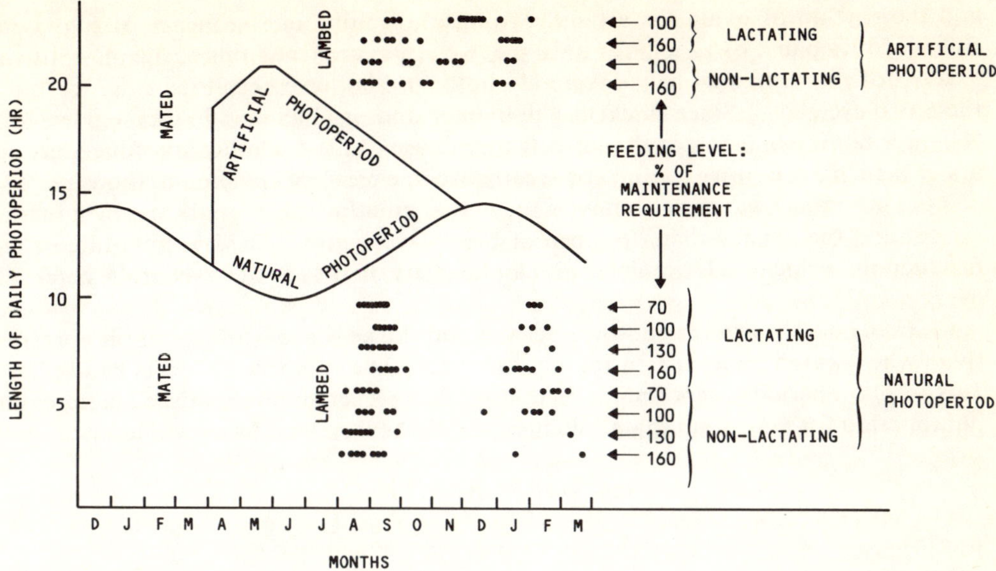

FIGURE 3. Mating, lambing, and first post-partum estrus in Mutton Merino ewes in relation to the time of year and the length of the respective daily photoperiods. Each observation of estrus is represented by a dot opposite the appropriate treatment listed on the right. (From Hunter, G. L. and Van Aarde, I. M. R., *J. Reprod. Fertil.*, 42, 208, 1975. With permission.)

and (3) species in which reproductive activity occurs on short- or long-day photoperiods because environmental information is of no significance in the control of the annual reproductive cycle. Domesticated ducks fall into the first category, whereas domesticated chickens fall into one of the last two categories. Light, rather than controlling the circennial cycle, affects the rate of sexual maturity and the rate of egg production in the chicken. Chickens will commence egg laying under short-day conditions or even in total darkness.

Morris[60] showed that in chickens, the age of sexual maturity varied inversely with the hours of light exposure, with 10 hr or more of light per day being sufficient to induce the maximum rate of sexual maturation. Below 10 hr the regression of sexual maturity is linear but inverse. Sexual development is associated with elevated gonadotrophin secretion. Morris[60] proposed the following equation for the prediction of sexual maturity in chickens:

$$y = \mu + 1.59 (\Delta D)$$

where y = average age in days at first egg, μ = a strain mean, and ΔD = the total change in daylength occurring between hatching and the time of sexual maturity. Changes in the photoperiod made during the brooding stage affect subsequent egg production.

Maximum stimulation of egg production in chickens is produced with continual lighting, either natural daylight or artificial lighting, for 10 to 12 hr. Less than 9 or 10 hr of light is not an adequate photoperiod for maximum egg production. Once sexual maturity is attained, decreasing photoperiods depress rate of egg production, while increasing photoperiods stimulate rate of reproduction.

The daily dark-light sequence is the primary cue for stimulation of ovulation-hormone (LH) release by the adenohypophysis. Evidence exists that the circadian rhythm of ovulation in most chickens is greater than 24 hr; thus, the daily dark-light sequence and the rhythm of ovulation are out of phase, resulting in a sequence of egg laying followed by a pause of 12 to 14 hr until the two cycles are synchronized again. Artificial "days" of more than 24 hr (adhemeral photoperiods) have been used to synchronize these two cycles.[61-63] Since chickens will ovulate and produce eggs in total darkness,[64-67] light is not the only factor that affects the release of the ovulating hormone. Secondary cues such as auditory stimuli apparently become primary in these situations.

Red and orange wavelengths have a greater stimulating effect on the neuroendocrine system and the gonads than do green or blue wavelengths.[68-71] Maximum rate of egg production in chickens is obtained with an intensity of 10 lx at the level of the chicken's eye.

Chickens do not exhibit photorefractivity, but turkeys show a form of photorefractivity when reared under increasing photoperiods. The response of turkeys and pheasants to photoperiodicity is similar to that of the chicken except that the length of the photoperiod for maximum egg production should be increased by several hours.

PHOTOREFRACTIVITY

In Birds

Photorefractivity occurs in many species during sustained photostimulation.[57,72] In species with photoperiodically regulated breeding cycles, photorefractivity is often considered an adaptive mechanism limiting propagation of offspring to periods during which environmental requirements are adequate.

In migratory birds, the refractory period terminates the breeding cycle in ample time to permit the deposition of fat, associated with hyperphagy during the autumn, while food is still abundant. The duration of the refractory period is such that it carries the animal into a declining photoperiod, which is nonstimulating. The breeding cycle does not recur until photoperiodic stimulation recurs in the spring.

Various methods have been attempted to reduce the photorefractive period. The most useful procedure has been to subject the animal to an artificially short photoperiod. The period of experimentally exposing the animal to a declining photoperiod depends upon the species. Ultimately, photosensitivity returns.

The physiological basis of this refractivity to photostimulation is not completely understood, but research has suggested an involvement of the hypothalamus-adenohypophysis pathway.

In Mammals

Like birds, ferrets show evidence of photorefractivity to continued long-day photoperiodic exposure. This can be terminated by exposing the animal to an artificially short photoperiod.[73]

Although sheep[42] and voles exhibit a fatigue of gonad functioning following photostimulation, there is not a refractory period comparable to that observed in birds and some mammals.[74]

EFFECT OF LIGHT ON PELAGE

It is clear that not all mammals are photoperiodically stimulated; nor is it true that the reproductive tract alone is altered by light. Skin and hair growth have been shown to respond to light stimuli in ferrets, mink, weasels,[75] hare,[76] fox,[77,78] sheep, cattle, and horses.

The effect of light on seasonal generations of hair, of which there is a spring and autumn molt in some species, was first studied in ferrets by Bissonette in 1935[79] and later in mink.[80,81] Despite the apparent circennian rhythm of fur molting and growth, these changes are capable of entrainment to shorter cycles by alternation of that photoperiod. Long-day photoperiods induce a spring molt and summer pelage, and short-day photoperiods during autumn induce autumn molt and winter pelage.[33] During the development of the normal winter pelage of mink, there is a concomitant period of fat deposition,[33] suggesting that the cue for the initiation of the winter pelage cycle also acts as a synchronizer for fat deposition. Whether this fat deposition is due to hyperphagia, as in migratory birds, is unknown. Hypophysectomy abolishes the molt pattern,[79] and the animal rapidly goes into a state of winter pelage. It has been suggested that the winter pelage is the dominant state and that the maintenance of summer pelage requires an inductive mechanism for its development and maintenance.[33] The result of hypophysectomy may be mediated through one or several hormones, including the gonads and the adrenal, or by the thyroid. The pineal gland may also be implicated in the control of changes in pelage.[82]

Burkhardt[17] stated that in horses, the shedding of the coat seems to be closely related to the date on which ovarian changes occur at the onset of reproductive activity. Mares exposed to a fixed continual light or 16L:8D shed their winter coat earlier than those on natural daylight or 9L:15D, indicating a positive role of the photoperiod on pelage.[21] These horses maintained a dense fuzzy coat throughout the year and did not display the seasonal shedding of their coat, a response similar to that reported in cattle on a fixed lighting of approximately 13 hr/day.[83]

The annual rhythm of wool growth in sheep from the temperate zone has been known for some time and occurs under conditions of constant nutrition. Sheep kept under conditions of continual light show an unchanged rhythm, but when kept in complete darkness by hooding, the rhythm slowly disappears.[84] Reversal of the photoperiodic rhythm changes the wool-growth rhythm. Modification by environmental influences other than light, such as temperature and nutrition, does occur.[85]

Development of the white winter pelage of the varying hare *Lepus americana* can be induced by short days, and the spring molt and summer pelage can be induced by long daily photoperiods. [86] Fox molt only once a year, in late fall, and can be primed prematurely by decreasing photoperiods.

Cattle in temperate climates molt seasonally in a wave pattern. In tropical photoperiods, the peaks of hair follicle activity and wave pattern disappear.[83]

INFLUENCE OF LIGHT ON GROWTH

In considering the influence of light on nutrition and growth in domestic species, one is immediately confronted with the ruminant- vs. the monogastric-stomached animal. The buffer on nutrition imposed by the rumen makes the study of diurnal variations imposed by light virtually impossible. Trials of long duration are the only useful tests, and these are limited.[87]

One such trial to determine the effect of corral lighting on milk production and feed intake of cows was conducted on three commercial drylot dairies.[88] Light apparently had little beneficial effect on production or feed intake in the summer and limited effect during the longer periods of darkness in winter. Belyeav and Gorbunova[89] reported a slight increase in milk production and a savings in feed when natural daylight was replaced with an 18-hr photoperiod. Tucker and co-workers have reported that maintenance of a 16L:8D artificial photoperiod stimulated body growth and milk yields of dairy cattle 6 to 15 percent in comparison with natural - length periods of 9 to 12 hours without requiring additional feed.[99-101] The effect of photoperiod on body-weight gains in sheep is inconsistent[90] and does not appear to be beneficial.

Environmental housing using artificial lighting is widely used in the production of monogastric animals such as swine and poultry. Photoperiodic control of the environment for pigs has failed to show any beneficial effects on growth or feed-efficiency performance.[91,91] Optically enucleated swine compared to intact animals show neither a change in daily gain nor feed required for gain. Age to attain puberty is delayed. Therefore, in swine production, data suggest that light plays no role in animal productivity.

In avian species, there is a definite nutritional response to changes in the photoperiod. In chickens, the greatest activity of feeding is soon after the onset of the photoperiod[93,94] and about 5 hr before the beginning of the scotoperiod.[95] Light intensity may have an influence on nutrition, since growth of broilers appears inversely proportional to the intensity of light.[60] Short-day photoperiods often give better chick growth than long-day photoperiods;[96] however, maximum growth rate in broilers is obtained with continual or near continual photoperiods.[97,98] Low-intensity or red lights are used to reduce the risk of cannibalism in poultry production.

From the above discussion, it can be concluded that for growth, both intensity and duration of the photoperiod plays a role in the daily rhythm of feeding activity, whereas in reproduction, once a threshold stimulus level of intensity is reached, only photoperiodic duration is of importance.

REFERENCES

1. **Bunning, E.,** *The Physiological Clock,* Academic Press, New York, 1964, 167.
2. **Marshall, F. H. A.,** Sexual periodicity and the causes which determine it, *Philos. Trans. R. Soc. London, Ser. B,* 226, 423—456, 1936.
3. **Brockway, B. F.,** Stimulation of ovarian development and egg laying by male courtship vocalization in budgerigars (*Melopsittacus undulatus*), *Anim. Behav.,* 13, 575—578, 1965.
4. **Matthews, L. H.,** Visual stimulation and ovulation in pigeons, *Proc. R. Soc. London,* 126B, 557—560, 1939.
5. **Hale, E. B.,** Visual stimuli and reproductive behavior in bulls, *J. Anim. Sci.,* Suppl. 25, 36—44, 1966.
6. **Bruce, H. M.,** Smell as an exteroceptive factor, *J. Anim. Sci.,* Suppl. 25, 83—87, 1966.
7. **van Tienhoven, A., Ed.,** *Reproductive Physiology of Vertebrates,* W. B. Saunders, Philadelphia, 1968, 498.
8. **Marshall, A. J.,** Environmental factors other than light involved in the control of sexual cycles in birds and mammals, in *La Photoregulation de la Reproduction Chez les Oiseaux et les Mammiferes,* Benoit, J. and Assenmacher, I., Eds., Editions du Centre National de la Recherche Scientifique, Paris, 1970, 53—69.
9. **Benoit, J. and Assenmacher, I., Eds.,** La Photo-regulation de la Reproduction Chez les Oiseaux et les Mammiferes, *Editions du Centre National de la Recherche Scientifique, Paris,* 1970, 588.
10. **Menaker, M.,** Synchronization with the photic environment via extraretinal receptors in the avian brain, in *Biochronometry,* Menaker, M., Ed., National Academy of Sciences, Washington, D.C., 1971.
11. **Quay, W. B.,** Epiphyseal responses to light and darkness in birds and mammals, in *La Photoregulation de la Reproduction Chez les Oiseaux et les Mammiferes,* Benoit, J. and Assenmacher, I., Eds., Editions du Centre National de la Recherche Scientifique, Paris, 1970, 549—564.
12. **Reiter, R. J.,** Comparative physiology: pineal gland, *Annu. Rev. Physiol.,* 35, 305—328, 1973.
13. **Menaker, M.,** Rhythms, reproduction and photoreception, *Biol. Reprod.,* 4, 295—308, 1971.
14. **Reiter, R. J.,** Pineal-anterior pituitary gland relationships, in *Endocrine Physiology,* Vol. 5, Guyton, A. C. and McCann, S. M., Eds., University Park Press, Baltimore, 1974, 277—308.
15. **Farner, D. S. and Lewis, R. A.,** Photoperiodic control mechanisms, in *Environmental Biology,* Altman, P. L. and Dittmer, D. S., Eds., Federation of the American Society of Experimental Biology, Bethesda, Md., 1966, 600.
16. **Ortavant, R., Mauleon, P., and Thibault, C.,** Photoperiodic control of gonadal and hypophyseal activity in domestic mammals, *Ann. N.Y. Acad. Sci.,* 117, 157—193, 1964.
17. **Burkhardt, J.,** Transition from anoestrous in the mare and the effects of artificial lighting, *J. Agric. Sci.,* 37, 64—68, 1947.

18. **Nishikawa, Y.,** *Studies on Reproduction in Horses,* Japan Racing Assoc., Tokyo, 1969, 340.
19. **Loy, R. G.,** Effects of artificial lighting regimes on reproductive patterns in mares, in *Proc. 14th Annu. Convention,* American Association of Equine Practitioners, Philadelphia, 1968, 159—169.
20. **Sharp, D. C. and Ginther, O. J.,** Stimulation of follicular activity and estrous behavior in anestrous mares with light and temperature, *J. Anim. Sci.,* 41, 1368—1372, 1975.
21. **Kooistra, L. H. and Ginther, O. J.,** Effect of photoperiod on reproductive activity and hair in mares, *Am. J. Vet. Res.,* 36, 1413—1419, 1975.
22. **Oxender, W. D., Noden, P. A., and Hafs, H. D.,** Estrous, ovulation, serum progesterone, estradiol, and LH concentrations in mares after an increased photoperiod during winter, *Am. J. Vet. Res.,* 38, 203—207, 1977.
23. **Nishikawa, Y. and Horie, T.,** Studies on the effects of day-length on the reproductive function in horses. II. Effect of daylength on the function of testes, *Nogyo Gijutsu Kenkyujo Bull. Ser. G,* 3, 45—52, 1952.
24. **Bissonette, T. H.,** Modification of mammalian sexual cycles. I. Reactions of ferrets (*Putorius vulgaris*) of both sexes to electric light added after dark in November and December, *Proc. R. Soc. London, Ser. B,* 110, 322, 1932.
25. **Vincent, D. S.,** Modification of the annual oestrous cycle of the ferret by various regimes of artificial light, *J. Endocrinol.,* 48, 3, 1970.
26. **Enders, R. K. and Pearson, O. P.,** Shortening gestation by inducing early implantation with increased light in the marten, *Am. Fur Breeder,* 15, 18, 1943.
27. **Canivenc, R.,** Photoperiodisme chez quelques mammiferes a nidation differee, in *La Photoregulation de la Reproduction Chez les Oiseaux et les Mammiferes,* Benoit, J. and Assenmacher, I., Eds., Editions du Centre National de la Recherche Scientifique, Paris, 1970, 453—469.
28. **Aulerich, R. J., Holcomb, L., Ringer, R. K., and Schaible, P. J.,** Influence of photoperiod on reproduction in mink, *Fur Trade J. Can.,* 41, 8—18, 1963.
29. **Klotchkov, D. V., Klotchkova, A. Ya., Kim, A. A., and Belyaev, D. K.,** Genotypic differences in photoperiodic reactivity of mink reproductive system out of breeding season, *Proc. 1st World Congr. Genetics Applied to Livestock Production,* Graficas Orbe, Madrid, 1974, 65—72.
30. **Bowness, E. R.,** Light and the pregnant mink, *Fur Trade J. Canada,* 46, 4—5, 1968.
31. **Belyaev, D. K., Klotchkov, D. V., Klotchkova, A. Ya., and Kim, A. A.,** Influence of photoperiod on embryonic mortality in minks and sows, *Congr. Int. Reprod. Anim. Insemination Artif.,* 1, 257—260, 1968.
32. **Aulerich, R. J., Holcomb, L., Ringer, R. K., and Schaible, P. J.,** Influence of lighting on mink reproduction, *Am. Fur Breeder,* 37(2), 10—11, 1964.
33. **Duby, R. T. and Travis, H. F.,** Photoperiodic control of fur growth and reproduction in the mink (*Mustela vison*), *J. Exp. Zool.,* 182, 217—226, 1972.
34. **Yeates, N. T. M.,** The breeding season of the ewe with particular reference to its modification by artificial means using light, *J. Agric. Sci.,* 39, 1, 1949.
35. **Hart, D. S.,** Photoperiodicity in Suffolk sheep, *J. Agric. Sci.,* 40, 143—149, 1950.
36. **Bissonette, T. H.,** Experimental modification of breeding cycles in goats, *Physiol. Zool.,* 14, 379—383, 1941.
37. **Eaton, O. N. and Simmons, V. L.,** Inducing extraseasonal breeding in goats and sheep by controlled lighting, *U.S. Dep. Agric. Circ.,* 933, 1—16, 1953.
38. **Nalbandov, A. V.,** Endocrine background of light action, in *La Photoregulation Chez les Oiseaux et les Mammiferes,* Benoit, J. and Assenmacher, I., Eds., Editions du Centre National de la Recherche Scientifique, Paris, 1970, 29—52.
39. **Pelletier, J. and Ortavant, R.,** Influence de la duree d'clairement sur le contenu hypophysaire en hormones gonadotropes FSH et ICSH chez le belier, *Ann. Biol. Anim. Biochim. Biophys.,* 4, 17—26, 1964.
40. **Pelletier, J. and Ortavant, R.,** Photoperiodic control of LH release in the ram. I. Influence of increasing and decreasing light photoperiods, *Acta Endocrinol. (Copenhagen),* 78, 435—441, 1975.
41. **Phillips, R. W., Schoot, R. G., Eaton, O. N., and Simmons, V. L.,** Seasonal variations in the semen of sheep and goats, *Cornell Vet.,* 33, 227—235, 1943.
42. **Pelletier, J. and Ortavant, R.,** Influence du photoperiodisme sur les activites sexuelles, hypophysaire et hypothalamique du Belier ile-de-France, in *La Photoregulation de la Reproduction Chez les Oiseaux et les Mammiferes,* Benoit, J. and Assenmacher, I., Eds., Editions du Centre National de la Recherche Scientifique, Paris, 1970, 483—496.
43. **Goot, H.,** Effect of light on spring breeding of Mutton Merino ewes, *J. Agric. Sci.,* 73, 177—180, 1969.
44. **Ducker, M. H. and Bowman, J. C.,** Photoperiodism in the ewe. IV. An attempt to induce sheep of three breeds to lamb every eight months by artificial daylength changes in a non-light-proofed building, *Anim. Prod.,* 14, 323—334, 1972.

45. **Orskov, E. R. and Robinson, J. J.**, Recent advances in ewe and lamb nutrition, *Rep. Rowett Res. Inst.*, 28, 116—129, 1972.
46. **Thibault, C., Courot, M., Martinet, L., Mauleon, P., du Mesnil du Buisson, F., Ortavant, R., Pelletier, J., and Signoret, J. P.**, Regulation of breeding season and estrous cycles by light and external stimuli in some animals, *J. Anim. Sci.*, Suppl. 25, 119—139, 1966.
47. **Hunter, G. L. and Van Aarde, I. M. R.**, Influence of age of ewe and photoperiod on the interval between parturition and first oestrus in lactating and non-lactating ewes at different nutritional levels, *J. Reprod. Fertil.*, 42, 205—212, 1975.
48. **Husnain, H. and Quddus, A.**, Photoperiodicity in Red Sindhi cows, *Agric. Pak.*, 14, 228—230, 1963.
49. **Koprowski, J. A. and Tucker, H. A.**, Serum prolactin during various physiological states and its relationship to milk production in the bovine, *Endocrinology*, 92, 1480—1487, 1973.
50. **Tucker, H. A., Koprowski, J. A., Britt, J. H., and Oxender, W. D.**, Serum prolactin and growth hormone in Holstein bulls, *J. Dairy Sci.*, 57, 1092—1094, 1974.
51. **Bourne, R. A. and Tucker, H. A.**, Serum prolactin and LH responses to photoperiod in bull calves, *Endocrinology*, 97, 473—475, 1975.
52. **Wadill, D. G., Chaney, C. H., and Dutt, R. H.**, Ovulation rate in gilts after short-time exposure to continuous light, *J. Reprod. Fertil.*, 15, 123-125, 1968.
53. **Klotchkov, D. V., Klotchkova, A. Ya., Kim, A. A., and Belyaev, D. K.**, The Influence of Photoperiodic Conditions on Fertility in Gilts, 10th Int. Congr. Animal Production, Paris, July 17—23, 1971, 1—8.
54. **Wolfson, A.**, Circadian rhythm and the photoperiodic regulation of the annual reproductive cycle in birds, in *Circadian Clocks*, Aschoff, J., Ed., North-Holland, Amsterdam, 1965, 370—378.
55. **Wolfson, A.**, Environmental and neuroendocrine regulation of annual gonadal cycles and migratory behavior in birds, *Recent Prog. Horm. Res.*, 22, 177—239, 1966.
56. **Lofts, B. and Murton, R. K.**, Photoperiodic and physiological adaptations regulating avian breeding cycles and their ecological significance, *J. Zool.*, 155, 327—394, 1968.
57. **Farner, D. S. and Lewis, R. A.**, Photoperiodism and reproductive cycles in birds, in *Photophysiology*, Vol. 6, Giese, A. C., Ed., Academic Press, New York, 1971, 325—370.
58. **van Tienhoven, A. and Planck, R. J.**, The effect of light on avian reproductive activity, in *Handbook of Physiology*, Vol. 2, American Physiological Society, Bethesda, Md., 1973, 79—107.
59. **Farner, D. S.**, Daylength as environmental information in the control of reproduction of birds, in *La Photoregulation de la Reproduction Chez les Oiseaux et les Mammiferes*, Benoit, J. and Assenmacher, I., Eds., Editions du Centre National de la Recherche Scientifique, Paris, 1970, 71—91.
60. **Morris, T. R.**, Light requirement of the fowl, in *Environmental Control in Poultry Production*, Carter, T. C., Ed., Oliver and Boyd, London, 1967, 15—39.
61. **Morris, T. R.**, The effects of ahemeral light and dark cycles on egg production in the fowl, *Poult. Sci.*, 52, 423—445, 1973.
62. **Melek, O., Morris, T. R., and Jennings, R. C.**, The time factor in egg formation for hens exposed to ahemeral light-dark cycles, *Br. Poult. Sci.*, 14, 493—498, 1973.
63. **Morris, T. R., Melek, O., and Cunningham, F. J.**, Luteinizing hormone concentration in the plasma of laying hens exposed to a 27-hour cycle of light and darkness, *J. Reprod. Fertil.*, 42, 381—384, 1975.
64. **Wilson, W. O. and Woodard, A. E.**, Egg production of chickens kept in darkness, *Poult. Sci.*, 37, 1054—1057, 1958.
65. **King, D. F.**, Egg production of chickens raised and kept in darkness, *Poult. Sci.*, 41, 1499—1503, 1962.
66. **Morris, T. R., Fox, S., and Jennings, R. C.**, The response of laying pullets to abrupt changes in daylength, *Br. Poult. Sci.*, 5, 133—147, 1964.
67. **Jochle, W.**, Trends in photophysiologic concepts, *Ann. N.Y. Acad. Sci.*, 117, 88—104, 1964.
68. **Bissonette, T. H.**, Studies on the sexual cycle in birds. VI. Effects of white, green, and red lights of equal luminous intensity on the testes activity of the European starling (*Sturnus vulgarus*), *Physiol. Zool.*, 5, 92—123, 1932.
69. **Benoit, J.**, The role of the eye and of the hypothalamus in the photostimulation of gonads in the duck, *Ann. N. Y. Acad. Sci.*, 117, 204—216, 1964.
70. **Harrison, P., Latshaw, J. D., Casey, J. M., and McGinnis, J.**, Influence of decreased length of different spectral photoperiods on testes development of domestic fowl, *J. Reprod. Fertil.*, 22, 269—275, 1970.
71. **Lake, P. E.**, The physical environment and reproduction in domesticated birds, *15th World Poultry Congress*, World Poultry Science Association, U.S. Branch, New Orleans, 1974, 2—13.
72. **Lofts, B. and Murton, R. K.**, Reproduction in birds, in *Avian Biology*, Vol. 3, Farner, D. S. and King, J. R., Eds., Academic Press, New York, 1973, 1—107.
73. **Donovan, B. T.**, The effect of light on reproductive mechanisms as illustrated by the ferret, *Ciba Found. Study Group*, 26, 43—52, 1967.

74. **Martinet, L.**, Role du photoperiodisme sur la biologie sexuelle du campagnol des Champs (*Microtus arvalis*), in *La Photoregulation de la Reproduction Chez les Oiseaux et les Mammiferes*, Benoit, J. and Assenmacher, I., Eds., Editions du Centre National de la Recherche Scientifique, Paris, 1970, 435—452.
75. **Wright, P. L.**, Correlation between the spring molt and spring changes in the sexual cycle in the weasel, *J. Exp. Zool.*, 91, 103—110, 1942.
76. **Lyman, C. P.**, Control of coat color in the varying hare by daily illumination, *Proc. N. Engl. Zool. Club*, 19, 75—78, 1942.
77. **Bassett, C. F., Pearson, O. P., and Wilke, F.**, The effect of artificially increased length of day on molt, growth and priming of silver fox pelts, *J. Exp. Zool.*, 96, 77—83, 1944.
78. **Bassett, C. F. and Llewellyn, L. M.**, The effect of increased or decreased length of daylight on pelt primeness in growing foxes, *Ann. N.Y. Acad. Sci.*, 48, 4, 1946.
79. **Bissonette, T. H.**, Relations of hair cycles in ferrets to changes in the anterior hypophysis and to light cycles, *Anat. Rec.*, 63, 156—168, 1935.
80. **Bissonette, T. H. and Wilson, E.**, Shortening daylight periods between May 15 and September 12 and the pelt cycle of the mink, *Science*, 89, 418—419, 1939.
81. **Adair, J. and Stout, F. M.**, Mink research: controlled light and furring, *Oreg. Agric. Exp. Str. Bull.*, 320, 1—26, 1971.
82. **Rust, C. C. and Meyer, R. K.**, Hair color, molt and testes size in male, short-tailed weasels treated with melatonin, *Science*, 165, 921—922, 1969.
83. **Yeates, N. T. M.**, The equatorial light environment and its effects on the coat of European cattle, *Aust. J. Agric. Res.*, 8, 733—739, 1957.
84. **Hutchinson, J. C. D.**, Photoperiodic control of the annual rhythm of wool growth, in *Biology of the Skin and Hair Growth*, Lyne, A. G. and Short, B. F., Eds., Elsevier, New York, 1965, 565—573.
85. **Slee, J.**, Seasonal patterns of moulting in Wiltshire Hornsheep, in *Biology of the Skin and Hair Growth*, Lyne, A. G. and Short, B. F., Eds., Elsevier, New York, 1965, 545—564.
86. **Lyman, C. P.**, Control of coat color in the varying hare *Lepus americanus Erxleben*, *Bull. Mus. Comp. Zool. Harv. Univ.*, 93, 394—461, 1943.
87. **Ringer, R. K.**, Effect of light and behavior on nutrition, *J. Anim. Sci.*, 35, 642—647, 1972.
88. **Murrill, F. D., Eide, R. N., Leonard, R. O., and Bath, D. L.**, Effect of Corral Lighting on Feed Intake and Milk Production of Dairy Cattle, paper presented at the American Dairy Science Association Meeting, Minneapolis, June 22—25, 1969.
89. **Belyaev, V. I. and Gorbunova, E. G.**, Effects of cowshed lighting on milk production of cows, *Veterinariya (Moscow)*, 11, 29—31, 1973.
90. **Hoersch, T. M., Reineke, E. P., and Henneman, H. A.**, Effect of artificial light and ambient temperature on the thyroid secretion rate and other metabolic measures in sheep, *J. Anim. Sci.*, 20, 358—362, 1961.
91. **Braude, R., Mitchell, K. G., Finn-Kelsey, P., and Owen, V. M.**, The effect of light on fattening pigs, *Proc. Nutr. Soc.*, 17, xxxviii—xxxix, 1958.
92. **Dufour, J. and Bernard, C.**, Effect of light on the development of market pigs and breeding gilts, *Can. J. Anim. Sci.*, 48, 425—430, 1968.
93. **Cherry, P. and Barwick, M. W.**, The effect of light on broiler growth. I. Light intensity and colour, *Br. Poult. Sci.*, 3, 31—39, 1962.
94. **Cherry, P. and Barwick, M. W.**, The effect of light on broiler growth. II. Light patterns, *Br. Poult. Sci.*, 3, 41—50, 1962.
95. **Ballard, P. D. and Biellier, H. V.**, The effect of photoperiod and oviposition on feed and water consumption by chicken laying hen, *Poult. Sci.*, 48, 1781—1782, 1969.
96. **Siegel, H. S., Beane, W. L., and Howes, C. E.**, Lighting regimes as an influence on maturity and productivity of Leghorn type layers, *Poult. Sci.*, 42, 1064—1971, 1963.
97. **Beane, W. L., Siegel, P. B., and Siegel, H. S.**, Interactions of lighting regimes, stock and feeding methods on broiler performance, *Poult. Sci.*, 42, 1255—1256, 1963.
98. **Beane, W. L., Siegel, P. B., and Siegel, H. S.**, Light environment as a factor in growth and feed efficiency of meat type chickens, *Poult. Sci.*, 44, 1009—1012, 1965.
99. **Peters, R. R., Chapin, L. T., Leining, K. B., and Tucker, H. A.**, Supplemental lighting stimulates growth and lactation in cattle, *Science*, 199, 911—912, 1978.
100. **Peters, R. R., Chapin, L. T., Emery, R. S., and Tucker, H. A.**, Growth and hormonal response of heifers to various photoperiods, *J. Anim. Sci.*, 51, 1148—1153, 1980.
101. **Tucker, H. A. and Oxender, W. D.**, Seasonal aspects of reproduction, growth, and hormones in cattle and horses, *Prog. Reprod. Biol.*, 5, 155—180, 1980.

EFFECTS OF COLD ON ANIMAL PRODUCTION

G. I. Christison and C. M. Williams

The overall ability of animals to resist cold depends upon several primary factors, including insulation, feed intake, and metabolic adaptation to cold, all of which are influenced by body size. These factors affect the animal's "critical temperature" and the temperature at which the animal exhibits maximum metabolic response to cold[1] (these interrelations are shown diagramatically in Figure 1). Critical temperature is the effective ambient air temperature below which physical methods alone become insufficient in maintaining thermostability; the animal must therefore increase heat production. Below the critical temperature, an unadapted animal must either consume more feed or produce less in order to counteract the environmental thermal demand. As adaptation to cold takes place over a period of weeks, animals may increase their insulation and resting metabolic rate, thereby decreasing the critical temperature. Critical temperatures of animals under a variety of conditions of body weight, pelage, and adaptation can be calculated[3-5] on the basis of their insulation and the rate of heat production (Table 1).

Although critical temperature and insulation give a general indication of the effect of cold on productivity of animals, depressed performance in cold conditions has been reported in cattle even though effective ambient temperature is above the critical temperature. The major reasons for the depressed performance are lower feed digestibility and higher resting metabolic rates in animals adapted to cold.[6] These changes occur progressively as environmental temperature declines. Performance of cattle does not, therefore, show an abrupt break point, as might be expected on the basis of critical temperature alone.[7]

BEEF CATTLE

Beef cattle, which are relatively large and well-insulated, are able to resist cold weather under most climatic conditions. Under the mild (10 to −10°C), wet, winter conditions in western Europe, temperature, rainfall, wind, and relative humidity do not affect liveweight gain or feed consumption.[8]

Under the more severe cold conditions of Canada and the northern U.S., cattle may grow at 70 to 90% of the rate of animals maintained indoors and may require as much as 40% more feed.[6,7,9-11]

Over the temperature range of 18 to −22°C, it was found that the average daily gain was reduced by 0.14 kg for every 10°C drop in environmental temperature, and that the metabolizable energy required to produce a 1 kg gain increased by 1.07 Mcal for every 10°C decline (Table 2).

Water consumption across the range 0 to −30°C was found to be consistently 2.4 kg of water per kilogram of dry feed.[12]

DAIRY CATTLE

Although environmental temperatures over 30°C have a pronounced effect on feed consumption and milk yield in high-producing dairy cows, the effects of cold are less marked (Table 3). Effects are more pronounced at extremely low temperatures. In the range 5 to −11°C, production dropped by 0.44 kg/10°C decline in ambient temperature, whereas in the range −11 to −20°C, production decreased 1.55 kg/10°C drop.[13]

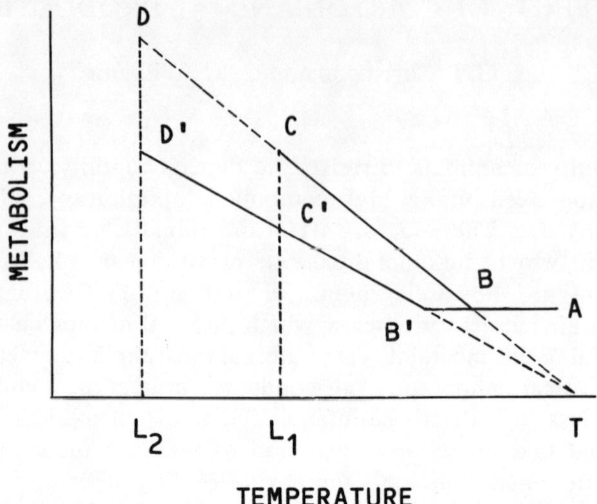

FIGURE 1. A diagram of the relationship between an animal's metabolic rate and the ambient temperature. As the animal's insulation increases, the slope moves from BC to B′C′, pivoting on the animal's deep body temperature, T. The critical temperature falls at the same time from that below B to B′, and the cold limit falls from L_1 to L_2, at the same maximum metabolism; this is insulative adaptation to cold. In "metabolic" adaptation, the curve BC is extended to BCD; at this point, the cold limit is extended from L_1 to L_2 by a rise in metabolic rate from C = D′ to D. Increased feed intake raises A and thus moves B down the temperature scale, decreasing the critical temperature. Similarly, variation in the level of minimum metabolism A would move B relative to the temperature scale and thus change the critical temperature. (From Barnett, S. A. and Mount, L. E., in *Thermobiology,* Rose, A. H., Ed., Academic Press, London, 1967, 414. With permission.)

Water consumption relative to feed intake remained constant across the temperature range at 4 kg of water per kilogram of dry feed.[17]

SWINE

The effects of cold have a greater depressing effect on swine productivity than on cattle, principally because of the poor thermal insulation of their pelage (Table 1). Although pregnant sows and gilts may be maintained outdoors with unheated but well-bedded shelter in regions where the mean monthly temperature is −20°C, young, lactating and growing-finishing swine need protection from the cold. The results of several experiments showing effects of decreasing ambient temperature on weight gain have been summarized in Figure 2.[4,18] The optimum ambient temperatures recommended for growing-finishing pigs are 21°C or 18°C for those weighing 10 to 45 or 45 to 95 kg, respectively.[19] Cold affects other measures of productivity to a greater extent than growth rates. Feed intake is increased more markedly, and there is a consequent pronounced increase in the feed required per unit gain (Table 4). Short-term changes in productivity in response to cold are marked, but over a period of weeks, swine, like all the productive domestic animals, are able to adapt to a considerable

Table 1
OVERALL THERMAL CONDUCTANCE, COMPONENTS OF THERMAL INSULATION, MINIMUM EVAPORATIVE HEAT LOSS, AND THERMONEUTRAL HEAT PRODUCTION, AND THE CALCULATED CRITICAL TEMPERATURES OF VARIOUS DOMESTIC ANIMALS[4,5]

Species and breed	Weight (kg)	Surface area (m²)	Overall conductance (kcal/m² × 24 hr)	Coat type	Insulation (°C × m² × 24 hr/Mcal)			Heat production (Mcal/m² × 24 hr)		Minimum evaporative heat loss (Mcal/m² × 24 hr)	Calculated critical temperature (°C)	
					Tissue	Coat	Air	At maintenance	Fully fed		At maintenance	Fully fed
Pig												
Large white	1.5	0.13	133	Normal	2.1	8.3[a]		1.6	2.8	0.16	27	18
Large white	4	0.23	100	Normal	—	—	—	1.6	2.8	0.09	23	11
Large while	8	0.36	100	Normal	—	—	—	1.6	2.8	0.10	23	11
Large white	10	0.42	100	Normal	—	—	—	1.6	2.8	0.11	23	11
Landrace	23	0.71	98	Normal	4.6	7.2		1.6	2.8	0.11	23	11
Large white	150	2.31	36	Normal	—	—	—	1.4	2.5	—	2	−28
Sheep												
Merino	5	0.26	58	Fine	8.2	8.5		1.2	1.6	0.48	26	19
Merino	5	0.26	43	Coarse	7.5	14.7		1.2	1.4	0.48	21	17
Down	45	1.14	31	Clipped	3.5	nil[b]	7.7	1.3	2.3	0.31	26	13
Down	45	1.14	31	5 cm	3.5	27.9		1.3	2.3	0.31	6	−26
Blackface	45	1.14	68	Clipped	5.7	nil	7.7	1.3	2.3	0.24	22	8
Blackface	45	1.14	29	5 cm	5.7	27.9		1.3	2.3	0.24	1	−33
Cattle												
Ayrshire	42	1.08	53	Normal	4.4	7.7	5.7	1.9	3.0	0.34	9	−12
Jersey	390	4.78	62	Normal	—	—	—	2.6	3.7	0.28	1	−17
Brahman	470	5.42	62	Normal	—	—	—	2.6	3.7	0.24	0	−18
Brown Swiss	550	6.02	52	Normal	—	—	—	2.6	3.7	0.21	−8	−29
Galloway	500	5.07	41	Normal	6.7	16.2		2.0	3.2	0.35	−2	−32
Hereford												
Steer	365	4.59	44	Severe winter	8.3	14.3		—	3.6	—	—	−48
Pregnant cow	500	5.78	36	Severe winter	12.7	15.3		2.2	—	—	−18	—
Calf	210	3.24	46	Severe winter	7.4	14.3		2.9[c]			−19[c]	

[a] The data in this column apply for combined coat and air insulation.
[b] nil = no coat.
[c] The data in this column apply to moderately fed animals.

Table 2
PERFORMANCE OF STEERS AND HEIFERS EXPOSED TO SEVERE COLD WITH VARYING DEGREES OF SHELTER[7,9]

Animals	Month	Weight (kg)	Mean temperature (°C)	Average daily gain (kg)	Feed intake (kg)	Feed/ gain
Feedlot steers[a]	December to February	419	−17	1.03	8.95	9.8
	March to May	390	2	1.33	9.18	7.2
	June to August	372	17	1.51	7.97	5.6
	September to November	431	3	1.57	10.68	6.9
Heifers						
Control[b]	November to March	230	20	0.63	4.73	—
Shelter[c]	November to March	225	−16	0.59	5.25	—
Exposed[d]	November to March	218	−16	0.54	5.14	—

[a] Outdoors: porous fence windbreak, manure-pack bedding.
[b] Heated barn.
[c] Outdoors: roofed open-front shed and dry lot, straw bedding.
[d] Outdoors: dry lot, straw bedding.

Table 3
EFFECT OF ENVIRONMENTAL TEMPERATURE ON MILK PRODUCTION AND FEED INTAKE OF LACTATING DAIRY COWS[13-16]

Breed	Mean ambient (°C)	Relative humidity (%)	Milk production (kg/day)	Digestible energy intake (Mcal/day)
Holstein[a]	−7	90—100	21.3	52.2
	−18	90—100	20.6	58.7
Holstein[b]	7	72—79	21.5	—
	−17	72—79	21.3	—
Holstein[c]	−10	64—67	15	49.3
	−13	60—68	14	45.8
Jersey[c]	10	64—67	7.6	30.0
	−13	60—68	3.5	32.6

[a] Unheated barn with manure pack. Concentrate fed for milk production, hay allowed *ad lib.*
[b] Same barn as [a], but with increased ventilation. Concentrate: fed for milk production, roughage fed for maintenance.
[c] Climatic laboratory: ambient temperature progressively decreased over a 2-month period. Concentrate fed for milk production, hay allowed *ad lib.*

extent (Table 5).[26] Young pigs are particularly susceptible to cold stress,[18,21] having a critical temperature of 33°C at birth. Cold resistance improves markedly in the first postnatal days largely because of improved metabolic capability. By the time the piglet weighs 10 kg, critical temperature has fallen to 19°C.

POULTRY

The production characteristics of poultry are more susceptible to temperature

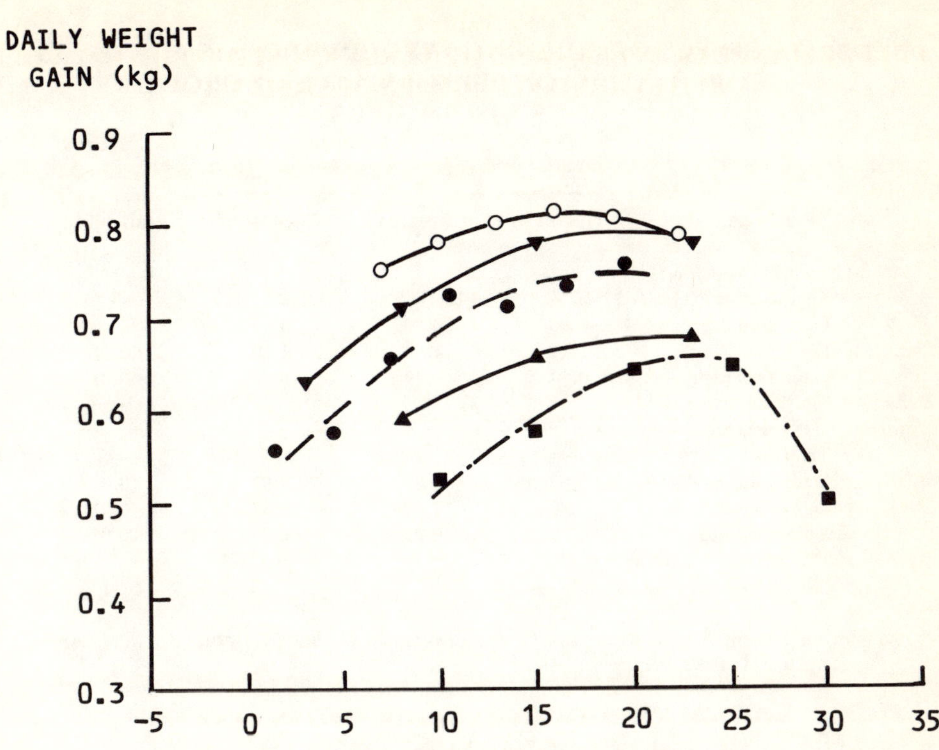

FIGURE 2. The daily weight gain of pigs as a function of environmental temperature. = pigs from 30 to 90 kg; ▼ – ▼ – and ▲–▲–▲ = pigs from 30 to 90 kg on two feeding regimes; ●— — ● = pigs from 30 to 110 kg; ■ —■ — = pigs from 2 to 10 weeks of age (4 to 40 kg). (Data from Comberg, *Zuchtungskunde,* 31, 462, 1959; Sorensen, *Tagungsber. Dtsch. Akad. Landwirtschaftswiss Berlin;* 23, 79, 1960; Siegl, *Arch. Tierz.*, 3, 188, 1960; and Fuller, *Br. J. Nutr.*, 19, 531, 1965.) (From Fuller, M. F., *Animal Growth and Nutrition,* Hafez, E. S. E. and Dryer, I. A., Eds., Lea & Febiger, Philadelphia, 1969, 98. With permission.)

changes than are those of other domestic animals. Both egg production (Figure 3)[22] and growth (Table 6)[23] are affected by small changes in environmental temperature.

Table 4
EFFECT OF BUILDING TYPE (ENVIRONMENTAL TEMPERATURE) ON PERFORMANCE OF GROWING-FINISHING PIGS

	Building			
Performance	Heated	Unheated	Open front	Probability
Growing (14—48 kg)				
Temperature, °C	22(16—24)[a]	10(1—5)[a]	−7(−23—15)[a]	—
Daily gain, kg	0.80	0.80	0.75	—
Daily feed, kg	1.47	1.64	1.80	<0.01
Gain/feed ratio	0.54	0.49	0.42	<0.01
Finishing (48—102 kg)				
Temperature, °C	21(16—25)[a]	15(2—24)[a]	1(−14—18)[a]	—
Daily gain, kg	0.82	0.82	0.92	<0.01
Daily feed, kg	2.89	2.87	3.35	<0.01
Gain/feed ratio	0.29	0.29	0.27	<0.05

[a] Mean with range in parentheses.

From Jensen, A. H., Kuhlman, D. E., Becker, D. E., and Harmon, B. G., *J. Anim. Sci.*, 29, 451, 1969. With permission.

Table 5
DAILY GAIN IN WEIGHT AND FEED CONVERSION RATIO IN GROWING PIGS (20—90 KG) AT CONSTANT AMBIENT TEMPERATURE AND FOLLOWING ABRUPT CHANGES OF AMBIENT TEMPERATURE

Temperature	Daily gain in weight (kg)	Scandinavian feed units (per kg gain)	Number of Pigs	Number of Periods
Constant temperature 3°C	0.58 ± 0.04	3.7 ± 0.15	4	
Constant temperature 19°C	0.72 ± 0.04	3.1 ± 0.02	4	
First 12 days following abrupt change from 19° to 3°C	0.26. ± 0.02	9.4 ± 1.12	8	16
13—28 days after change of temperature	0.59 ± 0.04	4.0 ± 0.16	8	14
First 12 days after abrupt change from 3° to 19°C	0.69 ± 0.03	3.0 ± 0.12	8	16
13—28 days after change of temperature	0.79 ± 0.05	3.0 ± 0.12	8	14

From Moustgaard, J., Nielsen, D. B., and Sorensen, P. H., Royal Veterinary and Agricultural College Sterility Research Institute, Annu. Rep. 173, Royal Veterinary and Agricultural College, Copenhagen, 1959. With permission.

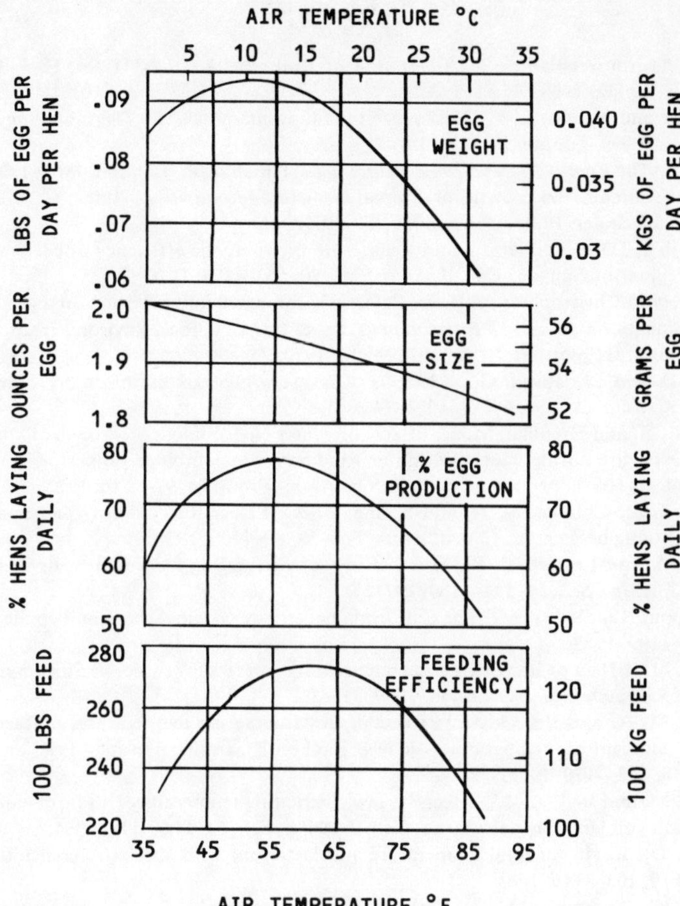

FIGURE 3. The effect of temperature on egg weight, egg size, egg production, and feed efficiency for hens. (From Esmay, M. S., *Principles of Animal Environment,* AVI Publishing, Westport, Conn., 1969, 248. With permission.)

Table 6
EFFECT OF VARIATION OF TEMPERATURE ON GROWTH OF BROILER CHICKS FROM 2—10 WEEKS OF AGE

House temperature range (°F)	House temperature average (°F)	Average liveweight at 10 weeks (g)	Food conversion at 10 weeks	Liveweight increase 6—10 weeks (g)	Food conversion 6—10 weeks
69—75	71	1345[a]	2.94	586[a]	3.83
61—66	64	1638[b]	2.73	808[b]	3.41
54—66	58	1678[b]	2.79	866[b]	3.41
50—66	55	1665[b]	2.78	854[b]	3.38

[a,b] Means in the same column with different superscripts differ ($p < .05$)

From Sorensen, P. H., in *Nutrition of Pigs and Poultry,* Morgan, J. T. and Lewis, D., Eds., Butterworths, London, 1962, 88. With permission.

REFERENCES

1. **Bianca, W.,** Thermoregulation, in *Adaptation of Domestic Animals,* Hafez, E. S. E., Ed., Lea & Febiger, Philadelphia, 1968, 97—118.
2. **Barnett, S. A. and Mount, L. E.,** Resistance to cold in mammals, in *Thermobiology,* Rose, A. H., Ed., Academic Press, London, 1967, 411—477.
3. **Blaxter, K. L.,** *The Energy Metabolism of Ruminants,* Hutchinson, London, 1967, 117—149.
4. **Fuller, M. F.,** Climate and growth, in *Animal Growth and Nutrition,* Hafez, E. S. E. and Dyer, I. A., Eds., Lea & Febiger, Philadelphia, 1969, 82—105.
5. **Webster, A. J. F.,** Direct effects of cold weather on the energetic efficiency of beef cattle production in different regions of Canada, *Can. J. Anim. Sci.,* 50, 563—573, 1970.
6. **Young, B. A. and Christopherson, R. J.,** Effect of prolonged cold exposure on digestion and metabolism in ruminants, in *Livestock Environment,* Proc. Int. Livestock Environ. Symp., American Society of Agricultural Engineers, St. Joseph, Mich., 1974, 75—80.
7. **Milligan, J. D. and Christison, G. I.,** Effects of severe winter conditions on performance of feedlot steers, *Can. J. Anim. Sci.,* 54, 605—610, 1974.
8. **McCarrick, R. B. and Drennan, M. J.,** Effects of winter environment on growth of young beef cattle. I. Effect of exposure during winter to rain or wind and rain combined on performance of 9-month-old Friesian steers fed on two planes of nutrition, *Anim. Prod.,* 14, 97—110, 1972.
9. **Webster, A. J. F., Chulmecky, J., and Young, B. A.,** Effects of cold environments on the energy exchanges of young beef cattle, *Can. J. Anim. Sci.,* 50, 89—100, 1970.
10. **Hidiroglou, M. and Lessard, J. R.,** Some effects of fluctuating low ambient temperatures on beef cattle, *Can. J. Anim. Sci.,* 51, 111—120, 1971.
11. **Knox, K. L. and Handley, T. M.,** The California net energy system: theory and application, *J. Anim. Sci.,* 37, 190—199, 1973.
12. **Williams, C. M.,** Effect of low fluctuating temperatures on feedlot cattle, in *Stockman's Day Report,* University of Saskatchewan, Saskatoon, 1969, 21—26.
13. **MacDonald, M. A. and Bell, J. M.,** Effects of low fluctuating temperatures on farm animals. III. Influence of ambient air temperature on feed intake of lactating Holstein-Friesian cows, *Can. J. Anim. Sci.,* 38, 148—170, 1958.
14. **Williams, C. M. and Bell, J. M.,** Effects of low fluctuating temperatures on farm animals. V. Influence of humidity on lactating dairy cows, *Can. J. Anim. Sci.,* 44, 114—119, 1964.
15. **Johnson, H. D.,** Environmental temperature and lactation: with special reference to cattle, *Int. J. Biometeorol.,* 9, 103—116, 1965.
16. **Ragsdale, A. C., Thompson, H. J., Worstell, D. M., and Brody, S.,** Milk production and feed and water consumption responses of Brahman, Jersey, and Holstein cows to changes in temperature, 50° to 105°F and 50° to 8°F, *Mo. Agric. Exp. Stn. Res. Bull.,* 460, 1950.
17. **MacDonald, M. A. and Bell, J. M.,** Effects of low fluctuating temperature on farm animals. II. Influence of ambient air temperature on water intake of lactating Holstein-Friesian cows, *Can. J. Anim. Sci.,* 38, 23—32, 1958.
18. **Mount, L. E.,** *Climatic Physiology of the Pig,* Williams & Wilkins, Baltimore, 1968, 229—243.
19. **Pond, W. G. and Maner, J. H.,** *Swine Production in Temperate and Tropical Climates,* W. H. Freeman, San Francisco, 1974, 472—493.
20. **Sorensen, P. H.,** Influence of climatic environment on pig performance, in *Nutrition of Pigs and Poultry,* Morgan, J. T. and Lewis, D., Eds., Butterworths, London, 1962, 88—103.
21. **Curtis, S. E.,** Environmental-thermoregulatory interactions and neonatal piglet survival, *J. Anim. Sci.,* 31, 576—587, 1970.
22. **Esmay, M. L.,** *Principles of Animal Environment,* AVI Publishing, Westport, Conn., 1969, 235—256.
23. **Payne, C. G.,** The relationship between climatic environment and poultry performance, in *Nutrition of Pigs and Poultry,* Morgan, J. T. and Lewis, D., Eds., Butterworths, London, 1962, 104—123.

EFFECT OF HEAT ON ANIMAL PRODUCTIVITY

William W. Thatcher and Robert J. Collier

INTRODUCTION

Since 1960 growth of the world population has been over 2% yearly, whereas the rate of increase in food production has been about 1.8%. Therefore, world food production per person is decreasing.[1] One of the main reasons for losing this critical balance is that many countries are not producing food to their potential. The region of the warm climates has been designated between latitudes 30° N and 30° S. This region contains approximately 50% of the world's potentially arable land. However, direct and indirect effects of the climates cause certain problems for crop and animal production.[2] Estimations are that 80% of the future population increase will occur in the developing countries of Latin America, Asia, and Africa. These are areas with the least capability to feed and support a growing population.

Production of more animal foods in tropical and subtropical areas will be important to meet future food needs. Animal foods are excellent sources of protein from the standpoint of both quantity and quality. Ruminant animals play an important role in the food chain because to a large degree they utilize feed products that cannot be eaten directly by humans, consume forages on land areas not ideal for production of cereal grains, and also utilize nonprotein nitrogen and by-products that are not suitable for human consumption. Furthermore, certain waste products in our environment can be recycled into the food chain via animal utilization. Both swine and poultry (nonruminants) also have been able to utilize by-product feeds in their rations.

Tropical and subtropical areas of the world will be providing a greater input into meeting the world food needs. However, animal productivity in these climatic areas is less than animals managed in temperate zones.[3] Higher temperatures and humidity contribute directly and indirectly to this inefficiency. Dynamics of animal responsiveness to heat, periods of thermal sensitivity that influence production, and management systems to improve animal productivity under these environments are the topics of this presentation.

THERMOREGULATION

Domestic animals all belong to the subgroup of vertebrates which are homeothermic. Homeothermic animals have developed successful strategies to maintain body core temperature within a narrow range. These strategies are termed thermoregulatory and can be divided into either voluntary (i.e., behavioral) or involuntary thermoregulation. A high priority is placed on thermoregulation by the mammalian system — so much so that the thermoregulatory system calls on and presents challenges to other regulatory systems such as the cardiovascular, respiratory, and endocrine systems. The reverse is seldom seen. Thus a greater priority is placed on thermoregulation than on any of the productive functions of domestic animals such as lactation, growth, and reproduction. This, therefore, is the basic cause of reduced performance of domestic animals during heat stress.

All homeotherms have a range of environmental temperatures which they can withstand without changes in basal metabolism. This range is termed the zone of thermal neutrality, which is bounded by the upper and lower critical temperatures. Within the zone, adjustments such as vascular distribution, pelage, or behavior are used successfully to maintain homeothermy. Productive functions of domestic animals are not decreased by ambient temperatures within the zone. As the critical temperature is exceeded, the physiological and metabolic adjustments needed to maintain body temperature are increasingly deleterious to productive functions.

Heat Loss

Animals exchange heat with their environment by means of conduction, convection, radiation, and evaporation. The first three are classified as sensible heat loss mechanisms which require a thermal gradient. The fourth is termed an insensible heat loss and does not require a thermal gradient to operate.

Conduction involves the passage of thermal energy from molecule to molecule according to the second law of thermodynamics. Convection is the transfer of thermal energy by circulation of a fluid or gas which is nonuniform in temperature. Thus blood flow is a major avenue of convective heat transfer to the body shell or skin surface. Radiation is the passage of thermal energy through space without heating the space through which it passes. Evaporative heat loss involves a reduction in thermal energy utilized when water is changed to the gaseous state.

Movement of heat to the surface and its dissipation are greatly affected by the insulative properties of the skin. This is affected by the amount of blood flow through surface vessels, thickness of the fat layer, thickness of hair coat, and piloerection. Thus in the thermoneutral zone, sensible heat loss is the major avenue of heat dissipation and metabolism proceeds independently of ambient temperature. At the upper critical temperature, sensible heat loss is maximal. When the thermoneutral zone is exceeded, the animal must rely on evaporative heat loss and reductions in heat of metabolism to maintain homeothermy.

Cardiovascular System

An early response to rising ambient temperature is an adjustment in the cardiovascular system. This response occurs within the thermoneutral zone before the upper critical ambient temperature.[4] Adjustments include an increase in cardiac output and blood volume,[5] and peripheral vasodilation.

Skin normally has a blood flow which far exceeds its nutritional needs.[6] Control of blood flow to the skin depends on tone and resistance of the skin capillary bed. Increases in ambient temperature result in vasodilation of skin vasculature and subsequent increases in blood flow. The sympathetic nervous system plays a significant role in regulation of cutaneous vascular resistance.[7] However, other factors such as bradykinen may be involved in regulating peripheral vascular resistance.[8]

Both sensible and insensible heat loss are increased by shifts in blood distribution to the skin. Sensible heat loss requires a gradient for heat to move down. Thus, by vasodilation of peripheral blood vessels, a greater amount of blood and therefore heat is brought to the body surface for dissipation by radiation, conduction, or convection. As long as the gradient is maintained the animal can rely on sensible heat loss as the primary mode of heat dissipation. However, as ambient air temperature and/or heat load increase, the gradient may disappear or actually reverse. Under these conditions the primary mode of heat dissipation becomes evaporative or insensible heat loss.

Another cardiovascular adjustment is the selective use of counter-current exchange mechanisms. Countercurrent exchange mechanisms are unique anatomical vascular arrangements which serve to conserve body core heat or selectively cool a portion of the body such as the brain or testis. They are characterized by an artery which is entwined with veins. Countercurrent exchange mechanisms have the general effect of returning heat to the body core via venous flow while cooling arterial blood flowing to the appendages, testis, or brain. During heat stress those countercurrent exchange mechanisms which are used to conserve heat during cold stress are discarded by shifting venous flow to surface vessels instead of those surrounding deep lying arteries.[9] In contrast, the countercurrent mechanisms which function to cool selected areas of the body are maintained. Baker and Hayward[10] demonstrated that as the sheep increases its respiration rate in response to a heat stress there is an increased loss of heat from cerebral arterial blood to venous blood from nasal and oral mucosa which prevents cerebral overheating. An additional example can be found in the testis where transfer of heat at the panpiniform plexus serves to drop arterial blood temperature approximately 5°C before it enters the testis.

Fluid Balance

Normally, increases in evaporative heat loss require an expansion of plasma volume to move more water to the body surface for evaporation. This is reflected in lower plasma protein and hematocrit percent. The plasma volume shift which occurs with changes in ambient temperature is rapid. Water requirements for expansion of plasma volume to increase evaporative heat loss is met by increasing fecal and renal water retention and activation of the thirst drive which increases water intake.

Two independent neurohumeral systems regulate body fluid balance. One is an antidiuretic system and the other the antinatriuretic system. Expansion of blood volume requires activation of both systems to regulate osmotic pressure and fluid volume. Additional work is required to document temperature effects on antidiuretic and aldosterone secretion in domestic animals.

Respiration

When ambient temperatures and solar heat loads increase there is a subsequent increase in respiratory frequency of cattle, chickens, sheep, and pigs.[13-16] This increase in respiratory rate increases evaporative heat loss from the upper respiratory passages or so-called "dead space". Panting is not as effective as sweating in increasing evaporative moisture loss,[17,18] and tends to alter alveolar ventilation, which subsequently alters blood CO_2, 0_2, and pH. In severe heat, when body temperature continues to rise, panting is replaced by "second phase breathing", characterized by low respiratory frequency and large tidal volume.[19] During this phase alveolar respiration increases dramatically which results in development of respiratory alkalosis.[20] Respiratory alkalosis has negative effects on animal performance, especially uterine and umbilical blood flow during pregnancy.[21]

Nutrition

Under thermoneutral conditions feed intake and metabolism proceed independently of ambient temperature. At higher temperature both feed intake and basal metabolism are reduced. This reduction is in a large part responsible for reduced performance of heat stressed animals. It also should be pointed out that in many areas of the world feed quality varies markedly with season and greatly influences animal productivity. Here, we shall address only the effects of hyperthermia on feed intake and metabolism.

Depression of voluntary feed intake by hyperthermia is believed to be due to several factors. One is a direct negative effect of temperature on the appetite center in the hypothalamus.[22] A second cause is reduced gut motility and rumination[23] which leads to increased gut fill. This in turn depresses appetite. Associated with decreased appetite is a lowered production of volatile fatty acids (VFA) in ruminants.[24] The reduction in VFA production is not entirely due to reduced feed intake because it is only partially restored when refused food is placed into the rumen via a fistula to restore feed intake to control levels.[25] Water intake of ruminants is dramatically increased during thermal stress.[26] The increased water intake substantially reduces rumen temperature, thus reducing heat load.[27] The relationship between feed intake and water intake in cows during thermal stress is negative,[28] as illustrated in Figure 1. Studies on the molar percentage of rumen VFA during thermal stress have been variable and require further examination.[29-31]

Heat production must balance heat loss if the domestic animal is to maintain homeothermy. Thus, when ambient temperatures exceed the zone of thermoneutrality a variety of mechanisms to reduce heat production come into play. Among these are reductions in feed intake, catabolic rate of ingested feed, and digestive tract performance. The heat of catabolism also is reduced by increased water intake. The reduced flow of nutrients from the digestive tract is reflected in lowered animal productivity. In addition, the cellular metabolism within the animal has been reduced via reductions in circulating levels of metabolic hormones such as thyroxine and growth hormone.[32]

Endocrine System

A complex neuroendocrine response is an integral part of the overall temperature regulating mechanism which permits endotherms to maintain constant body temperature in the face of acutely varying environmental and body conditions.[33] Unfortunately, a great deal of confusion exists regarding heat stress effects on domestic animal neuroendocrine systems for two reasons. One is that there have been few experiments directed at the problems. Also, studies performed in climatic chambers often give results which are not duplicated in long-term experiments under natural conditions. Available information will be discussed as acute stress responses when performed in a chamber and a chronic stress response when performed under natural conditions.

Some monoamines such as dopamine, epinephrine, norepinephrine, and serotonin are implicated in molecular control of neurotransmission within the thermoregulatory center of the hypothalamus as well as having peripheral effects on blood flow and sweat rate.[34] Plasma epinephrine and norepinephrine are elevated following acute heat exposure in steers, cattle, and chickens.[34-36] Also, cattle maintained at 35°C for 24 days had elevated concentrations of plasma epinephrine and norepinephrine.[34] Sweat glands of cattle are activated by catecholamines.[37,38] Since these glands are not innervated,[39] increased catecholamine concentrations may be involved in regulating sweat gland activity. The effect of centrally administered monomaines on thermoregulation are quite variable. Bligh et al.[40] summarized several experiments that demonstrated differences in thermoregulatory responses that may be attributable to species, route and site of administration, dosage, environmental temperature or sampling time. Additional work is required before definitive conclusions may be drawn on the specific roles of the various monoamines in central control of thermoregulation in domestic animals.

Anterior pituitary function is altered by environmental heating. Primary effects of increased heat load on pituitary function are related to those hormones involved in basal metabolism such as thyroid stimulating hormone, growth hormone, prolactin, and adrenocorticotropic hormone.

Exposure to heat and subsequent increases in body temperature reduce hormone secretions by the thyroid gland in rams,[41] poultry,[42] pigs,[43] and cattle.[50] Reduced thyroid function is preceded by reductions in secretion of TSH by the pituitary.[44,45] The decline in thyroid gland activity reduces metabolic rate of the animal and thereby reduces metabolic heat load.

Heat stressed cows and steers have a reduced plasma growth hormone concentration.[46,47] This has been demonstrated in the laboratory rat after 34°C for up to 48 hr by Krulich and co-workers.[45] These investigators also detected a significant rise in pituitary growth hormone concentrations implicating a negative effect of heat stress on

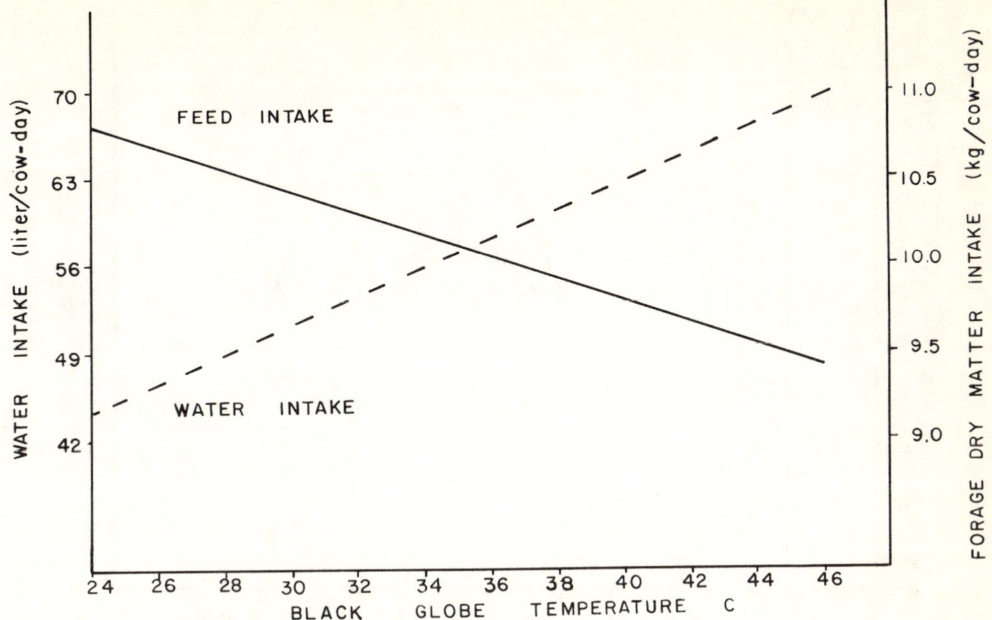

FIGURE 1. Least squares regressions of black globe temperature on water intake and forage dry matter intake in dairy cows.

GH release rather than synthesis. Since GH is involved in control of basal metabolism, a reduction in its secretion would lower metabolic heat production. Injection of growth hormone (200 to 300 mg/cow IV) increases heat production.[48]

When environmental temperatures change at a rapid rate or when preoptic temperature in the hypotholamus is acutely raised or lowered by means of an implanted electrode, there is a sudden rise in plasma glucocorticoid concentrations.[12,49] When cattle are maintained at elevated environmental periods for several days, an initial rise in plasma glucocorticoid concentrations is detected, followed within a few hours by a return to pretreatment levels, and eventually glucocorticoid concentrations are depressed in these animals.[34,50,51] Furthermore, cattle which have acclimatized to warm summer conditions have a reduced responsiveness to an injection of ACTH.[52] Cattle exposed to the natural environment are exposed to marked changes in environmental temperatures within a 24-hr period.[12] Under these conditions there is a daily rate change in both environmental temperature and glucocorticoid secretion as shown in Figure 2. Thus, as stated by Chowers, the hypothalamo-hypophyseal-adrenal axis is more sensitive to rate of change of environmental temperature than it is to the absolute temperature of the surroundings.[33]

Prolactin secretion is greatly influenced by changes in photoperiod and temperature.[53,54] There is a marked seasonal pattern in basal and milking-stimulated release of prolactin in ruminants.[55-57] Wettemann and Tucker[54] demonstrated that the response of serum prolactin to change in ambient temperature occurs within 3 to 4 hr, which is much faster than the response to a change in photoperiod.[53] The response of serum prolactin concentrations to change in ambient temperature is similar to the glucocorticoid response with one exception. Rapid changes of temperature either up or down increases serum glucocorticoid concentrations. In contrast, prolactin concentrations are elevated if temperature increases and decline during cold stress.[54,58] Since basal and TRH or milking stimulated prolactin release are increased by elevation of ambient

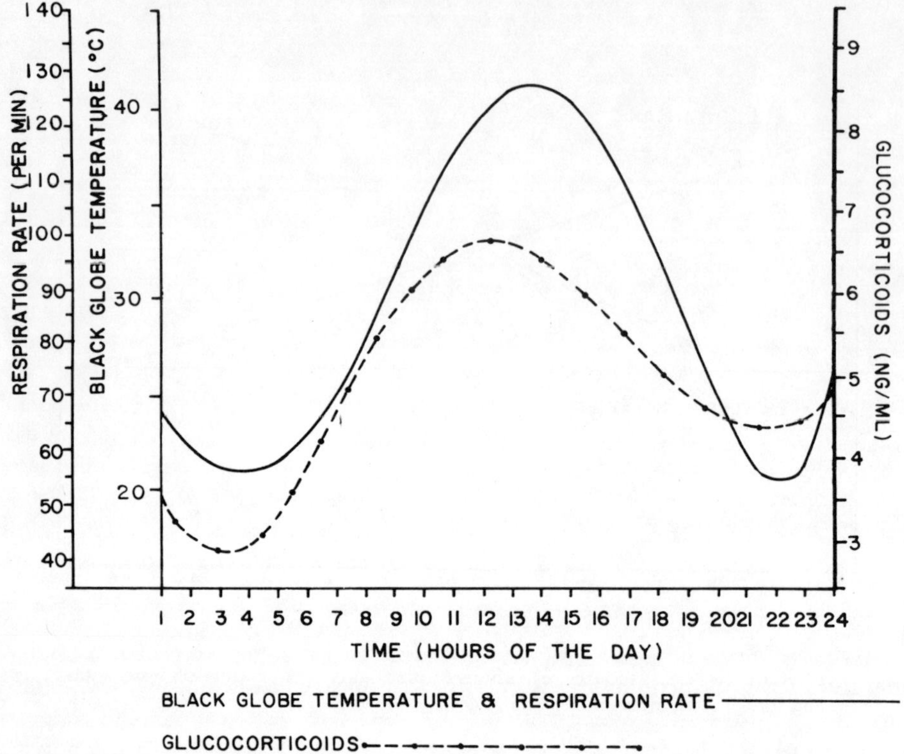

FIGURE 2. Least squares regressions of circadian patterns of black globe temperature, respiration rate, and plasma glucocorticoids concentrations in Jersey cattle during summer.

temperature and/or photoperiod, synthesis and secretion of prolactin appear to be influenced.

Thus prolactin concentrations in domestic animals are quite sensitive to changes in temperature. The effect of these changes in serum prolactin on animal physiology are presently unknown. Prolactin is essential for onset and maintenance of milk secretion.[59,60] However, the influence of prolactin on these processes in response to environmental modification is not known presently.

Behavioral Thermoregulation

Environmental conditions influence animal behavior. These alterations in behavior have physiological significance since they are directed at thermoregulation. The role of the hypothalamus in behavioral thermoregulation has been most often studied by means of localized thermal stimulation of the preoptic region of the hypothalamus using implanted electrodes. Most of these experiments involved effects of cooling animals and evaluating their behavior to obtain warm air by pressing bars or panels.[61-63]

Other studies have been directed at examining animal behavior under varying environmental conditions. Cattle exposed to heat frequently sprinkle water over their bodies,[64] seek shade,[65] and shift grazing or feeding to nighttime hours.[66] In addition the spontaneous activity of most animals decreases during periods of high ambient temperature. Pigs, which do not actively sweat, seek a wallow,[67] or wallow in their own urine to achieve evaporative cooling.[68]

A widely recognized effect of heat stress on farm animals is a decreased libido and expression of estrus which has been misinterpreted as an interruption of normal estrous cycles.

ENVIRONMENTAL EFFECTS ON LACTATION

Milk Yield

The dairy cow has been one of the main species used during the last 40 years to evaluate the effects of climatic factors on lactation. This is not surprising since milk is a high quality protein food produced in large quantities from consumption of a diet comprised largely of food sources that don't compete with components of the human diet.

Regan and Richardson[69] studied the influence of environmental temperature on high-producing dairy cattle over a temperature range of 4 to 37.8°C. Temperatures above 26.6°C decreased milk yield, casein content, and solids-not-fat (SNF) level. A great input of knowledge in this area came from the intensive research program carried out at the University of Missouri since 1948. This program was directed toward studying physiological and production responses of dairy cattle exposed to different thermal stress conditions.[70] Ragsdale and co-workers[71] first reported the effects of gradual increases in environmental temperature from 10 to 40°C on milk production, feed consumption, and body weight of Holstein and Jersey cows. Decreases in milk production and feed intake were observed in Holstein and Jersey cows at high temperatures, starting at 26.6 in Holsteins and at 29.4°C in Jerseys. Increasing environmental temperatures above these temperatures rapidly depressed feed intake and milk production so that at 40.6°C both virtually stopped. A later report indicated that the optimal air temperature for milk production of dairy cows appeared to be about 10°C; milk yield begins to decline above 21.1°C and below 4.4°C.[72] The decline with rising temperature was earlier in Holsteins than Jerseys. Yeck and Stewart[73] reviewed the Missouri studies and concluded that milk yield declines as air temperatures exceed 23.9°C.

Worstell and Brody[74] presented a summary of critical temperatures for various physiological reactions of lactating dairy cows. Rising temperatures affected European cattle markedly above the level of 15.6°C when respiration rate was suddenly accelerated. Rectal temperature began to rise in high-producing European cows at about 21.2°C followed by a depression of feed consumption, milk yield, heat production, and pulse rate. Lactating Brahman cows were more heat tolerant; however, these cows produced only 20% as much milk as Holsteins. The main difference in thermoequilibrium between Red-Sindhi-European breed crosses (F_1) and European breeds of cows was in heat production.[75] A lower heat load of the crosses was attributed to lower basal metabolic rates. The heat increment per kg of 4% fat-corrected-milk (FCM) was the same for both breed groups. However, milk production was lower for the crossbreds. Consequently, the tendency for crossbreds to maintain lower respiration rates and rectal temperatures was due to the lower heat load. A heat-tolerant animal is not necessarily the most productive food-producing animal when exposed to a thermal stress.

The influences of humidity and its interaction with temperature on thermoregulation responses and production are well recognized. Above 18.3°C higher humidities caused losses in milk production for Holstein cows.[76] Johnson et al.[77] observed that all combinations of temperature and humidity above 18.3°C adversely affected milk production and that humidity played an important role in animal comfort. In a subsequent report[78] significant temperature and humidity effects on total digestible nutrient (TDN) consumption were found at several temperature humidity combinations from 4.4 to 35°C. It was found that humidity at constant environmental temperatures above 18.3°C, particularly above 26.7°C dry bulb, became a critical factor in maintenance of heat balance and, thus in feed intake and milk production. TDN intake, water consumption and milk yield were related to the temperature-humidity-index (THI = 0.55 [DBT] + 0.2 [DP] + 17.5). In this equation, DBT represents dry bulb and DP represents dewpoint temperatures in °F. A THI value of 77 appeared to be the upper limit at which higher values resulted in decreases in TDN intake, water consumption, and milk yield of cows. At 50% RH, it was found that a constant environmental temperature of 31.1°C was necessary to cause a 1.1°C rise in rectal temperature. For each 0.6°C rise in rectal temperature there was a loss of 1.4 kg in TDN intake and a loss of 1.8 kg in milk yield.

A practical question is whether the decrease in milk yield associated with high environmental temperature is due solely to decreased feed intake. Johnson et al.[79] found that a decline in feed intake was a major factor associated with the decline in milk production due to heat. The effect of controlling feed intake (forced-fed through a rumen fistula) at 31°C environmental temperature was significant in maintaining lactation although full production was not supported. Recently in New Zealand, Bandaranayaka and Holmes[80] observed that Jersey cows exposed to a 30°C-air temperature, with controlled feed intake through a rumen fistula, had higher rectal temperatures and respiration rates, and lower milk yields than cows exposed to 15°C air temperature. McDowell[81] reported that high environmental temperatures decreased efficiency of utilization of digestible energy (DE) for milk yield. At 21°C, the efficiency was 60%; but after 7 days at 32°C, efficiency was only 40%, and was 31% by day 14. Average daily consumption of DE declined about 16% at 32°C, but the daily output of milk energy declined over 22%. Therefore, cows consumed more energy than needed for maintenance and milk production under heat stress but produced a poorer return. The cows undoubtedly increased their expenditure of energy to maintain homeostasis, such as energy spent towards an increased respiration rate or other processes of heat dissipation.

Brody et al.[82] reported detrimental effects of radiation combined with high temperature on milk production. Reduction in milk production after radiation exposure (250 BTU/ft^2/hr) varied in Holsteins from 7 to 25% and from 4 to 35% in Jersey cows. Wind at high temperatures was found to be beneficial to milk production in Holstein, Brown Swiss, and Jersey cows.[83] At 26.7°C and 0.8 km/hr wind, production of Holstein cows was approximately 85% of normal. However, at 35°C and the same wind speed, milk production dropped 37, 26, and 17% from normal in Holstein, Jersey, and Brown Swiss cows, respectively. Increasing wind speed up to 16 km/hr at 35°C further improved milk production in the three breeds.

Evidence for the direct effects of climate on milk production comes from the quantitative studies conducted in climatic chambers. Most of these studies were done at constant temperatures and quantitative interrelationships were characterized. Level of temperature at which significant depressions in milk yield will occur is dependent on various factors such as: level of milk production, size of the cow, breed, previous acclimation, and type of nutrition. Controlled laboratory studies cannot be relied upon in total because it is difficult to duplicate daily climatic and management conditions such as changing air temperatures, variable wind speeds, solar radiation, variability in feed supplies, management practices, and various other factors. Furthermore, in practice the cow is not exposed to constant temperatures but to circadian temperature patterns.

Thermal stress effects on milk production have been quantified under more natural conditions. In most of these studies the interactions of nutritional management and thermal stress on milk production have been investigated. In Louisisana,[84] diurnal variations in air temperature and solar radiation had a marked effect on behavioral grazing patterns of lactating cows. During the summer in Texas,[85] dairy cattle production and physiological performance can be improved by feeding lactating cows high-energy rations. Johnson et al.[86] in Georgia reported that environmental elements could explain

40% of the variation observed in feed intake during the summer months. In Arizona, during the summer season, a low roughage ration was superior and resulted in 0.8 kg more 4% fat-corrected milk per cow per day.[87] Evaluation of production performance of dairy cows fed high levels of fat under controlled environmental temperatures of 15.2 and 32.2°C were studied by Moody et al.[88] They observed that elevated temperatures resulted in a marked depression in milk yield, milk fat, and feed intake, and an increase in water intake and rectal temperature. Environmental effects were independent of ration effects in which level of fat was varied.

Maust and McDowell[89] studied summer effects on milk yield and feed intake of Holsteins cows. Cows which calved during July-August produced an average of 11% less milk than those calving in January-February. Changes in milk yield and feed intake depended largely on stage of lactation. Midlactation cows (100 to 180 days) were most adversely affected; late (180 to 260 days), intermediate, and early (less than 100 days), least. However, early lactation cows catabolized more of their body reserves. Across stage of lactation, percentages of variation attributable to weather conditions for milk yield, milk fat, feed intake, and rectal temperature were 9, 13, 5 and 65%, respectively.

Lactation milk yield for Holstein cows in five Louisiana herds calving in the hot season of the year was consistently 200 to 300 kg (5 to 8%) less than in cows calving during cool and mild seasons. Yields during the first 90 days of lactation were 10 to 14% less.[90] Hassan and Roussel[91] reported that with a high protein diet lactating dairy cows improved both feed intake and milk production under a high ambient temperature. Cows fed a 14.3% crude protein ration produced 7% less milk and consumed 11% less dry matter than cows fed a 20.8% crude protein ration.

Studies of thermal stress effects on milk production also have been conducted in other areas of the world. Payne and Hancock[92] did a direct comparison of two climatic environments. They selected eight pairs of identical twins, Jersey and Shorthorn heifers, and kept one set in the temperature environment on the island of New Zealand while the other set was reared in the tropics of Fiji from 7 months of age. Both groups consumed the same ration. Results showed that average milk (44%) and milk fat (56%) productions were lower in the twins at Fiji where temperatures were about 11°C higher at any given time of the year.

Climatic effects exert both direct and indirect effects on milk yield. For example, environmental temperature and rainfall largely control both the quantity and quality of feed that will be available. Furthermore, these factors also influence disease and parasite conditions in hot-humid climates. Providing a diet with sufficient available energy throughout the year is a major management factor to partially reduce indirect climatic effects. Cows managed under more severe environments require additional husbandry practices (reduced pasture, increased dry lot feeding, frequent feeding) to maximize their production and to partially overcome indirect climatic effects. Such factors as shade, a good water supply, and high quality feed contribute to reducing direct climatic effects.

Under natural subtropical conditions at Gainesville, Florida various climatic measurements have been quantitatively related to milk yield and composition.[93] These relationships were developed over a 16-year period from 7998 milk yields from 866 Holstein cows. Curvilinear relationships of milk yield with maximum dry bulb temperature and relative humidity are presented in Figure 3. Relative humidity and maximum and minimum temperatures accounted for 1 to 6% of variability in milk yield. Maximum daily temperature effects on milk yield were slight, between 7 and 27°C, but milk yield declined appreciably above 27°C. This is surprisingly close to the 23.9°C air temperature above which milk yield decreases based on climatic chamber studies at Missouri.[73] The quantitative relationship presented in Figure 3 was established under natural con-

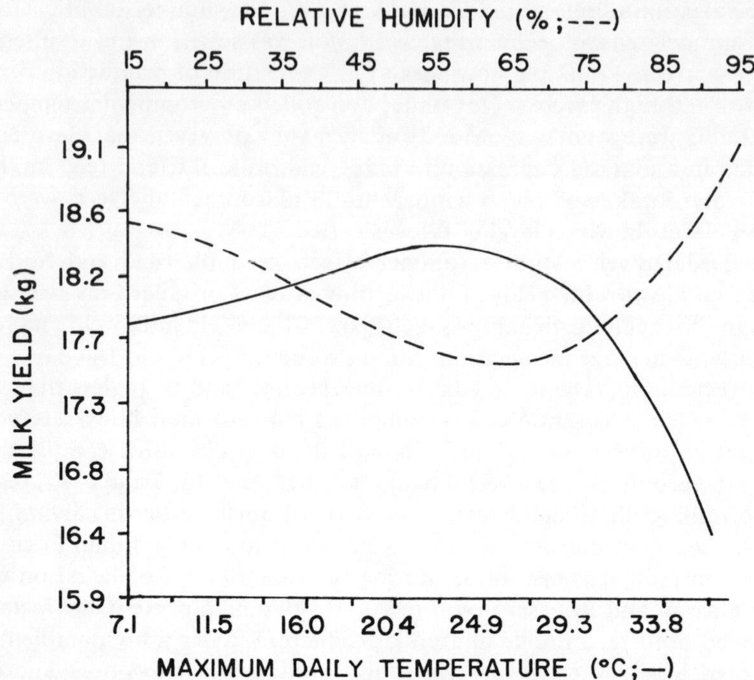

FIGURE 3. Least squares regressions of relative humidity and maximum daily temperature effects on milk yield in dairy cows.

ditions in which cows were exposed to cyclic climatic rhythms (yearly, monthly, and circadian).

Milk Composition

Climatological factors as well as stage of lactation, and feeding and management practices influence the composition of milk. Pronounced seasonal variations occur in the composition of milk with percentages of fat, SNF, and total solids being highest during the winter months and lowest in summer months.[94-96] Protein and mineral contents of milk are lower in summer than in winter. The major portion of SNF variation due to season was found in protein.[97] Seasonal effects on milk composition are partially due to feeding and management changes. However, studies in large California herds in which feeding changes during a 14-month period were minimized indicated that changes in fat and protein concentrations were parallel.[98] Concentrations were higher for winter milk (November to February) than summer (May to August). Monthly variation in lactose was less.

Majority of studies on effects of climate on milk composition and yield have been done in relation to temperature. Variations in environmental temperatures from −1 to 23.9°C have little influence on milk composition. However, between 29.5 and 40.6°C SNF, protein and lactose contents decreased and fat content increased.[99] Specific gravity of milk was lowered by high temperatures. Changes which occurred when temperatures were elevated were due in part to a lower feed intake (loss of appetite) and the stressing effects associated with high body temperature. Quantitative temperature trends also have been determined under natural climatic conditions in the subtropical area of Gainesville, Florida.[93] Daily maximum temperature influenced fat and protein content of milk in that content decreased throughout the range of 7.8 to 34.5°C. These temperature trends were estimated after adjustment for stages of lactation and pregnancy. Consequently, when animals are acclimatized and exposed to daily circadian temperature changes, fat percentage decreased with elevated maximum temperatures.

Month of parturition has a pronounced effect on subsequent milk yield and composition. Cows that begin their lactation in winter and spring produce more milk than those beginning during the summer.[100] This suggests that the detrimental effect of thermal stress occurs in early lactation. However, summer weather effects on established milk yield were more adverse for cows in midlactation than those in early lactation.[89] Collectively these results infer that perhaps part of the temperature effects associated with month of calving may be due to thermal stress effects on development of the mammary gland during the dry period before birth of the calf. Hormones produced by the conceptus which stimulate the mammary gland may be sensitive to environmental temperature. Perhaps production rate of conceptus hormones is altered under stressful environmental conditions. Uterine and umbilical blood flow decreased in pregnant sheep in response to induced maternal hyperthermia.[21] Consequently, the hypothesis that thermal stress may affect hormonal production rates from the conceptus which may influence subsequent function of the maternal mammary gland warrants additional investigation. Lactational performance of rats was depressed if they were exposed to heat during the last two thirds of pregnancy.[101] Tentative evidence that thermal stress may partially influence milk yield via the conceptus is presented in Figure 4 in which month of parturition influenced both calf birth weight and the dam's subsequent milk yield. Thus factors associated with calf birth weight such as placental function (production of estrogens, placental lactogen; nutrient exchange) also may be associated with subsequent milk yield. These trends were comprised of 975 parturitions in Holstein cows for a 23-year period at the Florida Agricultural Experiment Station, Gainesville, Florida.[195]

Genotype by Environmental Interactions

Climatic chamber studies indicate that there are breed differences in the temperature which reduces milk yield in cattle. Of extreme importance also are the relative magnitude of genotype by environment interactions (GEI), especially if they represent changes of rank of genotypes in different environments. Breed by environment, and sire within breed by environment, are two GEI of particular importance. The first would determine which breed should be selected for any given climate, area, system of nutritional and/or management conditions. Knowledge of the second is necessary to determine if, within a breed, those sires proven genetically superior in good environments also would be superior in less desirable environments. Again, whether or not interactions represent changes in rank of breeds or sires is of major practical importance.

Under the relatively high levels of management provided the U.S. dairy cow, there seem to be few if any changes in rank of breeds regardless of climatic and other environmental conditions. Though breed by temperature interactions were demonstrated clearly by Rodriguez et al.[93] in that Holsteins declined more in milk yield and less in fat and protein percentages than did Jerseys with increasing maximum daily temperatures, the breeds did not change ranks. In a humid tropical area of Venezuela, Verde et al.[102] demonstrated major differences (974 kg) in lactation milk production of breed groups consisting of various percentages of Holstein breeding (50 to 100%), and between yields of cows freshening at different seasons of the year (290 kg range for three seasons). Yet no breed by season interaction could be detected.

Sire by environment interactions have been studied extensively, and in general been shown to be of little importance in milk yield of the dairy cow. North Central and Southeastern U.S. represent wide environmental differences (climate, management,

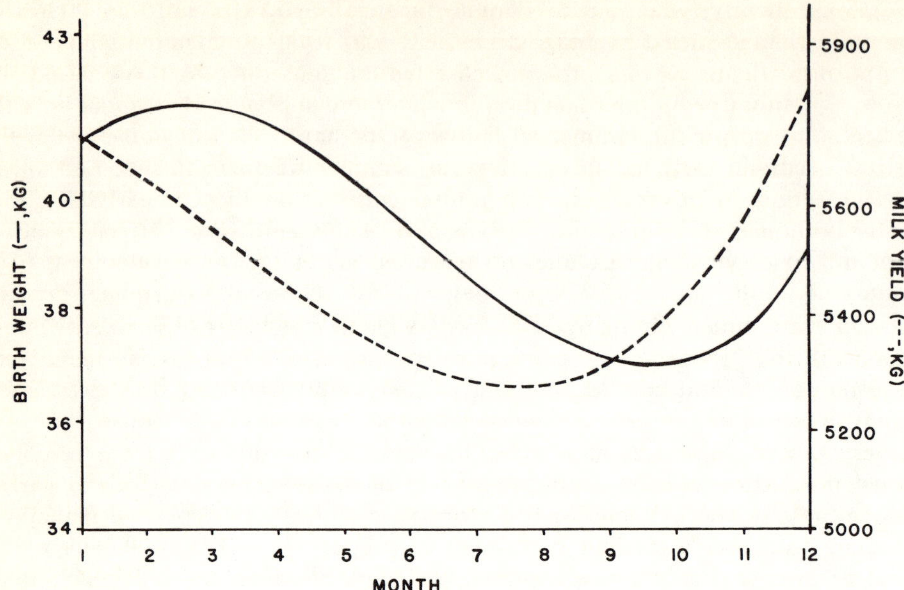

FIGURE 4. Least squares regressions of calf birth weight and dam's milk yield for the lactation following parturition by month of year (975 Holstein parturitions).

and nutrition), but Lytton and Legates[103] were unable to detect noteworthy sire by region interactions for region. Likewise, McDowell et al.[104] suggested that effects of sire by temperate or tropical environment should be small, after examining performance of daughters of Holstein sires of U.S., Canada, Mexico, and Puerto Rico.

Environmental Modification

The cow's sensitivity to heat, as evidenced by the decrease in production, indicates that environmental modification should be a means of increasing food production. However, consideration of environmental modification should be complemented with better feeding and management systems. Such alterations with cattle of good genetic potential will allow considerable future increases in both production and efficiency of production in arid, subtropical, and tropical areas of the world. This is supported by the high levels of milk production obtained by certain dairy herds and systems in Arizona, California, Israel, and Florida.

Various practical and economical systems to modify the micro-climate of the cow are needed to improve production responses. Arizona workers have been very successful in reducing air temperature 10 to 12°C with the use of evaporative cooling under practical farm conditions in large herds.[105] Both milk production and fertility are improved in cows exposed to cooled shades.

Environmental conditions in tropical and subtropical areas are not ideally suited for evaporative cooling systems due to the high relative humidity. Evaporative cooling requires the addition of moisture to the air, and its effectiveness is limited by the ability of air to absorb additional water. Consequently, evaporative cooling systems cool more effectively in dry arid climates than in areas with higher relative humidities. Several alternative systems combined with proper management are useful in these environments. In a Florida project, daily total air conditioning or partial air conditioning during different portions of the day allowed for gradient increases, up to 9.4% in production of 4% FCM.[106] Cows cooled either during daylight hours or cooled throughout a 24-hr period produced more milk. The increases in milk production agreed with those reported by Johnston et al.[107] and with those predicted by Hahn[108] for the Florida area based on climatological records. Establishment of a good relationship between laboratory production data and commercial herd production enables projection of expected production losses for cows in any area with climatological records. Estimates of these predicted losses allow producers to evaluate from an economic standpoint the merit of environmental control or other modification alternatives. In the air conditioned study in south Florida, the producer felt that the benefits of increased milk production were indeed not sufficient to pay for the expense of operating the unit.

Perhaps the simplest environmental modification is use of shade structures. The principal function of shade is to reduce the heat load of animals by reducing incident solar radiation. If this reduction is sufficient to maintain a body temperature more conducive for production of food, then increases in production should be detected. However, type of shade and associated management of animals will be critical in obtaining a production benefit. Exposure of cows managed as a group to an insulated shade structure in which cows also had access to feed, water, and an adjacent sod area for loafing resulted in a distinct alteration of the animals microenvironment, lowered respiration rate, and rectal temperatures, and improved milk yield and reproductive performance. Cows exposed to the shade management system produced 10.7% more milk.[109]

As cited by Roman-Ponce et al.[109] environmental modifications such as air conditioning, evaporative cooling, zone cooling, and various shade structures have been used with different degrees of success to reduce the detrimental effects of heat stress. However, use of various systems to alter the environment should be coupled with management that provides an adequate feed supply (quantity and quality) and readily available drinking water. Use of a particular system to alter the environment depends on the severity of that environment, characteristics of the climate, and economical considerations.

EFFECT OF HEAT ON ANIMAL REPRODUCTION

Environmental Factors Associated with Fertility

Dairy producers are very aware that heat stress decreases milk production, but they do not immediately recognize the financial losses associated with seasonal infertility. The consequences of a thermal stress induced infertility are not evident until a distant future date when the cow has extended periods of no milk production while waiting for birth of a calf that should have arrived much earlier. However, the cow had experienced a seasonal period of infertility that delayed conception and therefore parturition.

In dairy cows low fertility during summer has been observed in arid, tropical, and subtropical areas. Although heat stress can affect both bulls and cows, the reduced fertility due to the bull can be eliminated through artificial insemination in which semen can be collected and frozen during cooler times of the year. This was shown by Stott[110] with liquid semen collected during the year from different localities (Phoenix, Arizona; Palo Alto, California; Columbus, Ohio) and used to inseminate cows in and out of Arizona. A significant seasonal depression in breeding efficiency paralleled high climatic temperatures and was comparable for all sources of semen used in Arizona. These results indicated that the female was the major contributor to summer depression of fertility.

A low rate of fertilization and a high rate of embryonic mortality are the major factors causing low seasonal breeding efficiency in lactating dairy cows associated with high ambient temperature and humidity.[111] It was suggested that changes in environmental temperature and humidity which affect fertility correspond closely to time of breeding, indicating that this is probably the critical period that fertility is affected. Low breeding efficiency in dairy and beef cattle during seasonal periods of high environmental temperature are well documented.[112-115]

High temperatures delayed puberty in Shorthorn and Brahman heifers when they were raised at 27°C as compared to those raised at 10°C or in an open shed, but Santa Gertrudis heifers were not affected, a breed by season interaction.[116] Length of the estrous cycle in heifers was slightly longer under hot climatic conditions,[117,118] but duration and intensity of estrus were decreased.[117-119]

Five experiments were undertaken to determine the long-term effects of thermal stress (32°C) on reproductive performance in heifers of several beef breeds.[120] When winter conditioned heifers were exposed to high temperature they became anestrous, with inactive ovaries, but later became acclimatized and reestablished their estrous cycles by the 16th week. In one trial heifers were bred after becoming acclimatized and five of six conceived and produced normal calves. Only one of six summer-conditioned heifers became anestrous when subjected to 32°C, but when exposed to 38°C, five of the six became anestrous. These experiments indicated that severe heat stress will cause "true" anestrous, but that the amount of heat stress required would seldom be encountered under natural conditions. In addition, beef heifers can become acclimatized to heat stress.

Longer estrous cycles[111] and higher frequency of anestrous[117,119] also have been associated with thermal stress in mature cows. High temperatures increase incidence of "quiet ovulations",[121] but perhaps the most consistent gross observation during thermal stress exposure is a reduction in length of estrus from a normal 18 hours to about 10 or less hours.[114,117,119,122] The lower intensity of estrous behavior and shorter estrous period which occur under hot climatic conditions makes estrous detection of paramount importance and may explain the longer estrous cycles and higher frequency of anestrous observed in heat stressed cows.

Of practical significance is whether specific climatic parameters can be quantitatively related to fertility on an insemination to insemination basis. Such associations would identify climatic factors that could be modified to improve reproductive performance within certain regional areas, and permit managers to make sound economic decisions. Both maximum environmental temperature the day after insemination ($\hat{Y} = 0.2434 + 0.0149X - 0.0003658X^2$; $\hat{Y}$ = conception rate %; X = maximum ambient temperature the day after insemination in centigrade) and solar radiation the day of insemination ($\hat{Y} = 0.3399 + 0.00035X - 0.0000005X^2$, $\hat{Y}$ = conception rate %; X = solar radiation measured as Langleys [1 g cal/cm^2]) had negative curvilinear relationships with conception rate in the subtropical environment of Gainesville, Florida.[115] For example, as maximum temperature increased from 21.1 to 35°C, conception rates declined from 40 to 31%. Estimates of these climatic effects were based on 3500 to 5000 inseminations over a 10-year period and were adjusted for various management and cow effects known to influence fertility such as inseminator, breed of cow, month of service, service number, and age of cow. When climatic effects were considered, such as maximum temperature or solar radiation, month to month differences in conception rates no longer occurred. Consequently, normal month effects were most likely related to climatological factors in this study rather than to nutrition or other management factors.

These studies emphasize the importance of ambient environmental conditions at the time of insemination on fertility. Lower conception rates were observed in cows with high body temperatures.[112,123,124] Besides a negative correlation between conception rate and rectal temperature (−0.51), a higher conception rate was observed in heifers exposed to 21.1°C (48%) than in heifers exposed to 32.2°C (0%) for 72 hr postbreeding.[125] Uterine temperatures recorded the day of insemination (UT_0) and the day after insemination (UT_1) were negatively related to conception rates.[124] An increase of 0.5°C above the mean UT_0 (38.6°C) and UT_1 (38.3°C) decreased conception rates 12.8 and 6.9% respectively.

Evidence is abundant that heat can influence reproductive performance in farm animals. An offspring at term represents the successful function of a series of sequential physiological events. The stress of heat could act by influencing sexual behavior, quality and quantity of sperm production, ova after fertilization, and/or elicit specific responses by the dam that perhaps could affect the embryo's environment and well being, fetal growth, and even postnatal development.

Influence of Heat on Reproductive Processes of the Female

High temperature does not have a very marked effect on ovarian function,[126-129] but rather on the uterus during the preparatory stages of pregnancy as well as during the initial development of the embryo. Yeates[129] studied the effects of high environmental temperatures (40.6°C) on reproduction of ewes. Ewes showed no adverse effects of temperature on occurrence of estrus but there was a significant reduction in the number of young produced.

Dutt et al.[130] reported that ewes subjected to high ambient temperature (32.2°C) at about the time of mating had lower fertilization and increased early embryonic death rates. Ewes exposed to high temperatures beginning on the 12th day of the cycle prior to breeding showed approximately one half the fertilization rate of control ewes. Embryo loss was estimated to be 92%. When ewes were not exposed to the treatment room until 8 days postbreeding, embryo losses were not significantly different from control ewes.

In pigs, prolonged increases in environmental temperatures during the first 15 days of gestation have a detrimental effect on embryo survival.[131] Warnick et al.[128] compared ovulation rate, conception rate and embryonic survival up to 25 days of pregnancy in five groups of gilts maintained under different environmental conditions of 15.6°C, 32.2°C or atmospheric conditions with shade. No significant differences were detected in ovulation rate, conception rate or number of live embryos at 25 days postbreeding. However, gilts maintained continuously at 32.2°C averaged 10.9 embryos, compared to 13.5 embryos for gilts at 15.6°C. High temperatures up to 3 days postbreeding had no effect on number of embryos; however, gilts maintained at 32.2°C from 3 days postbreeding had 11.3 embryos compared to 13.6 for gilts at 15.6°C. Tompkins et al.[132] found that exposure of sows to 35°C for 24 hr on day 1 of gestation significantly reduced embryo survival at 27 to 51 days of gestation. The difference in results between these two studies in swine could have been due to a higher temperature stress in the later study. Omtvedt et al.[133] found that the greatest reduction in number of viable embryos was among gilts heat stressed 8 to 16 days postbreeding. However, 42% of the gilts exposed to heat between 0 to 8 days postbreeding failed to conceive, whereas 100% of the controls were pregnant. Recently, Wildt et al.[134] confirmed that pigs stressed during the period of 2 to 13 days of pregnancy had a high embryonic mortality rate.

Alliston and Ulberg,[135] using embryo transfers, studied the time during which the detrimental effects of high temperature were exerted upon the sheep embryo. Transfers were performed approximately 72 hr after onset of estrus and successful transfers were verified by a laparotomy performed 25 to 30 days later. When both donor and recipient were maintained at 21.2°C, 56.6% of the transfers were successful compared to 9.5% when donors were maintained at 32.2°C and recipients at 21.2°C. They concluded that some detrimental action had occurred by 3 days after onset of estrus in ewes at 32.2°C. It also was observed that embryonic death occurred at a later stage of development in utero. When donors were maintained at 21.1°C and recipients at 32.2°C, 24% of the transfers were successful.

Dutt[136] exposed ewes to 32°C at the time of breeding and at 1, 3, and 5 days after breeding. Results showed no significant differences in fertility rate in the different groups. Exposure to heat resulted in an increase in morphologically abnormal ova; embryo loss, estimated as the percentage of fertilized ova that failed to survive, was significantly higher in all the treated groups. Embryo loss for the combined 0- and 1-day groups was significantly higher than in the 3- and 5-day ewes. They concluded that the sheep zygote is most sensitive to the harmful effects of high ambient temperatures during the initial stages of cleavage while in the oviduct. Eighty-five percent of the control ewes lambed, compared to 10% for the ewes in the 0- and 1-day groups, 35% for the 3-day group and 40% in the 5-day group. Dutt[137] recently reported that the period of sensitivity may extend to the period of 10 to 22 days of pregnancy. Exposure to higher elevated environmental temperatures (35°C) for 1 week reduced number of ewes lambing. Furthermore, ewes exposed to this thermal stress at 16 days had lambs with significantly shorter tail lengths. Perhaps, the thermal stress altered development of the embryo.

High air temperature does not adversely affect the ovum prior to fertilization.[138] When sheep ova were recovered from donors at 21°C or 32°C shortly after ovulation and transferred to mated recipients, there were just as many embryos 30 days postmating in recipients which received ova from animals maintained at 32°C as those which received ova from animals maintained at 21°C. Alliston et al.[139] demonstrated that fertilized ova grown in vitro through the first cell division at 40°C had a lower rate of embryo survival than those grown at 38°C. As the period of culture at 40°C was delayed to either the second, third, or fourth cell division, differences in postimplantation death losses disappeared.

Since an increase in temperature surrounding the embryo at the time of first cell divisions reduces survival, body temperatures of females following insemination should be associated with conception rates. As previously described, rectal and uterine temperatures near the time of insemination indeed are related to conception rates in cattle. Collectively, these studies in the female indicate that heat stress of the ovum immediately after fertilization causes the resulting conceptus to perish some time later in its development. In contrast to these effects of heat on early embryogenesis, experimental results tend to indicate that once the embryo undergoes the initial stages of placentation it will survive a moderate heat stress in midpregnancy.

Several reports indicate that thermal stresses applied during late gestation decrease fetal growth in sheep.[140-142] When sheep are heated from midgestation until delivery, birth weight of lambs was approximately 50% that of control lambs.[140] Placenta weights also were reduced. Brown et al.[14] reported that heat stress during the last month of pregnancy was sufficient to induce stunting or dwarfing of the lamb. Studies indicate that birth weights of lambs are influenced by breed-temperature interactions.[140,143] Sensitivity to fetal stunting varied among breeds when exposed to various periods of elevated environmental temperatures during the day. Elevated environmental temperatures decrease feed intake. However, ewes housed at prevailing spring temperatures with feed intake restricted to that of heat stressed ewes produced lambs similar in weight to lambs of range ewes.[141] In another study, ewes that were unheated and fed to maintain the same body weight as heated ewes produced lambs with a greater birth weight.[142] Thus the adverse effect of heat on fetal growth is due to factors other than just nutrient intake of the mother.

Pigs exposed to high ambient temperatures during late gestation (102 to 110 days postbreeding) produced fewer live pigs and more stillborn pigs than controls.[133] Chicken embryos also are stunted when exposed to elevated incubation temperatures.[144] Critical periods exist both at the beginning and end of gestation when reproductive competence of the female is affected by heat stress.

Influence of Heat on Reproductive Processes of the Male

It is well recognized that heat has a detrimental effect upon the reproductive function of male farm animals. Puberty, as measured by time of sperm production, is delayed in bull calves placed in hot environmental chambers,[145] or in boars exposed to a tropical environment.[146] In rams sexual libido is decreased with elevations in ambient temperatures. Breed differences exist, and Merino rams often are able to maintain sexual activity at high temperatures.[147]

One obvious response variable to high environmental temperatures is semen quality, and it is adversely affected in the bull.[148,149] The first observed abnormalities are decreases in sperm mobility and an increase in percentage of morphologically abnormal spermatozoa. These effects can be experimentally induced by locally heating the testis or placing the animal in a hot chamber. Detrimental effects appeared in the second week post-treatment in the bull,[149] ram,[150,151] and boar.[152-154] Of practical importance is that the decrease in semen quality induced with short-term high temperature also is correlated with decreased fertility in females inseminated with this semen.[150,151,155] A gradual return to normal semen quality and fertility rate takes approximately 60 days after a heat stress but is dependent upon the duration and intensity of the stress.

Freezability of Zebu bull sperm was impaired when animals were exposed to environmental temperatures greater than 30°C at 36 to 54 days before semen collection.[156] As little as 6 hr of total body heating at 41°C may be sufficient to induce seminal degeneration in rams.[155] Acclimatization to a high thermal environment may occur, since Egbunike and Steinbach[146] were unable to detect any limiting effects of tropical climate on spermatogenesis in boars.

Stages of spermatogenesis susceptible to heat have been studied by evaluating the germinal epithelium at short intervals after local heating.[157] Waites[158] summarizes that spermatogonia are relatively resistant with the exception of B-type spermatogonia of rams and bulls. Primary spermatocytes of all species examined pass through a thermally sensitive stage. Dividing spermatocytes and spermatids become involved if testicular temperature remains high for longer periods. These cytological effects were reviewed extensively by vanDenmark and Free.[159] Evaluation of testicular outflow of sperm and fluid from the rete testis after short periods of scrotal heating confirmed that a precise stage in the meiotic prophase of spermatocytes must be particularly sensitive to heat.[158]

In addition to heat effects on sperm production and quality in the male, there are direct heat effects on sperm after its delivery into the female that influence fertility. Howarth et al.[160] capacitated sperm for 6 hr in uteri of rabbits kept at two different air temperatures (32°C and 21°C). The sperm were recovered and used to inseminate females maintained at 21°C. The rate of fertilization was the same. However, the ability of the resulting embryo to survive and form an implantation site was significantly reduced in rabbits fertilized by heat stressed sperm. Most implantation sites contained normal embryos indicating that death had occurred prior to implantation.

Burfening and Ulberg[161] studied the direct effect of high temperature on rabbit sperm in vitro. Each ejaculate was split and cultured for 3 hr at either 38°C or 40°C and placed in opposite uterine horns of females previously mated to vasectomized males. No significant effects of temperature on either semen quality or fertilizing capacity could be found. However, the rate of continued embryonic development to the point of implantation was greatly reduced for those ova fertilized by sperm cultured at the higher temperature. These data suggested that spermatozoa could be influenced before fertilization by a 2°C increase in temperature which caused a decrease in subsequent preimplantation embryo survival. First et al.[162] postulated that embryo loss, as a result of elevated ambient temperatures on sperm via the uterine environment, may be related to aging of sperm. Perhaps the elevated ambient temperature speeds up the sperm aging process.

Heat-Sensitive Mechanisms Contributing to Decreased Reproductive Performance

Mechanisms by which heat stress depresses fertility have received intense investigation in the male and female using various species for models. Responses of the animal to thermal stress that compromise fertility are multifold, interrelated, and undoubtedly involve direct effects of temperature, altered nervous system regulation, water balance, hormonal alternations, nutritional influences, and biochemical alterations. The so called "infertility heat stress syndrome" probably is a result of a combination of responses associated with the animal's attempt to thermoregulate in the face of either acute, chronic, circadian, monthly, or seasonal heat stresses. Reproductive processes are sensitive at all stages including gamete production, sexual behavior, early and late pregnancy.

As previously cited, in vitro experiments indicate that high temperatures modify the ability of sperm or fertilized ova to produce viable embryos. This emphasizes the importance of factors regulating the microenvironment of the zyzote or the subsequent conceptus during pregnancy. This is evident by the observation that a rise of 0.5°C above the mean uterine temperature on the day of and the day after insemination was associated with decreases in conception rates of 12.8 and 6.9%, respectively, in cattle.[124] The uterine temperature always is higher than the arterial blood supplying the uterus,[163] and the dissipation of uterine metabolic heat depends on uterine blood flow. Consequently, an increase in uterine temperature during thermal stress may be due to an obvious increase in blood temperature, an increase in uterine metabolic heat associated with a rise in body temperature, or perhaps a decline in uterine blood flow associated with the animal's thermoregulatory response.

Two steroid hormones known to regulate uterine blood flow are estrogens and progesterone. Injection of estrogens in cows,[164] sheep,[165] and sows[166] increases uterine blood flow, whereas progesterone injection with estrogen decreases the uterine blood flow response compared to estrogen alone.[167] The effects of heat stress on uterine blood flow of nonpregnant-ovariectomized sheep and cows were evaluated after injection of estradiol.[164,165] In cows exposed to the sun with no shade during the summer, the increase in uterine blood flow after injection of estradiol was less than with the same animals exposed to an effective shade structure. A release of catecholemines into the peripheral plasma was detected when cattle were exposed to acute heat stress in a chamber.[34] In ovariectomized ewes, a heat stress reduced the estradiol-induced increase in uterine blood flow by 37%, and a combination of heat stress plus epinephrine infusion reduced the flow by 55%.[165] Consequently, uterine blood flow is sensitive to heat stress and undoubtedly contributes to the elevation in uterine temperature. Decreases in uterine blood flow also may affect availability of water, nutrients, and hormones to the uterus. Such thermal stress responses may contribute to the higher rate of embryo death in early pregnancy.

Alterations in hormonal levels during the estrous cycle and early pregnancy in response to heat stress may alter uterine blood flow and the environment of the uterus. Hormonal changes in response to thermal stress have not been consistent among various studies. This may be due to differences between chamber studies and natural field experiments, intensity of thermal stress and its duration (continuous, acute, circadian), experimental design, hormonal procedures, sensitivity of statistical analysis and perhaps acclimatization of experimental animals. Thermal induced changes or lack of a change in hormonal concentrations, such as LH, progesterone, estradiol, corticoids, and norepinepherine, are not sufficient to cause cattle to cease cycling under mild heat stress conditions (32°C).

Measurement of plasma progesterone concentrations under natural climatic conditions of circadian temperature changes indicate that cows in a hyperthermic condition have elevated progesterone concentrations throughout the estrous cycle.[28,196] In an experiment conducted in the subtropical environment of Gainesville, Florida, daily plasma concentrations of progesterone, LH and corticoids were higher throughout the estrous cycle of cows not exposed to a shade structure during the summer months.[28] Daily hormonal measurements were made between 1300 and 1500 hr during the period of maximum temperature (Figure 1). Time of sampling needs to be well controlled since hormonal circadian rhythms exist in association with temperature change (Figure 1).[12] The proestrus rise in estradiol was less for cows exposed to no shade. Such a heat stress effect on estradiol concentrations also was demonstrated previously under control chamber conditions.[169] It is suggested that such alterations in endogenous hormonal concentrations (increase in progesterone, and decrease in ratio of estradiol/progesterone) supplying the uterus may contribute to a decrease in uterine blood flow of heat stressed animals, Figure 5. Endogenous adrenocortical hypersecretion has been identified as having negative influences on estrogen actions such as expansion of the uterine microcirculation.[170] Thus the higher concentrations of corticoids of heat stressed cows exposed to no shade also may contribute to a hypothesized reduction in uterine blood flow.

Fetal stunting after heat stress in late pregnancy of sheep is associated with a marked reduction in size of fetal cotyledons and maternal caruncles.[140] The decrease in placentome size should result in decreased nutrient availability to the fetus. Furthermore, production of placental hormones in heat stressed ewes also may be reduced due to the decrease in placentome mass. Contributing to this dilemma of the fetus is the observation that induced hyperthermia in late pregnant ewes caused a 53% reduction in uterine blood flow in association with respiratory alkalosis. Umbilical flow was decreased 30%.[21] Collectively, these observations in late pregnancy indicate that thermal stress reduces nutrient availability to the developing fetus, and/or perhaps reduces conceptus production of hormones (i.e., estrogens, ovine chorionic somatomammotropic hormone) involved either in fetal growth or regulation of the maternal unit for mobilization of nutrients to the conceptus.

The adverse effects of heat on sperm production are related to local thermoregulatory control of the testis.[158] Spermatogenesis in mammals is decreased when the testis is at deep body temperature. However, testicular temperature is maintained approximately 5°C lower in two distinct ways. The cremaster and dartos muscles allow the testis to descend when temperatures are high and hold testes closer to the body when environmental temperatures are low. A countercurrent heat exchange also takes place between the highly convoluted spermatic artery within the pampiniform plexus of veins draining the testis. Temperature of the blood decreases as it passes through the convoluted artery that is in close contact with the cooler venous blood of the pampiniform plexus. The mechanism of countercurrent exchange aids the scrotum in dissipating heat. Heat also may be dissipated through the scrotal wall and body tissues adjacent

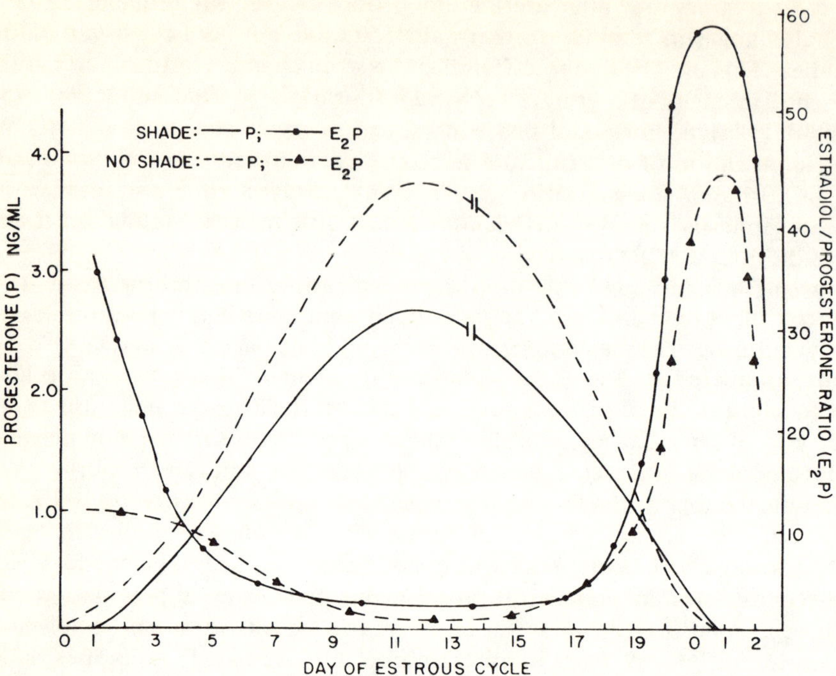

FIGURE 5. Least squares regressions of plasma progestin and estradiol concentrations during the estrous cycle in shade and unshaded cattle during summer.

to the testes. As expected, if blood flow decreases then testicular function is compromised. In the ram, localized heating of the scrotum at 37 or 40°C[171] or on the first day of total body exposure at 32°C,[172] an initial increase in testicular blood flow is followed by a significant reduction lasting several days after treatment. After 1 week of entire body exposure at 32°C, the wall of the spermatic artery within the pampiniform plexus had thickened and arterial lumenal diameter had decreased. Since $PGF_{2}\alpha$ content of the testis had increased, it may be that high levels of $PGF_{2}\alpha$ may constrict the spermatic artery within the region of the pampiniform plexus region and reduce blood flow to the testis.

Gomes et al.[173] concluded that elevated ambient temperature is detrimental to Leydig cell function in the ram. This was based on an evaluation of various endocrine responses in which testosterose decreases were detected in testicular tissue concentrations, spermatic venous concentrations and in vitro biosynthesis of testosterone.

Therefore the testicular response to heat is multifold in which spermatogenesis, semen quality, steroid production, and testicular blood flow are decreased in response to heat. It is not surprising that a temporary infertility follows exposure of the testis or whole animal to heat.

Environmental Modification to Improve Reproductive Efficiency

The various studies reviewed indicate that prevention of severe heat stress is one of the major modifications of the external environment which can be conducted to improve reproduction. Daily total air conditioning or partial air conditioning during daylight hours improved conception rates (39.4 vs. 28.3%) compared to non air-conditioned control cows or cows cooled only at night.[106] Coupled with the ability of air conditioning to reduce the usual summer period of infertility was increased milk production. However, air conditioning was not economically feasible. Evaporative cooling also has been used in regions with a hot and dry atmosphere to improve reproductive efficiency and milk production of dairy cows.[105] The physical principle of heat exchange with evaporative cooling is such that it has less application in tropical and subtropical areas with high relative humidity.

Since solar radiation contributes to the animal's heat load and is quantitatively related to conception rate,[115] benefits would be expected with suitable environmental modification and management to reduce the net solar radiation load on the animals. In the subtropical environment of Gainesville, Florida, shade-managed dairy cows had lower respiration rates and rectal temperatures than cows exposed to no shade. Improvement in conception rate for shaded cows was comparable to the response achieved with air conditioning.[106,109]

Future utilization of hormonal techniques to control estrous cycles will allow producers to avoid the hot seasonal period for breeding.[169] As the precision of ovulation control improves, artificial insemination at an appointed time after treatment will avoid the problems of poor estrous detection during hot seasons.

Wettemann et al.[174] demonstrated that shade combined with sprinklers reduced the stressful effects of high ambient temperature. Sperm quality of shaded boars was comparable to that of boars maintained in cool chambers.

It is clear that environmental modification can improve fertility during heat stressing periods of the year. However, it is important to consider the nature of the environment, economics of the system, and the associated degree of management to obtain practical benefits. In most instances, temperature effects are confounded with gradual change in length of photoperiod. Endocrine responses to the environment may be tuned to temperature and/or photoperiod changes. Certain species such as the sheep and horse are markedly influenced by photoperiod relative to control of reproductive rhythms during the year. Regulation of photoperiod may become an integral part of future management systems to improve efficiencies of reproduction, lactation and growth.[175]

GROWTH

Thermal stress reduces prenatal and postnatal growth rate in domestic animals. Prenatal growth is reduced by decline in substrate utilization such as albumen in chicken eggs.[144] Fetal stunting due to heat stress in late pregnancy is well established[140-142] and probably related to decreased uterine blood flow,[21] substrate availability, and placental mass.[140]

Body weight gain in growing animals is more severely affected than adults. Reductions in growth rate are associated with decreased feed intake,[176,177] reduced metabolic rate,[178] and increased catabolism.[179] The reduced feed intake is mediated via the hypothalamic satiety center. Cooling the anterior hypothalamus and preoptic areas initiated feeding in satiated goats, while heating inhibited feed consumption by a fasted goat.[180] As feed intake declines, total heat production drops and a greater proportion of the energy consumed goes for maintenance resulting in a decline of gross efficiency.[181]

Age, weight, size,[177] and breed[179] have significant effects on growth rate during thermal stress. In addition, level of feeding[181] and type of feed[182] influence feed intake in response to heat stress. Primary causes of reduced growth rate are related directly to decreasing heat production and shifting energy utilization to heat dissipation. In addition to changes in growth rate, changes in body conformation occur in animals growing in hot climates. Holstein cows were shorter in body length and height at withers in

Louisiana compared to paternal half-sibs in Maryland.[11] Pigs raised at 35°C for 8 weeks had longer extremities and less hair than controls raised at 25°C.[183]

DISEASE

Environmental conditions can influence susceptibility of domestic animals to disease. A high incidence of clinical mastitis in dairy cattle occurs during the hot summer months.[184,185] Within a herd management system,[109] either air-conditioned cows[106] or cows exposed to a shade management system[109] had a lower frequency of clinical mastitis than cows exposed to their natural environments. Thus the stress of heat and other associated environmental factors predispose the animal to develop clinical mastitis. Paape and co-workers[186] reported that neither heat stress nor injection of ACTH increases the number of somatic cells in milk produced from healthy mammary glands (no pathogenic organisms). The higher incidence of milk somatic cells during the summer months is apparently due to development of clinical mastitis from infected cows in the subclinical stage. Stress conditions apparently predispose the infected animal so that its defense mechanism is not most efficient to prevent development of clinical mastitis.[187,188]

Final completion of the fetal life cycle is the initiation of lactation synchronized with parturition (under fetal control) to provide continued nourishment of the calf after delivery from its in-utero environment. The sheep, cow, pig, and goat belong to a group of animals which do not confer passive immunity in utero during pregnancy.[189] Rather, passive immunity is acquired via colustrum or first milk which is rich in immunoglobulins. During the first few hours after parturition the immunoglobulins are actively absorbed across the gut wall rather than digested.[190] The process whereby the gut loses the ability to transfer immunoglobulins into the blood stream is called gut closure. Failure to obtain or to absorb adequate amounts of colostrum results in neonatal septicemia or diarrhea.[191-193] Stott and co-workers[194] presented evidence that high environmental temperatures interfere with immunoglobulin transfer by accelerating the process of gut closure. They hypothesized that elevated plasma glucocorticoids due to heat stress may influence passive immunity of the calf, incidence of disease and calf mortality via its effect on gut closure. Various calf management systems to reduce environmental heat load were related to calf viability, plasma glucocorticoid concentrations, and absorption of immunoglobulins. Further research is required to establish a direct link between elevated plasma glucocorticoid concentrations and precocious gut closure.[189]

REFERENCES

1. **Van Horn, H. H., Cunha, T. J., and Harms, R. H.,** The role of livestock in meeting human food needs, *BioScience,* 22, 710—714, 1972.
2. **McDowell, R. E.,** The role of livestock in the warm climates, in *Improvement of Livestock Production In Warm Climates,* W. H. Freeman & Co., San Francisco, 1972, chap. 1.
3. **Branton, C.,** The effects of climatic factors on milk production in the tropical and subtropical areas of the world, *Congr. Mundial Medicina Veterinaria Zootecnia Mexico,* 19, 1—41, 1971.
4. **Horvath, S. M. and Howell, C. D.,** Organ systems in adaptation: the cardiovascular system, in *Handbook of Physiology, Adaptation to the Environment,* Vol. 4, American Physiological Society, Washington D.C., 1964, 153—166.
5. **Hertzman, A. B.,** Vasomotor regulation of the cutaneous circulation *Physiol Rev.,* 39, 280—306, 1959.

6. **Rowell, L. B.**, The cutaneous circulation, in *Physiology and Biophysics*, Vol. 2, Ruch, T. C., Patton, H. D., and Scher, A. M., Eds., W. B. Saunders, Philadelphia, 1974, chap. 12.
7. **Cooper, K. E., Johnson, R. H., and Spalding, J. M. K.**, The effects of central body and trunk skin temperatures on reflex vasodilation in the hand, *J. Physiol. London*, 1974, 46—54, 1964.
8. **Fox, R. H. and Hilton, S. M.**, Bradykinen formation in human skin as a factor in heat vasodilation, *J. Physiol. London*, 142, 219—232, 1958.
9. **Schmidt-Nielsen, K.**, Heat conservation in countercurrent systems, in *Temperature, its Measurement and Control in Science and Industry*, Hardy, J. D., Ed., Reinhold, New York, 1954, 143—148.
10. **Baker, M. A. and Hayward, J. N.**, The influence of the nasal mucosa and the carotid rete upon hypothalamic temperature in the sheep, *J. Physiol. London*, 198, 561—579, 1968.
11. **Conley, C. L. and Nickerson, J. L.**, Effects of temperature changes on the water balance of man, *Am. J. Physiol.*, 143, 373—378, 1945.
12. **Israel, L. A., Collier, R. J., Stover, D. G., Eley, R. M.**, Buffington, D. E., and Wilcox, C. J., Effect of Shade on Physiological Patterns in Jersey Cattle over a 24 hr period, Proc. 70th Annu. Meet. Am. Soc. Anim. Sci., Michigan State University, East Lansing, July 9 to 13, 1978, 369.
13. **Thompson, G. E.**, Climatic physiology of cattle, *J. Dairy Res.*, 40, 441—473, 1973.
14. **Hutchison, J. C. D.**, Evaporative cooling in fowls, *J. Agric. Sci.*, 45, 48—59, 1954.
15. **Bligh, J.**, The receptors concerned in the thermal stimulus to panting in sheep, *J. Physiol. London*, 146, 142—151, 1959.
16. **Ingram, D. L. and Legge, K. F.**, The effect of environmental temperature on respiratory ventilation in the pig, *Respir. Physiol.*, 8, 1—12, 1970.
17. **McLean, J. A. and Calvert, D. T.**, Influence of air humidity on the partition of heat exchanges of cattle, *J. Agric. Sci.*, 78, 303—307, 1972.
18. **Macfarlane, W.**, Terrestrial animals in dry heat: ungulates, in *Handbook of Physiology, Adaptation to the Environment*, Vol. 4, American Physiological Society, Washington, D .C., 1964, chap. 33.
19. **Bianca, W.**, Thermoregulation, in *Adaptation of Domestic Animals*, Hafez, E. S. E., Ed., Lea & Febiger, Philadelphia, 1968, 97—118.
20. **Bianca, W. and Findlay, J. D.**, The effect of thermally-induced hyperpnea on the acid-base status of the blood of calves, *Res. Vet. Sci.*, 3, 38—49, 1962.
21. **Oakes, G. K., Walker, A. M., Ehrenkranz, R. A. Cefalo, R. C., and Chez, R. A.**, Uteroplacental blood flow during hyperthermia with and without respiratory alkalosis, *J. Appl. Physiol.*, 41, 197—201, 1976.
22. **Baile, C. A. and Forbes, J. M.**, Control of feed intake and regulation of energy balance in ruminants, *Physiol. Rev.*, 54, 160—214, 1974.
23. **Robinson, K. W. and Klemm, G. H.**, A study of heat tolerance of grade Australian Illawarra Shorthorn Cows during early lactation, *Aust. J. Agric. Res.*, 4, 224—234, 1953.
24. **Gengler, W. R., Martz, F. A., Johnson, H. D., Krause, G. F., and Hahn, L.**, Effect of temperature on food and water intake and rumen fermentation, *J. Dairy Sci.*, 53, 434—437, 1970.
25. **Kelly, R. O., Martz, F. A., and Johnson, H. D.**, Effect of environmental temperature on ruminal volatile fatty acid levels with controlled feed intake, *J. Dairy Sci.*, 50, 531—533, 1967.
26. **Ingram, D. L. and Mount, L. E.**, Animals in hot environments, in *Man and Animals in Hot Environments*, Springer-Verlag, Basel, 1975, chap. 9.
27. **Bianca, W.**, Thermoregulatory responses of the dehydrated or to drinking cold and warm water in a warm environment, *Res. Vet. Sci.*, 5, 75—80, 1964.
28. **Roman-Ponce, H., Thatcher, W. W., Wilcox, C. J., and van Horn, H. H.**, Hormonal interrelationships and physiological responses of dairy cattle to a shade structure, *J. Dairy Sci.*, 60, 104, 1977.
29. **Lippke, H.**, Digestibility and volatile fatty acids in steers and wethers at 21 and 32°C ambient temperature, *J. Dairy Sci.*, 58, 1860—1864, 1975.
30. **Martz, F. A., Mishra, M., Campbell, J. R., Daniels, L. B., and Hildebrand, E.**, Relation of ambient temperature and time postfeeding on ruminal, arterial and venous volatile fatty acids, and lactic acid in Holstein steers, *J. Dairy Sci.*, 54, 520-525, 1971.
31. **Weldy, J. R., McDowell, R. E., van Soest, P. J., and Bond, J.**, Influence of heat stress on rumen acid levels and some blood constituents in cattle., *J. Anim. Sci.*, 23, 147—153, 1964.
32. **Whittow, G. C.**, Ungulates, in *Comparative Physiology of Thermoregulation*, Vol. 2, Whittow, G. C., Ed., Harvard University Press, Cambridge, Mass., 1971, 192—273.
33. **Chowers, I., Conforti, N., and Siegel, R. A.**, Interrelationships between the central nervous system and pattern of adrenocorticotropic secretion following acute exposure to severe environmental conditions, *Isr. J. Med. Sci.*, 12, 1010—1018, 1976.
34. **Alvarez, M. B. and Johnson, H. D.**, Environmental heat exposure on cattle plasma catecholamine and glucocorticoids, *J. Dairy Sci.*, 56, 189—194, 1973.
35. **Robertshaw, D. and Whittow, G. C.**, The effect of hyperthermia and localized heating of the anterior hypothalamus on the sympathoadrenal system of the ox *(Bos taurus)*, *J. Physiol.*, 187, 351—360, 1967.

36. **Yu-Chang, L. and Sturkie, P. D.**, Effect of environmental temperature on the catecholamines of chickens, *Am. J. Physiol.*, 214, 237—240, 1968.
37. **Joshi, B. C., McDowell, R. E., and Sadhu, D. P.**, Surface evaporation from the normal body surface and with sweat glands inactivated in Indian cattle, *J. Dairy Sci.*, 51, 915—917, 1968.
38. **Allen, T. E. and Bligh, J.**, A comparative study of the temporal patterns of cutaneous water vapor loss from some domesticated mammals with epitrichial sweat glands, *Comp. Biochem, Physiol.*, 31, 347—363, 1969.
39. **Jenkinson, D. M., Sengupta, B. P., and Blackburn, P.S.**, The distribution of nerves, monoamine oxidase and cholinesterase in the skin of cattle, *J. Anat.*, 100, 593—613, 1966.
40. **Bligh, J., Cottle, W. H., and Maskray, M.**, Influence of ambient temperature on the thermoregulatory responses to 5-hydroxytryptamine, noradrenaline and acetycholine injected into lateral cerebral ventricles of sheep, goats, and rabbits, *J. Physiol. London*, 212, 377—392 1971.
41. **Brooks, J. R., Pipes, G. W., and Ross, C. W.**, Effect of temperature on the thyroxine secretion rate of rams, *J. Anim. Sci.*, 21, 414—417, 1962.
42. **Hoffman, E. and Shaffner, C. S.**, Thyroid weight and function as influenced by environmental temperature, *Poult. Sci.*, 29, 365—376, 1950.
43. **Ingram, D. L. and Slebodzinski, A.**, Oxygen consumption and thyroid gland activity during adaptation to high ambient temperature in young pigs, *Res. Vet. Sci.*, 6, 522—530, 1965.
44. **Anderson, B.**, Hypothalamic temperature and thyroid activity, in brain-thyroid relationships, *Ciba Found. Study Group*, 18, 35—50, 1964.
45. **Krulich, L., Hefco, E., and Illner, P.**, Effect of exposure to cold or heat on the activity of the pituitary thyroid system, *Isr. J. Med. Sci.*, 12, 1090—1098, 1976.
46. **Mitra, R., Christison, G. I., and Johnson, H. D.**, Effect of prolonged thermal exposure on growth hormone (GH) secretion in cattle, *J. Anim. Sci.*, 34, 776—779, 1972.
47. **Mitra, R. and Johnson, H. D.**, Growth hormone response to acute thermal exposure in cattle, *Proc. Soc. Exp. Biol. Med.*, 139, 1086—1089, 1972.
48. **Yousef, M. K. and Johnson, H. D.**, Calorigenesis of cattle as influenced by growth hormone and environmental temperature, *J. Anim. Sci.*, 25, 1076—1082, 1966.
49. **Chowers, I., Hammel, H. T., Eisenman, J., Abrams, R. M., and McCann, S. M.**, Comparison of effect of environmental and preoptic heating and pyrogen on plasma cortisol, *Am. J. Physiol.*, 210, 606—610, 1966.
50. **Bianca, W.**, Reviews of the progress of dairy science. Section A. Physiology. Cattle in a hot environment, *J. Dairy Res.*, 32, 291—345, 1965.
51. **Christian, G. I. and Johnson, H. D.**, Cortisol turnover in heat-stressed cows, *J. Anim. Sci.*, 35, 1005—1010, 1972.
52. **Shayanfar, F., Head, H. H., Wilcox, C. J., and Thatcher, W. W.**, Adrenal responsiveness in lactating Holstein cows, *J. Dairy Sci.*, 58, 870—878, 1975.
53. **Bourne, R. A. and Tucker, H. A.**, Serum prolactin and LH responses to photoperiod in bull calves, *Endocrinology*, 97, 473—475, 1975.
54. **Wetteman, R. P. and Tucker, H. A.**, Relationship of ambient temperature to serum prolactin in heifers, *Proc. Soc. Exp. Biol. Med.*, 146, 908—911, 1974.
55. **Koprowski, J. A. and Tucker, H. A.**, Serum prolactin during various physiological states and its relationship to milk production in the bovine, *Endocrinology*, 92, 1480—1487, 1973.
56. **Hart, I. C.**, Seasonal Factors affecting the release of prolactin in goats in response to milking, *J. Endocrinol.*, 64, 313—322, 1975.
57. **Thatcher, W. W.**, Effects of season, climate, and temperature on reproduction and lactation, *J. Dairy Sci.*, 57, 360-368, 1974.
58. **Mueller, G. P., Chen, H. T., Dibbit, J. A., Chen, H. J., and Meites, J.**, Effects of warm and cold temperatures on release of TSH, GH, and prolactin in rats, *Proc. Soc. Exp. Biol. Med.*, 147, 698—700, 1974.
59. **Collier, R. J., Bauman, D. E., and Hays, R. L.**, Lactogenesis in explant cultures of mammary tissue from pregnant cows, *Endocrinology*, 100, 1192—1200, 1977.
60. **Tucker, H. A.**, General endocrinological control of lactation in *Lactation: A Comprehensive Treatise*, Vol. 1, Larson, B. L. and Smith, V. R., Eds., Academic Press, 1974, 200—235.
61. **Baldwin, B. A.**, The effects of intra-ruminal loading with cold water on thermoregulatory behavior in sheep, *J. Physiol. London*, 249, 139—152, 1975.
62. **Baldwin, B. A. and Ingram, D. L.**, The effects of heating and cooling the hypothalamus on behavioral thermoregulation in pigs, *J. Physiol. London*, 191, 375—392, 1967.
63. **Baldwin, B. A. and Lipton, J. M.**, Central and periperal temperatures and EEG changes during behavioral thermoregulation in pigs, *Acta Neurobiol. Exp.*, 33,433—447, 1973.

64. **Ragsdale, A. C., Thompson, H. J., Worstell, D. M., and Brody, S.,** Influence of increasing temperatures, 40 to 105°F on milk production in Brown Swiss cows and on feed and water consumption, and body weight in Brown Swiss and Brahman cows and heifers, *Mo. Agric. Exp. Sta. Res. Bull.* 471, 1951.
65. **Seath, D. M. and Miller G. D.,** Effect of warm weather on grazing performance of milking cows, *J. Dairy Sci.,* 29, 199—206, 1946.
66. **Payne, W. J. A., Laing, W. I., and Raivoka, E. N.,** Grazing behavior of dairy cattle in the tropics, *Nature (London),* 167, 610—611, 1951.
67. **Ingram, D. L.,** Evaporative cooling in the pig, *Nature (London),* 207, 415—416, 1965.
68. **Mount, L. E.,** Adaptation to the thermal environment in the growing pig, in *Climatic Physiology of the Pig,* Williams & Wilkins, 1968, 97—130.
69. **Regan, W. M. and Richardson, G. W.,** Reactions of the dairy cow to changes in environmental temperature, *J. Dairy Sci.,* 21, 73—79, 1938.
70. **Brody, S.,** Environmental physiology, I. Physiological backgrounds, *Mo. Agric. Exp. Sta. Res. Bull.,* 423, 1—43, 1948.
71. **Ragsdale, A. C., Brody, S., Thompson, H. J., and Worstell, D. M.,** Influence of temperature, 50 to 105°F, on milk production and feed consumption of dairy cattle, *Mo. Agric. Exp. Sta. Res. Bull.,* 425, 1—27, 1948.
72. **Ragsdale, A. C., Thompson, H. J., Worstell, D. M., and Brody, S.,** Environmental physiology. IX. Milk production and feed and water consumption responses of Brahman, Jersey, and Holstein cows to changes in temperature, 50 to 105°F and 50 to 8°F, *Mo. Agric. Exp. Sta. Res. Bull.,* 460, 5—28, 1950.
73. **Yeck. R. G. and Stewart, R. E.,** A ten-year summary of the psychroenergetic laboratory dairy cattle research at the University of Missouri, *Trans. ASAE,* 2, 71—77, 1959.
74. **Worstell, D. M. and Brody, S.,** Environmental physiology. XX. Comparative physiological reactions of European and Indian cattle to changing temperature, *Mo. Agric. Exp. Sta. Res. Bull.,* 515, 1—42, 1953.
75. **Johnston, J. E., Hamblin, F. B., and Schrader, G. T.,** Factors concerned in the comparative heat tolerance of Jersey, Holstein and Sindhi-Holstein F cattle, *J. Anim. Sci.,* 17, 473—479, 1958.
76. **Ragsdale, A. C., Thompson, H. J., Worstell, D. M., and Brody, S.,** Environmental physiology and shelter engineering. XXI. The effect of humidity on milk production and composition, feed and water consumption, and body weight in cattle, *Mo. Agric. Exp. Sta. Res. Bull.,* 521, 1—23, 1953.
77. **Johnson, H. D., Ragsdale, A. C., Berry, I. L., and Shanklin, M. D.,** Environmental physiology and shelter engineering. LXII. Effect of various temperature-humidity combinations on milk production of Holstein cattle, *Mo. Agric. Exp. Sta. Res. Bull.,* 791, 1—39, 1962.
78. **Johnson, H. D., Ragsdale, A. C. Berry, I. L., and Shanklin, M. D.,** Environmental physiology and shelter engineering. LXVI. Temperature-humidity effects including influence of acclimation in feed and water consumption of Holstein cattle, *Mo. Agric. Exp. Sta. Res. Bull.,* 846, 1—43, 1963.
79. **Johnson, H. D., Kibler, H. H., Berry, I. L., Wayman, O., and Merilan, C. P.,** Environmental physiology and shelter engineering. LXX. Temperature and controlled feeding effects on lactation and related physiological reactions of cattle, *Mo. Agric. Exp. Sta. Res. Bull.,* 902, 1—27, 1966.
80. **Bandaranayaka, D. D. and Holmes, C. W.,** Changes in the composition of milk and rumen contents in cows exposed to a high ambient temperature with controlled feeding, *Trop. Anim. Health Prod.,* 8, 38, 1976.
81. **McDowell, R. E.,** Physiological approaches to animal climatology, *J. Hered.,* 49, 52—61, 1958.
82. **Brody, S., Ragsdale, A. C., Thompson, H. J., Worstell, D. M.,** Environmental physiology and shelter engineering. XXVIII. The thermal effects of radiation intensity (light) on milk production, feed and water consumption, and body weight in Holstein, Jersey and Brahman cows at airtemperatures 45°, 70° and 80°F, *Mo. Agric. Exp. Sta. Res. Bull.,* 556, 1—20, 1954.
83. **Brody, S., Ragsdale, A. C. Thompson, H. J., and Worstell, D. M.,** Environmental physiology and shelter engineering. XXV. The effect of wind on milk production, feed and water consumption and body weight in dairy cattle, *Mo. Agric. Exp. Sta. Res. Bull.,* 545, 1—20, 1954.
84. **Johnston, J. E.,** The effects of high temperature on milk production, *J. Hered.,* 49, 65—68, 1958.
85. **Rupel, J. W., Leighton, R. E., and Harris, R. R.,** High-fiber, high-fat and restricted roughage diets in relation to hot weather performance of dairy cows, *Int. Dairy Congr.,* 1, 319, 1958.
86. **Johnson, J. C., Southwell, B. L., Givens, R. L., and McDowell, R. E.,** Interrelationships of certain climatic conditions and productive responses of lactating dairy cows, *J. Dairy Sci.,* 45, 695, 1962.
87. **Stott, G. H. and Moody, E. G.,** Tolerance of dairy cows to high climatic temperatures on low roughage ration, *J. Dairy Sci.,* 43, 871, 1960.
88. **Moody, E. G., van Soest, P. J., McDowell, R. E., and Ford, G. L.,** Effect of high temperature and dietary fat on performance of lactating cows, *J. Dairy Sci.,* 50, 1909—1916, 1967.

89. **Maust, L. E., McDowell, R. E., and Hoover, N. W.,** Effect of summer weather on performance of Holstein cows in three stages of lactation, *J. Dairy Sci.,* 55, 1133—1139. 1972.
90. **Branton, C., Rios, G., Evans, D. L., Farthing, B. R., and Koonce, K. L.,** Genotype-climatic and other interaction effects for productive responses in Holsteins, *J. Dairy Sci.,* 57, 833—841, 1974.
91. **Hassan, A. and Roussel, J. D.,** Effect of protein concentration in the diet on blood composition and productivity of lactating Holstein cows under thermal stress, *J. Agric. Sci.,* 85, 409—415, 1975.
92. **Payne, W. J. A. and Hancock, J.,** The direct effect of tropical climate on performance of European-type cattle. II. Production, *Emp. J. Exp. Agric.,* 25, 321—338, 1957.
93. **Rodriguez, L. A., Wilcox, C. J., Bachman, K. C., Thatcher, W. W., and Martin, F. G.,** Climatological, physiological and genetic effects on milk composition and yield, *J. Dairy Sci.,* 60 (Suppl. I), 80, 1977.
94. **Spike, P. W. and Freeman, A. E.,** Environmental influences on monthly variation in milk constituents, *J. Dairy Sci.,* 50, 1897-1904, 1967.
95. **Wilcox, C. J., Pfau, K. O., Mather, R. E., and Bartlett, J. W.,** Genetic and environmental influences upon solids-not-fat content of cows milk, *J. Dairy Sci.,* 42, 1132—1145, 1959.
96. **Parkhie, M. R., Gilmore, L. O., and Fechheimer, N. S.,** Effect of successive lactations, gestation, and season of calving on constituents of cows' milk, *J. Dairy Sci.,* 49, 1410—1415, 1966.
97. **Waite, R., White, J. C. D., and Robertson, A.,** Variations in the chemical composition of milk with particular reference to the solids-not-fat. I. The effect of stage of lactation, season of year and age of cow, *J. Dairy Res.,* 23, 65—81, 1956.
98. **Brun, J. C. and Franke, A. A.,** Monthly variations in gross composition of California herd milks, *J. Dairy Sci.,* 60, 696—700, 1977.
99. **Cobble, J. W. and Herman, H. A.,** The influence of environmental temperatures on the composition of milk of the dairy cow, *Mo. Agric. Exp. Sta. Res. Bull.,* 485, 1—18, 1951.
100. **McDowell, R. E., Hooven, N. W., and Camoens, J. K.,** Effect of climate on performance of Holsteins in first lactation, *J. Dairy Sci.,* 59, 965—973, 1976.
101. **Benson, G. K. and Morris, L. R.,** Foetel growth and lactation in rats exposed to high temperatures during pregnancy, *J. Reprod. Fertil.,* 27, 369—384, 1971.
102. **Verde, O., Wilcox, C. J., Koger, M., Plasse, D., and Martin, F. G.,** Influencias genéticas, ambientales y sus interacciones sobre la producción lechera en Venezuela, *Asociatión Latinoamericana de Producion Animal Memoria,* 7, 117—135, 1972.
103. **Lytton, V. H. and Legates, J. E.,** Sire by region interaction for production traits in dairy cattle, *J. Dairy Sci.,* 49, 874—878, 1966.
104. **McDowell, R. E., Wiggans, G. R., Camoens, J. K., Van Vleck, L. D., and St. Luis, D. G.,** Sire comparisons for Holsteins in Mexico versus the United States and Canada, *J. Dairy Sci.,* 59, 298—304, 1976.
105. **Stott, G. H. and Wiersma, F.,** Response of Dairy Cattle to an Evaporative Cooled Environment, *Proc. Int. Livestock Environment Symp.,* ASAE SP09174, American Society of Agricultural Engineers, St. Joseph, Mich., 1974, 88—95.
106. **Thatcher, W. W., Gwazduaskas, F . C., Wilcox, C. J., Toms, J., Head, H. H., Buffington, D. E., and Fredriksson, W. B.,** Milking performance and reproductive efficiency of dairy cows in an environmentally controlled structure, *J. Dairy Sci.,* 57, 304—397, 1974.
107. **Johnston, J. E., Stone, E. J., and Frye, J. B., Jr.,** Effects of hot weather on the productive function of dairy cows. I. Temperature control during hot weather, *La. Agric. Exp. Sta. Bull.,* 608, 1—16, 1966.
108. **Hahn, L.,** Predicted versus measured production differences using summer air-conditioning for lactating dairy cows, *J. Dairy Sci.,* 52, 800—802, 1969.
109. **Roman-Ponce, H., Thatcher, W. W., Buffington, D. E., Wilcox, C. J., and van Horn, H. H.,** Physiological and production responses of dairy cattle to a shade structure in a subtropical environment, *J. Dairy Sci.,* 60, 424-430, 1977.
110. **Stott, G. H.,** Female and breed associated with seasonal fertility variation in dairy cattle, *J. Dairy Sci.,* 44, 1698—1704, 1961.
111. **Stott, G. H. and Williams, R. J.,** Causes of low breeding efficiency in dairy cattle associated with seasonal high temperatures, *J. Dairy Sci.,* 45, 1369—1375, 1962.
112. **Vincent, C. K.,** Effects of season and high environmental temperature on fertility in cattle: a review, *J. Am. Vet. Med. Assoc.,* 161, 1333—1338, 1972.
113. **Ingraham, R. H., Gillette, D. D., and Wagner, W. D.,** Relationship of temperature and humidity to conception rate of Holstein cows in subtropical climate, *J. Dairy Sci.,* 57, 476—481, 1974.
114. **Monty, D. E. and Walff, L. K.,** Summer heat stress and reduced fertility in Holstein-Freisian cows in Arizona, *Am. J. Vet. Res.,* 35, 1495—1500, 1974.
115. **Gwazdauskas, F. C., Wilcox, C. J., and Thatcher, W. W.,** Environmental and managemental factors affecting conception rate in a subtropical climate, *J. Dairy Sci.,* 58, 88—92, 1975.

116. **Dale, H. E., Ragsdale, A. D., and Cheng, C. S.,** Effect of constant environmental temperatures 50° and 80°F, on appearance of puberty in beef calves, *J. Anim. Sci.,* 18, 1363—1366, 1959.
117. **Gangwar, P. D., Branton, C., and Evans, D. L.,** Reproductive and physiological responses of Holstein heifers to controlled and natural climatic conditions, *J. Dairy Sci.,* 48, 222—227, 1965.
118. **Madan, M. L. and Johnson, H.D.,** Environmental heat effects on bovine lutenizing hormone, *J. Dairy Sci.,* 56, 1420—1423, 1973.
119. **Hall, J. G., Branton, C., and Stone, E. J.,** Estrus, estrous cycles, ovulation time, time of service, and fertility of dairy cattle in Louisiana, *J. Dairy Sci.,* 42, 1086—1094, 1959.
120. **Bond, J. and McDowell, R. E.,** Reproductive performance and physiological responses of beef females as affected by a prolonged high environmental temperature, *J. Anim. Sci.,* 35, 820—829, 1972.
121. **Labhsetwar, A. P., Tyler, W. J., and Casida, L. E.,** Genetic and environmental factors affecting quiet ovulations in Holstein cattle, *J. Dairy Sci.,* 46, 843—845, 1963.
122. **Wolff, L. K. and Monty, D. E.,** Physiologic response to intense summer heat wave and its effect on the estrous cycle of nonlactating and lactating Holstein-Friesian cows in Arizona, *Am. J. Vet. Res.,* 35, 187—192, 1974.
123. **Ulberg, L. L. and Burfening, P. J.,** Embryo death resulting from adverse environment on spermatozoa or ova, *J. Anim. Sci.,* 26, 571—577, 1967.
124. **Gwazdauskas, F. C., Thatcher, W. W., and Wilcox, C. J.,** Physiological, environmental, and hormonal factors at insemination which may affect conception, *J. Dairy Sci.,* 56, 873—877, 1973.
125. **Dunlap, S. E. and Vincent, C. K.,** Influence of postbreeding thermal stress on conception rate in dairy cattle, *J. Anim. Sci.,* 32, 1216—1218, 1971.
126. **Ryle, M.,** Early reproductive failure of ewes in a hot environment. I. Ovulation rate and embryonic mortality, *J. Agric. Sci.,* 57, 1—9, 1961.
127. **Ryle, M.,** Early reproductive failure of ewes in a hot environment. IV. The ovary, *J. Agric. Sci.,* 60, 101—104, 1963.
128. **Warnick, A. C., Wallace, H. D., Palmer, A. I., Sasa, E., Duerre, D. J., and Coldwell, V.E.,** Effect of temperature on early embryo survival in gilts, *J. Anim. Sci.,* 24, 89—96, 1965.
129. **Yeates, N. T. M.,** The effect of high air temperature on reproduction in the ewe, *J. Agric. Sci.,* 43, 199—203, 1953.
130. **Dutt, R. H., Ellington, E. F., and Carlton, W. W.,** Fertilization rate and early embryo survival in sheared and unsheared ewes following exposure to elevated air temperature, *J. Anim. Sci.,* 18, 1308—1318, 1959.
131. **Edwards, R. L., Omtvedt, I. T., Turman, E. J., Stephens, D. F., and Mahoney, G. W. A.,** Reproductive performance of gilts following heat stress prior to breeding and in early gestation, *J. Anim. Sci.,* 27, 1634—1637, 1968.
132. **Tompkins, E. C., Heidenreich, C. J., and Stob, M.,** Effect of postbreeding thermal stress on embryonic mortality in swine, *J. Anim. Sci.,* 26, 377—380, 1967.
133. **Omtvedt, I. T., Nelson, R. E., Edwards, R. L., Stephens, D. F., and Turman, E. J.,** Influence of heat stress during early, mid and late pregnancy of gilts, *J. Anim. Sci.,* 32, 312—317, 1971.
134. **Wildt, D. E., Riegle, G. D., and Dukelow, W. R.,** Physiological temperature response and embryonic mortality in stressed swine, *Am. J. Physiol.,* 229, 1471—1475, 1975.
135. **Alliston, C. W. and Ulberg, L. C.,** Early pregnancy loss in sheep at ambient temperatures of 70° and 90°F as determined by embryo transfer, *J. Anim. Sci.,* 20, 608—613, 1961.
136. **Dutt, R. H.,** Critical period for early embryo mortality in ewes exposed to high ambient temperatures, *J. Anim. Sci.,* 22, 713—719, 1963.
137. **Dutt, R. H. and Jabara, C. D.,** Gestation stage and embryo loss in ewes heat stressed during early placentogenesis, *J. Anim. Sci.,* 43, 282, 1976.
138. **Woody, C. O. and Ulberg, L. C.,** Viability of one-cell sheep ova as affected by high environmental temperature, *J. Reprod. Fert.,* 7, 275—280, 1964.
139. **Alliston, C. W., Howarth, B., Jr., and Ulberg, L. C.,** Embryonic mortality following culture in vitro of one- and two-cell rabbit eggs at elevated temperatures, *J. Reprod. Fert.,* 9, 337—341, 1965.
140. **Alexander, G. and Williams, D.,** Heat stress and development of the conceptus in domestic sheep, *J. Agric. Sci.,* 76, 53—72, 1971.
141. **Brown, D. E., Harrison, P. C., Hinds, F. C., Lewis, J. A., and Wallace, M. H.,** Heat stress effects on fetal development during late gestation in the ewe, *J. Anim. Sci.,* 44, 442—446, 1977.
142. **Cartwright, G. A. and Thwaites, C. J.,** Foetal stunting in sheep. I. The influence of maternal nutrition and high ambient temperatures on the growth and proportions of Merino foetuses, *J. Agric. Sci.,* 86, 573—580, 1976.
143. **Yeates, N. T. M.,** The effect of high air temperature on pregnancy and birth weight in Merino sheep, *Aust. J. Agric. Res.,* 7, 435—439, 1956.
144. **Thinh, N. X., Cumming, R. B., and Thwaites, C. J.,** The effects of high incubating temperature on the growth of the chick embryo, *Aust. J. Agric. Res.,* 28, 551—555, 1977.

145. **de Alba, J. and Riera, S.**, Sexual maturity and spermatogenesis under heat stress in the bovine, *Anim. Prod.*, 8, 137—144, 1966.
146. **Egbunicke, G. N. and Steinbach, J.**, Comparative studies of sperm production in boars raised in temperate and tropical climates, *Pros. 8th Int. Congr. Anim. Reprod. Artif. Insem.*, 3, 42—45, 1976.
147. **Lindsay, D. R.**, Sexual activity and semen production of rams at high temperatures, *J. Reprod. Fert.*, 18, 1—8, 1969.
148. **Casady, R. B., Myers, R. M., and Legates, J. E.**, The effect of exposure to high ambient temperature on spermatogenesis in the dairy bull, *J. Dairy Sci.*, 36, 14—23, 1953.
149. **Johnston, J. E., Naelapaa, H., and Frye, J. B., Jr.**, Physiological responses of Holstein, Brown Swiss and Red Sindhi crossbred bulls exposed to high temperatures and humidities, *J. Anim. Sci.*, 22, 432—436, 1963.
150. **Williamson, P.**, The fine structure of ejaculated ram spermatozoa following scrotal heating, *J. Reprod. Fert.*, 40, 191—195, 1974.
151. **Howarth, B., Jr.**, Fertility in the ram following exposure to elevated ambient temperature and humidity, *J. Reprod. Fert.*, 19, 179—183, 1969.
152. **McNitt, J. I. and First, N. L.**, Effects of 72-hour heat stress on semen quality in boars, *Int. J. Biometeorol.*, 14, 373—380, 1970.
153. **Roller, W. L., Teague, H. S., Christenson, R. K., and Grifo, A. P.**, Effect of Ambient Heat Exposure upon Swine Reproduction, Annu. Meet. ASAE, No. 73-416, American Society of Agricultural Engineering, St. Joseph, Mich., 1973, 1—17.
154. **Wettemann, R. P., Wells, M. E., Omtvedt, I. T., Pope, C. E., and Turman, E. J.**, Influence of elevated ambient temperature on reproductive performance of boars, *J. Anim. Sci.*, 42, 664—669, 1976.
155. **Smith, J. F.**, The effect of temperature on characteristics of semen of rams, *Aust. J. Agric. Res.*, 22, 481—490, 1971.
156. **Da Silva, R. G. and Casagrande, J. F.**, Influence of high environmental temperatures on some characteristics of Zebu bull semen, *Proc. 8th Int. Congr. Anim. Reprod. Artif. Insem.*, 4, 939—942, 1976.
157. **Waites, G. M. H. and Ortavant, R.**, Effets précoces d'une brève élévation de la temperature testiculaire sur la spermatogenèse du bélier, *Ann. Biol. Anim. Biochim. Biophys.*, 8, 323, 1968.
158. **Waites, G. M. H.**, Temperature regulation and fertility in male and female mammals, *Isr. J. Med. Sci.*, 12, 982—993, 1976.
159. **Van Demark, N. L. and Ree, M. J.**, Temperature effects, in *The Testis*, Vol. 3, Johnson, A. D., Gomes, W. R., and van Demark, N. L., Eds., Academic Press, New York, 1970, chap. 7.
160. **Howarth, B., Jr., Alliston, C. W., and Ulberg, L. C.**, Importance of uterine environment on rabbit sperm prior to fertilization, *J. Anim. Sci.*, 24, 1027—1032, 1965.
161. **Burfening, P. J. and Ulberg, L. C.**, Embryonic survival subsequent to culture of rabbit spermatozoa at 38° and 40°C, *J. Reprod. Fertil.*, 15, 87—92, 1968.
162. **First, N. L., Stratman, F. W. S., and Casida, L. E.**, Effect of sperm age on embryo survival in swine, *J. Anim. Sci.*, 22, 135—138, 1963.
163. **Gwazdauskas, F. C., Abrams, R. M., Thatcher, W. W., Bazer, F. W., and Caton, D.**, Thermal changes of the bovine uterus following administration of estradiol-17β, *J. Anim. Sci.*, 39, 87—92, 1974.
164. **Roman-Ponce, H., Thatcher, W. W., Caton, D., Barron, D. H., and Wilcox, D. J.**, Thermal stress effects on uterine blood flow in dairy cows, *J. Anim. Sci.*, 46, 175—180, 1978.
165. **Roman-Ponce, H., Thatcher, W. W., Caton, D., Barron, D. H., and Wilcox, C. J.**, Effects of thermal stress and epinephrine on uterine blood flow in ewes, *J. Anim. Sci.*, 46, 167—174, 1978.
166. **Dickson, W. M., Basc, M. J., and Locatelli, A.**, Effect of estrogen and progesterone on uterine blood flow of castrate sows, *Am. J. Physiol.*, 217, 1431—1434, 1969.
167. **Anderson, S. G., Hackshaw, B. T., Still, J. G., and Greiss, J. C.**, Uterine blood flow and its distribution after chronic estrogen and progesterone administration, *Am. J. Obstet. Gynecol.*, 127, 138—142, 1977.
168. **Vaught, L. W., Monty, D. E., and Foote, W. C.**, Effect of summer heat stress on serum luteinizing hormone and progesterone values in Holstein-Friesian cows in Arizona, *Am. J. Vet. Res.*, 38, 1027—1030, 1977.
169. **Thatcher, W. W. and Chenault, J.R.**, Reproductive physiological responses of cattle to exogenous prostaglandin $F_{2}\alpha$, *J. Dairy Sci.*, 59, 1366—1375, 1976.
170. **Lippe, M. B. and Szego, C. M.**, Participation of adrenocortical hyperactivity in the suppressive effect of systemic actinomycin D on uterine stimulation by oestrogen, *Nature (London)*, 207, 272—274, 1965.

171. **Fowler, D. G. and Setchell, B. P.,** Selecting merino rams for ability to withstand infertility caused by heat. II. The effect of heat on scrotal and testicular blood flow, *Aust. J. Exp. Agric. Anim. Husb.,* 11, 143—147, 1971.
172. **Dutt, R. H., Sand, R. J., and Singh, B.,** Changes in testis blood flow, the spermatic artery and prostaglandin $F_{2}\alpha$ content in testis tissue of heat stressed rams, *Int. J. Biometeorol.,* 21, 75—84, 1977.
173. **Gomes, W. R., Butler, W. R., and Johnson, A. D.,** Effect of elevated ambient temperature on testis and blood levels and in vitro biosynthesis of testosterone in the ram, *J. Anim. Sci.,* 33, 804—807, 1971.
174. **Wettemann, R. P., Wells, M. E., Brock, L. W., Johnson, R. K., Harp, R., and Vencl, R.,** Recovery of normal semen quality after heat stress of boars, *Okla. Agric. Exp. Sta. Misc. Publ.,* 101, 152—156, 1977.
175. **Ortavant, R. and Loir, M.,** The Environment as a Factor in Reproduction in Farm Animals, World Congr. Anim. Prod., Buenos Aires, August 1978.
176. **Blaxter, K. L.,** Nutrition and climatic stress in farm animals, *Proc. Nutr. Soc.,* 17, 191—197, 1958.
177. **Heitman, H., Jr. and Hughes, E. H.,** The effects of temperature and relative humidity on the physiological well being of swine, *J. Anim. Sci.,* 8, 171—181, 1949.
178. **Brody, S.,** Temperature in life processes, in *Bioenergetics and Growth,* Hafner Press, New York, 1945, chap. 11.
179. **Colditz, P. J. and Kellaway, R. C.,** The effect of diet and heat stress on feed intake, growth and nitrogen metabolism in Friesian, F_1 Brahman × Friesian, and Brahman heifers, *Aust. J. Agric. Res.,* 23, 717—725, 1972.
180. **Andersson, B. and Larsson, B.,** Influence of local temperature changes in the preoptic area and rastral hypothalamus on the regulation of food and water intake, *Acta Physiol. Scand.,* 52, 75—89, 1961.
181. **McDowell, R. E.,** The role of livestock in the warm climates, in *Improvement of Livestock Production In Warm Climates,* W. H. Freeman & Co., San Francisco, 1972, chap. 4.
182. **Vohnout, K. and Bateman, I. V.,** Effects of crude fiber upon feeding efficiency of cattle in "warm" environments, *J. Agric. Sci.,* 78, 413—416, 1972.
183. **Ingram, D. L.,** Adaptations to ambient temperature in growing pigs, *Pflügers Arch.,* 367, 257—264, 1977.
184. **Macleod, P., Anderson, E. O., and Plastridge, W. N.,** Cell counts of platform samples of herd milk, *J. Dairy Sci.,* 37, 919—923, 1954.
185. **Paape, M. J., Schultze, W. D., Miller, R. H., and Smith, J. W.,** Thermal stress and circulating erythrocytes, leucocytes and milk somatic cells, *J. Dairy Sci.,* 56, 84—91, 1973.
186. **Paape, M. J., Kral, A. J., Desjaredins, C., Schultze, W. D., and Miller, R. H.,** Failure of either corticosteroids, or ACTH to increase the leukocyte concentration in milk, *Am. J. Vet. Res.,* 34, 353—356, 1973.
187. **Wegner, T. N., Schuh, J. D., Nelson, F. E., and Stott, G. H.,** Effect of stress on blood leucocyte and milk somatic cell counts in dairy cows, *J. Dairy Sci.,* 59, 949—956, 1976.
188. **Paape, M., Wergin, W. P., Guidry, A. J., and Pearson, R. E.,** Leukocytes — the second line of defense against invading mastitis pathogens, *J. Dairy Sci.,* 61, 1510—1522, 1978.
189. **Patt, J. A., Jr.,** Factors affecting the duration of intestinal permeability to macromolecules in newborn animals, *Biol. Rev.,* 52, 411—429, 1977.
190. **Sasaki, M., Davis, C. L., and Larson, B. L.,** Immunoglobulin IgGI metabolism in newborn calves, *J. Dairy Sci.,* 60, 623—626. 1977.
191. **Boyd, J. W.,** The relationship between serum immune globulin deficiency and disease in calves. A farm survey, *Vet. Rec.,* 90, 645—649, 1972.
192. **McGuire, T. C., Pfeiffer, N. E., Weikel, J. M., and Bartsch, R. C.,** Failure of colostral immunoglubulin transfer in calves dying from infectious disease, *J. Am. Vet. Med. Assoc.,* 169, 713—718, 1976.
193. **Naylor, J. M., Kronfeld, D. S., Bech-Nielsen, S., and Bartholomew, R. C.,** Plasma total protein measurement for prediction of disease and mortality in calves, *J. Am. Vet. Med. Assoc.,* 171, 635—638, 1977.
194. **Stott, G. H., Wiersma, F., Menefee, B. E., and Radwanski, F. R.,** Influence of environment on passive immunity in calves, *J. Dairy Sci.,* 59, 1306—1311, 1976.
195. **Collier, R. J., Thatcher, W. W., and Wilcox, C. J.,** unpublished observations.
196. **Vaught, L. W., Monty, D. E., Jr., and Foote, W. C.,** Effect of summer heat stress on serum luteinizing hormone and progesterone values in Holstein-Friesian cows in Arizona, *Am. J. Vet. Res.,* 38(7), 1027—1030, 1977.

AIR ENVIRONMENT AND ANIMAL PERFORMANCE

S. E. Curtis and J. G. Drummond

Rearing domestic animals under conditions of complete confinement subjects them to surroundings quite unlike their natural environments. Complete confinement limits the animal's opportunity to seek more favorable environs, thus intensifying animal-environmental factors. The trend toward enclosed housing has led to the recognition of air quality as a potentially critical element in animal production.[1]

Air pollutants of most importance to animal production differ from those of greatest concern to human health. Pollutants arising from industrial processes and internal-combustion engines are of prime concern to public health workers. Most air pollutants related to animal production result from normal animal functions, production practices, or both. Thus, many air factors affecting animals originate in the animals themselves.

In addition to normal atmospheric components, air in animal quarters contains exotic substances, as well as natural components in excess. They may be gases, liquid droplets, or solid particles; organic or inorganic; viable or nonviable; noxious, pathogenic, or inert — and there are several feasible permutations of these characterizations. Enclosure of animals lessens dilution of these atmospheric factors, especially when other considerations such as energy conservation and economics dictate low ventilation rates.

Air pollutants may exert both direct and indirect effects on animal performance. Indirect effects seem to be more important, but animal homeokinesis may be more directly coupled with air environment than is now appreciated. The respiratory tract is, of course, a prime target of air pollutants, and some effects on performance could owe indirectly to effects on this system. If certain pollutants reach the animal's circulation, they might affect metabolism, function, and health — and, hence, nutrient requirements and performance of the animal.

Hazen[2] noted that criteria for air quality in animal quarters are unestablished, despite the animal-house designer's need for them. Although speculation abounds regarding deleterious air-pollutant effects on animal performance, there exists no definitive knowledge of any.[3] Not enough specific data have accumulated to permit formulation of design guidelines.

Since poultry confinement preceded livestock confinement, poultrymen encountered confinement-induced constraints on performance before livestock producers did. This holds for air environment just as it does for other factors of production. Available recommendations for air-factor limits in poultry environments[3] do not necessarily apply to livestock environments. Interspecific inferences are tempting but impermissible. (It is fortunate that animal scientists can use pertinent species experimentally.) Further reservations accompany application of limits established for human workers to domestic animals. Workers confront industrial environments for relatively short, intermittent periods, whereas confined animals are exposed to polluted air environments almost continuously. In addition, food animals must oftentimes face more than one potentially harmful air factor simultaneously.

Air pollutants may affect animal performance, but definitive experimental elucidation of their roles remains to be carried out. We recognize effects of acutely noxious levels of certain factors, but such high levels occur infrequently — usually only in cases of electrical or mechanical failure. The effects of more or less continuous exposure of animals to levels and combinations of air pollutants practically encountered are of much greater significance to the animal producer.

IDENTIFYING AIR FACTORS

Animals' air environments contain dusts, liquid droplets, microbes, gases, "odors," and ions. Industrial hygienists have developed techniques for measuring these pollutants in the field.[4]

Airborne particles are either solid or liquid. Dust particles range in diameter from more than 0.1 mm — that is, visible — to less than 1 μm; most are larger than 10 μm. They arise from feed, bedding, excreta, concrete, skin, and skin secretions. The period during which a particle remains airborne is determined by its settling velocity, which is inversely related to particle surface to mass ratio, and hence directly related to size.[5]

Droplets result from passage of an airstream over a liquid: a wave is caught up, a ligament forms, it breaks, and the detached mass coheres to form a droplet. In a sneeze, air speed reaches 100 m/sec. As many as 40,000 droplets are formed per sneeze. Most have an initial diameter of around 10 μm, but quickly evaporate to form smaller "droplet nuclei."[5] Droplet nuclei are potentially dangerous because particles less than 10 μm in aerodynamic diameter (the diameter of an aerodynamically equivalent sphere of unit density) remain suspended in the air for hours and can settle deep in the respiratory tree.[6]

Airborne dusts and droplets may be collected by filtration, surface or liquid impingement, electric or thermal precipitation, settling, or centrifugation. Various sampling devices are commercially available.[7]

Dusts and droplets often carry microbes that can invade the respiratory system. Many samplers have been devised for measuring the concentration of viable bacteria in air.[8] Especially useful are the Andersen sampler, which sizes as well as counts viable bacteria-carrying particles, and the Greenburg-Smith impinger, which estimates total viable airborne-bacterial count, since particles containing more than one bacterium disintegrate upon impingement in this system.

Gaseous pollutants — especially CO_2, CH_4, NH_3, and H_2S — arise in enclosed animal houses from excreta decomposition and respiratory excretion. Numerous other compounds have also been identified in the atmosphere of enclosed animal houses (Table 1).

Odor is a physiological response to airborne compounds; thus, the most reliable meter is the nose of the pertinent species. Odor thresholds for many compounds — mostly hydrocarbons containing sulfur or nitrogen — have been determined in humans,[9] but they will be more difficult to ascertain directly in livestock. Many of the constituents of animal-house odors have been identified (Table 2).

Air ions are negatively or positively charged molecules (usually O_2^- and CO_2^+) or molecular groups (an ion surrounded by neutral molecules of the same element or compound). They may be gaseous or particulate. Small ions (0.001 to 0.005 μm in diameter) are formed by forces — such as solar or cosmic radiation or mechanical stress — capable of displacing electrons from atomic orbits. Several small ions combine with an airborne particle to form a large ion (0.015 to 0.10 μm). Ion content of air can be measured by specialized equipment.[15]

SURVEY STUDIES

Available evidence regarding levels of air pollutants found in enclosed animal houses is limited and fragmentary. Aerial dust levels measured over a 15-month period in 5 swine houses at an agricultural experiment station were generally lower than those observed in 11 houses at five commercial operations.[16] Dust level in the houses was significantly and negatively correlated with median outside temperature. Of course,

Table 1
COMPOUNDS IDENTIFIED IN THE AIR FROM THE ANAEROBIC DECOMPOSITION OF LIVESTOCK AND POULTRY MANURE

Alcohols	Isobutyraldehyde
Methanol	Hexanal
Ethanol	Acetone
2-Propanol	3-Pentanone
n-Butanol	Formaldehyde
n-Propanol	Heptaldehyde
Isobutanol	Valeraldehyde
Isopentanol	Octaldehyde
	Decaldehyde
Acids	
Butyric	Esters
Acetic	Methyl formate
Propionic	Methyl acetate
Isobutyric	Isopropyl acetate
Isovaleric	Isobutyl acetate
	Isopropyl propionate
Amines	Propyl acetate
Methylamine	*n*-Butyl acetate
Ethylamine	
Trimethylamine	Sulfides
Triethylamine	Dimethyl sulfide
	Diethyl sulfide
Fixed gases	
Carbon dioxide	Disulfides
Methane	
Ammonia	Mercaptans
Hydrogen sulfide	Methyl mercaptan
Carbonyls	Nitrogen heterocycles
Acetaldehyde	Indole
Propronaldehyde	Skatole

From J. R. Miner, Odors from Confined Livestock Production, EPA-660/2-74-023 Environ. Prot. Agency Techn. Ser., 1974, 125 pp.

Table 2
IMPORTANT CONSTITUENTS OF ANIMAL HOUSE ODORS

Compounds	Ref.
Ammonia, hydrogen sulfide	10
Butyric acid	11
Amines, sulfides	12
Indole, skatole, mercaptans, sulfides	13
Dimethyl sulfide	14

fluctuations in aerial dust level probably owed only indirectly to the outside temperature; they probably resulted from variation in building-ventilation rate in response to weather changes.[17] Aerial dust in swine houses appears to be mainly feed dust,[18,19] while in poultry houses, it appears to be composed to a greater extent of feather and skin debris.[20] Animal-house dust is usually considered to be "inert." When inhaled, "inert dust" causes no change in air-space architecture, no significant formation of collagen, and no irreversible tissue reactions.[21] The human threshold-limit value* for inert aerial dust is 10 mg m^{-3}.

Measurements of aerial bacterial colony-forming particles (BCFP) have been made in various animal houses (Table 3). In the animal houses studies, aerial BCFP levels were generally higher at ground level and animal respiratory level than at human respiratory level.[25,27]

Lebeda[28] found no significant difference between the level of aerial BCFP in the morning and afternoon in the swine house he studied, but samples were collected only twice daily. Continuous monitoring of aerial BCFP numbers within two swine houses indicated that aerial BCFP concentration tended to increase in the afternoon, but the concentration at a given hour was unpredictable even within a building.[16] Aerial BCFP levels are affected by activity of the animals within the house.[22,29,30] Agitation of bedding in a hog house increased aerial BCFP counts from 10^5 m^{-3} to 10^6 m^{-3} in one case.[22] In general, daily variation in aerial BCFP concentration has been found to be less than the variation observed during studies of longer duration (e.g., a farrowing period or 1 year).[16]

Annual fluctuations of aerial BCFP levels observed in the experiment-station swine houses discussed earlier were similar to the observed fluctuations in aerial dust levels. In general, the lower the outside temperature, the higher the aerial BCFP levels in the swine houses. This probably was due in large part to different ventilation rates during periods of cool and warm weather.

Aerial humidity and bacterial levels in swine houses are inversely related.[22,31,32] A direct relation exists between bacterial concentration on surfaces and in the air in poultry hatcheries.[33] Hence, time changes in aerial BCFP level may reflect changes in bacterial contamination of surfaces in other animal houses as well. Aerial BCFP level increased linearly in farrowing rooms over farrowing periods lasting several weeks.[34] The rooms were emptied and cleaned between farrowing periods. Aerial BCFP level increased at a faster rate in a broiler-chicken house after introduction of birds than in the farrowing rooms.[35] Goodrich et al[30] found that the high levels of aerial BCFP in two enclosed cattle units could be attributed almost entirely to the presence of the animals. When the animals were removed from the buildings, aerial BCFP levels fell within 1 hr to levels closely approximating those of the outside environment even though the oxidation ditch remained in operation.

Staphylococci have been reported to be the predominant aerial bacteria found in animal houses, while aerial coliforms appear to be scarce.[19,22,25,26,30,35,36] Elliot et al.[25] found that only 458 of 1112 colonies (41%) isolated on a staphylococcus special medium were actually staphylococci when tested biochemically. Only 5 of their 458 staphylococcal isolates were coagulose-positive. Fecal streptococci are found in much greater numbers in animal-house air than are fecal coliforms; the ratio in feces is much closer.[23] Hence, fecal streptococci may be better able to survive the rigors of aerosolization than are the coliforms.

Important air pollutants that have been identified in enclosed animal quarters include NH_3, H_2S, CH_4, and CO_2.[10] In the particular swine houses sampled, CO_2 level was less than 1000 ppm,[37-39] NH_3 level varied from 6 to 35 ppm,[38-40] and H_2S level was less than 10 ppm.[38,39,41] Ammonia level was higher in swine houses with solid floors than in those with slotted floors.[42] Average levels of non-ammonia-N compounds in

* Airborne concentrations of substances which represent conditions under which it is believed that nearly all workers may be repeatedly exposed day after day without adverse effect.[21]

Table 3
AERIAL BACTERIAL COLONY FORMING PARTICLE (BCFP) LEVELS IN ANIMAL HOUSES

Type of house	Common logarithm of aerial BCFP level (no/m³)		Ref.
	Range	Mean ± SE	
Swine			
Enclosed	4.21—5.36	4.77 ± 0.07	22
	2.78—3.33	3.12 ± 0.07	23
	—	5.87	24
	3.77—6.05	5.01 ± 0.03	16
	4.45—6.45	—	25
Modified open-front	3.52—5.08	4.33 ± 0.06	16
Various commercial	4.46—6.20	5.45 ± 0.07	16
Dairy cow			
Enclosed	—	4.54	26
Beef cattle			
Enclosed	—	5.21	27

the air ranged from two to several times higher than ammonia-N levels.[39] Non-ammonia-N compounds include amines and amine-related compounds, which are important constituents of animal-house odor. Gaseous air-pollutant concentrations decrease with distance above the manure pit.[39] The noxious-gas content of animal-house air depends, of course, upon ventilation rate.[38]

DEPOSITION STUDIES

The nature of deposition of air pollutants in the respiratory tract has not been systematically studied in livestock, but results with other species probably hold in general. Slow, deep breathing (hyperpnea) favors deep penetration and impingement of air in alveoli; rapid, shallow breathing (polypnea) favors deposition in the upper respiratory tract. The level within the respiratory tract at which a particle deposits also depends upon the particle's aerodynamic diameter. Those with aerodynamic diameters on the order of 10 μm or larger — such as most aerial dusts in animal houses — are efficiently removed from inspired air in the nose by either settling or impinging onto mucosal surfaces.[43] Bacteria deposited in the nose can infect that region or be subsequently aspirated into the lungs. Smaller particles deposit maximally in progressively lower portions of the respiratory tree. Many of the particles less than 5 μm in aerodynamic diameter reach terminal bronchioles and alveoli, and many are retained there.[6,44]

Results obtained when particle deposition was studied in chickens parallel the observations in mammals.[45] The largest particles (3.7 to 7 μm) deposited in the head and anterior trachea, 1.1-μm particles deposited mainly in the lung and posterior air sacs, 0.3-μm particles tended to pass through the posterior sacs to the anterior sacs, and the smallest particles tended to deposit in the caudal region of the air-sac system.

Gases, odoriferous molecules, and ions contact the respiratory tract along its entire length. Their concentrations in inspired air decrease as the lung is approached, depending upon their relative solubilities in mucus. Ammonia, for example, readily dissolves in water and thus in mucus.[46] Soluble factors absorbed into mucus deep in the tract more readily diffuse into capillaries.

RESPIRATORY TRACT DEFENSES

The mechanisms by which the respiratory tract defends itself against impinging air factors have recently been reviewed.[47] Although respiratory tract linings are susceptible to various noxious agents, two vigorous defense mechanisms ordinarily maintain the integrity of these tissues: the mucociliary apparatus and alveolar phagocytes.

The mucociliary apparatus comprises a blanket of mucus atop ciliated epithelium extending from nose to bronchioles. Mucus contains bactericidins such as lysozyme. Particles or molecules entrapped in the mucus are transported by ciliary beating[48] — either down from the nose or up from the lower tract — toward the pharynx, where the mucus collects before being swallowed.

Coughing aids in delivering secretions from the lower tract. The epiglottic reflex helps prevent aspiration of contaminated mucus from the upper tract into the lungs.

Secretion rate and viscosity of mucus, as well as ciliary activity, determine mucociliary-clearance rate. Mucus both dilutes irritating substances and aids in their transport. Upon irritation, respiratory-mucosal surfaces generally increase mucus production and flow rate in defensive reaction. Somewhat ironically, however, very large amounts of mucus have been believed to increase the chances of lung infection.[49] Goblet cells produce mucus, and chronic irritation leads to hyperplasia and hypertrophy of bronchial goblet cells.

Free phagocytes[50] engulf particles, including bacteria, that reach alveoli. Alveolar phagocytosis thus comprises the prime defender of the lungs against infection and disease.[51] Phagocytes either eventually arrive with their contents at the mucus to be escalated to the pharynx or enter pulmonary lymphatics.[52] Many factors are known to influence the rate of bacterial clearance from the lung, including animal species,[53] bacterial species[54] and strain,[53] hypoxia, cold stress, ethanolic intoxication,[54] NO_2 exposure,[55] starvation,[56] and concurrent viral infection.[57,58] In experiments dealing specifically with livestock — particularly pigs — cold stress, age of pig, and exposure to aerial NH_3 depressed pulmonary clearance.[59,60] Pulmonary bacterial clearance in calves followed a pattern similar to that observed in laboratory animals.[61] Induced pulmonary edema decreased pulmonary bacterial clearance, while immunization led to increased clearance.[58]

EFFECTS OF AIR FACTORS — EXPERIMENTAL EXPOSURES

Few experiments have examined the effects of air factors on performance and health of livestock in practical environments. Infectious respiratory disease deleteriously affects performance.[62] Under certain experimental conditions, air factors have damaged respiratory tissues[63] and impaired resistance to lung disease[64] in laboratory animals.

Although not an important animal-house air pollutant, the effect of sulfur dioxide on the respiratory tract has been studied in swine. Results were conflicting, however; one group reported the development of pulmonary lesions following SO_2 exposure,[65] while another reported no lesions.[66] Interestingly, while SO_2 exposure increased goblet-cell density in rats,[67] exposure of young pigs led to the disappearance of tracheal and turbinate goblet cells.[66]

More common animal-house air pollutants such as NH_3 and H_2S are of greater concern to livestock producers. In laboratory animals, exposure to aerial NH_3 increased respiratory mucus output[68] and impaired mucociliary activity.[69] Exposure of healthy pigs to atmospheric NH_3 at concentrations of 50 or 75 ppm had little or no effect on rate of body-weight gain and respiratory tract structure.[70] Aerial HN_3 alone at 100 ppm both did[71] and did not[72] affect respiratory tissues in pigs in separate experiments.

In the former study, it was noted that the thickness of nasal and tracheal epithelium increased and goblet-cell numbers decreased. However, no changes were observed in the bronchial epithelium or in the alveoli of exposed pigs. These researchers found no adverse effect of NH_3 at 100 ppm on appetite or daily gain. On the other hand, Stombaugh et al.[72] did find an adverse effect of such treatment on performance. Aerial NH_3 at concentrations of 100 ppm or more decreased feed consumption and average daily gain, but did not affect the efficiency of feed conversion. Similarly, Drummond et al.[107] found a 12% reduction in growth rate of pigs subjected to NH_3 at an aerial concentration of 50 ppm, 2nd 30% at 100 or 150 ppm.

Poultry appear to be more sensitive to the effects of atmospheric NH_3 than are pigs. Exposure to 20-ppm aerial NH_3 for 6 weeks produced gross and histopathologic damage to the respiratory tract of chickens.[73] Chickens exposed to aerial NH_3 at 100 ppm also had depressed growth and feed consumption.[74] Exposure to aerial NH_3 at 25 or 50 ppm coupled with infectious bronchitis vaccination led to reduced body weights and feed efficiencies in chicks.[75,76] Weights of bursac of Fabricius and lungs, as well as number of air-sac lesions, were higher in ammonia-exposed birds.[75] Aerial NH_3 is thought to be the cause of a variety of ocular lesions in chickens kept on litter.[77]

Hydrogen sulfide levels (8.5 ppm) higher than those routinely encountered in commercial swine houses had little or no effect on the pigs' rate of gain.[70] Aerial H_2S may have important, even lethal, secondary effects, but the levels of aerial H_2S known to induce such effects[65] are much higher than those in the above study. Hydrogen sulfide at 2 ppm in combination with aerial NH_3 at 50 ppm also had little effect on pig growth rate.[70]

Particulate air pollutants, either alone or in combination with gases, also concern livestock producers. Exposure to swine-house dust at levels as high as or higher than those usually encountered in practice had little or no effect on rate of gain or respiratory tract structure in pigs.[70] This substantiated earlier work in which pigs were exposed to either aerial corn dust[78] or aerial cornstarch.[71] In the latter study, however, the concentration of dust particles less than 3 μm in diameter (particles able to reach the lung) was about the same in the control and dust-treatment chambers. The increased aerial dust load in the experimental atmosphere owed to particles in the 3 to 10 μm range — particles which impinge on upper respiratory surfaces. In the Illinois study,[70] on the other hand, about half of the dust particles added to the air in the dust-treatment chambers were 5 μm or less in diameter and thus able to reach and deposit in the lower respiratory tract. In still another study, dust particles (of which approximately 90% were larger than 10 μm) increased the incidence and severity of air sacculitis in turkeys.[74] The dust exposure in this study led to loss of tracheal cilia and increased density of tracheal goblet cells.

Jericho and Harries[79] attempted to relate an outbreak of acute respiratory disease to the dusty feed being given the pigs. However, an attempt to experimentally reproduce this respiratory disease via controlled exposure to dusty feed failed.[80]

The respiratory tract lining normally is covered with aqueous mucus. Thus, gases that are highly soluble in water (such as NH_3) are absorbed from the inspired air by the upper respiratory tract mucus. Hence, gaseous NH_3 rarely penetrates to the lungs. However, aerial dust in animal houses absorbs and carries gases.[10,81] Aerial gases may thus be transported to the lungs by dust particles small enough to be carried into them.[46]

When particles containing compounds such as NH_3 deposit on respiratory linings, they serve to increase the concentration of the absorbed compounds at that point.[82] This may be unfortunate, as when the particles are small enough to penetrate to alveoli; but it may also be advantageous, as when the particles are quite efficient in absorbing the gas and large enough to deposit in relatively well-protected regions such as the nose. When particulate penetration exceeds vapor penetration, toxicity is increased, and vice versa.[46]

A combination of aerial NH_3, CO_2, and dust (half or more of the particles were larger than 10 μm) did not increase chickens' susceptibility to Newcastle disease virus,[83] whereas aerial NH_3 alone did.[84] Aerial NH_3 plus dust did not increase the incidence or severity of air sacculities in turkeys; dust alone did.[73] While aerial NH_3 (100 ppm) alone altered tracheal linings in pigs, aerial NH_3 plus dust (no particles less than 2 or 3 μm) did not.[71] Only when aerial dust was applied at a very high level (300 mg m^{-3}) did it affect the performance of pigs.[70] The effects of aerial dust and NH_3 in this study tended to be additive, but they did not interact; in particular, aerial dust apparently did not increase the assault of aerial ammonia on the pigs.

Another possible avenue of air-factor-related damage is by exacerbation of respiratory diseases. Air factors in swine houses may influence the incidence and severity of chronic pneumonia in pigs.[85,86] Ehrlich[87] felt that in cases where air-pollutant concentrations were low, respiratory tract damage might be inapparent unless the subject were challenged by an infectious microbe. Exposure to 30-ppm aerial NH_3 increased the susceptibility of chickens to Newcastle disease virus.[84] Multiplication of *Mycoplasma gallisepticum* was enhanced in tracheas of chicks inoculated with that agent and subsequently exposed to aerial NH_3 at 50 to 100 ppm.[88] Chicks exposed to aerial NH_3 had more severe histopathological changes of the trachea than did control birds, but no such changes were noted in the lungs. In the same study, chicks exposed to 20- or 50-ppm aerial NH_3 for 3 days prior to intratracheal inoculation with *M. gallisepticum* also showed enhanced multiplication of the agent within the trachea. This tendency was reduced in birds exposed to only 20-ppm NH_3. Aerial NH_3 has also been found to influence courses of *Bordatella bronchoseptica* and *Ascaris suum* infections in swine.[108,109]

Air factors may also influence the course of diseases outside of the respiratory tract. Broiler chickens infected with coccidia *Eimeria acervulina* and exposed to 50- or 100-ppm aerial NH_3 had decreased body-weight gains, but not different feed efficiencies, than infected, non-NH_3-exposed birds.[89] In another study, chickens were contact-exposed to birds infected with Marek's disease and then subjected to atmospheres with either high or low levels of "airborne decomposition products."[90] Atmospheric level of these products was monitored by measuring aerial NH_3, which ranged from as high as 70 ppm in the experimental cubicles to less than 15 ppm in the control cubicles. Atmospheric composition did not influence the incidence of Marek's disease lesions. In a similar study, the infection rate of chickens with Marek's disease was not altered by short-term (two 2-hr periods) aerial-NH_3 exposures (200 ppm).[91]

AIR FACTORS — EFFECTS ON RESPIRATORY ACTIVITY

Aerial NH_3, ordinarily considered a respiratory stimulant, elicited rapid, shallow breathing when present at high levels.[92] In contrast, NH_3 at 50 or 100 ppm lowered respiratory rate in rabbits by about 33%[93] and by 7 to 24% in chickens.[74] If, under practical conditions, respiratory activity decreased as a result of aerial NH_3, then respiratory evaporative rate might drop and thus alter heat balance in species dependent on respiratory evaporation (as opposed to sweat evaporation) in hot environments. Hence, metabolic rate might be decreased, which in turn might lower energetic efficiency for production.[74] Conversely, if the work of respiration increased, maintenance requirement would also increase, again perhaps decreasing productive efficiency.

AIR FACTORS — EFFECTS ON REPRODUCTIVE ACTIVITY

Swine in enclosed housing commonly display impaired reproductive performance.

While space restriction might be a crucial factor in this situation,[94] it is of interest that olfactory bulbectomy adversely affected reproductive function in 15 of 24 sows.[95] Thus, apart from possible indirect effects of air factors, olfactory stimuli necessary for normal reproduction[96] may be altered by air factors in enclosed animal quarters.

AIR FACTORS — EFFECTS OF AIR IONS

Particulate challenge to animals held within enclosed houses is great. One means of reducing this pollutant load is air ionization. In general, one would expect that the air-ionization process would be most useful and effective in relatively dusty animal houses. Nevertheless, in relatively low-dust-level swine houses, a commercially available air-ionization system was found to reduce aerial dust level by about two thirds and aerial-bacterial level by about one half.[97] In a study using experimentally generated bacterial aerosols, negatively ionized air reduced the concentration of airborne microbes.[98] Levels of airborne *Serratia marcescens* and *Escherichia coli* were reduced on the average of 84% and 89%, respectively. However, despite the reduced air-pollutant levels, no performance differences were noted between pigs held in ionized atmospheres and those held in nonionized atmospheres.[99]

In addition to possible indirect effects of air ionization on animal performance, small negative air ions may have direct beneficial effects on animal function and behavior. Improved growth rate and reduced aggressiveness have been observed when other species of animals have been exposed to negative air ions, yet this remains a controversial subject. Furthermore, it is doubtful whether, in practical animal-production systems and using the ionization equipment now available, many of the small negative air ions actually reach the animals. One beneficial result of reducing air pollution by air ionization that has been noticed by many animal producers has been an improvement in working conditions in the animal house. Again, this effect would be most apparent in houses with especially dusty atmospheres.

AIR FACTORS — FUTURE RESEARCH

The significance of the topic — air environment and animal performance — is still controversial. Practically occurring levels and combinations of air factors need further characterization. This information is needed to facilitate the design of experiments to ascertain the effects of air factors on livestock. Here again we can benefit from the experience of industrial hygienists. Necessary techniques have been developed by scientists in other disciplines, but they will require specific adaptation to problems in animal science. Perhaps the most critical element is exposure-chamber design, particularly as regards animal volume in relation to total exposure-zone volume, which should be 5% or less, and homogeneity of pollutant concentrations in that space. Inadequate chamber design, of course, jeopardizes inferences from all results. U.S. Public Health Service personnel have thoroughly discussed chamber design.[100] The dynamic-type chambers they have developed[101] can be used to expose animals to all air factors except ions.[102] Auxiliary equipment is needed to condition supply air and to aerosolize dusts,[103] liquids, and bacterial suspensions;[104] to prepare gaseous test atmospheres;[105] introduce odoriferous compounds; or to generate airborne ions.[106]

CONCLUSION

One can conclude from the preceding discussion that the potential for air-pollutant effects on the health and productivity of food animals exists, but as yet, no such effects have been clearly defined. As more knowledge of the relations between food animals and the air environments they face in practical management systems accumulates, designers and operators of modern animal facilities will gain better guidelines for satisfactory air quality.

REFERENCES

1. **Curtis, S. E.,** *J. Anim. Sci.,* 35, 628—634, 1972.
2. **Hazen, T. E.,** *J. Anim. Sci.,* 32, 584—589, 1971.
3. **Lillie, R. J.,** *Air Pollutants Affecting the Performance of Domestic Animals, U.S. Dep. Agric. Agric. Handb. No. 380,* 1970, 14.
4. **Anon.,** *Air Sampling Instruments for Evaluation of Atmospheric Contaminants,* 3rd ed., American Conference of Governmental Industrial Hygienists, Cincinnati, 1966, A-1-1—B-10-48.
5. **Wells, W. F.,** *Airborne Contagion and Air Hygiene,* Harvard University Press, Cambridge, 1955, 13—19.
6. **Hatch, T. F.,** *Bacteriol. Rev.,* 25, 237—240, 1961.
7. **Silverman, L.,** in *Air Sampling Instruments for Evaluation of Atmospheric Contaminants,* 3rd ed., American Conference of Governmental Industrial Hygienists, Cincinnati, 1966, A-1-1—A-1-16.
8. **Wolf, H. W., Skaliy, P., Hall, L. B., Harris, M. M., Decker, H. M., Buchanan, L. M., and Dahlgren, C. M.,** Sampling microbiological aerosols, *U.S. Publ. Health Serv. Publ. Health Monogr.,* 60, 18—53, 1959.
9. **Byrd, J. F. and Phelps, A. H., Jr.,** in *Air Pollution,* Vol. 2, Stern, A. C., Ed., Academic Press, New York, 1968, 305—327.
10. **Day, D. L., Hansen, E. L., and Andersen, S.,** *Trans. Am. Soc. Agric. Eng.,* 8, 118—121, 1965.
11. **Deibel, R. H.,** in *Agriculture and the Quality of Our Environment,* Brady, N. C., Ed., American Association for the Advancement of Science, Washington, D.C., 1967, 395—399.
12. **Merkel, J. A., Hazen, T. E., and Miner, J. R.,** *Trans. Am. Soc. Agric. Eng.,* 12, 310—315, 1969.
13. **Burnett, W. E.,** *Environ. Sci. Technol.,* 3, 744—749, 1969.
14. **White, R. K., Taiganides, E. P., and Cole, G. D.,** in *Livestock Waste Management and Pollution Abatement. Proceedings of the International Symposium on Livestock Waste Management,* American Society of Agricultural Engineers, St. Joseph, Mi., 1971, 110—113.
15. **Corn, M.,** in *Air Pollution,* Vol. 1, Stern, A. C., Ed., Academic Press, New York, 1968, 47—94.
16. **Curtis, S. E., Drummond, J. G., Kelley, K. W., Grunloh, D. J., Meares, V. J., Norton, H. W., and Jensen, A. H.,** *J. Anim. Sci.,* 41, 1502—1511, 1975.
17. **Bresk, B. and Stolpe, J.,** *Monatsh. Verterinaermed.,* 30, 572—576, 1975.
18. **Hovmand, H. C. and Slot, P.,** *Acta Vet. Scand.,* 9, 86—89, 1968.
19. **Curtis, S. E., Drummond, J. G., Grunloh, D. J., Lynch, P. B., and Jensen, A. H.,** *J. Anim. Sci.,* 41, 1512—1520, 1975.
20. **Rollo, C. A., Howes, J. R., and Grub, W.,** *Dust Production of Poultry Litter Materials,* Circ. 169, Auburn University Agricultural Experimental Station, Auburn, Alabama, 1969, 1—15.
21. **Anon.,** *Industrial Ventilation: A Manual of Recommended Practice,* 11th ed., American Conference of Governmental Industrial Hygienists, Cincinnati, 1970, 13-1—13-2.
22. **Gordon, W. A. M.,** *Br. Vet. J.,* 119, 263—273, 1963.
23. **Hill, I. R. and Kenworthy, R.,** *J. Appl. Bacteriol.,* 33, 299—316, 1970.
24. **Fiser, A.,** *Acta Vet. (Brno),* 39, 273—286, 1970.
25. **Elliot, L. F., McCalla, T. M., and DeShazer, J. A.,** *Appl. Environ. Microbiol.,* 32, 270—273, 1976.
26. **Benham, C. L. and Egdell, J. W.,** *J. Soc. Dairy Technol.,* 23, 91—94, 1970.
27. **Goodrich, P. R., Spier, S. L., Diesch, S. L., and Will, L. A.,** in *Livestock Environment. Proceedings of the International Livestock Environment Symposium,* American Society of Agricultural Engineers, St. Joseph, Mi., 1974, 189—194.
28. **Lebeda, D. L.,** *Air Pollutants in Swine Buildings,* M. Sci. thesis, University of Illinois at Urbana-Champaign, 1964.
29. **Magwood, S. E.,** *Poult. Sci.,* 43, 441—449, 1964.
30. **Goodrich, P. R., Diesch, S. L., and Jacobson, L. D.,** in *Managing Livestock Wastes. Proceedings of the 3rd International Symposium on Livestock Wastes,* American Society of Agricultural Engineers, St. Joseph, Mi., 1975, 7—10.
31. **Tonks, H. M. Smith, W. C., and Bruce, J. M.,** *Vet. Rec.,* 90, 531—537, 1972.

32. Beer, K., Melhorn, G., and Arnold, H., *Monatsh. Veterinaermed.*, 30, 406—409, 1975.
33. Magwood, S. E., and Marr, H., *Poult. Sci.*, 43, 1558—1566, 1964.
34. Grunloh, D. J., Curtis, S. E., Jensen, A. H., Simon, J., and Harmon, B. G., *J. Anim. Sci.*, 33(Abstr.), 1139, 1971.
35. Carlson, H. C. and Whenham, G. R., *Avian Dis.*, 12, 297—302, 1968.
36. LeBars, J., *Rech. Vet.* 1, 141—166, 1968.
37. Lebeda, D. L., Day, D. L., and Hayakawa, I., *Paper 64—940, American Society of Agricultural Engineers, St. Joseph, Mi., 1964.*
38. Robertson, A. M. and Galbraith, H., *Farm Building R and D Studies* (1), Scottish Farm Buildings Investigation Unit, Craibstone, Scotland, 1971, 17—28.
39. Elliot, L. F., DeShazer, J. A., Peo, E. R., Jr., Travis, T. A., and McCalla, T. M., in *Livestock Environment. Proceedings of the International Livestock Environment Symposium,* American Society of Agricultural Engineers, St. Joseph, Mi., 1974, 189—194.
40. Miner, J. R. and Hazen, T. E., *Paper 68—910, American Society of Agricultural Engineers, St. Joseph, Mi., 1968.*
41. Lebeda, D. L. and Day, D. L., *Ill. Res.*, 7, 15, 1965.
42. Day, D. L., *Ill. Agr. Exp. Sta. Publ., AS -624, 1965.*
43. Boyland, E., Gaddum, J. H., and McDonald, F. F., *J. Hyg.*, 45, 290—296, 1947.
44. Hatch, T. F. and Gross, P., *Pulmonary Deposition and Retention of Inhaled Aerosols,* Academic Press, New York, 1964, 61—67.
45. Hayter, R. B. and Besch, E. L., *Poult. Sci.*, 53, 1507—1511, 1974.
46. LaBelle, C. W., Long, J. E., and Christofano, E. E., *Arch. Ind. Health,* 11, 297—304, 1955.
47. Cohen, A. B. and Gold, W. M., *Annu. Rev. Physiol.*, 37, 325—350, 1975.
48. Litt, M., *Arch. Intern. Med.*, 126, 417—423, 1970.
49. Nungester, W. J. and Klepser, R. G., *J. Infect. Dis.*, 63, 94—102, 1938.
50. Brain, J. D., *Arch. Intern. Med.*, 126, 477—487, 1970.
51. Green, G. M., *Annu. Rev. Med.*, 19, 315—336, 1968.
52. Courtice, F. C., *Br. Med. Bull.*, 19, 76—79, 1963.
53. Southern, P. M., Jr., Pierce, A. K., and Sanford, J. P., *Appl. Microbiol.*, 21, 377—378, 1971.
54. Green, G. M. and Kass, E. H., *Br. J. Exp. Pathol.*, 46, 360—366, 1965.
55. Ehrlich, R., *Bacteriol. Rev.*, 30, 604—614, 1966.
56. Green, G. M. and Kass, E. H., *J. Clin. Invest.*, 43, 769—776, 1964.
57. Jakab, G. J. and Green, G. M., *J. Clin. Invest.*, 51, 1989—1998, 1972.
58. Gilka, F., Thomson, R. G., and Savan, M., *Can J. Comp. Med.*, 38, 251—259, 1974.
59. Curtis, S. E., Kingdon, D. A., Simon, J., and Drummond, J. G., *Am. J. Vet. Res.*, 37, 299—301, 1976.
60. Drummond, J. G., Curtis, S. E., Simon, J., and Jensen, A. H., *J. Anim. Sci.*, 39, 967 (Abstr.), 1974.
61. Lillie, L. E. and Thomson, R. G., *Can. J. Comp. Med.*, 36, 129—137, 1972.
62. Huhn, R. G., *Am. J. Vet. Res.*, 31, 1097—1108, 1970.
63. Gross, P., *Arch. Environ. Health,* 14, 883—891, 1967.
64. Rylander, R., *Arch. Intern. Med.*, 126, 496—499, 1970.
65. O'Donoghue, J. G. and Graesser, F. E., *Can. J. Comp. Med. Vet. Sci.*, 26, 255—263, 1962.
66. Martin, S. W. and Willoughby, R. A., *J. Am. Vet. Med. Assoc.*, 159, 1518—1522, 1971.
67. Lamb, D. and Reid, L., *J. Pathol. Bacteriol.*, 96, 97—111, 1968.
68. Boyd, E. M., MacLachlan, M. L., and Perry, W. E., *J. Indust. Hyg. Toxicol.*, 26, 29—34, 1944.
69. Dalhamn, T., *Acta Physiol. Scand. Suppl.*, 36, 1—161, 1956.
70. Curtis, S. E., Anderson, C. R., Simon, J., Jensen, A. H., Day, D. L., and Kelley, K. W., *J. Anim. Sci.* 41, 735—739, 1975.
71. Doig, P. A. and Willoughby, R. A., *J. Am. Vet. Med. Assoc.*, 159, 1353—1361, 1971.
72. Stombaugh, D. P., Teague, H. S., and Roller, W. L., *J. Anim. Sci.*, 28, 844—847, 1969.
73. Anderson, D. P., Wolfe, R. R., Cherms, F. L., and Roper, W. E., *Am. J. Vet. Res.*, 29, 1049—1058, 1968.
74. Charles, D. R. and Payne, C. G., *Br. Poult. Sci.*, 7, 177—187, 1966.
75. Kling, H. F. and Quarles, C. L., *Poult. Sci.*, 53, 1161—1167, 1974.
76. Quarles, C. L. and Kling, H. F., *Poult. Sci.*, 53, 1592—1596, 1974.
77. Wright, G. W. and Frank, J. F., *Can. J. Comp. Med. Vet. Sci.*, 21, 225—227, 1957.
78. Martin, S. W. and Willoughby, R. A., *Arch. Environ. Health,* 25, 158—165, 1972.
79. Jericho, K. W. F. and Harries, N., *Can. Vet. J.*, 16, 360—366, 1975.
80. Jericho, K. W. F., *Vet. Pathol.*, 12, 415—427, 1975.
81. Burnett, W. E., *Poult. Sci.*, 48, 182—185, 1969.

82. **Dalhamn, T. and Reid, L.**, in *Inhaled Particles and Vapours*, 2nd Ed., Davies, C. N., Ed., Pergamon Press, New York, 1966, 209—308.
83. **Anderson, D. P., Beard, C. W., and Hanson, R. P.**, *Avian Dis.*, 10, 177—188, 1966.
84. **Anderson, D. P., Beard, C. W., and Hanson, R. P.**, *Avian Dis.*, 8, 369—379, 1964.
85. **Jericho, K. W. F.**, *Vet. Rec.*, 82, 507—517, 1968.
86. **Kovács, F., Nagy, A., and Sallai, J.**, *Magy. Allatorv. Lapja*, 22, 496—505, 1967; *Vet. Bull. (London)*, 38, 727, 1968.
87. **Ehrlich, R.**, *Arch. Environ. Health*, 6, 638—642, 1963.
88. **Sato, S., Shoya, S., and Kobayashi, H.**, *Natl. Inst. Anim. Health Q.*, 13, 45—53, 1973.
89. **Quarles, C. L., Ransom, J. A., Fagerberg, D. J., and Migaki, T. T.**, in *Research Results*, Department of Animal Science, Colorado State University, Fort Collins, 1975, 31—32.
90. **Lapen, R. F. and Kenzy, S. G.**, *Poult. Sci.*, 54, 659—663, 1975.
91. **Brewer, R. N. and Koon, J.**, *Avian Dis.*, 17, 851—854, 1973.
92. **Banister, J., Fegler, G., and Hebb, C. Q.**, *J. Exp. Physiol.*, 35, 233—250, 1949.
93. **Mayan, M. H. and Merilan, C. P.**, *J. Anim. Sci.*, 34, 448—452, 1972.
94. **Jensen, A. H., Yen, J. T., Gehring, M. M., Baker, D. H., Becker, D. E., and Harmon, B. G.**, *J. Anim. Sci.*, 31, 745—750, 1970.
95. **Thibault, C., Courot, M., Martinet, L., Mauleon, P., du Mesnil du Buisson, F., Ortavant, R., Pelletier, J., and Signoret, J. P.**, *J. Anim. Sci.*, Suppl. 25, 119—139, 1966.
96. **Bruce, H. M.**, *J. Anim. Sci.*, Suppl. 25, 83—87, 1966.
97. **Curtis, S. E., Grunloh, D. J., Jensen, A. H., Simon, J., and Harmon, B. G.**, *J. Anim. Sci.*, 35(Abstr.), 187, 1972.
98. **Songer, J. R., Bundy, D. S., Braymen, D. T., and Mathis, R. G.**, in *Proc. Int. Pig Veterinary Congr.*, 4th ed., American Association of Swine Practitioners, Ames, Iowa, 1976, C-2.
99. **Jensen, A. H. and Curtis, S. E.**, *J. Anim. Sci.*, 42, 8—11, 1976.
100. **Fraser, D. A., Bales, R. E., Lippmann, M., and Stokinger, H. E.**, Exposure chambers for research in animal inhalation — design, construction, operation, and performance, *U.S. Public Health Serv. Public Health Monogr.*, 57, 1—53, 1959.
101. **Hinners, R. G., Burkart, J. K., and Punte, C. L.**, *Arch. Environ. Health*, 16, 194—206, 1968.
102. **Krueger, A. P. and Levine, H. B.**, *Int. J. Biometeorol.*, 11, 279—288, 1967.
103. **Crider, W. L., Barkley, N. P., and Strong, A. A.**, *Rev. Sci. Instrum.*, 39, 152—155, 1968.
104. **Rosebury, T.**, *Experimental Air-Borne Infection*, Williams & Wilkins, Baltimore, 1947, 6—72.
105. **Lodge, J. P.**, in *Air Pollution*, Vol. 2, Stern, A. C., Ed., Academic Press, New York, 1968, 465—483.
106. **Krueger, A. P., Kotaka, S., Reed, E. J., and Turner, S.**, *Int. J. Biometeorol.*, 14, 247—260, 1970.
107. **Drummond, J. E., Curtis, S. E., Simon, J., and Norton, H. W.**, *J. Anim. Sci.*, 50, 1085—1091, 1980.
108. **Drummond, J. E., Curtis, S. E., Meyer, R. C., Simon, J., and Norton, H. W.**, *Am. J. Vet. Res.*, 42, 963—974, 1981.
109. **Drummond, J. E., Curtis, S. E., Simon, J., and Norton, H. W.**, *Am. J. Vet. Res.*, 42, 969—974, 1981.

GRAVITY AND ANIMAL PRODUCTIVITY

Arthur H. Smith

Because man lacks the ability to alter the earth's gravitational field, concepts of its effects on organisms have been derived indirectly. Classically, the biological effects of gravity have been inferred from differences observed between different sized animals, since the influence of gravity upon a system is generally dependent upon its size.[1] More recently, information has been added from procedures which limit the effectiveness of gravity, e.g., water immersion and chronic recumbency. Particularly important is information, only now becoming available, on animals removed from gravitational influence in Earth-orbital weightlessness. Observations in augmented gravity fields, produced by protracted centrifugation, also are useful in resolving gravitational effects. The kinetics of acceleration relationships can be estimated with findings from animal exposures to several field strengths.

TERRESTRIAL GRAVITY AND SCALE EFFECTS

Energy Metabolism

Among homoiotherms, energy is required for the maintenance of body temperature and for the support of posture, locomotion, etc. Theoretically, thermoregulatory heat should be proportional to the body surface — the surface rule[2] — which is proportional to the two thirds power of the body size. However, direct observations[3,4] have indicated that the basal heat production of homoiotherms (H; in kilocalories per day) is proportional to the three fourths power of body mass (M; in kilograms). This is known as the *metabolic size rule* (Table 1):

$$H = 70\,M^{3/4}$$

Recently, Kleiber[5] has proposed that the maintenance requirement is a complex function, combining the thermoregulatory requirement (proportional to the power of body mass, $M^{2/3}$), and essential antigravity work, e.g., postural maintenance, which would necessarily be directly proportional to body mass (M^1). Consequently, the influence of body size on the metabolic rate should be intermediate, which may account for its proportionality to the power of body mass ($M^{3/4}$). Kleiber's hypothesis is supported by the decreased energy requirement (about −8% for basal and −40% for normal maintenance) of human males during forced bed rest,[6] which removes the work requirements for maintenance of posture and for ambulation. Similarly, unloading of the antigravity muscles through counterweighting[7,8] was found to have only a minor effect on resting metabolism, but it greatly reduced the energy requirements for locomotion. Contradictory evidence regarding the contribution of gravity to the resting metabolism is seen in the conformance of aquatic mammals to the metabolic size rule.[9] Because their buoyant existence relieves them from an equivalent effect of gravity, it might be anticipated that their basal metabolic requirements would be essentially thermoregulatory and proportional to their body surface ($M^{2/3}$).

Organ Size

Sizes of load-bearing organs in terrestrial animals are strongly influenced by body size. Body weight approximates body volume, which is proportional to the cube of some dimension. However, strength of load-bearing elements, bone or muscle, is proportional to the functional cross-sectional area, the square of some dimension. There-

Table 1
METABOLIC RATE AND BODY MASS[4]

Animal	Body weight (kg)	Metabolic rate per day (kcal)
Mouse	0.021	3.6
Rat	0.282	28.1
Guinea pig	0.410	35.1
Rabbit	1.52	83
	2.46	119
	2.98	167
	3.57	164
	4.33	191
	5.33	233
Cat	3.00	152
Monkey (macaque)	4.2	207
Dog	6.6	288
	14.1	534
	24.8	875
	23.6	872
Goat	36.0	800
Chimpanzee	38.0	1090
Sheep	46.4	1254
	46.8	1330
Human (female)	54.8	1224
	57.2	1368
	57.9	1320
Cow	300	4221
	435	8166
Beef heifers	482	7754
Cow	600	7877

Note: This sample supports the metabolic size rule. A log-log regression of these data yields the equation:

$$H = 68\ M^{0.76}$$

but the more generally accepted relationship is cited in the text.

fore, if body size were increased symmetrically, at some limit the load would exceed the strength and the system would fail. Terrestrial species of increasing size avoid this hazard by having a relatively greater component of load-bearing organs:[10,11]

$$\text{Skeleton}_{(kg)} = 0.082\ M_{(kg)}^{1.15}$$

$$\text{Skeletal muscle}_{(kg)} = 0.235\ M_{(kg)}^{1.05}$$

The scale effect, the functional relationship to increasing body size, is indicated by the exponential proportionality coefficient. Loading with weighted packs has an effect on

Table 2
ORGAN SIZE AND BODY MASS

Organ	Rats	Dogs	Horses	All mammals (interspecies)
Blood	70.0 $M^{0.98}$	72.0 $M^{0.95}$	72.0 $M^{0.93}$	50.7 $M^{0.99}$
Brain[a]	734.0 $M^{0.17}$	44.0 $M^{0.25}$	141.0 $M^{0.24}$	10.0 $M^{0.70}$
Heart	3.2 $M^{1.00}$	10.0 $M^{0.93}$	13.0 $M^{0.91}$	5.9 $M^{0.98}$
Kidney	6.5 $M^{0.82}$	11.5 $M^{0.70}$	24.3 $M^{0.66}$	7.3 $M^{0.85}$
Liver	42.0 $M^{0.89}$	64.0 $M^{0.71}$	137.0 $M^{0.61}$	33.3 $M^{0.88}$
Lung	3.8 $M^{0.75}$	13.8 $M^{0.82}$	133.0 $M^{0.58}$	11.3 $M^{0.99}$

Note: Organ sizes (g) are ordinarily related parabolically to body mass (kg) with this general equation:

$$\text{Organ size} = a\,(\text{body size})^{b}$$

Typical relationships for several organs during late development in various species of mammals are listed above.

[a] The general dissimilarity of *intra-* and *interspecies* equations for brain size reflects this organ's rapid early growth.

bone size that is similar to the effect of increasing body mass.[12] Greater body size also requires an earlier skeletal maturation in large animals, e.g., cows, because the developing bone contains tissues of low mechanical strength (cartilage). In small animals, e.g., hamsters, the loads are so small that cartilage is not disadvantageous, and skeleton and body weight mature together.

Increasing load also induces appropriate changes in bone conformation, a principle known as *Wolff's Law* which was formalized in 1892.[13] (More recent discussions also are available.[1,14]) Enlargement of bone thickness, which determines bone strength, is not accompanied by a proportionate increase in length, and the bones become "stubby". This relationship also maintains a low center of gravity, promoting mechanical stability.

Nonload-bearing organs are not particularly affected by gravity, and their sizes appear to reflect only functional requirements.[15] Within species, the scale effect of body size on the size of the developing organ tends to be similar to the interspecies scale effect of organ size as a function of mature body size (Table 2). However in larger species, e.g., horses, the proportionality coefficient for a viscus in the later stages of growth is generally less than in smaller species, e.g., rats. This change in scale effect on visceral size is merely a reflection of the larger late growth development rate of the complemental load-bearing organs in larger animals as body size matures.

DIMINISHED GRAVITY EFFECTS

A variety of procedures have been employed to limit gravitational effects, including counterweighting[7,16,17] and chronic recumbency or bed rest.[6,18,19] Their effect, however, is selective in that some parts of the organism are unloaded (particularly the antigravity skeletal muscles) while others (viscera, sensory organs, etc.) are unaffected. Consequently, the information derived is less useful than other procedures in which the effect is symmetrical.

Earth-Orbital Weightlessness

Objects in earth orbit produce a centrifugal force equal and opposite to the earth's gravity, and the net effect — weightlessness — simulates a gravity-free state.[20-23] The biological effect of this condition is one of unloading, and the remaining physiological activity represents a mass-determined function. Differences between observations made in Earth orbit and under normal terrestrial conditions represent the biological consequences of earth gravity, weight-determined functions. At present, information on the biological effects of residence in weightlessness is largely limited to observations of man, particularly those made during the Skylab series[24] and the Apollo program.[25] A summary of the physiological responses of the three astronauts on Skylab 4 for 84 days is provided in Table 3. These data are contrary to the generally anticipated diminished metabolic function with the unloading of orbital weightlessness. For example, during bed rest[6] the resting metabolism decreases 8%. The greater metabolic activity observed in the 84-day Skylab mission may be the result of the great amount of spontaneous exercise, which alleviated problems resulting from fluid distribution.[24] Reloading, by exercise at 75% of aerobic capacity, restored the terrestrial metabolic levels.

Food intake data for all Skylab missions, reported by Thornton and Ord[24b], supports the increased metabolic function indicated by the Skylab 4 respiratory observations. Regressions of body mass lost (Δbm, gram per kilogram of mass per day) on the caloric intake (H, kilocalorie per kilogram of mass per day), indicates a rectilinear relationship (Table 4):

$$\Delta bm = 0.079\,H - 4.22\ [n = 9;\ r = 0.717;\ p < 0.02]$$

Taken literally, this would indicate a high maintenance requirement (H, where $\Delta bm = 0$) of 53.4 kcal/kg/day equivalent to the energetic requirement for walking at a rate of 3 mph (4.8 km/hr) on Earth. It was generally expected that the energetic requirement for a weightless existence would be comparable to that for bedrest under Earth gravity, about 27 kcal $kg^{-1}d^{-1}$. Anticipated selective losses of body water[24d] were not encountered; therefore, the large maintenance energy cannot be explained as a dehydration artifact.

Similarly, high maintenance requirements were also reported for the Apollo astronauts[25] with those of the Moon landers being considerably higher:

$$\text{Moon landers } (n = 12):\ \Delta bm = 0.293\,H - 10.28\ [r = 0.417;\ p = 0.13\ \text{ns}]$$

$$\text{Nonlanders } (n = 21):\ \Delta bm = 0.369\,H - 14.35\ [r = 0.720;\ p < 0.01]$$

These data indicate a maintenance requirement of 48.4 kcal $kg^{-1}d^{-1}$ for the Moon landers and 38.9 kcal $kg^{-1}d^{-1}$ for the nonlanders (equivalent to the requirement for standing under Earth gravity). Among the Apollo nonlanders, no significant difference in maintenance requirement was apparent between inexperienced (first trip) and experienced astronauts (at least one previous orbital flight):

$$\text{Inexperienced } (n = 9):\ \Delta bm = 0.514\,H - 18.73\ [r = 0.908;\ p < 0.001]$$

$$\text{Experienced } (n = 12):\ \Delta bm = 0.416\,H - 14.81\ [r = 0.612;\ p = 0.04]$$

Consequently, maintenance requirements are 36.5 kcal $kg^{-1}d^{-1}$ for the experienced and 37.6 kcal $kg^{-1}d^{-1}$ for the inexperienced Apollo astronauts.

There is no explanation for the remarkably high energy turnover by astronauts except for the energetic exercise of the Skylab crews. Equally difficult to understand is the difference in kinetics between Skylab and Apollo series, the energy-body substance coefficient (k) being about fourfold greater for the latter.

Table 3
PHYSIOLOGICAL CHANGES IN WEIGHTLESSNESS AND RETURN TO EARTH GRAVITY[24e]

	Resting			Level 3—exercise			Exercise recovery		
	Preflight	Δ% In flight	Δ% Post flight	Preflight	Δ% In flight	Δ% Post flight	Preflight	Δ% In flight	Δ% Post flight
Heart rate (beats/min)	61.3 ± 5.2	−1.7 ± 0.09	17.1 ± 1.7[a]	156.0 ± 7.0	−0.7 ± 1.3	3.9 ± 1.2	110.0 ± 4.3	−18 ± 3.3	−0.4 ± 1.9
$\dot{V}_{O_2}$ (cc/min)	248 ± 15	15.2 ± 3.9	−3.4 ± 6.0	2730.0 ± 343	−4.7 ± 2.4	−5.2 ± 1.6	709.0 ± 103	1.3 ± 6.4	10.6 ± 5.6
O_2 pulse (cc O_2/beat)	4.07 ± 0.35	17.2 ± 3.1	−17.6 ± 4.1[c]	17.5 ± 2.2	−4.0 ± 2.9	−8.8 ± 2.7	6.44 ± 0.85	23.6 ± 6.8[c]	11.3 ± 7.7
$\dot{V}_{CO_2}$ (cc/min)	235 ± 16	17.5 ± 5.8[c]	−10.2 ± 6.8	2580.0 ± 318	0.7 ± 2.3	−1.6 ± 1.5	911.0 ± 221	6.7 ± 10.3	8.4 ± 10.5
RQ (CO_2/O_2)	0.95 ± 0.04	2.0 ± 3.0	−7.0 ± 2.7	0.95 ± 0.01	5.6 ± 1.8[c]	3.9 ± 1.9	1.27 ± 0.12	5.0 ± 3.9	−2.5 ± 4.7
SBP (mmHg)	113 ± 13	−2.8 ± 2.3	5.3 ± 4.2	200 ± 6	−0.8 ± 1.2	1.0 ± 2.1	174 ± 18	−6.6 ± 3.2	8.1 ± 3.6
DBP (mmHg)	74 ± 7	−12.6 ± 0.3[a]	1.1 ± 4.3	62 ± 7	−13.9 ± 4.5[c]	−4.9 ± 1.7[c]	66 ± 0.5	−7.9 ± 0.03[a]	6.6 ± 6.6
Pulse P (mmHg)	38 ± 7	18.1 ± 7.6	13.5 ± 4.4[c]	138 ± 12	5.9 ± 4.7	3.8 ± 2.6	109 ± 18	−6.4 ± 5.7	8.5 ± 1.8[b]
$\dot{V}_E$ (L/min)	7.7 ± 0.9	30.6 ± 2.0[a]	34.0 ± 16.3	82.3 ± 14.0	1.3 ± 7.2	3.9 ± 9.1	30.5 ± 7.4	2.5 ± 13.0	20.3 ± 9.1

Note: Data from Skylab 4 (84[d] mission) is summarized as mean (± SD) for three astronauts, preflight, and as the percentage change in flight and after return. Individual astronaut data used in the summary were means of eight measurements in 6 months for the preflight data and of twelve measurements for the flight data. Post flight data were those obtained on the second day after Earth return. Resting data were determined over a 5-min period prior to exercise, and exercise data, for the last 3 min of a 5-min period at 75% of aerobic capacity. Exercise recovery data were collected over the second minute after exercise.

[a] $p < 0.001$.
[b] $p < 0.01$.
[c] $p < 0.05$.

Table 4
BODY MASS AND CALORIC INTAKE IN SPACE[24b]

	Body mass (kg)			Mean caloric intake (kcal/day)
	At launch	At recovery	Change	
Skylab 2 (28[d])				
Commander	62.0	60.3	−1.7	2850
Pilot	79.8	76.1	−3.7	2812
Scientist	77.4	74.3	−3.1	2936
Skylab 3 (59[d])				
Commander	68.5	64.7	−3.8	2792
Pilot	88.5	84.3	−4.2	3866
Scientist	61.9	58.3	−3.6	2850
Skylab 4 (84[d])				
Commander	68.0	67.9	−0.1	3176
Pilot	67.7	66.2	−1.5	3457
Scientist	71.3	69.8	−1.5	2962

Weightlessness also induces negative mineral and nitrogen balances[24a] for the 84-day Skylab mission. Calcium loss in the second month of weightlessness was 4 g/month, about 0.3 to 0.4% monthly loss of total skeletal calcium. This was not significantly reduced in the third month. At these depletion rates, it was considered that irreversible changes, e.g., a loss of trabecular structure, would occur after 6 to 7 months of weightlessness. Negative nitrogen and phosphate balances also existed throughout the flight; the net effect was evident in the atrophic changes in muscle mass.[24c] The vigorous exercise performed by the astronauts on the 84-day Skylab mission did not reduce the net loss of mineral or nitrogen.

Buoyancy

Although the weightlessness of water immersion removes the antigravity work aspect for postural maintenance and locomotion, it does not provide a good procedure for long-term studies with terrestrial animals because it also produces a marked dehydration.[27,27] This results from a central displacement of body fluids by the high-density external medium, which activates the Gauer-Henry reflex.[29] It is interesting that aquatic mammals lack this reflex and apparently do not produce antidiuretic hormone.[30]

Among equatic mammals, body size has much less influence on skeletal size than it does in terrestrial mammals (see Table 5). Bones become more slender with increasing size (as first discussed by Galileo in 1638[31]) a result of the reversal of mechanical forces on the bones of terrestrial and aquatic animals. In terrestrial animals, the bones bear the load of the soft tissues with a compressive force. However, in aquatic animals, the less dense soft tissues buoyantly bear the load of the denser bone and with a tension on the bone. In whales, there is a relative decrease in muscle mass with increasing body size. This decrease is reasonable because blubber provides the antigravity load-bearing function (Table 5).

A comparison of the maximum sizes of terrestrial and aquatic mammals also indicates that gravity may determine the extent of body size development. The largest entirely land animal that ever lived was a type of rhinocerous estimated to have attained a mass of 16 t. The largest living terrestrial animals, male African elephants, have been recorded to reach 11 ton body mass. However, blue whales routinely reach 100 t; the largest one captured was 203 t. Earth gravity would appear, therefore, to

Table 5
BODY AND ORGAN SIZE IN AQUATIC AND TERRESTRIAL ANIMALS[3,111]

	Whales		Terrestrial	
	a	b	a	b
Skeleton	137	1.024	230	1.15
Skeletal muscle	752	0.830	357	1.05
Blubber	122	1.194	—	—
Heart	3.56	1.003	5.27	0.984
Kidney	6.42	0.856	2.53	0.846
Liver	33.62	0.705	13.29	0.867
Lung	8.22	0.949	10.26	0.986
G I tract	59.34	0.697	49.63	0.941

Note: The relationship between organ size (kg mass) and body size (t mass) is summarized as the constants for the equation:

$$\text{Organ} = \text{a body size}^{\text{b}}$$

limit the body size of terrestrial mammals to 5 or 10% of their biological potential, that achieved by aquatic mammals.

AUGMENTED GRAVITY EFFECTS

Enhancement of the effects of gravity under terrestrial conditions is readily arranged by having an animal carry a loaded pack. It is possible to increase the effect of gravity, i.e., the normal load, by perhaps 50%.[12] Because this loading is asymmetric, however, the results, like those of bed rest (an asymmetric unloading), have limited usefulness. Symmetrical loading can be arranged artifically by summation of gravitational and inertial fields, the latter being generated by centrifugation. According to *Einstein's Principle of Equivalence*[32-34] the effects of inertial and gravitational forces are indistinguishable; therefore, it is reasonable to interpret the results of centrifugation studies generally, as a representation of changes that would be encountered in an increased gravity field. A detailed account of the physiological changes associated with long-term increases in acceleration has been reported elsewhere.[35]

Metabolic Effects

Chronic acceleration imposes greater energy requirements for an equivalent locomotion and postural maintenance, thereby increasing the maintenance requirements. This has been demonstrated for chickens (Table 6)[35] and rationalized as an arithmetic relation between the maintenance feed requirement (F_G grams of feed per kilogram of body mass^{-l} per day^{-1}, and the acceleration field strength (G) over the range of 1 to 2.5 G:

$$F_G = 26.6 + 9.6\,G$$

A similar relationship applies to metabolizable feed,[4] the feed intake less the excreta:

$$F_G = 17.3 + 6.5\,G$$

On this basis, it appears that 27% of the terrestrial maintenance requirement of chickens is determined by Earth gravity. In absolute terms, this is equivalent to 16 kcal/kg

Table 6
GRAVITATIONAL DETERMINATION OF NUTRITIVE REQUIREMENTS OF CHICKENS[36]

	Field strength (G)				
	1	1.5	2	2.5	3
Number of determinations	10	6	6	5	4
Body mass (kg)	1.93 ± 0.07	1.90 ± 0.07	1.81 ± 0.02	1.70 ± 0.05	1.57 ± 0.03
Maintenance feed requirement (g feed/kg body mass^{-1}/day^{-1})	35.6 ± 3.4	43.4 ± 2.4	46.5 ± 4.4	49.5 ± 1.4	44.7 ± 3.2
Feed utilization ratio (g body mass/g feed^{-1})	0.41 ± 0.15	0.28 ± 0.11	0.32 ± 0.05	0.57 ± 0.31	0.62 ± 0.32
Feed metabolizability (%)	65.5 ± 2.0	72.7 ± 2.1	65.2 ± 2.0	72.5 ± 3.4	69.5 ± 4.8
Maintenance metabolizable feed requirement (g metabolizable feed/kg body mass^{-1}/day^{-1})	23.8 ± 2.9	28.7 ± 2.6	30.2 ± 2.4	32.7 ± 1.1	28.7 ± 2.7
Metabolizable feed utilization ratio (g body mass/g metabolizable feed^{-1})	0.52 ± 0.23	0.37 ± 0.14	0.46 ± 0.07	0.67 ± 0.33	0.92 ± 0.25

Note: Mean data (± SD) are listed for maintenance requirements and feed metabolizability at several acceleration field strengths. The utilization ratio is the slope of the regression of change in body mass upon feed intake (Δ grams body mass per Δ gram feed).

body mass^{-1} per G^{-1} per day^{-1}. As a physically determined requirement, this should apply equally to all animals, irrespective of body size. For large animals, gravity would require a larger part of the metabolic activity, which is proportional to $M^{3/4}$. On this basis, Kleiber[5] has estimated that 40% of the maintenance metabolism of a mammal weighing 75 kg is expended against gravity. This amount is approximately the decrease in the maintenance requirement observed in man during bed rest.[6] The influence of gravity upon energetics reflects only the increased work required for antigravity processes. The efficiency for the performance of such work is unaffected.[37]

Changes in intermediate metabolism also have been observed in rats[38-40] and chickens.[41,42] In rats at 4.7 G, there is an increased incorporation of acetate into nonsaponifiable lipids, which accompanies a decreased lipid content in the tissue. There is also a greater incorporation of acetate C-2 carbon atoms into lipids. At normal gravity, C-1 and C-2 atoms are equally involved in fat synthesis. Acceleration also enhances both the uptake and oxidation of glucose by diaphragm tissue in vitro.[40] A variety of changes in enzyme activities was observed in the liver of chronically accelerated chickens and interpreted to indicate an increased mobilization and a decreased synthesis of lipid during acceleration stress. With physiological adaptation, normal lipid utilization and synthesis are restored, but an increased carbohydrate utilization persists.

Body Composition

Chronically accelerated small homoiotherms (mice,[43] rats,[44] hamsters,[45] and chickens[46]) characteristically become incapable of accumulating depot fat. The degree of defatting is generally arithmetically related to field strength. By periodic fasting of centrifuging animals,[47] it can be demonstrated that this lesser body fat is a regulated phenomenon and not merely the result of an inability to acquire feed or a diminished synthetic capacity. A summary of body composition for several kinds of birds exposed to several field strengths is provided in Tables 7 and 8, indicating that the apparent degree of this gravitational effect is proportional to body size.

The selective defatting of small homoiotherms during chronic acceleration resembles the human syndrome lipodystrophy,[48,49] which results from an oversecretion of a hormonal agent, the fat mobilizing substance (FMS). This material is also released in the urine of small mammals in response to low temperature exposure or fasting.[50,51] It appears to be a small polypeptide[52] produced in the pituitary of mammals and the hypothalamus of birds.[53] Urine of centrifuging rabbits has been found to have anorexogenic[73] as well as lipotropic activity.[74] The possibility that FMS is produced in response to a mechanical stimulus to the brain has also been considered.[35] An exception to the general acceleration-induced defatting of homoiotherms is found in monkeys[54] (Table 9). Although centrifuged monkeys exhibit a loss of lean body mass, they actually accumulate fat and subsequently lose it at Earth gravity. This difference in simian acceleration response is associated with a normally low body fat and also an unusual brain geometry, which, speculatively, might provide a load-bearing function and limit an FMS-provoking mechanical stimulus.[54]

Growth

The influence of augmented gravity upon animal growth is generally consistent with concepts derived from scale effects under terrestrial gravity and those from buoyant weightlessness. Early growth of most animals follows an exponential relationship:[3]

$$M_t = M_o e^{kt}$$

Where M is body mass, M_0 at birth and M_t at time t, and k is the proportionality coefficient, the relative increase in body size per unit of time. When rats were centri-

Table 7
CHRONIC ACCELERATION AND BODY COMPOSITION OF BIRDS[46]

	Field (G)	(n)	Body mass	Carcass composition (%) Water	Fat	Lean
Quail (*Coturnix japonica*)	1	(10)	116.1 ± 7.5 g	65.0± 3.5	10.90 ± 4.15	24.12 ± 1.86
	2	(5)	122.6 ± 6.7 g	66.0 ± 4.6	10.64 ± 4.53	23.36 ± 1.30
	2.5	(6)	106.7 ± 2.7 g	70.2 ± 2.4	5.60 ± 2.30	24.35 ± 0.79
	4	(2)	99.6 ± 0.7 g	71.5 ± 0.27	1.21 ± 0.05	27.26 ± 0.22
Leghorn chickens	1	(13)	2.29 ± 0.19 kg	54.2 ± 3.7	22.94 ± 4.70	22.88 ± 1.75
	1.5	(5)	1.94 ± 0.36 kg	62.2 ± 5.0	13.34 ± 6.88	24.44 ± 2.02
	2	(7)	1.90 ± 0.15 kg	69.2 ± 2.3	3.40 ± 1.50	27.43 ± 1.04
	2.5	(10)	1.87 ± 0.17 kg	70.0 ± 1.1	2.61 ± 1.08	27.38 ± 0.68
Arbor Acre chickens	1	(14)	5.39 ± 0.54 kg	61.6 ± 4.8	14.94 ± 5.53	23.71 ± 1.47
	2	(5)	4.02 ± 0.31 kg	72.1 ± 3.4	2.66 ± 1.38	25.12 ± 2.33

Note: The results of chemical analysis of carcass samples are summarized by groups as the mean ± SD.

Table 8
ACCELERATION RELATIONSHIPS[46]

		Body mass		Carcass water (%)		Carcass fat (%)	
	(n)	A_o	$-k_m$	W_o	k_w	F_o	$-k_f$
Quail (1—4 G)	(4)	127.2 g	−6.93	62.67	2.32	15.35	−3.48
Leghorn chickens (1—2.5 G)	(4)	2.46 kg	−0.260	44.84	10.89	35.40	−14.19
Arbor Acre chickens (1—2 G)	(2)	6.76 kg	−1.37	51.12	10.47	27.22	−12.28

Note: Body mass, carcass water, and carcass fat concentrations all appear to vary arithmetically with field strength (G) and can be described by the equation:

$$y = y_o + kG$$

Regressions of group mean data upon acceleration field strength are summarized above for several parameters by the appropriate constants for the general equation.

Table 9
BODY COMPOSITION OF CHRONICALLY ACCELERATED MONKEYS[54]

Period of treatment	Body mass[a] (kg)	Body fat[a] (kg)	(%)	Lean body mass[a] (kg)	(%)
Preacceleration	12.23 ± 1.54	0.55 ± 0.18	4.10 ± 1.10	11.68 ± 1.49	95.9 ± 1.1
4 weeks at 1.5 G	11.29 ± 1.38	0.57 ± 0.13	5.00 ± 0.84	10.72 ± 1.27	95.0 ± 0.8
4 weeks at 2.0 G	11.11 ± 1.09	0.54 ± 0.16	4.80 ± 1.97	10.57 ± 0.99	95.2 ± 1.9
16 weeks at 2.0 G	11.38 ± 0.71	0.69 ± 0.25	6.02 ± 2.10	10.69 ± 0.66	94.0 ± 2.2
8—34 days at 2.5 G	11.07 ± 0.97	1.04 ± 0.34	9.47 ± 2.77	10.03 ± 1.05	90.5 ± 2.8
Recovery, 50—67 days at Earth gravity	11.78 ± 1.26	1.00 ± 0.34	8.35 ± 2.24	10.78 ± 1.06	91.6 ± 2.2

[a] Mean ± SD.

fuged during early growth,[55] there was a slowing of the growth rate, k (with M in grams and time in days), that is proportional to field strength:

$$k \times 100 = 2.45 - 0.086\,G$$

Late growth also is exponential, but with decreasing increments towards a mature body size:

$$M_t = A - Be^{-kt}$$

where A is the mature size, the genetically determined growth potential (mathematically an asymptote); B is an arbitrary constant; and −k is a proportionality coefficient indicating maturation rate, the relative decrease in remaining growth potential ($A - M_t$) per unit of time. With increasing field strength, there is a decrease in the mature body mass, A, which is largely a matter of decreased body fat but also includes a decreased lean body mass (Table 10). The maturation constant, −k, also changes with acceleration, but not consistently among species. In chickens, it increases (becoming a larger negative number) in stronger fields,[47] which indicates a more rapid maturation. However, the reverse situation occurs in rats.

Organ Size

Developing organs respond to artifical acceleration fields much as they do to Earth gravity. Load-bearing organs are generally considered to increase in size, with the response being proportional to field strength. It has been demonstrated that isolated osteogenic tissue responds to compressive forces in a way that promotes calcification.[57] Several reports of bone growth during chronic acceleration provide conflicting conclusions, which may result from lack of a reasonable basis for comparison. Generally, the treatment slows growth so that bone sizes are diminished, but body sizes also decrease, and the scale factors for comparison are not obvious. In addition, experimental treatment is necessarily limited to moderate acceleration fields because any significant overloading of developing bone will lead to its deformation,[55,58,59] with undefined pathological consequences.

A relative increase in femur size and a change in cross-section to a circular shape, improving load-bearing function, have been reported for chronically accelerated mice.[60] Relative increases in femur size were also reported for chronically accelerated rats at several acceleration intensities.[56] In chronically accelerated chickens, relative bone size was also increased; it increased equally for the femur (load bearing) and the humerus (nonload bearing), indicating the bone growth stimulus to be a whole-animal rather than a local response.[61] Contrary observations, i.e., that chronic acceleration does not affect bone growth, have also been offered.[62,63] Centrifugation of late chick embryos (which are aquatic, and with a tensile force on the bone) leads, appropriately, to an opposite effect — the bones become longer and more slender.[64]

Qualitative examination of bones of centrifuged rats have revealed histological changes that indicate an increased rate of ossification.[65] An increased density of bone was induced in female (but not male) rats by centrifugation.[66] No changes in chemical composition were found in the bone ash of the centrifuged rats.[59]

Muscles also respond to an increased load (or overload), with a characteristic hypertrophy.[67] However, with gravitational loading, the effect is limited to the extensor, antigravity muscles, and the reverse may occur in the antagonistic flexors. Because most muscle masses contain both extensor and flexor elements, their size measurement is not necessarily informative under altered gravity conditions. Comparisons of isolated extensor and flexor muscles not only avoid this difficulty, but they also eliminate

Table 10
ACCELERATION AND MATURE BODY MASS IN MAMMALS

Species	A_o	−b	I (%)	Ref.
Mice				
Female	38.5 g	−0.33	−0.9	53
Male	40.5 g	−0.33	−0.8	53
Rats				
Female	307 g	−17.	−5.5	54
Rabbits				
Male Polish	1.76 kg	−0.33	−18.6	—
Male New Zealand	4.70 kg	−0.66	−14.0	—

Note: The potential mature size (A_o) is reduced arithmetically by increasing acceleration fields, with a proportionality coefficient, ^{-k}m:

$$A_G = A_o - k_m G$$

Comparisons of the inhibitory effect of acceleration (I) can be made by the ratio of the two coefficients, literally indicating the percentage size reduction from exposure to Earth gravity:

$$I = (-K/A_o) \times 100$$

uncertainties arising from scale effects of coincident changes in body size and composition.[68] In chronically accelerated chickens, the changes induced in the leg muscles proceeded hyperbolically and slowly, requiring 1 year to elicit 85% of the indicated maximum effect:

$$\text{Field strength, 2 G E:F} = 1.17 - 0.33e^{-0.157\,t}$$

$$\text{Field strength, 0 G E:F} = 0.62 + 0.22e^{-0.490\,t}$$

where 0 G represents extrapolated intercept data from observations involving several field strengths; E:F is the mass ratio of extensor to flexor muscles; and, t is the time in months. The maximum E:F ratio appears to be arithmetically related to acceleration field strength (G):

$$E{:}F_{max} = 0.59 + 0.28\,G$$

Functional properties of the muscles also change after chronic acceleration. After 1-year exposure to 3 G, rat leg muscles exhibited a marked decerebrate extensor tonus.[69] Gastrocnemius muscles from chronically accelerated hamsters were more fatigue resistant during tetanic contraction.[70] After 7 months at 1.75 G, exercise capacity of chickens, measured by treadmill running to exhaustion, was three times greater than that of the controls.[71]

CONCLUSION

Gravity is obviously an important factor in animal productivity, being a major determinant of body size, form, and composition, as well as of the material and energy

Table 11
RELATIVE FOOD CAPACITY OF ANIMALS[4]

Animal	Body weight (kg)	Maximum daily intake of food energy: kcal per animal	Maximum daily intake of food energy: kcal per kg$^{3/4}$	Fasting energy loss (kcal/kg$^{3/4}$)	Relative food capacity
Chick	0.078	53.5	360	81	4.4
Rabbit	2.36	480	253	50	5.1
Sheep	50	5730	305	69	4.4
Swine	130	13980	363	64	5.7
Steer	427	42429	452	81	5.6
	444	36026	373	88	4.2

Table 12
EXAMPLE OF THE INDEPENDENCE OF BODY SIZE AND FOOD UTILIZATION[4]

	Animals tested: 1 steer	Animals tested: 300 rabbits
Total body weight	1,300 lb	1,300 lb
Food consumption per day	16⅔ lb	66⅔ lb
Duration of 1 ton of food	120 days	30 days
Heat loss per day	20,000 kcal	80,000 kcal
Gain in weight per day	2 lb	8 lb
Gain from 1 ton of food	240 lb	240 lb

requirements for maintenance. However, utilization of this information is difficult due to man's inability to control gravity. The possibility of reducing gravitational susceptibility by breeding smaller homoiothermic animals is counterbalanced by their greater thermoregulatory requirements. In fact, the efficiency of food utilization for animal productivity is the ratio of the capacity of food intake to the basal metabolism,[4] and, as formalized by Kleiber's Law, this is independent of body size (Table 11). An example of this relationship with respect to food utilization and growth is provided in Table 12. Perhaps the only available way to frustrate gravity in animal production is to utilize poikilothermic animals in a buoyant existence — aquaculture.[72]

REFERENCES

1. **Thompson, D'A. W.,** *On Growth and Form,* 2nd ed., Cambridge University Press, New York, 1942, 1116.
2. **Voit, E.,** Über die Grösse des Energiebedarfs der tiere in Hungerzustande, *Z. Biol. Munich,* 41, 113—154, 1901.
3. **Brody, S.,** *Bioenergetics and Growth,* Reinhold, New York, 1945, 1023.
4. **Kleiber, M.** *Fire of Life,* John Wiley & Sons, New York, 1961, 454.
5. **Kleiber, M.,** Further consideration of the relation between metabolic rate and body size, in *Energy Metabolism of Farm Animals,* Blaxter, K. L., Kielanowski, J., and Thorbeck, G., Eds., Oriel Press, Newcastle on Tyne, England, 1969, 505—511.

6. **Bernauer, E. M. and Adams, W. C.,** The Effect of Nine Days Recumbency With and Without Exercise on the Redistribution of Body Fluids and Electrolytes, Renal Function and Metabolism, NASA Publication No. CR-73664, National Aeronautics and Space Administration, Washington, D.C., 1968, 172.
7. **Wortz, E. C.,** Effects of reduced gravity environments on human performance, *Aerosp. Med.,* 39, 963—966, 1968.
8. **Newsom, B. D.,** A Lurian simulator for metabolic studies, *Aerosp. Med.,* 40, 672—673, 1969.
9. **Tenney, S. M.,** Respiration in mammals, in *Dukes' Physiology of Domestic Animals,* 8th ed., Swenson, M. J., Ed., Comstock Press, Ithaca, N.Y., 1970, 295.
10. **Keyser, Ch. and Heusner, A.,** Étude comparative due mẽtabolisme energẽtique dans la sẽrie animale, *J. Physiol. (Paris),* 56, 489—524, 1964.
11. **Smith, A. H. and Pace, N.,** Differential component and organ size relationships among whales, *Environ. Physiol.,* 122—136, 1971.
12. **Tulloh, N. M. and Romberg, B.,** An effect of gravity on bone development in lambs, *Nature (London),* 200, 438—439, 1963.
13. **Wolff, J.,** *Des Gesetz der Transformation der Knochen,* Hirshwald, Berlin, 1892.
14. **Ham, A. W.,** *Histology,* 5th ed, Lippincott, Philadelphia, 1965, 1041.
15. **Günter, B.,** Dimensional analysis and theory of biological similarity, *Physiol. Rev.,* 55, 659—699, 1975.
16. **Fox, E. L., Bartels, R. L., Chaloupka, E. C., Klinzing, J. E., and Houche, J.,** Oxygen cost during exercise in simulated sub-gravity environments, *Aviat. Space Environ. Med.,* 46, 300—303, 1975.
17. **Robertson, W. C. and Wortz, E. C.,** Effect of lunar gravity on metabolic rates, *Aerosp. Med.,* 39, 799—805, 1968.
18. **Browse, N. L.,** *The Physiology and Pathology of Bed Rest,* Charles C Thomas, Springfield, Ill., 1965, 221.
19. **Vernikos-Danellis, J., Winget, C. M., Leach, C. S., and Rambaut, P. C.,** Circadian, endocrine and metabolic effects of prolonged bedrest: two 56-day bedrest studies, *NASA Tech. Memo.* X-3051, 1974, 42.
20. **Gauer, O. H. and Zuidema, G. D.,** *Gravitational Stress in Aerospace Medicine,* Churchill Livingstone, Edinburgh, 1961, 278.
21. **Hardy, J. C.,** *Physiological Problems in Space Exploration,* Charles C Thomas, Springfield, Ill., 1964, 333.
22. **McCally, M.,** *Hypodynamics and Hypogravics,* Academic Press, New York, 1968, 306.
23. **Calvin, M. and Gazenko, O.,** The Foundations of Space Biology and Medicine, Vol. 3, National Aernautics Space Administration, Washington, 1975.
24. **Johnson, R. S. and Dietline, L. F., Eds.,** Biomedical Results from Skylab, *NASA SP-377, 1977, 491.*
24a. **Whedon, G. D., Lutwak, L., Rambaut, P. C., Whittle, M. W., Smith, M. C., Reid, J., Leach, C., Stadler, C. R., and Sanford, D. D.,** Mineral and nitrogen metabolic studies, experiment MO71, Biomedical Results from Skylab, Johnson, R. S. and Dietline, L. F., Eds, *NASA SP-377,* 1977, 164—174.
24b. **Thornton, W. E. and Ord, J.,** Physiological mass measurements in Skylab, Biomedical Results from Skylab, Johnson, R. S. and Dietline, L. F., Eds., *NASA SP-377,* 1977, 175—182.
24c. **Whittle, M. W., Herron, R., and Cuzzi, J.,** Biostereometric analysis of body form, Biomedical Results from Skylab, Johnson, R. S. and Dietline, L. F., Eds., *NASA SP-377,* 1977, 198—202.
24d. **Thornton, W. E., Hoffler, G. W., and Rummel, J.,** Anthropometric changes and fluid shifts, Biomedical Results from Skylab, Johnson, R. S. and Dietline, L. F., *NASA SP-377,* 1977, 330—338.
24e. **Michel, E. L., Rummer, J. A., Sawin, C. F., Buderer, M. C., and Lem, J. D.,** Results of Skylab medical experiment M171 — metabolic activity, Biomedical Results from Skylab, Johnson, R. S. and Dietline, L. F., Eds., *NASA SP-377, 1977, 372—387.*
25. **Johnson, R. S., Dietline, L. F., and Berry, C. A.,** Biomedical Results of Apollo, NASA Publication No. SP-368, Washington, D.C., 1975, 592.
26. **Burton, R. R. and Smith, A. H.,** Hemotological findings associated with chronic acceleration, *Space Life Sci.,* 1, 501—513, 1969.
27. **Graveline, D. C. and Jackson, M. M.,** Diuresis associated with prolonged water immersion, *J. Appl. Physiol.,* 17, 519—524, 1962.
28. **Hunt, N. C.,** Immersion diuresis, *Aerosp. Med.,* 38, 176—180, 1967.
29. **Gauer, O., Henry, J. P., and Behn, C.,** The regulation of extracellular fluid volume, *Annu. Rev. Physiol.,* 32, 547—595, 1970.
30. **Malvin, R. L, Bonjour, J. P., and Ridgeway, S.,** Antiduretic hormone levels in some cetaceans, *Proc. Soc. Exp. Biol. Med.,* 136, 1203—1205, 1971.
31. **Galilei, G.,** *Dialogues Concerning Two Sciences,* translated by Crew, H. and DeSalvio, A., MacMillan, New York, 1914.

32. **Rosser, W. G. V.,** *An Introduction of the Theory of Relativity,* Butterworths, London, 1964.
33. **Witten, L.,** *Gravitation, An Introduction to Current Research.* John Wiley & Sons, New York, 1962.
34. **Weinberg, S.,** *Gravitation and Cosmology: Principles and Applications of the General Theory of Relativity,* John Wiley & Sons, New York, 1972, 657.
35. **Smith, A. H.,** Physiological changes associated with long-term increases in acceleration, *COSPAR Life Sci. Space Res.,* 14, 91—100, 1976.
36. **Smith, A. H., Burton, R. R., and Kelly, C. F.,** Influence of gravity on the maintenance requirement of chickens, *J. Nutr.,* 101, 13—24, 1971.
37. **Bjurstedt, H., Rosenhamer, G., and Wigertz, O.,** High-G environment and response to graded exercise, *J. Appl. Physiol.,* 25, 713—719, 1968.
38. **Feller, D. C. and Neville, E. D.,** Conversion of acetate to lipids and CO_2 by liver of rats exposed to acceleration stress, *Am. J. Physiol.,* 208, 892—895, 1965.
39. **Feller, D. C., Neville, E. D., Oyama, J., and Averkin, E. G.,** Chemical and metabolic changes of hepatic lipids from rats exposed to chronic radial acceleration, *Proc. Soc. Exp. Biol. Med.,* 19, 522—525, 1965.
40. **Daligcon, B. C. and Oyama, J.,** *In vitro* stimulation of glucose uptake and utlization by diaphragm of rats exposed to chronic centrifugation, *Physiologist,* 13, 174, 1970.
41. **Evans, J. W., Smith, A. H., and Boda, J. M.,** Fat metabolism and chronic acceleration, *Am. J. Physiol.,* 216, 1468—1471, 1969.
42. **Evans, J. W. and Boda, J. M.,** Glucose metabolism and chronic acceleration, *Am. J. Physiol.,* 219, 893—896, 1970.
43. **Keil, L. C.,** Changes in growth and body composition of mice exposed to chronic centrifugation, *Growth,* 33, 83—88, 1969.
44. **Pitts, G. C., Bull, L. S., and Oyama, J.,** Effect of chronic centrifugation on body composition in the rat, *Am. J. Physiol.,* 223, 1044—1048, 1972.
45. **Briney, S. R. and Wunder, C. C.,** Comparative study of effects of gravity on the growth of hamsters and mice, *Proc. Iowa Acad. Sci.,* 67, 495—500, 1960.
46. **Smith, A. H., Sanchez P. O., and Burton, R. R.,** Gravitational effects on body composition in birds, *COSPAR Life Sci. Space Res.,* 14, 21—27, 1975.
47. **Smith, A. H. and Burton, R. R.,** The influence of the ambient accelerative force on mature body size, *Growth,* 31, 317—329, 1967.
48. **Chalmers, T. M.,** Lipid-mobilizing activity during fasting, in *Handbook of Physiology,* Sect. 5, Adipose tissue, Renold, A. E. and Cahill, G. F., Eds., Waverly Press, Baltimore, 1965, 542—549.
49. **Senior, B.,** Lidodystrophy, in *Handbook of Physiology,* Sect. 5, Adipose tissue, Renold, A. E. and Cahill, G. F., Eds., Waverly Press, Baltimore, 1965, 662—667.
50. **Beaton, J. R., Borre, A. J., and Stevenson, J. A. F.,** Diet and temperature effects on excretion of fat mobilizing substances, *Proc. Soc. Exp. Biol. Med.,* 118, 362—365, 1965.
51. **Stevenson, J. A. F., Box, B. M., and Szlavko, A. J.,** A fat mobilizing and anorectic substance in the urine of fasting rats, *Proc. Soc. Exp. Biol. Med.,* 115, 424—429, 1964.
52. **Beaton, J. R. and Stevenson, J. A. F.,** Purification by ultrafiltration of a fat mobilizing substance extracted from the urine of fasting rats, *Can. J. Physiol. Pharmacol.,* 44, 701—709, 1966.
53. **Nir, I., Dimick, M. K., and Lepkovsky, S.,** A fat mobilizing substance in chicken urine, *Can. J. Physiol. Pharmacol.,* 47, 535—543, 1969.
54. **Smith, A. H., Rahlmann, D. F., Kodama, A. M., and Pace, N.,** Metabolic responses of monkeys to increased gravitational fields, *COSPAR Life Sci. Space Res.,* 14, 129—132, 1974.
55. **Oyama, J. and Platt, W. T.,** Effects of prolonged centrifugation on growth and organ development of rats, *Am. J. Physiol.,* 209, 611—615, 1965.
56. **Oyama, J. and Platt, W. T.,** Reproduction and growth of mice and rats under conditions of simulated increased gravity, *Am. J. Physiol.,* 212, 164—166, 1967.
57. **Glucksman, A.,** The role of mechanical stresses in bone formation *in vitro, J. Anat.,* 76, 231—239, 1942.
58. **Burton, R. R. and Smith, A. H.,** Chronic acceleration sickness, *Aerosp. Med.,* 36, 39—44, 1965.
59. **Oyama, J. and Zeitman, B.,** Tissue composition of rats exposed to chronic centrifugation, *Am. J. Physiol.,* 213, 1305—1310, 1967.
60. **Wunder, C. C., Briney, S. R., Kral, M., and Skaugstad, C.,** Growth of mouse femurs during continual centrifugation, *Nature (London),* 188, 151—152, 1960.
61. **Smith, A. H. and Kelly, C. F.,** Influence of chronic acceleration upon growth and body composition, *Ann. N.Y. Acad. Sci.,* 110, 410—424, 1963.
62. **Amptmann, E. and Oyama, J.,** Changes in functional contruction of bone in rats under conditions of simulated increased gravity, *Z. Anat. Entwicklungsgesch.,* 139, 307—318, 1973.
63. **Jankovich, J. P.,** Structural Development of the Bone in the Rat Under Earth-Gravity, Simulated Weightlessness, Hypergravity and Mechanical Vibration, *NASA Publication No. CR-1823,* 1971, 141.

64. **Redden, D. R.,** Chronic acceleration effects on bone development in the chick embryo, *Am. J. Physiol.,* 218, 310—313, 1970.
65. **Smith, S. D.,** Effect of long-term rotation and hypergravity on developing rats fermurs, *Aviat. Space Envrion. Med.,* 46, 248—253, 1975.
66. **Fosse, G.,** The radiodensity of skeletal parts in animals growing and living in a constant artificially increased gravitational field, *Growth,* 35, 35—53, 1971.
67. **Clarke, D. H.,** Adaptations in strength and muscular endurance resulting from exercise, *Exercise Sport Sci. Rev.,* 1, 73—102, 1973.
68. **Burton, R. R., Besch, E. L., Sluka, S. J., and Smith, A. H.,** Differential effect of chronic acceleration upon skeletal muscles, *J. Appl. Physiol.,* 23, 80—84, 1967.
69. **Matthews, B. H. C.,** Adaptation to centrifuge acceleration, *J. Physiol. (London),* 122, 31p, 1953.
70. **Canonica, P. C.,** Effects of Prolonged Hypergravity Stress on the Myogenic Properties of the Gastrocnemius Muscle, M.S. thesis, University of South Carolina, Columbia, 1966, 61.
71. **Burton, R. R. and Smith, A. H.,** Proc. 16th Int. Congr. Aviat. Space Med., Lisbon, 1967.
72. **Bardach, J. E.,** Aquaculture, *Science,* 161, 1098—1106, 1968.
73. **Katovich, M.,** Response and Physiological Adaption to Chronic Acceleration, Ph.D. thesis, University of California, Davis, 1976, 137.
74. **Horwitz, B. A.,** unpublished data.

HOUSING AND ANIMAL PRODUCTIVITY*

B. C. Stenning

DEFINITIONS

At the outset it is necessary to explain the meaning of the three keywords in the above title.

Housing — Affords artificial protection against the elements, possibly with provision for controlling air temperature, relative humidity, ventilation rate, air speed at any point, illumination level, day length, and availability of feeding-stuffs and water. Housing does not necessarily imply complete enclosure; open fronted buildings, pole barns with no wall-cladding, and even structures comprising walls but no roofs, all qualify. Facilities and fitments within the structure all contribute to the general "housing" of stock. However equipment for milking, egg handling, and manure handling arrangements, together with amenities for the well-being of the stockman are omitted from this chapter.

Animal — In the present farming context, this term is used to cover poultry, pigs, cattle, and sheep. Rarer or more exotic creatures such as goats, rabbits, mink, and fish are excluded. A distinction is made between young stock, for which survival and good health are the farmer's criteria, and mature stock to which the word productivity applies.

Productivity — A measure of the mass of output — be it in terms of eggs, milk, meat, wool, or offspring — for a given input. Input may be measured in cash, food, heat energy or total energy.

THE MORALS AND AESTHETICS OF INTENSIVE LIVESTOCK HOUSING

It is appropriate that the moral issues of so called "factory farming" be discussed here. Conferences[1] and inquiries[2] have been convened by governments and other bodies to enable the humanitarian, economic, and operational aspects of intensive livestock production to be discussed openly. In general the extreme "pro" and "con" views of these farming practices have consequently become moderated, and a reasonable state of satisfaction appears to exist among all parties concerned — perhaps influenced by the argument that "animals have to be treated well if they are to pay". In Britain the Brambell Report[2] influenced subsequent legislation.[3]

The use of drugs in animal production, and the drug residues which are often consequent in animal products, are outside the terms of reference of this chapter. Again, however, considerable attention[4,5] has been given to the subject and legislation exists[6] to minimize the risk to consumers.

THE ANIMAL

Farm animals are warm blooded and maintain an approximately constant deep body temperature. There is a continuous energy exchange between an animal and its surroundings, the physical phenomena of radiation, convection, conduction, and evaporation all being involved.

Bodily movement — a natural and necessary phenomenon — gives rise to changes in the energy output. Energy loss or expenditure by the animal must be offset by its

* Tables follow text, beginning on page 147.

intake of food. The difference between food energy input and physical energy output appears as change in body weight, in desired products (eggs, milk, etc.), or as excreta, since an overall energy balance must exist.

The housing of animals is seen as a convenient means of optimizing, or at least improving, the overall energy balance which would occur under natural conditions. Temperature is the most important of the environmental parameters and it is found that for a limited range of effective air temperature, normally termed the thermoneutral zone, the heat production of the animal is largely independent of its surroundings. Above the upper limit (the Upper Critical Temperature) and below the lower limit (the Lower Critical Temperature) of this zone of neutrality, the animal responds to the rigors of the environment with reduced or increased appetite, respectively. Both situations result in loss of food conversion efficiency.

Prolonged periods of high temperature can lead to heat prostration, abortion of litters, and death. Low temperature, particularly if attended by high humidity or high airflow (draft) conditions, is well known to aggravate conditions of pneumonia. The physical "discomfort" experienced by animals housed under adverse conditions also may contribute to aggression which is manifest, for example, as tail biting in pigs and cannibalism in hens.

ASPECTS OF GENERAL HOUSING

Economic and managerial factors are usually the major influences in the siting of stock buildings. Consideration should, however, be given to the effects of the immediate surroundings upon the performance of the building. Ventilation is affected significantly by obstructions sited upwind of a building and the profile of the building itself is of importance. Wind tunnel investigations of building models having simulated extractor fan ventilation have revealed that the internal pressure varies according to the ratio of spacing, L, to the height, h, of adjacent buildings.[7] For an isolated building it was found that the fan dominated the flow direction through the building only for windspeeds of less than 4 m/sec. Where another building was sited to windward of the test building, even though the windspeed was high (8.4 m/sec) the fan dominated the flow for the range $0.2 \leqslant L/h \leqslant 2$. Above this range the flow direction was reversed through the leeward opening (See Figure 1). As already mentioned, the type, size and siting of the building are usually determined very largely by economic and operational considerations. However, manufacturers of prefabricated units necessarily offer restricted ranges of dimensions. In Britain the publication of British Standards has assisted in the trend towards uniformity of building components and assemblies. These Standards have been of particular value in the process of conversion, to metric units, of the British building industry.

Recent trends in farm buildings, have been away from small units, to very much larger ones. It is appropriate, therefore, that some consideration be given to the way in which these new structures fit into the landscape. Thus the overall appearance, the type and color of the materials used, and the compatibility of the building shape with its surroundings should be borne in mind.

Matters of taste and esthetics cannot easily be quantified or tabulated, except by general agreement as to what is good and what is not. One important factor in modern building design, however, is color and attempts have been made in the U.K. to select appropriate colors and shades which fit well with the widely differing types of countryside (see Table 1).

Most modern buildings are of single-story construction comprising a structural frame, selected from a range of standard sizes, and suitable cladding material for the walls and roof. Large single-story buildings of single span construction typically have shallow pitched roofs. The overall appearance of the modern building gives an impres-

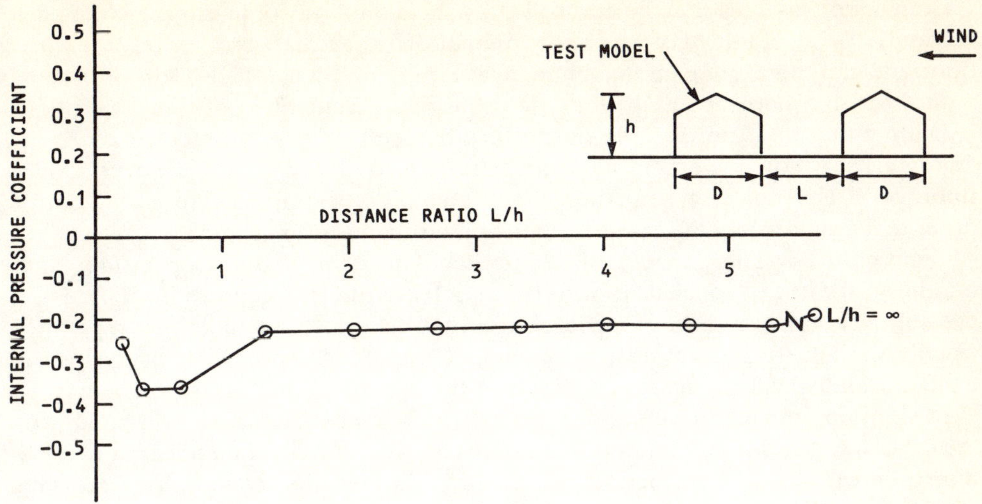

FIGURE 1. Variation of internal pressure coefficient with distance ratio. Model to leeward. (From Abdel-Reheem, A. H. A. and Douglass, M. P., *Agric. Eng.*, 31(4), 74, 1976. With permission.)

sion of "ground-hugging comfort" and this can often be used to advantage when sympathetically matched with local topography and trees.

An attempt has been made to coordinate the size of buildings on an international basis. The Construction Index/SfB manual, published in 1968 by the Royal Institute of British Architects, was a revision of the 1947 report from the Swedish Coordinating Committee for the Building Industry.

Durability of building materials in the face of corrosion is important, and steps must be taken to protect exposed steelwork with nontoxic coatings. Where silage effluent is likely to come into contact with concrete, a higher cement content than normal should be used in the mix.

Minimum content ordinary Portland cement	330 kg/m^3
Minimum compressive strength at 28 days	22.5 MN/m^2
Maximum size of aggregate	20 mm

Where buildings are provided with an electrical supply, particular care must be taken to minimize risk of shock. Animals are normally in very good electrical contact with the ground, which is usually damp, so that accidental bodily contact between a beast and an exposed, "live", conductor can easily lead to damage or death. An alternating voltage of 40 V is accepted as a safe level of exposure for human being. Animals, however, have often been found to react adversely to much lower values — perhaps as little as 20 V in some circumstances. The use of very sensitive protection devices, in the form of appropriate types of circuit breaker, is therefore to be encouraged. Particular care is also necessary in the siting of earthing electrodes; significant earth leakage currents, flowing in a resistive soil, can lead to potential differences which would be intolerable to an animal standing close to the electrode.

Thermal Properties and Ventilation of Buildings

Temperature experience by housed stock is a function of the four main factors: conduction (between the animal and, probably, the floor on which it lies), convection (usually resulting from ventilation), radiation exchange (between the animal and its immediate surroundings), and evaporation of moisture (from the skin or respiratory tract).

Conduction — This may be controlled by the animal to some extent by the posture it adopts. Lying completely prone, the animal offers greatest area of contact with the floor and can therefore gain maximum heat input from a warmed floor, or lose maximum heat to a cool or damp floor. If it adopts a crouching position, the animal is indicating that the floor is at an uncomfortable temperature. Straw or other dry bedding material allow the animal to arrange its own conditions to some extent. Concrete floors with electrical, or sometimes hot water pipe heating require close control in order that a suitable match between comfort and economy are achieved.

Convection — The purpose of ventilation is to control the temperature, relative humidity, toxic gas concentration (arising often from decomposition of feces), and possibly the concentration of airborne solid particles in the building. Temperature is usually thought to be the most important of these and, happily, if adequately controlled, usually leads to acceptable levels of the other "contaminants". There is, however, a minimum rate of ventilation below which the contaminants will build up. On the other hand, ventilation at a rate greater than a certain maximum leads to very little improvement of house temperature, even under hot weather conditions. Accordingly, maximum and minimum limits to ventilation rates are normally recommended (Table 2).[8]

Where artificial (fan) ventilation is used, the propellor type of fan is normally employed (Table 3). Usually available for operation at a static pressure of up to 5 mm (2 in.) water gage, such fans are available in various sizes and with 3 slightly different types of mounting.[8]

Building heat loss by a combination of ventilation and structural heat conduction can easily be determined for a range of housing conditions (Figure 2).[9]

Radiation — This heat exchange between animal skin and surrounding surfaces depends upon the difference of the fourth powers of the respective absolute temperatures. Under cold ambient conditions the wall and ceiling temperatures of a poorly insulated house can adopt low temperatures which may lead to a large radiant heat loss from an exposed animal skin. Conversely, radiant heating units are of value in maintaining satisfactory skin temperatures, particularly of young stock.

The temperature of the interior surface of a building is largely dependent upon the heat conduction properties of the structure and its degree of exposure to the elements (Table 4).[10]

Evaporation — In a bare-skinned animal, such as man or pig, evaporative heat loss from the skin can constitute a large part of the temperature control mechanism of the body. Evaporation of water from the respiratory tract also makes a significant contribution and experiments by Mount have yielded interesting results with young pigs (Table 5).[11]

Heat loss from the skin surface is often increased artificially, by pigs, by the process of wallowing. Normal evaporation from the pig's skin results from diffusion, without glandular secretion. A pig smeared with mud or water increases its evaporative heat loss to a level comparable with that achieved by sweating in man.

The various modes of heat loss from an animal contribute to the total loss in proportions which vary with the ambient environment, with the building surroundings and with the species, size and health of the animal. Examples for pigs and man are given (Figure 3, Tables 6 and 7).[11,12]

Disposal of feces is an ever-present problem in all animal housing situations. The approximate amounts of excreta produced by various types of stock are summarized in Table 6. The amount to be collected and dealt with will depend upon the degree of dilution and the addition of any bedding or litter. No allowance is made in the data for any rainwater or washing water.

Gaseous products of both animals and feces, already referred to briefly, are not

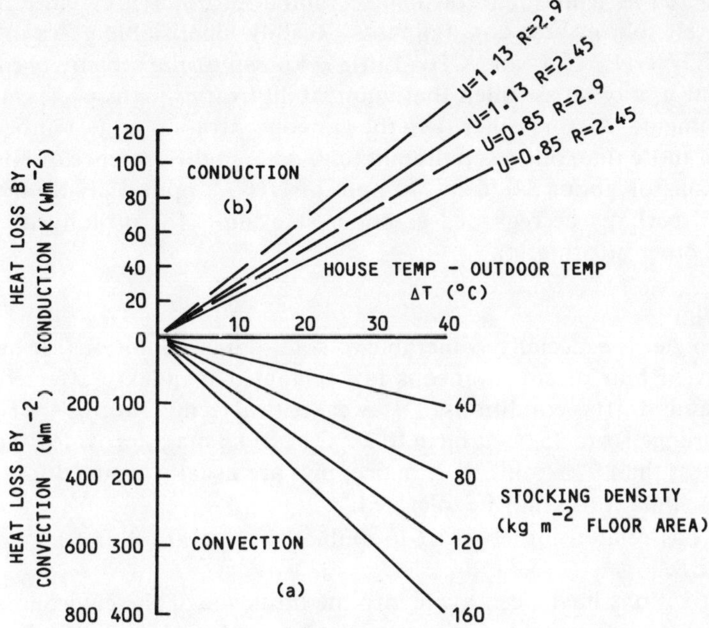

FIGURE 2. (a) Loss of heat by convection as a function of stocking density, ventilation rate, and the difference between house and air temperature. The vertical scales refer to ventilation rates of 0.372 m^3 h^{-1} kg^{-1} (left hand column) and 0.186 m^3 h^{-1} kg^{-1} (right hand column). (b) Loss of heat by conduction as function of R and U value of structure and the difference between house and air temperature, where R = ratio of surface area of house to floor area, and U = heat transfer coefficient. (From Stenning, B. C., in *Heat Loss from Animals and Man,* Monteith, J. L. and Mount, L. E., Eds., Butterworths, London, 1973. With permission.)

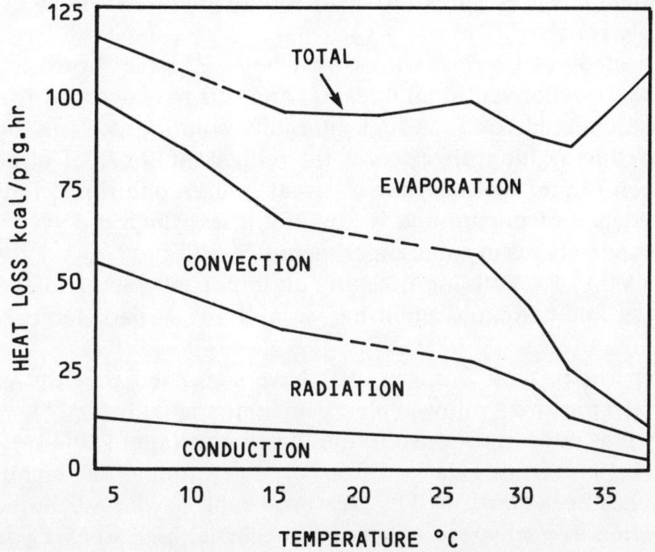

FIGURE 3. The effect of environmental temperature on heat loss and its partition for an average pig of a group, with body weight ranging from 26 to 37 kg. (From Bond, T. E., Kelly, C. F., and Heitman, H., Jr., *Agric. Eng.,* 33, 148, 1952. With permission.)

usually considered as a major hazard since ventilation rates may easily be achieved which adequately dilute these contaminants. Readily identifiable gases in stockbuildings include CO_2, NH_3, H_2S, and CH_4. Little is known of the sensitivity of animals to these gases, but it may be assumed that vulnerability varies with species, stage of maturity, environmental factors other than the gas concentration (e.g., temperature), and the presence of more than one gas pollutant (e.g., CO_2 in the presence of NH_3).

Concentrations of about 5% CO_2, 70 ppm of NH_3, 8 ppm of H_2S, and 1000 ppm of CH_4 should perhaps be regarded as upper safe limits for prolonged exposure, in the absence of other information.

Housing the Pig

The young piglet is especially vulnerable to cold, damp conditions. It has little protection by way of hair or subcutaneous fat, so that it is quickly affected by low air temperature and drafty conditions. "Lower critical temperatures" of single (ungrouped) pigs range from 35°C at birth to 24°C at 10 kg mass, provided that air movement is slow (less than 9 m/min). In practice, pigs are usually grouped together so that slightly lower temperatures may be tolerated.

Sainsbury[13] has related pig comfort to ambient temperature and air movement as shown in Table 8.

Many investigations have been made into the influence of the environment within a house upon the food conversion rate, the rate of growth and the general well-being of the housed stock. Classical work by Heitman, Kelly, and Bond[14] showed well-defined interaction among liveweight, ambient air temperature, and rate of liveweight gain (Table 9).

These data and others relating to swine production have been published by Dale (see Figures 4 and 5).[15]

While many environmental factors do, in some way, influence productivity, experiments by Braude et al.[16] have indicated that daylength has no significant effect (Table 10).

Disease among stock has a significant effect, not surprisingly, upon production. Enzootic pneumonia has been shown to delay weight gain by as much as 50% in newly weaned pigs (Table 11).[17]

Perhaps unexpectedly, pigs raised in "sweat houses" have shown less incidence of lesions than those from conventional housing, and this may account for the improved production record claimed for such high humidity conditions. It is thought that the major factor in reducing lung disorders is the reduced number of airborne particles, within the 1 to 3 μ range, which occur in sweat house conditions. It is well known, too, that the incidence of pneumonia is low in houses which are very well ventilated and stocked only sparsely, as in some experimental conditions.

Density of stocking of a building is clearly an important factor in economic animal production. Hazen and Mangold published some typical space requirements (Tables 12, 13, and 14.)[18]

Subsequent experiments by Bond et al.[19] have suggested that the greatest weight gains occurred when pigs were allowed plenty of floor space (Table 15).

The number of pigs per pen was also found to be important (Table 16).

That fatteners benefit from plenty of floor area per animal and small pen size (i.e., few pigs per pen) has been confirmed by Gehlbach et al.,[28] who attributed the improvement to the reduction of heat stress which often occurs at high stocking densities.

Building environment has been shown to have a real effect on the breeding performance of swine. Teague et al.[20] conducted experiments which are summarized in Table 17. In their experiments, 240 gilts were exposed to constant dry bulb temperatures of 26.7, 30.0, and 33°C (Table 17).

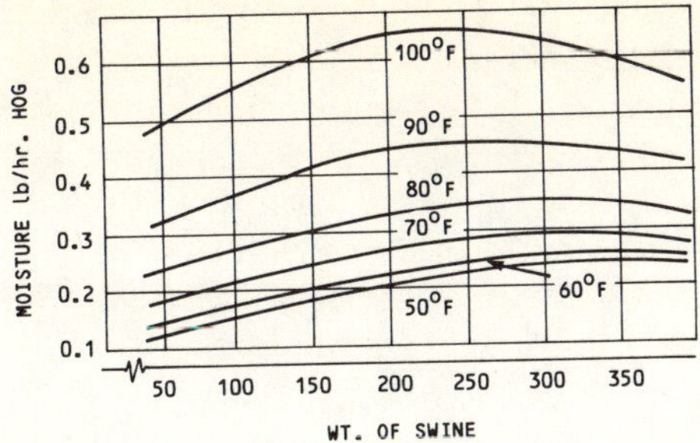

A

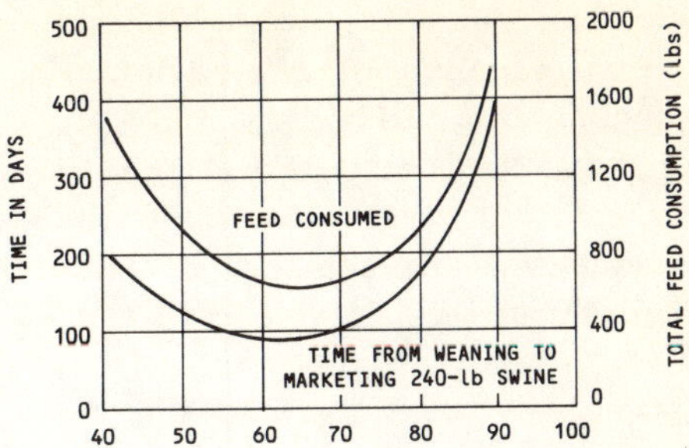

B

FIGURE 4. (A) Moisture production of swine. (B) Effect of temperature on feed consumption and time to market. (From Dale, A. C., *National Hog Farmer Swine Information Service Bull.*, F 21, Purdue University, Lafayette, Ind., October 1964. With permission.)

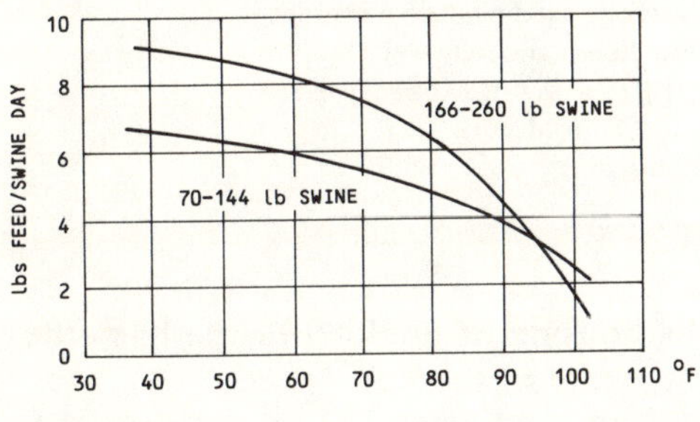

A

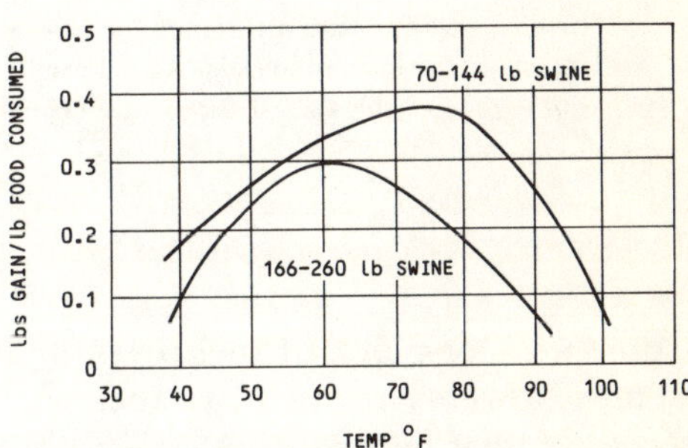

B

FIGURE 5. (A) Effect of temperature on feed consumption by swine. (B) Effect of temperature on feed efficiency. (From Dale, A. C., *National Hog Farmer Swine Information Service Bull.*, F 21, Purdue University, Lafayette, Ind., October 1964. With permission.)

Floors are of major importance in pig production as in any other form of stockrearing. Poorly designed and constructed floors, perhaps with poor drainage, may lead to abrasions of feet, knees, etc., may act as sources of bacterial infection, and may behave as gross conductors of heat, leading to chilling of stock in cold weather.

Well-designed slatted floors are successful in many situations, sometimes being used as a route for air extraction in forced ventilation systems.

Floors of flattened expanded metal of 5/8 × 1½ in. have proved satisfactory for small animals, but lack durability when used with stock over 50 lb.

Experiments by Kite[21] suggest that many designs of slat would prove acceptable, the major criteria being that the animal is not exposed to possible physical damage, either by abrasion or by becoming trapped in the slot, and that the slats are self-cleaning. Results of particular designs are shown in Table 18.

Insulated concrete floors, or floors covered with bedding material are usually successful. Uninsulated concrete, however, should be viewed with suspicion, as indicated by Mount's results (Figure 6).[22]

Poultry Housing

In 1975, there were 286 million chickens in the U.S. Most of these would be housed

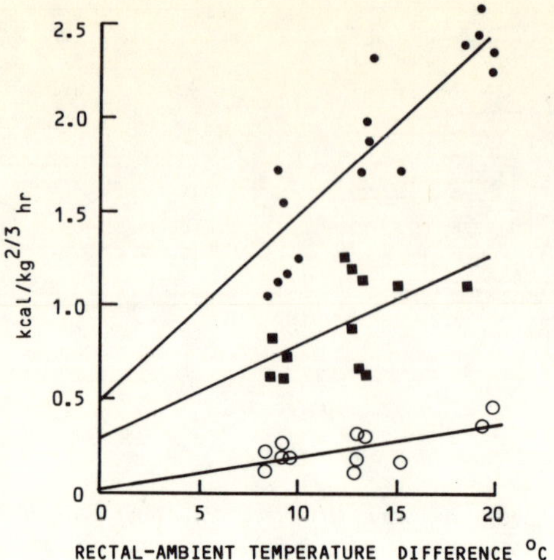

FIGURE 6. Heat loss to the floor against the rectal-ambient temperature difference for new-born pigs in a relaxed posture on three floor materials. Calculated regression lines: concrete (•) (H = 0.098T + 0.50); wood (■) (H = 0.049T + 0.30); expanded polystyrene (O) (H = 0.017T + 0.023). (From Mount, L. E., *Res. Vet. Sci.*, 8, 176—186, 1967. With permission.)

in some way for much of their lives. Indeed the housing of poultry was perhaps the first move towards intensive livestock production of any sort.

As with other housed stock, the criteria for successful farming change slightly with animal maturity. In the early days after hatching, survival and good health are the major considerations. Ideal air temperatures at this stage are a matter of some dispute, but provided that an appropriate range of conditions is available to the chick at any time, it will adapt its posture or location to best suit its own comfort. A temperature range of 70° to 100°F is appropriate and can conveniently be achieved by confining the chicks on the floor within the region covered by an artificially (radiant) heated hover.

Brooding may also be achieved by convective space heating, although the thermal efficiency of this process, expressed as a percentage of the heat ultimately arriving at bird level, is lower.

	Direct fired efficiency (%)	Indirect fired efficiency (%)
Radiant	95	80
Convected	40	33

After the brooding stage, temperatures can be reduced. Experiments by Ota and McNally[31] at Beltsville, over a 9-week period of broiler production, using air temperatures of 41, 50, 59, 68, 77, and 86°F yielded the following results. Airflow was maintained between 0.10 ft^3/min per bird at the beginning, to 1.7 ft^3/min at the end of the trial. Relative humidity was maintained at 75% (see Figure 7).

For laying hens, a U.S. Department of Agriculture publication relates egg production and feed consumption to ambient temperature (Figure 8).

These results are again based on tests conducted at Beltsville.

The rate of air movement is important in any consideration of animal comfort, and

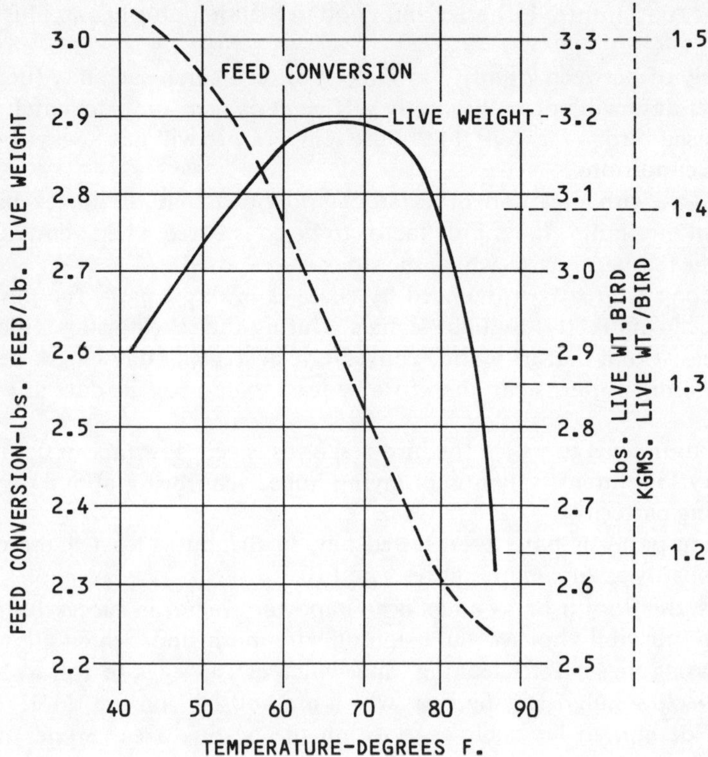

FIGURE 7. Nine-week average live weight and feed conversion data for Athens randombred broilers grown at various environmental temperatures. (U.S. Department of Agriculture.)

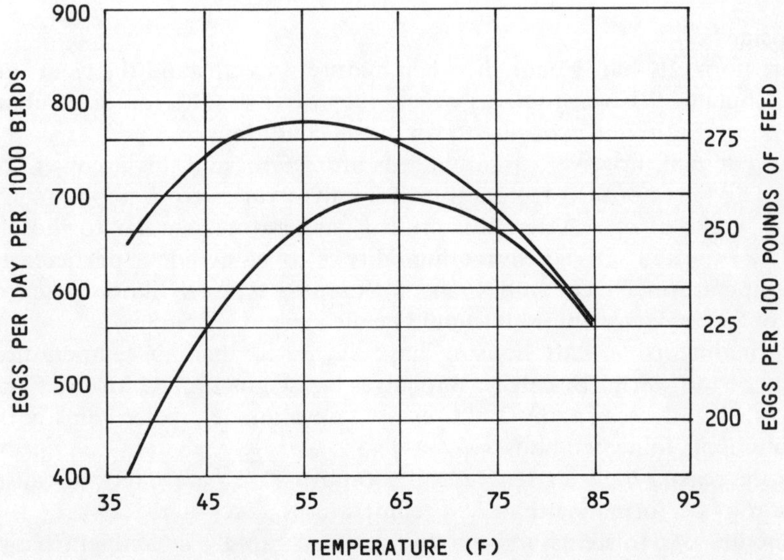

FIGURE 8. Egg production (upper curve) and feed efficiency (lower curve) at various house temperatures. (U.S. Department of Agriculture.)

the Ministry of Agriculture, Fisheries and Food in Britain publishes an illustrative table (Table 19).[30]

An air supply of between 7 and 13 m^3/hr/kg of feed eaten each day (i.e., 2 to 4 ft^3/min/lb feed per day) will normally supply sufficient oxygen and adequately dilute toxic wastes for housed birds — *except* that house temperature will not always be taken care of under these conditions.

Thus again, as with pigs and other stock, provided that the air-exchange rate is above a certain minimum, the major factor to be considered when ventilation is being controlled is the temperature to which the stock are exposed.

Egg production is greatly influenced by changes in day length, the pituitary gland being influenced (indirectly) by light signals. During the rearing stage, increasing day length advances sexual maturity and, conversely, decreasing day length delays it. The response to lighting patterns can therefore be used to control the date at which pullets come into lay.

The illumination level to which the bird responds is very low (about 0.4 lux), so that the use of very low intensity lamps in laying houses can bring about very economic control of laying patterns.

Many lighting patterns have been tested but, in Britain at least,[30] the most widely accepted is probably as shown in Figures 9 and 10.

As with pigs, the floor used by a hen is an important factor in successful production. Caged hens are normally housed on a sloping wire-mesh floor which allows easy passage of ventilating air, is self-cleaning, and which causes eggs to roll away from the hen into a collecting gully. Laying hens which are housed "on the floor" are encouraged, by nest design, to lay their eggs within the nesting area. Some "floor eggs" however, are almost inevitable, and this has resulted in a design of sloping mesh floor, for the whole house, which minimizes losses of such eggs and is beneficial in house hygiene and stockman comfort.

The density of stocking of poultry varies greatly according to the housing system used. Sainsbury[23] quotes the range shown in Table 20 as being appropriate.

Cattle Housing

Cattle are normally hardy enough, when mature, to withstand the rigors at least of the British climate. Where problems occur, they often result from a combination of poor diet, poor health, and exposure to wind chill conditions.

The young animal, however, usually needs protection, and this involves housing of some sort. The lower critical temperature for calves varies from about 14°C at birth to 8°C at 3 weeks of age. After this, critical temperatures similar to those of older cattle can be expected. High relative humidity is to be avoided, particularly at low ambient temperatures, since chilling and pneumonia types of illness often result. A maximum of 85% relative humidity should be the aim.

British experiments on calf housing have suggested that air temperatures above 15.5°C may be too warm for calves. But calves housed at 15.5°C for the first 3 weeks of their lives, then decreasing by 2.8°C every 3 days, made greater gains in the first 5 weeks than those in unheated houses.

For mature beasts, high air temperatures (above 75°F) are likely to cause greater deterioration of performance than low temperatures. Yeck and Stewart[27] found that milk production of Holsteins and Jerseys declined rapidly at ambient temperatures above 75°F. Hosteins tolerated subfreezing temperatures without loss of production, but yield of Jerseys began to decline below 40°F. Other authors have found that yarded (and therefore shielded) cattle subjected to temperatures even down to 20°F performed as well as those housed at 50°F.

Some reduction in nutrient conversion, on the other hand, may be expected, and

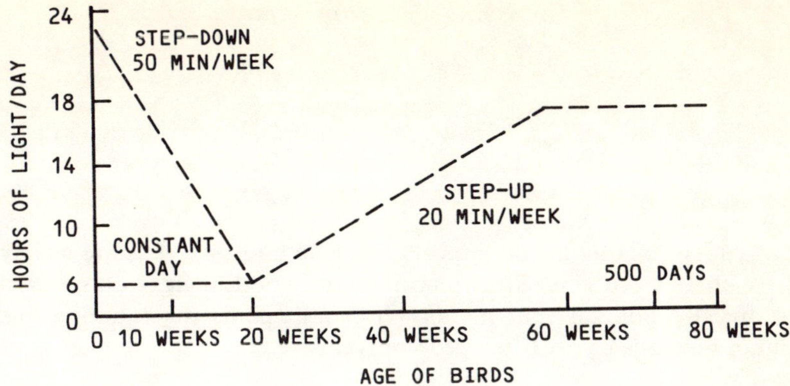

FIGURE 9. Lighting patterns for windowless houses. (From MAFF Bull. No. 212, Ministry of Agriculture, Fisheries, and Food, Her Majesty's Stationery Office, London, 1976.

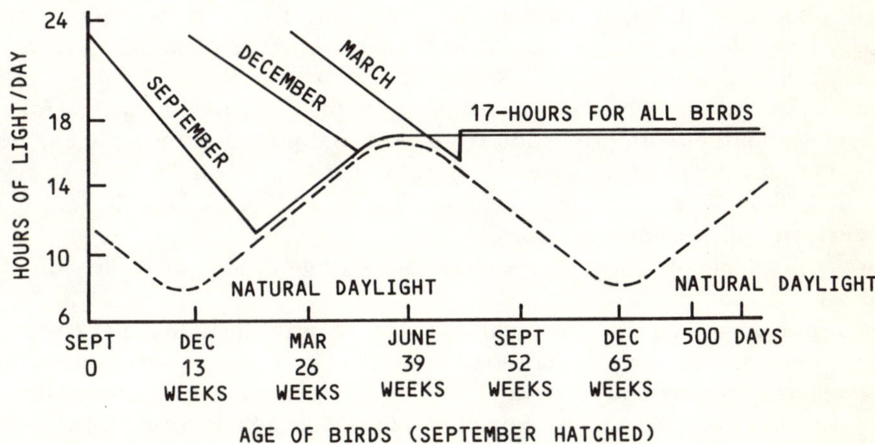

FIGURE 10. Step-down system for winter-hatched birds in houses with windows. (From MAFF Bull. No. 212, Ministry of Agriculture, Fisheries, and Food, Her Majesty's Stationery Office, London, 1976.)

Young and Christopherson[24] reported lower digestibility of dry matter among sheep, calves, and cows housed at low temperatures. The average windspeed at animal height was less than 30 m/min (Table 21).

Experiments by J. T. Morgan[25] in England in the 1960s led to the adoption of the following specification for ventilation and temperature in intensive beeflots (Table 22).

Recent preliminary investigations into roofless buildings or "slatted yards" for beef cattle, in Scotland, reveal that animal behavior is not substantially different from that observed under roofed conditions. A smaller volume of feces and urine were produced, however, than was anticipated. No obvious deterioration of animal condition or performance was reported from these trials. A topless unit has been reported in use on a Scottish farm for dairy herd followers. Stocking densities as follows have been proved satisfactory.

Weight		Space per head	
kg	cwt	m²	ft²
200	5	1.3	14
300	6	1.5	16
400	8	1.8	19
500	9¾	2.0	22

Floors, of course, again play an important role in housing. Slats are widely used for beef cattle, with great success. Straw, sawdust, or woodshavings on an earth or concrete floor are also popular, but manpower requirements for handling this bedding into and out of the housing are often prohibitive.

Sheep Housing

This matter is receiving more attention at the present time than has hitherto been thought justified. Glimp and Ames in the U.S. expressed their dissatisfaction, in 1974, with the state of knowledge regarding sheep and their interaction with their environment.[29] In Britain, the farmers' attitude to the apparent improvement in performance of inwintered sheep has largely been one of scepticism because of the cost of buildings.

Lately, however, the picture may have changed, because of improvements in the market.

Buildings can generally be constructed along the lines of covered yards as for cattle. Adequate ventilation, with protection from wind and precipitation are the important criteria. Perhaps the most important feature of a successful sheep shed, however, is the floor. This must be self-cleaning, and predominantly dry. A suitably designed slatted system is usually the most satisfactory.

Space requirements for housed ewes have been recommended by Robertson (Tables 23 and 24).[26]

It is customary under British conditions also to provide rudimentary shelter for lambing. This may comprise a series of pens about 5 ft square, arranged to form a hollow square. Roofing and rear walls must be adequate to provide protection from weather for the newly born lambs. Sometimes the whole area is covered, for improved protection and improvement of working conditions for the shepherd.

CONCLUSIONS

It will be seen, from the foregoing paragraphs, that farm animals are housed primarily for reasons of good health and productivity. Clearly, however, financial considerations are of prime importance to the practicing farmer, so that building materials, building hardware such as pens, feeding equipment, ventilation gear, and so on, must be effective and reliable, but as inexpensive as possible.

It is clear that in many situations the productivity of the stock and the profit for the farmer are both optimized only when animals are housed intensively. This means that, while things are "going right", the farm will thrive. But as with all concentrated production enterprises, small deviations from the ideal conditions can be disastrous.

Particular care is therefore necessary in setting up intensive housing systems. And careful maintenance of the hardware is essential at all times.

Table 1
COLORS SELECTED BY THE COUNCIL FOR INDUSTRIAL DESIGN ADVISORY PANEL ON FARM BUILDINGS, FROM THE RANGE OF BRITISH STANDARD BS2660 COLORS

Color	Code	Color	Code
Browns	3—036 to 3—039	Grey greens	5—059 and 5—060
Grey-browns	4—048 to 4—051	Greys to near black	7—078 9—095 to 9—098 9—100, 9—101 and 9—103

Table 2
MAXIMUM AND MINIMUM VENTILATION RATES

Livestock	Weight (kg)	Ventilation rate Max (m^3/sec kg × 10^{-4})	Min (m^3/sec kg × 10^{-4})
Pullets and hens	1.8	16	1.3—2.0
	2.0	16	1.8
	2.5	15	1.7
	3.0	13	1.6
	3.6	12	1.6
Broilers	0.045	—	6.3
	0.36	—	3.9
	0.9	—	2.1
	1.4	—	1.7
	1.8	16	2.0
	2.3	16	2.1
Turkeys	0.45	37	4.2
	2.3	14	1.4
	4.5	9.4	0.94
	6.8	8.3	0.83
	11.3	6.7	0.67
Ducks	0.45	37	—
	1.4	20	—
	2.3	17	—
	4.5	14	—
Geese	0.45	42	—
	2.3	16	—
	4.5	10	—
	6.8	9.0	—
	9.1	8.8	—
Fattening pig	20—100	5.3	0.53
Sow and litter	150—200	5.3	0.53
Dry sow	125—200	5.3	0.53
Calf	45—200	5.3	1.1
Cattle	200 +	4.0	0.8
Sheep	20—100	11	2.2

Table 3
THE PERFORMANCE OF PROPELLER FANS AT 5 MM WATER GAUGE[a]

Diameter (mm)	Speed (r/min)	Mounting arrangement	Volume (m^3/sec)	Area (m^2)	Mean air speed (m/sec)
315	1380	B	0.38	0.078	4.9
		D	0.31		4.0
355	1380	B	0.68	0.099	6.9
		D	0.58		5.9
400	1360	B	1.03	0.126	8.2
		D	0.89		7.1
450	1350	B	1.6	0.16	10.0
		D	1.4		8.8
500	900	B	1.0	0.20	5.0
		D	0.9		4.5
	1360	B	2.1		10.5
		D	1.8		9.0
630	700	R	1.6	0.32	5.0
		D	1.5	0.33	4.5
	920	B	2.7	0.33	8.2
		R	2.5	0.32	7.8
		D	2.5	0.33	7.6
	1440	R	4.1	0.32	12.8
		D	4.0	0.33	12.1
800	700	R	3.8	0.50	7.6
		D	3.7		7.4
	920	R	5.3		10.6
		D	5.2		10.4
1000	570	R	7.1	0.79	9.0
		D	6.9		8.7
	710	R	9.2		11.6
		D	9.0		11.4

[a] B, Bellmouth; D, diaphragm; R, ring.

From Randall, J. M., Handbook on the Design of a Ventilation System for Livestock Buildings, Using Step Control and Automatic Vents, *NIAE Rep. No. 29,* National Institute of Agricultural Engineers, Silsoe, England, 1977.

Table 4
THERMAL TRANSMITTANCE OF STRUCTURES (*U*) (W/M² °C)

Material	Construction and finish	U-values[a]		
		S	N	E
Walls				
Brick	112 mm	2.84	3.12	3.34
	225 mm	2.21	2.38	2.5
	255 mm + rendering	2.04	2.15	2.32
	275 mm cavity	1.65	1.76	1.88
Brick and block	Brick cavity 100-mm clinker, plastered	1.14	1.25	1.36
	Similar but foamed slag block	1.02	1.14	1.25
Solid concrete	100 mm	3.12	3.4	3.74
	200 mm	2.55	2.72	2.95
Hollow block	150-mm gravel aggregate	2.55	2.65	2.78
	150-mm lightweight	1.88	1.98	2.1
	225-mm gravel	2.38	2.5	2.61
Weatherboard	21 mm on building paper, 100 × 50 mm studs	2.5	2.84	3.17
Windows	Single glass on wood frame	3.96	5.1	6.25
Roofs				
Claytiles	On battens, felt, rafters	3.57	3.96	4.42
Felt	Three-ply on 25-mm boards, purlins, 12-mm fiberboard	1.02	1.14	1.25
	three-ply on 50-mm straw-board	1.19	1.36	1.53
Corrugated	On purlins	6.8	7.95	9.65
Asbestos-cement	As above, with 25 mm glass fiber combined sheet	0.8	0.97	1.14
Corrugated	On purlins	7.1	8.5	10.2
Galvanized sheet	As above with 12 mm fiberboard	2.21	2.38	2.61

[a] S, sheltered; N, normal — average conditions; E, exposed — coast, hill.

From Moore, I., Ed., *The Agricultural Notebook,* Butterworths, London, 1976, 837. With permission.

Table 5
THE TOTAL HEAT OF VAPORIZATION OF WATER IN THE BABRAHAM PEN CALORIMETER[a]

Calorimeter temperature (°C)	9	20	30
Calorimeter relative humidity	90	60	45
Evaporation at skin surface (kcal/g water)	0.614	0.612	0.612
Evaporation in respiratory tract (kcal/g water)	0.621	0.616	0.611
Evaporation from floor (kcal/g water)	0.595	0.602	0.606
Weighted mean heat of vaporization (kcal/g water)	0.616	0.605	0.609

[a] Includes mean values weighted for evaporation from the skin, respiratory tract, and floor for the three temperatures of operation.

From Mount, L. E., A direct calorimeter for continuous recording of heat loss from groups of growing pigs over long periods, *J. Agric. Sci.*, 68, 47, 1967. With permission of the Cambridge University press.

Table 6
EXCRETA PRODUCTION BY AGRICULTURAL STOCK

	Amount per week			
	Dung		Urine	
Stock	ft³	cwt	ft³	gal
Mature cattle	6	4	24	4
Young cattle	3	2	12	2
Bacon pigs	0.5	0.3	3.5	0.5
100 hens	0.75	0.4	—	—

Table 7
RADIANT AND CONVECTIVE COMPONENTS OF NONEVAPORATIVE HEAT LOSS FOR THE 2-kg PIG AND FOR MAN

	Radiant			Convective		
Wind-speed cm/sec	Pig 20°C	Pig 30°C	Man 25°C	Pig 20°C	Pig 30°C	Man 25°C
5	50	59	59	50	41	41
34	25	37	35	75	63	65
82	14	29	26	86	71	74
158	8	27	21	92	73	79

From Mount, L. E., *The Climatic Physiology of the Pig*, Edward Arnold, London, 1968, 189. With permission.

Table 8
THE RELATIONSHIP BETWEEN PIG COMFORT AND COMBINED AMBIENT AIR TEMPERATURE AND MOVEMENT

Temperature	Air movement below 0.15 m/sec	Air movement from 0.15—0.25 m/sec	Air movement from 0.25—0.38 m/sec
21°C	Pigs of all ages comfortable	Pigs of all ages comfortable	Young piglets uncomfortable (1—8 weeks)
18°C	Pigs below 1 week uncomfortable	Pigs below 5 weeks uncomfortable	Pigs below 12 weeks uncomfortable
15°C	Pigs below 10 days uncomfortable	Young piglets (approx. 1—3 weeks old) uncomfortable	Pigs below 12 weeks uncomfortable
13°C	Pigs below 8 weeks uncomfortable	Pigs below 12 weeks uncomfortable	Pigs below 14 weeks uncomfortable
10°C	Pigs below 15 weeks uncomfortable	Pigs below approx. 16 weeks uncomfortable	Pigs below 16 weeks uncomfortable
7°C	Pigs below 20 weeks uncomfortable	Pigs below 14 weeks uncomfortable	Pigs below 20 weeks uncomfortable
4°C	Pigs below 20 weeks uncomfortable	Pigs below 20 weeks uncomfortable	Pigs below 20 weeks uncomfortable
2°C		All fattening pigs uncomfortable	

From Sainsbury, D., *Pig Housing,* Farming Press, Ipswich, England, 1976, Chap. 2. With permission.

Table 9
EFFECT OF AMBIENT AIR TEMPERATURE AND MEAN LIVEWEIGHT ON RATE OF GAIN OF SWINE[a]

Mean liveweight, lb	Air temperatures°F 40	50	60	70	80	90	100	110
100	—	1.37	1.58	2.00	1.97	1.40	0.39	−132
150	1.27	1.47	1.75	2.16	1.82	1.14	−0.19	−2.60
200	1.19	1.57	1.91	2.22	1.67	0.88	−0.77	
250	1.10	1.67	2.08	2.14	1.51	0.62	−1.36	
300	1.02	1.77	2.24	2.06	1.36	0.36	−1.95	
350	0.94	1.87	2.41	1.98	1.21	0.10	−2.53	

[a] Average daily gain in pounds per pig.

From Heitman, H., Jr., Kelly, C. F., and Bond, T. E., *Trans. ASAE,* 1(1), 1, 1959. With permission.

Table 10
EFFECT OF LIGHT ON SWINE PERFORMANCE

	Dark 24 hr	14 hr L[a] 10 hr D	10 hr L[a] 10 hr D	Light, 24 hr
Group I (9—19 weeks)				
Final weight, lb	129.0	124.2	125.9	127.8
Daily gain per pig, lb	1.3	1.2	1.3	1.3
Feed per pound gain, lb	2.8	2.9	2.8	2.9
Group II (9 weeks to market)				
Final weight, lb	205.2	201.2	203.5	202.0
Daily gain per pig, lb	1.4	1.3	1.3	1.3
Feed per pound gain, lb	3.3	3.4	3.4	3.4

[a] L, light; D, dark.

From Braude, R., Mitchell, K. G., Finn-Kelcey, P. G., and Owen, V. M., *Proc. Nutr. Sci.*, 17, 38, 1958. With permission

Table 11
TRIAL OF PIGS AFFECTED WITH ENZOOTIC PNEUMONIA COMPARED WITH UNAFFECTED CONTROL GROUPS

	Summer		Winter	
	Unaffected	Affected	Unaffected	Affected
Weight difference between largest and smallest at start of trial	10 lb	6 lb		
Weight difference between the first pig to reach 200 lb and the smallest pig	29 lb	66 lb		
First pig to reach 100 lb	113 days	121 days		
Last pig to reach 100 lb	133 days	203 days		
Average daily weight gain	1.29 lb	1.11 lb	1.19 lb	0.92 lb
Food conversion ratio	3.39 lb	4.25 lb	3.85 lb	4.90 lb

From Betts, A. O., Whittlestone, P., Beveridge, W. I. B., Taylor, J. H., and Campbell, R. C., *Vet. Rec.*, 67, 61, 1955. With permission.

Table 12
SPACE REQUIREMENTS FOR SWINE IN SQUARE FEET PER ANIMAL[a]

		Open Shed	
	Enclosed confinement	Concrete lot	Shelter
Sow and litter	35	30	40
10 to 40 lb	4	4	2
40 to 80 lb	5	5	3
80 to 120 lb	6	6	4
120 to 160 lb	8	8	6
160 to 200 lb	10	10	8

[a] Does not include space allowance for alleys. These recommendations are based on current practices in confinement production.

From Hazen, T. E. and Mangold, D. W., *Agric. Eng.*, 41(9), 586, 1960. With permission.

Table 13
SPACE REQUIREMENTS FOR MATURE SWINE IN SQUARE FEET PER ANIMAL[a]

	On Concrete		Dirt Lots	
	Shelter	Lot	Shelter	Lot
Gilts	10	15	15	100
Sows	12	15	20	150

[a] Based on current practices in confinement production.

From Hazen, T. E. and Mangold, D. W. *Agric. Eng.*, 41(9), 586, 1960. With permission.

Table 14
FEED AND WATERING SPACE

Weight (lb)	Hand-fed or watered (lineal foot per animal)	Automatic waterers (animals per cup)	Self-feeders (animals per lineal foot)
12—50	½	25—30	6—8
50—100	¾	25—30	5—6
100—150	1	20—25	5—6
150—200	1¼	20—25	4—5
Sows	2	15—20	—[a]

[a] Self-feeding not normally recommended because of inability to control weight.

From Hazen, T. E. and Mangold, D. W., *Agric. Eng.*, 41(9), 586, 1960. With permission.

Table 15
WEIGHT GAIN BY PIGS

Space per pig (m^2)	Gain during experiment (kg)	Average daily feed (kg)	Feed (kg) per unit gain
0.46	40.4	2.4	4.09
0.92	42	2.37	3.86
1.8	45	2.36	3.69

From Bond, T. E., Kelly, C. F., and Heitman, H., Jr., *Agric. Eng.*, 33, 148, 1952. With permission.

Table 16
NUMBER OF PIGS IN RELATIONSHIP TO WEIGHT GAIN

Number of pigs per pen	Gain (kg)	Average daily gain	Feed per unit gain
3	42.7	2.56	4.15
6	42.5	2.32	3.79
12	42.2	2.26	3.71

From Bond, T. E., Kelly, C. F., and Heitman, H., Jr., *Agric. Eng.*, 33, 148, 1952. With permission.

Table 17
A SUMMARY OF MEASUREMENTS OBTAINED IN THE CONTROLLED TEMPERATURE ROOMS AND OBSERVATIONS AT SLAUGHTER 25 DAYS AFTER BREEDING.[a]

Dry-bulb temperature, °C	26.7	30.0	33.3
Average daily feed intake, kg	2.11	2.03	1.86
Average daily gain, kg	0.47	0.46	0.35
Average rectal temperature, °C	38.4	39.3	39.9
Breeding and reproductive performance			
Number returning to estrus after breeding	2	8	8
Number failing to come into estrus in rooms	0	2	7
Number not pregnant at slaughter (Did not return to heat after breeding)	5	2	3
Number pregnant (25 days)	67	67	62
Average number corpora lutea (25 days)	14.2	13.6	13.1
Average number live embryos (25 days)	10.3	9.7	9.8
Percent pregnant at 25 days	90.5	84.8	77.5

[a] Adjusted for differences in age and initial weight.

From Teague, H. S., Roller, W. L., and Grifo, A. P., Jr., *J. Anim. Sci.*, 27, 408, 1968. With permission.

Table 18
EFFECTS OF SLAT WIDTH AND SPACING ON DAILY GAIN OF GROWING-FINISHING SWINE

Floor	Slats[a]		Pig weights (lb)		Average daily gain (lb)
	Width (in.)	Spacing (in.)	Initial	Final	
Solid concrete	—	—	40	200	1.42
Concrete slats	5	1	41	205	1.45
Wood slats	4	1	41	199	1.40
Wood slats	1¼	½	40	204	1.45
Wood slats	1¼	1	40	170	1.15

[a] Totally slotted floors.[11]

From Kite, G. D., *ASAE Paper 67-401,* American Society of Agricultural Engineers, St. Joseph, Mich., 1967. With permission.

Table 19
TEMPERATURES LIKELY TO RESULT IN SIMILAR RATES OF BODY HEAT LOSS AT DIFFERENT AIR SPEEDS

	Brooder temperature		House temperature		Air speed (ft/min)		Air speed (m/sec)	
	°C	°F	°C	°F	Sleeping birds	Active birds	Sleeping birds	Active birds
Day-old	32	90	16	60	—	40	—	0.2
	32	90	21	70	—	70	—	0.4
	32	90	24	75	—	100	—	0.5
4 weeks old			16	60	55	60	0.3	0.3
			21	70	100	110	0.5	0.6
			24	75	150	200	0.8	1.0
10 weeks old			16	60	60	70	0.3	0.4
			21	70	150	210	0.8	1.0
			24	75	—	500+	—	2.5+

From the climatic environment of poultry houses, MAFF Bull. No. 212, Ministry of Agriculture, Fisheries, and Food, Her Majesty's Stationery Office, London, 1976.

Table 20
STOCKING DENSITY AND COMPARATIVE COSTS OF HOUSING WITH DIFFERENT SYSTEMS

System	Floor space per bird	Minimum cost per bird £	s.	d.
Layers				
Deep litter	3 ft^2	2	0	0
Deep litter and slats in ratio 2:1	2 ft^2	1	10	0
Deep litter and slats in ratio 1:2	1½ ft^2	1	0	0
All slats or welded mesh	1 ft^2		17	6
Multi-bird battery cages and house	½ ft^2		15	0
Rearing				
Tier brooders	36 $in.^2$ at 3 weeks		18	0
Floor rearing	1—2 ft^2		15	0
		to 1	10	0
Haybox brooder	50 $in.^2$ to 8 weeks plus run		8	0
Sussex night ark	70 $in.^2$ to point-of-lay plus pasture		10	0
Range shelter	100 $in.^2$ to point-of-lay plus pasture		7	0
Fold units	100 $in.^2$ plus pasture		15	0

From Sainsbury, D., *Animal Health and Housing*, Balliere, Tindall, and Cassell, London, 1967. With permission.

Table 21
APPARENT DIGESTIBILITY OF RATION DRY MATTER (DM) IN WARM AND COLD ENVIRONMENTS

Animal	Ration	Exposure temp. (C)	Apparent DM dig. (C)	Change in % DM dig. per 1°C
Sheep	Alfalfa pellets	21	52.0	
		−6.5	44.5	−0.27
	Alfalfa-grass	20	55.3	
	pellets	−8	48.4	−0.25
	Grain and alfalfa	20	69.0	
	pellets	−8	57.9	−0.40
Calves	Grain and chopped	18	70.4	
	alfalfa	−10[a]	65.1	−0.19
	Grain and chopped	18	69.8	
	alfalfa	−9[a]	60.7	−0.34
Cows	Alfalfa-grass	21	61.3	
	long hay	−11	61.6	−0.01
			mean ± SE	0.24 ± 0.06

[a] Average temperature of outdoor environment.

From Young, D. A. and Christopherson, R. J., in *Proc. Livestock Environment Symp. ASAE,* American Society of Agricultural Engineers, St. Joseph, Mich., 1974. With permission.

Table 22
VENTILATION AND TEMPERATURE SPECIFICATIONS IN INTENSIVE BEEFLOTS[25]

Liveweight (lb)	Ventilation rate (ft^3/min) "Minimum"	"Maximum"	Optimum temperature (°F)
85	7	40	60, falling to 55
250	15	87	50—55
300	16	97	50—55
350	18	107	50—55
400	20	117	50—55
450	22	126	50—55
500	23	135	50—55
550	25	145	50—55
600	26	153	50—55
650	28	162	50—55
700	29	170	50—55
750	31	178	50—55
800	32	186	50—55
850	33	193	50—55
900	35	200	50—55
1,000	37	215	50—55

Table 23
FLOOR SPACE FOR SHEEP

Type	Space allotment (m^2) Slatted floor	Solid floor
Large ewe (68—70 kg)	0.95—1.1	1.2 —1.4
Large ewe and lamb	1.2 —1.7	1.4 —1.85
Small ewe (45—69 kg)	0.75—0.95	1.0 —1.3
Small ewe and lamb	1.0 —1.4	1.3 —1.75
Ewe hogg	0.45—0.75	0.65—0.95

From Robertson, A. M., *Farm Building Progress*, 51, 1978.

Table 24
RECOMMENDED TROUGH LENGTHS

Type of sheep	Trough length (mm)[a]
Large ewes	475—500
Small ewes	375—425
Hoggs	350—400

[a] On self-feed silage 100—250 mm is adequate for all sheep.

From Robertson, A. M., *Farm Building Progress*, 51, 1978.

REFERENCES

1. **Bellerby, J. R., Ed.,** Factory Farming, Proc. Symp. on Behalf Br. Assoc. Advancement Sci., Educational Services, London, 1970.
2. **Brambell, F. W. R.,** Report of the Technical Committee to Report into the Welfare of Animals Kept Under Intensive Husbandry Livestock Systems, Cmnd 2836, Her Majesty's Stationery Office, London, 1965.
3. Agriculture (Miscellaneous Provisions) Act, Great Britain, 1968.
4. Report of the Agricultural and Medical Research Council's Joint Committee on Antibiotics in Animal Feeding, Her Majesty's Stationery Office, London, 1962.
5. **Swann M.,** Rep. of Jt. Committee on Use of Antibiotics in Animal Husbandry and Veterinary Medicine, Cmnd 4190, Her Majesty's Stationery Office, London, 1969.
6. Food, Drug, and Cosmetics Act, U.S.A.
7. **Abdel-Reheem, A. H. A. and Douglass, M. P.,** Effect of adjacent structures on farm building ventilation, *Agricultural Engineer (U.K.),* 31(4), 74—79, 1976.
8. **Randall, J. M.** A Handbook on the Design of a Ventilation System for Livestock Buildings Using Step Control and Automatic Vents, NIAE Rep. No. 29, National Institute of Agricultural Engineering, Silsoe, England, 1977.
9. **Stenning, B. C.,** Some economic aspects of the heating of pig houses, in *Heat Loss from Animals and Man,* London, Monteith, J. L. and Mount, L. E., Eds., Butterworths, London, 1973.
10. **Moore, I., Ed.,** The Agricultural Notebook, Newnes-Butterworth, London, 1976, 837.
11. **Mount, L. E., Holmes, C. W., Start, I. B., and Legge, A. J.,** A direct calorimeter for continuous recording of heat loss from groups of growing pigs over long periods, *J. Agric. Sci.,* 68, 47—55, 1967; Mount, L. E., *The Climatic Physiology of the Pig,* Edward Arnold, London, 1968, 189.
12. **Bond, T. E., Kelly, C. F., and Heitman, H., Jr.,** Heat and moisture loss from swine, *Agric. Eng.* 33, 148—152, 1952.
13. **Sainsbury, D.,** The environmental needs of the pig, *Pig housing,* Farming Press, Ipswich, England, 1976, Chap. 2.
14. **Heitman, H., Jr., Kelly, C. F., and Bond, T. E.,** Hog house conditioning and ventilation data, *Trans. ASAE,* 1(1), 1, 1959.
15. **Dale, A. C.,** National Hog Farmer Swine Information Serv. Bull. F21, Purdue University, Lafayette, Ind., October, 1964.
16. **Braude, R., Mitchell, K. G., Finn-Kelcey, P. G., and Owen, V. M.,** The effect of light on fattening pigs, *Proc. Nutr. Soc.,* 17, 38, 1958.
17. **Betts, A. O., Whittlestone, P., Beveridge, W. I. B., Taylor, J. H., and Campbell, R. C.,** *Vet. Rec.,* 67, 61, 1955.
18. **Hazen, T. E., and Mangold, D. W.,** Functional and basic requirements of swine housing, *Agric. Eng.* 41, (9), 586, 1960.
19. **Bond, T. E., Heitman, H., Hahn, L. and Kelly, C. F.,** *Calif. Agric.,* 9—11, 1962.
20. **Teague, H. S., Roller, W. L., and Grifo, A. P., Jr.,** Influence of high temperature and humidity on the reproductive performance of swine, *J. Anim. Sci.,* 27, 408—411, 1968.
21. **Kite, G. D.,** Slatted Floor Swine Farrowing and Nursery Buildings, ASAE Paper 67—401, American Society of Agricultural Engineers, St. Joseph, Mich., 1967.
22. **Mount, L. E.,** The heat loss from new-born pigs to the floor, *Res. Vet. Sci.,* 8, 176—186, 1967.
23. **Sainsbury, D.** The housing of poultry, *Animal Health and Housing,* Balliere Tindall and Cassell, London, 1967.
24. **Young, B. A. and Christopherson, R. J.,** Effect of Prolonged Cold Exposure on Digestion and Metabolism in Ruminants, *Proc. of Livestock Environment Symp.,* American Society of Agricultural Engineers, St. Joseph, Mich., 1974.
25. **Morgan, J. T.,** The Control of Climatic Environment in Intensive Beeflots, Proc. of Conf. Intensive Housing of Beef Cattle, Farm Buildings Association, U.K., 1964.
26. **Robertson, A. M.,** Sheep housing, Farm Building Progress, 51, 1—4, 1978.
27. **Yeck, R. G. and Stewart, R. E.,** A ten-year summary of the psychroenergetic laboratory dairy cattle research at the University of Missouri, *Trans. ASAE,* 2, 71, 1959.
28. **Gehlbach, G. D., Becker, D. E., Cox, J. L., Harmon, B. G., and Jensen, A. H.,** Effects of floorspace allowance and number per group on performance of growing-finishing swine, *J. Anim. Sci.,* 25, 386—391, 1966.
29. **Glimp, H. A. and Ames, D.,** Sheep and their environment — new knowledge needed, *Proc. of Livestock Environment Symposium,* ASAE, St. Joseph, Mich., 1974.
30. The climatic environment of poultry houses, MAFF Bull. No. 212, Ministry of Agriculture, Fisheries, and Food, Her Majesty's Stationery Office, London, 1976.

31. **Ota, H. and McNally, E. H.,** Preliminary Broiler Heat and Moisture Data for Designing Poultry Houses and Ventilation Systems, ASAE Paper 65—411, American Society of Agricultural Engineers, St. Joseph, Mich., 1965.

Physiological Factors

BEHAVIOR OF LIVESTOCK IN RELATION TO THEIR PRODUCTIVITY

J. J. Lynch

INTRODUCTION

Climate and social customs have resulted in a wide variety of animal production systems throughout the world. This chapter reviews the relevance of behavior to production in *intensive systems* where animals are fed in sheds, milked daily, or given supplementary feed, and in *pastoral systems* where animals are grazing throughout the year. In intensive systems much of the reduced productivity originates from animals being kept at a high density. In pastoral systems, lowered productivity is most frequently associated with sexual and maternal behavior. The review begins with the recent history of behavioral research, and deals with mother young relations, critical periods, the behavior of young and mature animals in normal and stressful environments, grazing and reproductive behavior, transport, and finally, behavior and selection. Examples have been taken from cattle, sheep, pigs, and poultry and have been considered under the most appropriate heading.

RECENT DEVELOPMENTS IN BEHAVIORAL RESEARCH

The development of production systems which cage poultry, tether sows, and feed large concentrations of housed beef or dairy cattle with processed food has led to considerable concern for the welfare of livestock. As a result of the British parliament appointment of a technical committee to inquire into the welfare of animals kept under intensive livestock systems, the Brambell Report was published in 1965.[1] This report has stimulated a great deal of research in animal behavior. Various facets have been reviewed by many authors.[2-15]

The Brambell Report indicated that there was little scientific basis for their recommendations and that the committee was often forced to give judgements based on opinions of a wide variety of people. Thorpe,[5] in summarizing a main conclusion of the committee, stated, "While accepting the need for much restriction (of animals), we concluded that on scientific grounds the line must be drawn at conditions which completely suppress most of the natural, 'innate' urges and behavior patterns characteristic of actions appropriate to the high degree of social organization which all domesticated farm animals share and which have been little, if at all, bred out in the process of domestication." In addition,[5] there was not necessarily a correlation between the degree to which the natural behavioral tendencies were thwarted or distorted and the physiological changes that ensue. These changes relate especially to those concerned with the adrenal gland, an organ whose responses have been widely accepted as indicative of stress.

The report has been the basis for stimulating much of the research on behavior and production of animals in intensive systems. The Brambell Report[1] considered that floors of poultry cages were inadequate to support the bird's feet and that the diameter of the wire should be changed from 2 mm to 3.25 mm. On the heavier floor, up to 64% of eggs would have cracked if some strains of hens were used,[16] and there was no evidence that birds were more comfortable on the heavier floors. It was shown later that birds did not have a marked preference for any particular floor type although the lighter the wire gauge the longer the birds spent on it when offered combinations of floors of different wire diameters.[8] Although the Brambell Report recommended that spectacles should not be used on poultry, with their use a substantial increase in egg production of 10% has been demonstrated.[17] This example highlights the question of whether high productivity was reliable evidence for the absence of severe stress.[5] In the absence of scientific evidence to the contrary, it does seem difficult to conclude that birds with spectacles are under greater stress than birds without spectacles. Restriction of space may not be nearly as important as the way space is designed.[18] By using baffles in a broiler breeder pen to break up the area into smaller units, the birds in the pen with baffles had an average gain which was 0.04 g per bird per day higher than the controls. This difference was seen only at the higher stocking density of one bird per 557 cm^2 and did not occur at the lower density of one bird per 696 cm^2.

These examples show the dangers of making recommendations about the welfare of animals without having adequate biological information to substantiate the recommendations. This does not imply that consideration of the matters raised by the Brambell Report[1] and subsequent Codes[19,20] is not worthwhile. In fact, if they had not been raised, a large phase of animal behavior and welfare studies might not have been initiated so rapidly.

MOTHER YOUNG BEHAVIOR

The first 14 days of the life of an animal is most important. Early in this period, close relationships are forged between the newborn and its mother and these last till weaning. The first 2 weeks is also a time of high death rates and of problems in fostering young animals.

In modern piggeries 20% of all piglet mortalities can be attributed to crushing by the sow,[21] with most deaths occurring in the first 2 days when piglets lie very close to the udder.[22] After this time, creep heaters attract the piglets away from the sow. It does not appear that the behavioral sequences associated with death of the piglets have been studied although examination of this facet of maternal behavior may well suggest different management techniques. One possibility is to make a substitute ''pig'' which will entice piglets from the mother except when feeding. Such a scheme would seem feasible provided crushing is actually related to the behavior which causes the sow and piglets to remain very close together.

The relatively poor growth rates[23] measured in an intensive system of calf-rearing may be a result of difficulties in social integration within the group. Cross sucking of ears, scrotum, and prepuce was observed in calves which had lowered weight gains. The high percentage of calves needing assistance in finding the artificial calf feeder (Table 1) even after 6 weeks is startling and illustrates the need to train calves during the period when they are most sensitive in learning to suck the teat, i.e., within the first week of life. In artificially reared lambs which were removed from their mother at 48 hours, some showed cross sucking of scrotum or navel which resulted in ill-thrift, infection, and removal of these lambs from the group. Stephens and Baldwin[24] also stated that the lambs go through a repertoire of sucking behavior but very little maternal reinforcement was received from the feeder. Nonnutritive sucking results in some oral stimulation of these young lambs, but as in thumb sucking of human infants, the reasons are obscure. Greater attention to the role of nonnutritive sucking may result in a feeder which more closely fits the needs of the young lambs. Puppies which sucked from bottles with freeflowing nipples or from cups also sucked on nonnutritive objects including the ears of their litter mates.[25] Puppies which could only suck through a slow-flowing nipple or from the dam did not show this behavior. If flow rates are important in the development of nonnutritive sucking, the teat size could be important in the design of automatic feeders for calves and lambs.

Merino sheep show several types of abnormal maternal behavior (Table 2)[26] which

Table 1
CALF GROWTH RATES UNDER INTENSIVE REARING SYSTEM

	Days 1—3 after arrival	Weeks pre-weaning					
		1	2	3	4	5	6
A. Calves needing guidance[a]	85 (71)	67 (56)	52 (43)	41 (34)	39 (32)	31 (26)	27 (22)
B. Calves cross-sucking from Group A[b]		5 (4)	3 (2)	2 (2)	2 (2)	2 (2)	2 (2)

Note: Observations from a total of 120 calves (8 groups of 15). Values in brackets are numbers as a percentage of the total calves under observation.

[a] Numbers of calves observed to require guidance in locating Nursette teat at least once per day.

[b] Number of calves from category A observed cross-sucking on more than three occasions during two 3-hr watches.

After Stephens D. B., *Anim Prod.*, 18, 23—34, 1974. With permission.

Table 2
ABNORMAL MATERNAL BEHAVIOR IN SHEEP AND SOME OF THE POSSIBLE CAUSES

Behavior	Desertion of single lamb
	Separation from twin
	Failure of primiparous ewes to stand still so the lamb can suck
	Failure of ewes to stand still after they have had a difficult birth
Causes	Inexperience
	Failure to realize the number of lambs born
	Weakness due to undernutrition
	Difficult birth

Note: Each form of behavior may have several causes.

often have a clearly identifiable cause. Abnormal lamb behavior is caused by chilling or birth injuries. Poor maternal behavior and chilling of lambs[27-29] result in the death of 20% of lambs in Australia each year. Recent research work has concentrated on attracting parturient ewes to shelter which would protect lambs from the chilling effects of wind, thus giving them a better chance for survival.[30,31] Lamb mortality has been reduced by as much as 75%.[195]

There is a short time immediately after birth when sheep and cattle establish the identity of their young, and thereafter the mother vigorously rejects alien young. This period is no longer than 24 hr and frequently is shorter [32,33] but it can be lengthened to 10 days [34] by enforced contact between the mother and young. Since the failure to foster orphan lambs may represent a considerable economic loss to farmers, adoption of twinning crates has developed as a practical result of the work on enforced contact between mother and alien young. As yet there are no data published on the rate of successful fostering of lambs. Tranquilizers have been used with apparent success[35] in fostering ewes to alien lambs but no further research on the technique appears to have been reported.

CRITICAL PERIODS AND EARLY EXPERIENCE

In 1945 Scott[36] described the social organization of a flock of sheep based on many observations of their behavior. He separated a female lamb from the flock at birth and returned it 9 days later. The lamb was butted off by the mother, and always remained relatively independent but returned to the flock at mating. After each lambing, this "orphan" ewe showed less maternal behavior and was not disturbed by separation from her lambs. The implications from these observations were that since no maternal young bond formed the lamb was never closely associated with its mother and the rest of the flock and its behavior did not quite conform with the social behavior of the flock. Scott[37] considered that the time immediately after birth was one *critical period* in a sheep's life.

Critical periods are defined[37] as times when a large effect can be produced by a smaller change in conditions than in other periods of life. Thus 5-min licking of calves[33] and kids[38] and 20 to 30 min licking of lambs[32] is sufficient for the mother young bond to form.

Scott[37] suggested "that any period in life when a major new relationship is being formed is a critical one for determining the nature of that relationship." Other critical periods may be related to the first experience of eating solid foods, being separated from the dam, being handled by man, exploring new paddocks, moving through stock yards, mating, and giving birth to young. All these periods represent times when "major" new relationships are being formed, and are periods when behavioral modifications may be influenced by man. There is little experimental work on the effects of any of these periods on later behavior except mating behavior. In sheep it has been shown that ewes mated for the first time at 6 to 7 months [39] did not stand or compete for the ram as 18- month-old ewes did. The young sheep's behavior was unchanged during the next two estrus cycles.

Experiences early in the life of some species other than domestic animals have been shown to have surprisingly long-term effects. Almost any daily routine of handling rats in early life resulted in a higher degree of "emotional stability" compared to unhandled rats.[40] Open-field tests have primarily been used. Other effects of extra stimulation of rats are said to include greater survival rates in stressful situations,[41] superior learning abilities,[42] and higher brain weights and corticosteroid levels.[43] Handled Siamese kittens were more docile[44] and handled dogs showed greater exploratory behavior, superiority in problem solving, and were more docile than the unhandled animals.[45] Whether such experiments have much relevance to the behavior of these species living in their natural environment is another matter. Perhaps it is important that some breeds of dogs be made more docile by handling. Extrapolation from these experiments to domestic animals would be unwise without prior experimentation.

There is little written about any effects of early experience on later behavior and production in the species discussed in this review. Different rearing treatments of calves[46] (1) fed separately — raised separately, (2) fed separately — raised in groups of three, (3) fed together (groups of three) — raised separately, (4) fed together (groups of three) — raised together (groups of three), affected their dominance order. Those animals in treatment (1) produced the most milk in the first lactation.[47] Animals raised together neglected their young, partially cleaned their calves, and were more reluctant to allow sucking. Those animals reared separately showed better maternal behavior. There were few differences in behavior at the second calving.

Calves removed from the mother at birth and fed milk from a bucket could not readily locate the teats when reintroduced to cows after 9 days.[48] Calves under 9 days could actively seek the teat or could be readily taught to suck from the teat. The behavior of calves which were reared on an artificial feeder after having had access to milk in a bucket for several weeks was observed.[23] Even after 6 weeks, 22% needed guiding to the teat. There were clear indications that lack of early experience in sucking behavior represented an economic loss because calves required constant supervision and had to be forced to the artificial feeder every day.

A similar problem to that described for calves has been described in artificially reared lambs.[49] Two of four lambs did not know how to drink from water containers after being weaned from a bottle. One lamb eventually dehydrated and needed replacement therapy. The labor component in the intensive lamb and calf rearing industry is so large that man should not have to teach young animals to use an artificial feeder. The young should have learned how to suck before being removed from their mothers.

The effects of vastly different geographical locations on grazing preferences, food intake, liveweight, and wool production of sheep brought to the same pasture at a central location were studied by Arnold and Maller.[50] In general there was little long-term effect on production, but there were marked differences in grazing preferences between sheep coming from the different areas of Australia. Adult sheep took longer to adjust to a new environment than did lambs.

There is a developing market for the export of live sheep from Australia to the Middle Eastern countries. Sheep are gathered in a feed lot and are provided with a pelleted ration. They are expected to have made the transition from eating grass to eating pellets in the 2 weeks before they are shipped overseas. There is little information concerning the number of sheep rejected because they failed to adapt to the ration, but it may be substantial. The situation may be improved by giving the sheep experience of pelleted food when they are young animals.

The ability of sheep to find their way through a maze is affected by early experience. Liddell[51] showed that 2-year old sheep which experienced the maze only as lambs solved it far more rapidly than sheep which experienced the maze only as 2-year-old animals. This may have some relevance to the ease with which sheep will travel through yards if they experience these yards as young animals.

Total isolation of boars from one another till puberty is undesirable[52] since boars raised either as a mixed sex group or as a male group had more active courting behavior and a higher number of copulations than boars reared in individual pens from 20 days to 30 weeks. This poor copulatory behavior persisted to 13 months and did not improve with sexual experience. Although these data suggest that these socially restricted animals may be ineffective sires, there were no data presented on the percentage of sows pregnant or the number of young born from boars in each of these groups.

Food preferences of chickens exposed to particular feeds immediately after hatching have been studied by Capretta.[53] The results suggest that the first experience of a food had an effect on selection of that particular food up to 14 days later.

Early experience and critical periods may be of some use in solving practical behavioral problems. Grain feeding early in life may overcome the problem of a group of sheep being reluctant to eat wheat.[54] The same problem of less than 100% acceptance of supplements in the form of liquids on solid blocks occurs in cattle.[54] If all cattle ate a supplement containing anthelmintic, then the time and cost of mustering beef cattle into yards could be overcome. It is possible that experience of yards and sheds may enable the flow of sheep and cattle to be much faster. Certainly, the factors impeding the flow of animals in yards should be studied to assist in design of better facilities for holding and working stock. Kilgour[56] has warned of the problems of allowing the multiple sucking of dairy heifers when it may be better that calves be handfed to ensure the greatest degree of interaction between man and calf. Man then has in his own hands the ability to produce a tractable milking cow. Buildings for rearing calves might simulate the design of the milking shed the calves will experience for most of their lives.[57]

Early experience may be a useful managerial technique in domestic animals but, as yet, it has rarely been used. In the few cases where experience might be expected to help, i. e., young maiden ewes[39] and socially restricted boars,[52] there was no evidence that it changed the animal's behavior. It is possible that effects of early experience are minimal or are confined to a brief period of adaptation. The use of critical periods and early experience in animal management needs further study.

DISTINCTION BETWEEN CROWDING AND DENSITY

If 30 sheep were held in a 3-ha paddock then the stocking rate would be 10 sheep/ha. The *density* would be one sheep in 0.1 ha; *crowding* would occur[54] if sheep were provided with supplementary feed in a trough 3 m long, i.e., 10 cm per sheep. Analogous situations can be seen with the design of watering troughs for cows and water nipples in pig or poultry units.

Density is purely associated with spatial parameters[58] while crowding depends on the absolute numbers present and occurs when there is interaction of spatial, social, and managerial factors. McBride[59] considers crowding to have occurred when one animal intrudes into the personal area of another. When this happens, there is an alerting response and an interaction of threat, overt aggression, or recognition of the intruder. Within a group of a few animals crowding may not occur, but with 100 animals at the same density, crowding may occur.[15] The likely reason is the failure of one animal to recognize another which results in dominance hierarchy breaking down because a subordinate animal does not give a submissive gesture.

Various research workers have provided examples of crowding:

1. A flock of seven male turkeys were held in an area which was gradually reduced in size till crowding and aggression occurred.[59] With further reduction in area to 1 m^2 the turkeys eventually all stood around the fence facing outwards and there was no further conflict!
2. As space per heifer was reduced from 100% of recommended pen area to 25%, the amount of agonistic behavior in the group and movement in the heifers low on the dominance rank increased markedly.[60] Increased crowding caused more frequent violation of the space of dominant animals.
3. Five steers were placed in both triangular and square pens (area 13.4 m^2).[61] In pens of both shapes, animals positioned themselves within 1 m of the perimeter in 85% of the observations. The main conclusion was that if the ratio of perimeter to area could be maximized it would lead to decreasing the effects of crowding.
4. McBride[62] (Figure 1) has illustrated the importance of providing sufficient space for egg production. If there is enough space, birds can disperse and there is a reduction of aggression. If space is inadequate there will be a reduction in the size and number of eggs produced with the subordinate animals being most affected.

It may be necessary to have a high density of animals together in a shed to produce an economically efficient management system but particular attention must be paid to feeding, drinking, and sleeping areas so that these places do not become localized areas of crowding.

Since such a large component of the behavioral literature relates to the effects of crowding animals, brief reference will be made to those authors who have discussed theoretical concepts of dominance, crowding, and stress.

Stress has been defined[63] as something which causes an animal to make abnormal

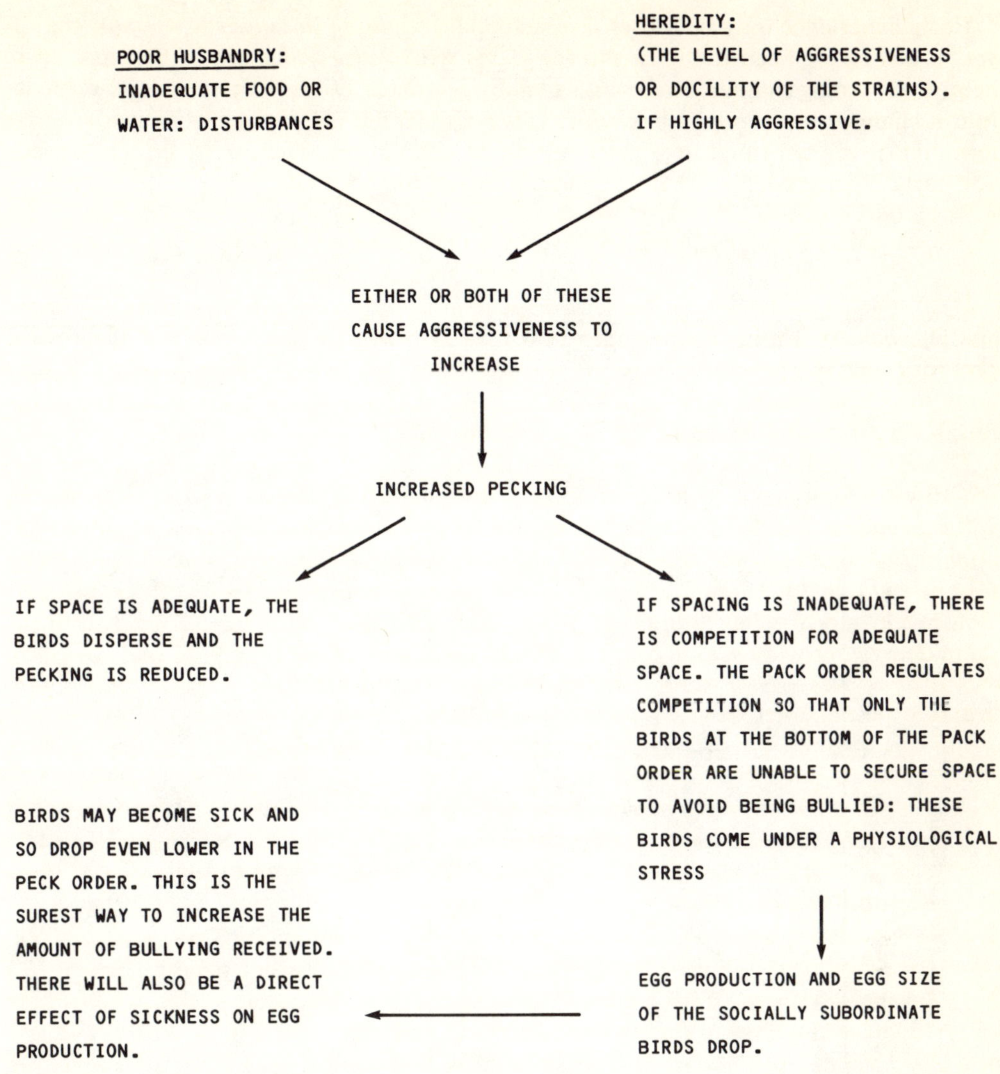

FIGURE 1. Consequences of crowding fowls. (After McBride, G., *Discovery*, 27, 16-19, 1966. With permission.)

or extreme adjustments to its physiology or behavior in order to cope with adverse effects of its environment. Environmental stresses include extremes of temperature, rain, wind, and humidity, while management stresses include transportation, alteration of routine, and physical injury.

Social Stress

Social stresses are those which come from conspecific animals in the immediate vicinity.[64] Animals are compelled to be close to each other in intensive piggeries, poultry units, milking sheds, feedlots, and during drenching, dipping, or other managerial procedures. An animal's responses to those stresses can be both physiological via the pituitary and adrenal glands, and behavioral via threat or submissive gestures. The responses are aimed at reducing the stress by adaptation. A theoretical explanation of the responses to social stress is given in McBride[64] (Figure 2).

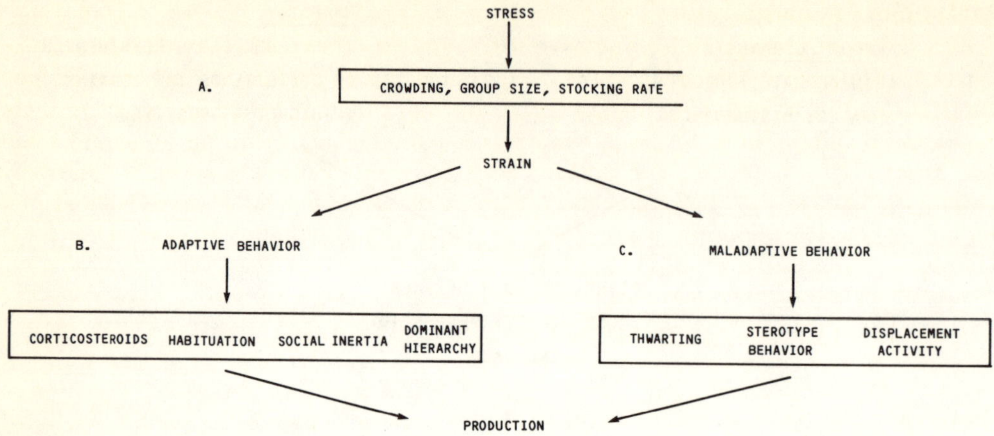

FIGURE 2. A summary of the major factors associated with stress and the animal's response to that stress.

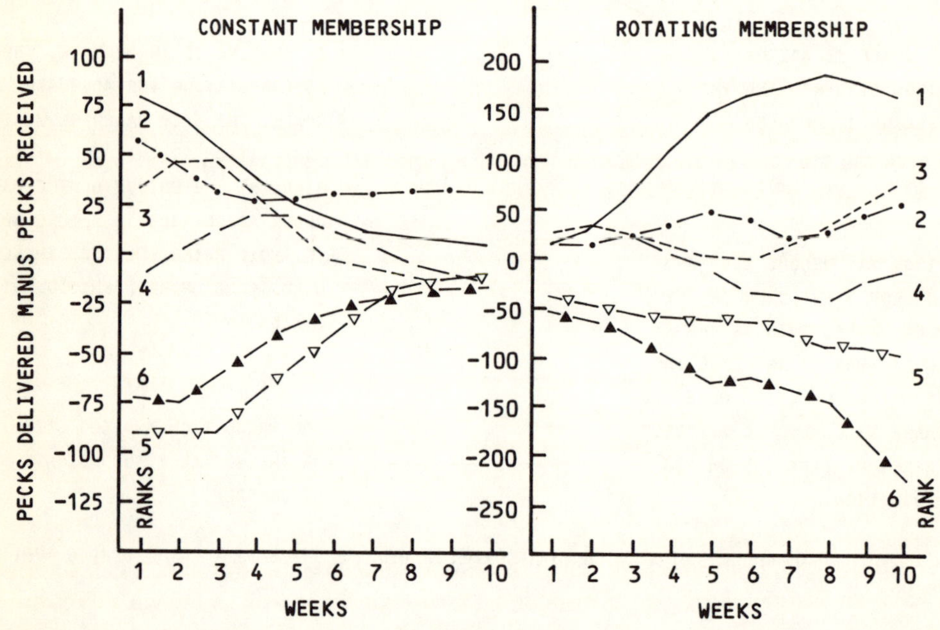

FIGURE 3. Weekly total interactions, pecks delivered minus pecks received, according to social ranks in a flock having a constant membership and another with a regular rotating membership. Note differences in scale on the vertical coordinates. (After Guhl, A. M., *Anim. Behav.*, 16, 219-232, 1968. With permission.)

Social Inertia

Two groups of six pullets were placed in separate pens and ranked according to pecks delivered and received.[65] In one group one bird was replaced every second day for the last 7 weeks of the 10-week experiment. The results in Figure 3 show the stability in the flock with constant membership and the level of agitation and instability in the flock with rotating membership. This illustrates the sequence of events which starts with the establishment of dominance hierarchy and leads to a stable social order. When one animal becomes habituated to another there is a state of *social inertia* with a resulting high level of social stability.

Maladaptive Patterns

If a group of animals fails to achieve social stability then there may be other consequences. Maladaptive patterns result from animals being in situations where they may be frustrated in trying to perform a full or normal range of behavior, or where there is a lack of stimulation.[66,67] Such examples include frequent shifting of weight from one front leg to the other, rattling feed buckets, wool chewing in sheep,[68] and many stereotype behaviors.[11] For fuller discussion of the development of adaptive and maladaptive behavior patterns as a response to social stimuli, Hinde,[69] Bryant,[6] Duncan,[11] Bareham,[12] and Wood-Gush[67] should be consulted.

DOMINANCE HIERARCHY AND PRODUCTIVITY

Poultry

Egg Production

In 1962 McBride[70] discussed the effects of dominance on a group of housed birds. With competition the age of sexual maturity was delayed and as competition increased, egg production, then egg weight and liveweight were reduced. Spectacles placed on birds' beaks so that forward vision was restricted have been shown to increase egg production and decrease feed intake whether the animals were in cages or in pens on the floor.[71,72] There was also a reduction in pecking, general activity and aggressiveness in these birds[72] and the adrenal glands were 50% of the size of those without spectacles. In general, there is some evidence that using spectacles has reduced the level of social stress in birds which were housed in cages or in floor pens.

Structure of Groups

Egg production was depressed when new hens were introduced into a socially organized laying flock.[73-75] However, if flocks were assembled before laying commenced the effect was minimal.[76] If birds which were strangers to each other were given a choice of cages containing 0 to 6 birds, they invariably chose a cage with no animals.[77] This was partly modified by group rearing when the birds preferred the cage with familiar animals to a cage with no animals. Once flocks are assembled and laying has commenced it is unwise to change the structure of the flock by adding new birds.

Effects of Group Size and Area

In poultry, increasing the numbers of animals placed in the one cage has been shown to have an influence on egg production. Although there was found no effect on egg weight, food consumption, or liveweight gain, egg production decreased and mortality increased in those cages where cannibalism occurred.[78] Bareham,[12] in summarizing the extensive literature of change in group size and area per bird, indicated that the more birds per cage the lower the egg production whether area per bird is held constant or decreased.

Pigs

Liveweight Gain

There was a positive relation between initial liveweight and dominance rank and both were positively correlated with rate of gain.[79-81] Within sex and litters, dominance was significantly related to weight at ages from birth to 154 days.[82] No correlation was found between weight and social rank in mixed groups of weaned pigs.[83] By contrast, Scheel et al.[80] found dominance was primarily determined by differences in weight rather than prior experience. The great care that Meese and Ewbank[83] took to make certain there was no contact between litters prior to mixing may have ensured no possibility of a dominance hierarchy forming prior to the experiments. That is not to say that once the hierarchy is established there is not a positive relation between dominance rank and rate of gain.[79-81]

Recognition in Groups of Pigs

If pigs low in the hierarchy were removed and then returned to the group after 3 days, many fights occurred. Dominant animals could be removed for up to 25 days and on returning there were few fights.[84]

This work indicates the importance of realizing that the development of social stability in a group of pigs depends on social rank. It is important practically to make sure that care is taken when adding to or substracting from a stable group of pigs. It is also important to study factors associated with recognition in pigs to further unravel the complex problem of the development and maintenance of dominance hierarchy in pigs. This research on recognition and maintenance of dominance in pigs has been continued by Ewbank and Meese,[85] Fraser,[86] and Meese and Baldwin.[87]

Effects of Group Size and Area

If the area per pig was less than 0.7 m² for a 50-kg pig there was likely to be a reduced liveweight gain for pigs fed *ad libitum*.[6] In 1974, Bryant and Ewbank[88] studied a group of eight pigs held at 0.56, 0.77 and 1.19 m² per pig. Liveweight gain and voluntary food intake were reduced at the highest density of pigs. In areas of 0.43 or 0.63 m² there was no effect on production of pigs weighing up to 68 kg, but from 68 kg to 100 kg there was a significant reduction in liveweight in the 0.43 m² per pig area ($p < 0.01$).[89] In the same experiment using areas of 0.43 and 0.63 m² per pig there was no difference between 10 vs. 15 pigs and 15 vs. 30 pigs in rate of gain. In reviewing this work one cannot but agree with Bryant and Ewbank[88] that there is a critical area per pig above which liveweight gain is depressed, but this level "is probably dependent on the genetic make-up of the pig, sex, size or weight, the group size and other environmental factors such as environmental temperature and ventilation rates."

Most research workers who have studied area per pig find the minimum area per pig is too big initially and then too small (Table 3). More frequent weights of pigs with calculated liveweight change may help identify those periods when crowding affects production.

A useful empirical formula has evolved from years of experience with raising pigs under intensive conditions and takes into account increasing pig size from weaning. It is[196]

$$\left[\frac{\text{number of pigs}}{4} \times \frac{(\text{age} + 4)}{\text{number of pigs}}\right] \times 0.093\ \text{m}^2$$

Age is calculated as the latest age that pigs stay in a particular pen (Table 3). It would be feasible to change pens at weaning (4 weeks), 12, 20, and 26 weeks. With 20 pigs the area per pig at 10 weeks of age is 0.32 m² from the formula which is well below the area shown by various authors (Table 3).

Overcrowding has been suggested as one of the many causes of gastric ulceration in pigs. The relationship of crowding to gastric ulcers has been reviewed,[6] but the effect of ulceration on production does not appear to be well documented. In a preliminary report, Blackshaw[91] found marked restriction of the esophageal entrance to the stomach in 9 of 107 pigs. All nine pigs failed to reach 60-kg liveweight in an acceptable time. At post-mortem there was no other evidence of disease which may have caused slow liveweight gain.

The work discussed in this section indicates the complex social orders that occur in

Table 3a
SUMMARY OF EXPERIMENTS RELATED TO AREA PER PIG AND NUMBER OF PIGS

No. of pigs	Age of pigs during experiment (weeks)	Area per pig (m^2)		Ref.
3	10—26	0.46	NB: Each density	191
6	10—26	0.93	was used for	
12	10—26	1.85	each group size	
10	No time given	0.64		192
15	No time given	0.42		
8	10—22	0.56		88
8	10—22	0.77		
8	10—22	1.19		
10	10—20; 20—26	0.43 and 0.63		89
15	10—20; 20—26	0.43 and 0.63		
30	10—20; 20—26	0.43 and 0.63		

Table 3b
AREA PER PIG CALCULATED FROM HOLDER'S FORMULA[196]

No. of pigs	Age (weeks when pigs shifted)	Area per pig (m^2)
20	4	0.19
20	10	0.32
20	12	0.37
20	16	0.46
20	20	0.56
20	22	0.60
20	26	0.69

$$\left[\frac{\text{Number of pigs}}{4} \times \frac{(\text{age} + 4)}{\text{Number of pigs}}\right] \times 0.093\ \text{m}^2$$

the life of pigs. The interactions between pigs, particularly related to recognition, are being studied, but the reasons for the effects of crowding need further investigation. Individual measurement of a pig's food intake and efficiency of conversion should be considered in pigs held in groups of various sizes.

Cattle

Milk Production

The role of dominance hierarchy in the social organization of groups of housed cattle and the relation of dominance to production has been studied over many years. There appears to be no relation between dominance and milk production.[92-97]

A 5% reduction in milk yield was measured when an additional animal was placed in a milking herd.[92] In another experiment,[98] 4 cows were added to a stable group of 24 in the later stages of lactation. There were twice as many conflicts on the first 7 days of the month compared to the last 3 weeks. There was a temporary reduction of 0.6 kg milk (average) on the first day of the month only.

Dominance rank was determined in two groups of 17 cows.[99] The cows with the highest, lowest, and middle ranking from each group were then exchanged. There was a change in milk yield of five of the six cows which sometimes was higher but more frequently lower than in the previous week. Another decrease in yield occurred when the cattle returned to their own groups and was greatest in the two most dominant animals.

When a group of cattle which were always milked on the left side of a herringbone shed were moved to the right side, it was found that milk production dropped 20% for 3 days and took 7 days to return to normal.[95]

These studies should make farmers aware that shifting milking cows into different groups can have unpredictable and perhaps detrimental effects on production.

Rate of Liveweight Change

When a grazing herd of mixed age Hereford cows was given supplementary feed,[100] the 2- and 3-year-old cattle had a higher liveweight loss compared to animals of the same age which were separated and fed by themselves. When 2- and 3-year-old Hereford steers were fed in small yards the dominant animals pushed others from feed troughs but no relation was found between dominance and weight gain.[101]

Warnick et al.[102] have studied the growth rate of calves kept in groups, as individuals where each calf could see the others, or in isolation. The isolated calves had lower rates of gain to 4 months than those receiving the other two treatments. There was little difference in growth rate between the other two groups though group-reared animals were dominant over all other animals.

In a study of the relationship of behavior to weight gain in young housed bulls, Borsi[103] found a negative correlation ($p < 0.001$) between walking and rate of weight gain and a negative correlation ($p < 0.05$) between group size and weight gain. There was no study of dominance. However, Brown[104] found no correlation between dominance values and any production measure in young bulls.

It is difficult to find any relationship between dominance hierarchy and liveweight change in cattle of similar ages except sometimes when the feed available is severely restricted and crowding occurs.

Restriction of Space

The restriction of housed dairy cows and steers to small areas is becoming a common management practice. The number of free stalls available to a group of housed cows was varied from one stall per cow to one stall to every three cows.[105] In the treatment of one stall per cow the amount of trough space was varied from 0.5 m to 0.1 m cow. The time spent resting and the number of resting periods per day changed when there were less than two stalls for three cows. When the trough space was less than 0.2 m per cow the time spent at the feeding area was reduced; as trough space became limiting there was an increase in fighting. Dominance was increasingly related to the mean length of eating periods as trough space decreased, but it had no effect on eviction of cows from stalls. Despite the conflicts, there was no effect of dominance on production.

For 30 weeks, Schmisseur et al.[106] held 20 cows in a free stall area and 24 in loose housing and separated the two areas by an electric fence. The fence was removed and cows were observed for 10 days. In that time only 10 cows were seen in the stall and they were seen only a total of 17 times.

The results indicate that though cows may fight more when stall and trough space are restricted, they would prefer to remain as a group rather than be housed in an area where individual stalls were available. Further, even though crowding increased fighting there was no apparent effect on production.

Other Social Orders

Social orders which are different from dominance hierarchy occur in cows and steers depending on the type of activity undertaken.[107-109] For example, different animals are likely to be first in moving to or from yards, leading the grazing cycle, moving through races or weighing scales, and coming to a feeding trough; but these orders had little correlation with production. There is some evidence[110] of heavier yielding cows coming in to be milked slightly earlier than others but dominant animals tended to come in about the middle of the group.

In cattle, dominance hierarchy may sometimes be related to production but there is little evidence that any other social orders have much effect.

Sheep

The presence of dominance and other social orders in grazing sheep has not been as well established as in cattle. There is little evidence of leadership hierarchies. Ewbank[111] and Arnold[112] concluded that leadership in sheep was more apparent than real. When supplementary feed was given to sheep[113] so that crowding occurred around the feeding area then there was a strong positive correlation between dominance and position (leadership) in the flock as the sheep moved to food. This is not an analogous situation to leadership when sheep were grazing since there is no obvious sense of competition between any members of the flock.

Dominant infertile rams reduced the fertility level of 66 to 133 ewes grazing in paddocks of 5 to 25 ha from 90% in the control to 72%.[114] The depression in fertility was not large and may have been due to ewes being with the dominant infertile ram during that part of estrus which was optimum for conception.[115] It is uncertain whether dominant animals would have this effect in paddocks of larger size where the dominant ram may not have so much influence on the other rams or the flock.

Other than the effect of dominant infertile rams, there appears to be little evidence of any social order affecting productivity of grazing sheep, except in the case of supplementary feeding which will be discussed separately in this review.

STRESS

Physiological Effects

Stress Related to New Environments

An elevated corticosteroid level has been associated with various managerial activities in sheep, including shearing.[116] Heart rate and corticosteroid levels were measured after exposing calves to some husbandry manipulations and "the responses seemed to depend largely on the magnitude and degree of noveltry inherent in the presented stimulus."[117] Four sheep were taken from pasture, placed in pens,[118] and were handled daily for 5 to 10 min by stroking the head and neck. Untamed sheep showed avoidance behavior and when caught displayed extreme muscular tension and tried to escape. When tamed, the sheep came forward and stood quietly, even when blood was being sampled. Corticosteroid levels of these sheep were elevated only for the first week. When repeated blood samples were taken over 1.5 hr, it took 5 weeks before the corticosteroid level was no longer elevated. This was the same time it took before sheep were judged tame from their behavioral reactions.

Most of the limited knowledge of the behavioral and endocrinological adjustment sheep make to new environments of housing, paddocks, and feed and specific stress of isolation, dogs, transport, and subclinical infection has been reviewed by Kilgour.[14,119]

There are three separate conclusions to be made from this work.

1. There is insufficient awareness by scientists of the lack of reliability when blood and other parameters are measured in animals not adjusted to new situations.

2. There is general lack of information on the effect of moving animals to new environments on any measure of animal production.
3. Most physiological measurements of stress have been associated with short-term stresses and very few have continued to study the adaptation phase of chronic stress.

Physiological Response to Psychological Stress

Few research workers have studied behavioral and physiological responses to "stress of a psychological origin."[12] No elevated corticosteroid level was found in pigs which were aware of an impending electric shock, but they squealed loudly. The results suggest that in these conditioning experiments "the behavior of the pig is a more sensitive indication of their emotional state than plasma cortiosteroids."[120]

The dominance ranking of a large number of dairy cattle was studied by Arave et al.[121] who subdivided cows into the most dominant and two subordinate groups. Body weight was the most important variable affecting dominance. There was no relation between total corticoids and dominance rank, body weight, or age and they concluded that in the experiment there was no relation between social stress as expressed by dominance hierarchy and total corticoids.

Elevation of plasma cortiosteroid levels may not be an accurate means of determining whether animals are suffering from psychological stress. It seems that the behavioral reactions may be a far better indicator.

Environmental Effects

Large differences in corticosteroid levels were measured between sheep killed under relatively quiet conditions at a research station and the environment of an abattoir.[122] The length of time sheep had been trucked the previous day was related to catecholamine level at slaughter, and travelling time of more than 1 hr doubled the cortisol level.[123]

Since stress occurs when animals are transported, unless there are good resting yards at the abattoirs where animals can recover, it is probable there will be a reduction in carcass quality.[124] The problem of stress related to transport and to selling stock in saleyards should be studied as they are important both from a welfare and an economic viewpoint.

Plasma corticosteroid levels prior to mating may be a reasonable measure of the fertility of cattle with the most highly fertile crossbred animals having lower plasma corticosteroid levels.[125] However, one should be particularly careful in interpreting the correlated results in this field. It is possible that the studies measure the inherent fertility of the different crossbred groups and not necessarily that related to plasma corticosteroid levels. The latter may be in some way related to the stress experienced by different crossbred groups in yarding and handling the animals.

Ewbank and Mansbridge[126] studied the effect of sudden noise on farm animals and indicated that dairy cattle and sheep showed little behavioral effect, but poultry showed a panic reaction though there was no death or decrease in egg yield.

It is possible to measure elevated corticosteroid levels in animals which are acutely stressed and those bear some relation to the eventual economic loss caused by downgrading of meat after slaughter. It is by no means clear that there are reasonable physiological measures of chronic stress situations. This is serious because some measure of stress is needed so it can be related to animal welfare as well as production.

Animal Health

The relationship of stress to infectious diseases has been seriously neglected. Gross and Colmano[127] showed that poultry maintained in stressful situations were more susceptible to viral diseases and less susceptible to bacterial diseases. Further, high levels of plasma corticosterone were positively related to resistance to *Escherichia coli*[128] infection. On the other hand, Thurley[129] showed that sheep experimentally infected with *Brucella ovis* and injected with ACTH showed more severe lesions than the control animals.

There is a relationship between stress associated with transport of sheep and cattle and salmonellosis. Sometimes there are severe disease outbreaks and some deaths. Even if there are no symptoms of the disease, the possibility of salmonella organisms in muscle of slaughtered animals has resulted in taking much greater care with animals in the days immediately prior to slaughter.

It could be expected that with intensive housing of animals, respiratory and enteric diseases may spread more rapidly. Ekesbo[130] found that there was a higher level of trampled teats among intensively housed dairy cows, particularly those without bedding or in stalls less than 1.85 m long.

Subclinical or clinical diseases may interact with stress and play an important role in increasing mortalities or reducing production under the crowded conditions of intensively housed animal management systems, but further research is needed.

ABNORMAL BEHAVIOR

Tail-Biting in Pigs

Tail-biting, a behavioral trait of unknown origin, can lead to a reduction in carcass quality due to multiple abscesses, which often extend up the spinal canal. Ewbank[131] failed to induce tail-biting by changing nutritional or climatic variables. A variety of causes for tail-biting have been suggested,[131,132] but the condition has never been produced experimentally, so its etiology cannot be specified.

Over a period of 12 months, 62 litters of various breeds of pigs were studied for tail-biting[133] and the animals graded from 0 to 4 with 0 being no tail-biting and 4 being three quarters of the tail removed. The average daily gain of all pigs was calculated as they increased in weight from 27 to 91 kg. Although numbers per litter were small, there were 59, 44, 16, 12, and 9 pigs in categories 0, 1, 2, 3, 4 and there were seven pigs so severely affected that they were removed and not included in the data. There was a significantly greater gain of approximately 0.09 g per head per day from pigs in categories 0 and 1 compared to 2, 3, and 4 ($p<0.01$).

The possible sequence of events leading to tail-biting has been described by Ewbank[3] who suggested that the problem has been resolved in the U.K. by cutting the tails off at an early age. Tail-biting remains a problem in Austrailia. If tails are removed, pigs tend to extensively damage the ears of other pigs.[197]

Feather-Pecking in Poultry

Feather-pecking leading to cannibalism and mortalities is an important factor in lowered productivity. The most important causes of feather-pecking were shown to be strain of birds, light intensity, and type of housing system.[134] More damage was found in cages with eight birds in them than with four. Hormones had a significant effect on the incidence of feather-pecking; progesterone and estrogen had a synergistic effect, and testosterone inhibited the rise seen as laying commences. The increased incidence of feather-pecking in caged birds compared with those in pens was significant.[8] Pecking in pens may be directed at the litter but with cages it was directed at other birds. Severe feather-pecking could be induced in pens if a large number of birds were present.

Stereotype Behavior

This type of behavior includes pacing behavior in birds, chain rattling in pigs, wool eating in sheep, and wood eating in horses. Its impact on production has never been assessed except in poultry where Arbi et al.[17] showed that more energy is used by those birds showing stereotype behavior.

Death from Stress

Sheep were given a restricted intake for several days and were placed singly in one corner of a fenced area 22 m by 22 m.[122] Food was available in the corner diagonally opposite. Initially, all sheep showed reluctance to move across the area. Some abnormal behavior was observed including lameness, displacement grazing above the level of the ground, and death in two sheep within 60 hr of the start of the trial. Later examination of the dominance ranking showed these sheep were two of the lowest in the hierarchy. Post-mortem examination did not reveal the cause of death and stress was considered to be a possibility.

BEHAVIOR DURING SUPPLEMENTARY FEEDING

In many areas it is necessary to supplement the food supply of grazing animals during some part of the year. The supplement may be in the form of roughage, or an energy- or protein-rich diet. During drought, which is common in Australia, it may be necessary to provide almost the whole daily intake. Franklin[135] placed the problem of drought in perspective when he stated that "...since 1892 drought has exacted a greater toll from the sheep industry than any other single factor." Amost 30 years later this would still be so for both sheep and cattle in Australia.

There are some behavioral problems associated with giving supplementary feed to sheep and cattle. Behavioral abnormalities such as coprophagia and geophagia were recorded in cattle being fed all grain diets in pens.[136-138] When initially offered a high energy diet, a few sheep[198] and cattle[137] ate excessively with resulting acidosis, laminitis, and sometimes death. A higher but extremely variable proportion of sheep[139,140] and cattle[55] will only eat small amounts of the supplement or none at all. Those animals that do not eat the supplement or eat only a little are known as "shy" feeders. This phenomenon is seen whether animals are supplemented while grazing at pasture, held in small areas for survival feeding, or in preparation for sea voyages.

Cattle

Since the individual intake of supplementary feed can be estimated by using tritiated water (TOH),[55] it is now possible to calculate the numbers of animals with little or no intake. The number of animals rejecting the supplement was extremely variable (Table 4) and ranged from 8 to 82%. The components of this variablility are not well known except from Nolan[199] when rain intervened and cattle preferred to graze the young green grass.

Sheep

Animals in Pens

The range of individual intakes of Scottish Blackface ewes given different feeding regimes were measured by Foot and Russell.[141] There were three treatments: (1) group penned, group fed; (2) group penned, individually fed; and (3) individually penned, individually fed. The food was pelleted concentrate which was not available *ad libitum*. The mean energy intake of three sheep with the highest intake was compared with the three lowest in each group and the difference was in excess of 80%. While no dominance ranking was calculated, the most aggressive sheep had lower than average in-

Table 4
SUMMARY OF EXPERIMENTS SHOWING PERCENTAGE OF TOTAL REJECTION OF SUPPLEMENTARY LICK OR BLOCK

Total number of animals	Percentage rejection	Other comments	Ref.
200	49	Sheep with urea molasses (liquid)	55
44	36	Weaner cattle, meat meal/ soy-bean meal (liquid)	193
33	33	Weaner cattle, meat meal/ molasses (liquid)	193
37	11	Weaner cattle, urea/ molasses (liquid)	193
39	8	Pregnant heifers, urea/ molasses (liquid)	199
38	82	Pregnant heifers, meat meal/molasses (liquid)	199
Trial 1: 25	40	18-month-old heifers, molasses solid block	202
Trial 2: 25	8	18-month-old heifers, molasses solid block	202
Trial 3: 25	60	18-month-old heifers, molasses solid block	202
Trial 4: 25	32	18-month-old heifers, molasses solid block	202

takes. The sheep more readily pushed out of the way did not have the lowest intakes. Since there was adequate trough space, 30-cm trough per sheep, Foot and Russell[141] suggest that time spent in aggression is time wasted when animals are given limited feed supply of an easily eaten food, such as oat pellets.

One would have expected that in the competitive situation described here, the more dominant animals would have obtained more food. The measurement of individual intakes, their production, and the dominance hierarchy may prove very interesting since this social order is often expected to be related positively to production.

Grazing Animals

The failure of some sheep to eat additional feed given to supplement the pasture available in a paddock has only been studied by Arnold and his co-workers.[54,140]

When oats were given to 270 Merino wethers grazing in a paddock, 37 sheep had eaten none after 8 days.[140] These sheep were removed from the flock to another area where they eventually all ate the supplement and were returned to the flock. Another group of nonfeeders developed but after being given similar treatment they were returned to the flock. All animals were eating oats 35 days after the start of the experiment.

In another experiment[54] Border Leicester × Merino ewes grazing in a paddock were given oats in a trough. The trough space initially was 24 cm per sheep but was gradually reduced to 4 cm per sheep. Below 16 cm per sheep there was an increasing number of nonfeeders until finally 31% of the sheep failed to feed.

There were also marked differences in competitive behavior between breeds of sheep with Merinos being least competitive. Within Merinos, young and old sheep were not as competitive as the other ages.

In the light of these observations a much more detailed study of the social behavior of sheep and cattle being given supplementary food at pasture is required. Apart from the problems produced by "shy" feeders, there is very little information on the behavior of those animals which eat excess supplementary food. The use of marker techniques together with studies on aggression should produce some interesting data on individual feed intake when costly supplements are being fed either for survival or increased production. Increasing the palatability of blocks and licks with additives or changing the texture of the material may help. Early experience of supplementary feeds may result in a much higher number of animals eating them from the first day.

The whole problem of increasing acceptance of supplementary foods needs much more attention than it has so far received.

BEHAVIOR OF GRAZING ANIMALS

Daily Behavior Cycle

Behavior and production are related, since walking and grazing result in treading, differential defoliation, changed plant growth, distorted cycling of nutrients, and altered energy and water expenditure. The gregarious nature of sheep and cattle results in translocation of nutrients in plants and seed dispersal. The daily behavior of sheep and cattle in the more arid areas of Australia and in some of the mountain areas of Northern America have been described in detail.[14,142-144] In these areas an animal's behavior is less likely to be changed by man's management or by fences.

Grazing

Reviews of grazing behavior have been produced frequently over the last 30 years.[142,145-148] While grazing behavior is one of the basic components of productivity there have been few recent developments.

The flexibility of an animal's grazing behavior should be emphasized. Hungry sheep living in an area with almost no grass completely disrupt their flocking behavior and any routine of grazing in preferred areas of a paddock.[149] Both sheep and cattle change to grazing mainly in the night during periods of hot weather in arid Australia.[142]

Grazing behavior of dairy cattle changes when eating some tropical pastures.[150] Dairy cows grazing pasture plants with low leaf yields or with relatively inaccessible leaves, may have difficulty in maintaining stable milk production. More recently it was shown that (1) size of bite fell sharply, (2) grazing time increased, and (3) number of bites per minute increased[151] when herbage available to calves and lambs decreased from 3500 to 2000 kg organic matter/ha.

There is almost no information on the behavior of calves and lambs learning to graze or to eat solid food in intensive systems. This learning behavior may be important in determining when lambs should be weaned, or if there is an optimal age at which sheep and cattle should be transported large distances to pastures foreign to them.

Camping (Resting on Preferred Areas of a Paddock)

One of the indirect effects of behavior on animal production is the way camping (resting) behavior of Merino sheep affects plant production. Merinos transferred up to one third of their feces to a camp which extended over a very small area of the paddock.[152] As a result, high concentrations of potassium and phosphorus were found in the area. After several years of continuous grazing the transfer of potassium was sufficient to cause a deficiency of potassium in plants over most of the paddock. There are substantial changes in plant species and herbage availability at increasing distances from the sheep camp (Table 5).

Table 5

PASTURE YIELDS AND COMPOSITION OF A PERENNIAL RYEGRASS (*Lolium perenne* L.)/WHITE CLOVER (*Trifolium repens* L.) PASTURE ALONG THE DIAGONAL TRANSECT FROM THE SHEEP CAMP (kg DM/HA)

Pasture component	Distance from camp (m)								
	1	4	6	10	23	46	68	90	133
Grass	0	0	162	243	573	581	849	544	808
Clover	0	0	3329	2491	1260	371	636	243	228
Weed	0	7172	0	0	162	22	213	44	48
Total	0	7172	3491	2734	1995	974	1698	831	1084

After Hilder, E. J., *Proc. Aust. Soc. Anim. Prod.*, 5, 241-248, 1964. With permission.

Behavioral Thermoregulation

The zone of physiological thermoregulation is very narrow compared to the zone of behavioral thermoregulation.

Cold Weather

Shelter can reduce lamb deaths from 24 to 5%. Yet, the relation between climate and shelter seeking behavior in grazing ruminants has been a neglected field. The strategic placement of shelter was suggested by Geytenbeek[153] to assist newly shorn sheep in surviving sudden weather changes with wind and rain. Shorn Merinos readily seek shelter except when grazing and if the weather is cold, wet, and windy even unshorn sheep may seek shelter.[31]

In another experiment 190 shorn sheep were placed in a paddock of 11 ha which contained five rows of grass shelter belts each 90 m long and 10 m apart. The same number of shorn sheep were also placed in an adjoining paddock with no shelter. The mortality of newborn lambs was halved in the paddock with shelter. Sheep in this paddock "sheltered" for 35 days before being exchanged with sheep in the next paddock. The new sheep did not use the shelter belts. After 8 days the sheep were exchanged again and sheep used the shelter. This finding needs further study but one possibility is that after sheep had become acclimatized in 14 to 21 days[154] they were camping rather than sheltering.[200]

Newborn pigs and newly hatched chickens are extremely sensitive to cold and can readily be seen to take advantage of additional heat.

Hot Weather

The provision of shade and iodine supplementation led to a marked increase in the level of fertility of Merino ewes in summer in a semiarid tropical environment.[155] However, the relative importance of iodine and shade could not be assessed from this experiment. Smith and Alexander[156] found 16% perinatal mortality in calves born in a large paddock in northwestern Queensland. They suggested neonatal hyperexia as a major source of calf death in Shorthorn cattle, although within the paddock there were several timbered areas which would provide shade. Shade-seeking behavior and maternal behavior could play an important part in reducing mortalities in these calves and should be examined further.

Sheep can be seen standing in shade in hot weather but there is very little information on the productivity of these animals compared to animals standing or lying in areas where no shade is available.

Behavior of Male Groups

Bulls are held in groups for the collection of semen, for eventual sale as stud bulls to improve beef production, and for the production of beef from young bulls. Groups of rams are run together as young animals and during periods when they are not being mated with ewes.

Fighting and Mounting

Fighting and homosexual behavior (mounting) are likely to seriously impair the productivity of bulls kept together in groups. Mounting behavior, resulting in injury to the penis and hematoma of the back in the mounted bull, is a natural consequence of groups of bulls running together. Mounting activity appeared to be similar in intensity to fighting and occurred around the same time.[157] Mounting and fighting behavior has been described by several workers.[157-160] A progression from amicable through aggressive to territorial behavior occurred as Friesian bulls increased in age from 3 to 6 years old.[157] In Boran × Sahiwal cattle, aggression was not seen until bulls were between 3 and 4 years old.[160] Fighting was seen in Hereford bulls aged 15 to 20 months when supplementary feed was given or the bulls were held in yards.[159] There was a positive correlation between dominance value and weight gain during the period when bulls were fed hay because there was not enough pasture available.[159] All animals lost weight, but the dominant animals lost less than the others. In spring when there was abundant pasture, no relationship was observed.

In Australia, graziers are most reluctant to grow bulls for beef production. This is due, in part, to a prejudice from the meat trade and in part to concern about being unable to manage the bulls. "Sterile" bulls have been produced by removing the tail of the epididymus in the hope that the "danger of unwanted pregnancies" would be removed and the graziers would be reassured.[161] The social behavior of sterile bulls was compared with steers at 10, 12, and 14 months.[162] All animals were grazing at 0.9 animals per ha. Fighting and mounting behavior was significantly greater ($p < 0.05$) in bulls than steers but was of such low incidence in the bulls that no different management strategy was warranted between the two groups.

In bulls less than 18 months old, two peaks of mounting and fighting activity were seen; one occurred early in the morning grazing period and the other in the late afternoon before grazing commenced.[201] Other published data has shown that in 3.5- to 4.5-year-old bulls, fighting and mounting reached a peak early in the afternoon.[157]

The skilful management of bulls by stockmen may pay large dividends. Hunter and Edwards[163] described the way new bulls were introduced into a group. This was done initially in housed areas and gradually the animals were mixed and allowed access to grazing areas. When they turned bulls loose for the first time it was into a field with very irregular boundaries since the irregular fenceline and hedges "provide shelter for timid bulls both from fighting and from being chased." Constant inspection, supervision, and movement of the bulls was practiced so that damage to the bulls was minimized. Since fighting and mounting are part of the normal social activities of adult bulls they should be subjected to more intensive behavioral observations. From detailed observations of individuals, it may be possible to assess the manner in which injury is occurring and perhaps suggest management procedures to help reduce the problem.

Reproductive Behavior

Sheep

Results of pen studies on male sexual behavior may not be applicable to grazing animals. When a nonworker dominant ram was located in the center of an area 22 × 22 m, the subordinate rams refused to serve ewes in estrus.[164] In 1966 Lindsay[165] stated that "...in confined conditions the position of a ram in the social order determines his activity while in an open paddock his natural sexual activity, unimpeded by dominance relationships, determines the number of ewes with which he mates." Nevertheless, three 20-min tests of rams with ostrus ewes in pens have been shown to adequately predict subsequent mating performance in paddocks.[166]

While rams which lack libido are a practical problem in a single sire mating system, because few lambs are born, most farmers would have two rams mating with every 100 ewes in the paddock so that more than one male is likely to inseminate a ewe. There were no significant differences in mating behavior between rams of different breeds but 15-month-old rams were not as fertile as mature rams.[167]

In a paddock mating system, more rams were needed per 100 primiparous ewes than for 100 multiparous ewes since the former did not stay as long in estrus as the latter and were not very active in seeking out the ram. It is strongly recommended that young and mature ewes should not be run together with rams at mating.[168,169]

Recent studies have investigated some problems of mating 6 to 8 month old ewes.[39,170,171] Lambs which were considered to have attained puberty were of less interest to rams than adults; their courtship behavior was deficient and only 86% of the lambs became pregnant even after mating in small paddocks where chances of contact between ewes and rams were high. In pen tests there was no improved mating behavior over three oestrus cycles.[171] Contrary to expectations experience associated with first oestrus did not modify the initial courtship behavior. This suggests an inadequacy of those hormones which are associated with sexual behavior. Further research work should investigate the hormonal and behavioral aspects of sexual maturity in both rams and ewes. There is strong evidence that if young animals are mated, then inadequate mating behavior is a significant component of reduced reproductive efficiency.

Cattle

Individuals in a group of 12 bulls, observed over 3 weeks of paddock mating, served between 2 and 85 cows.[172] Since variation between bulls in the number of cows served was so large, Blockey[173] proposed a test to try to rapidly assess in hours the likely field performance of bulls. He called it a serving capacity test. Bulls which had been sexually stimulated by being held in a yard but allowed to observe other bulls mating with restrained heifers were then put with the heifers. The number of services each bull achieved over 20 min was counted. These were highly correlated ($r = 0.95$) with the number of services a bull achieved in the first 3 weeks of paddock mating.[172] The calving percentage in a herd of 4000 cows was increased by 15% by including the serving capacity test in an annual soundness examination of bulls.[174]

There may be a problem of estrous detection in dairy cows.[7,175] As herd size increased there was a disproportionately increasing number of animals showing a short estrous cycle,[176] and when it occurred, the cycle was not necessarily detected by the farm staff.[177] If marker bulls were used they were relatively more efficient at detecting estrous in dairy cows than farmers but an appreciable number of cows in estrous were missed when compared with per rectum palpation in cows to determine ovarian activity (Table 6). These behavioral and endocrinological problems together may result in a wasted estrous cycle.

DIRECT EFFECT OF MAN ON BEHAVIOR AND PRODUCTION

If normal behavior patterns are not considered, a possible result can be an immediate and major drop in production. One man can open a poultry shed door and have birds explode to the far walls in panic while another can walk through a shed with birds barely getting out of his way.[178] Similarly, it is time-wasting and exasperating when driving a flock of sheep through yards if an assistant stands in the wrong position and no sheep moves past him.

Table 6
RELATIONSHIP OF AGE AND ESTRUS DETECTION TECHNIQUE WITH THE RELATIVE INCIDENCE OF OVARIAN ACTIVITY IN 14 HERDS IN THE MANAWATU AND WAIRARAPA AREA DURING THE 1971—72 BREEDING SEASON

Age and ovarian status	Detection technique used	
	Marker bulls	Farmer observation
2 years		
Number	68	64
% inactive	91	94
3 years		
Number	23	44
% inactive	87	80
4 years and over:		
Number	91	80
% inactive	63	41

After Fielden, E. D. and McMillan, K. L., *N. Z. Soc. Anim. Prod.*, 33, 87-93, 1973. With permission.

Two hundred birds were briefly handled each day from day 2 to 16 weeks and another 250 were raised normally.[179] This and subsequent experimental treatments are shown in Table 7. During Phase 1 (28 weeks) all eggs were examined on 3 successive days; during Phase 2 (35 weeks) eggs from the nonhandled birds were examined for 2 days and then 2 days after handling commenced. Egg production, which was recorded daily, was similar in both groups but was reduced in that group of hens unused to handling. Handling (1) reduced the avoidance reaction (flightiness) in the young birds but the effect declined as the birds grew older and (2) increased the incidence of equatorial bulges and cracks in eggs. It was concluded that handling can be regarded as causing stress to the birds.

A commercial cattle producer, Hassall[180], discussed the consequences of the handling of cattle by stockmen who had little knowledge of the behavior of *Bos indicus* cattle. He suggested that "...lack of understanding, tolerance, and knowledge may lead to real difficulties in management, and consequent production losses."

In 1975 Kilgour[181] reviewed the various methods that research workers used in assessing the relation of temperament to production in cattle and concluded that the methods have not been successful. He used the open-field test to assess objectively the temperament of dairy cattle and related this both to production and to two technician's assessment of temperament of the same cattle. There was a poor correlation between technicians in their ranking of a cow's temperament. There was no relation between placid cows as assessed by the technicians and high or low milk production, but the nervous cows tended to be the best producers. These cows would probably have been culled if they had not been good producers! He concluded that the open-field testing system was not a useful method of measuring the temperament of a dairy cow. In this regard, open-field areas were not dissimilar to yards and other enclosures. Any objective tests such as ambulation and vocalization were not useful indications of temperament in dairy cattle.

Assessing temperament remains an intractable behavioral problem. Difficult tem-

Table 7
SUMMARY OF THE EXPERIMENTAL DESIGN

Time (weeks)	Group handled		Group nonhandled	
0	•[a]		•	
	•		•	
8	AR[b]		AR	
	•		•	
	•		•	
16	AR		AR	
18	Handled	Nonhandled	Nonhandled	Handled
	•	•	•	•
	•	•	•	•
	•	•	•	•
26	Phase 1 SQ[c]	Phase 1 SQ	Phase 1 SQ	Phase 1 SQ
	•	•	•	•
	•	•	•	•
	•	•	•	•
	•	•	•	•
34	AR	AR	AR	AR
35		Phase 2 SQ		
		•		
		•		
		•		
		Handled		
		•		
		•		
		•		
		Phase 2 SQ		

[a] Dots indicate the time of each treatment
[b] AR indicates that the birds were tested for their avoidance responses to a strange stimulus.
[c] SQ indicates that eggs were examined for shape, "strength", and texture.

After Hughes, B. O. and Black, A. J., *Br. Poult. Sci.*, 17, 135-144, 1976. With permission.

perament and inability to handle cattle are major reasons why cattle producers in Northern Australia are likely to raise cattle with three quarters *Bos indicus* blood rather than using the pure breeds with their greater heat adaptation and tick resistance.

TRANSPORT

The behavior of sheep and cattle which are shipped long distances has been described by many authors.[182-186] Provision of flooring and bedding which reduced soilage and slip would aid the comfort of these animals. Cattle adapt themselves to the movement of the truck by arranging themselves parallel to each other and at right angles to the direction of movement.

The effects of transporting animals on subsequent production have not been measured. These may be important since experience of particular plant species is an important factor in sheep eating the plants.[50] Lack of experience of different plant communities may well result in a slower recovery from a long trip.

Regulations for transporting animals are framed to prevent any cruelty to the animals but more observations on the behavior of animals at loading, during the trip, and afterwards may suggest methods of reducing stress.

Handling, loading, and transporting sheep and cattle result in bruising and salmonellosis. The costs in deaths and rejection or downgrading of carcasses are severe.[187] Greater consideration must be given to the normal behavior of animals when designing stock crates or large holding yards. If costs of bruising are to be reduced, stockmen moving or loading animals must substitute some behavioral understanding for brute force.

BEHAVIOR AND SELECTION

Some behavioral parameters are related to production and lend themselves to genetic selection. The species with the greatest potential for rapid genetic change are birds. Strains of birds were selected for high and low aggressiveness and under crowded conditions, egg production was higher in the less aggressive birds.[188] In individual cages, egg production was equal to or slightly higher in the highly aggressive strain. Hence, the relation between aggressiveness and egg production may be related to the conditions under which the experiments are done. Under crowded conditions, aggressive strains may not produce as many eggs as more docile animals.

Hens have been selected for high and low plasma corticosterone as a response to social stress. Birds with low corticosterone levels were more resistant to Marek's disease and *Mycoplasma gallisepticum,* but were more susceptible to *Escherichia coli* infection than birds with high levels of corticosterone. The latter showed resistance to a variety of other viral diseases and susceptibility to a variety of bacterial diseases.[127] Selection for low corticosterone level may confer resistance to one disease but was not necessarily related to a general resistance. Resistance was not absolute and differences between high and low corticosterone strains were more easily demonstrated in a low stress environment.

Hopes were held that turkeys could be selected for low responses to stress as measured by low plasma corticosterone levels,[189] since Brown and Nestor[190] showed that reduction in steroid level in birds given a standard stress was almost 50% by the sixth generation. Further, the resistant strain was significantly heavier at all ages than the more susceptible strain. Freeman[189] saw no reason why similar results should not hold for hens in view of the wide range of temperament in different breeds of fowls, but clearly selection for different corticosterone levels are correlated with different infectious diseases; different corticosterone levels can influence disease patterns.

Complex ancillary problems arising from genetic selection for a particular trait can occur and should serve as a warning to be careful in selecting animals on behavioral parameters without a full understanding of the consequences. Some chickens were selected for high and low bodyweight at 8 weeks.[13] Plasma corticosterone levels were lower in the high bodyweight strain. When the birds were held in floor pens the mortality from Marek's disease in the S_{13} generation was 5% in the high bodyweight strain and 15% in the other. Some male birds were removed to individual cages with metal partitions and within 3 weeks mortality caused by *Staphylococcus* sp. was 3% in the low bodyweight group and 45% in the high bodyweight group.

There do not appear to be many other well-documented accounts of selecting behavioral characteristics with a view to increasing production. This is not to deny their importance. In the studies done so far, selecting for a particular behavioral parameter has had other consequences which have taken some time to become manifest.

CONCLUSIONS

The twin topics of welfare and stress keep recurring throughout this review. It is clear that behavioral and physiological measurements must be made in chronic stress situations. Wherever possible these measurements must be made *simultaneously* and must be related to measures of productivity. The relation of stress to clinical and subclinical infections will need much further attention.

There is inadequate knowledge concerning early experience and whether it has any effect on adult productivity. Early experience may be important in grazing behavior and supplementation of grazing animals. It seems likely that the relation of hormones to behavior will receive considerable attention, particularly those associated with sexual behavior in young animals.

Specific behavioral problems involving detection of estrous in synchronized groups of animals, mortalities of young piglets, and tail-biting in pigs stand out as important topics to be researched.

Finally, greater consideration must be given to man's place in affecting production through altering animals' behavior. More attention must be given to measures of an animal's temperament and to the behavioral consequences of designing intensive production systems and of selecting animals for special behavior traits which may be related to production. Technology will have to consider animals as well as efficiency in the future.

ACKNOWLEDGMENTS

The extensive comments by Drs. G. Alexander, B. Siebert, and D. Fowler on the draft manuscript are gratefully acknowledged. R. Elwin and G. Green have assembled and checked the references and manuscripts. It is a pleasure to thank Mrs. M. Henderson for typing the manuscript.

REFERENCES

1. **Brambell, F. W. R.,** Report of the Technical Committee to Enquire into the Welfare of Animals Kept under Intensive Livestock Husbandry Systems, Cmnd 2836, Her Majesty's Stationery Office, London, 1965.
2. **Ewbank, R.,** Behavioural implications of intensive animal husbandry, *Outlook Agric.,* 6, 41—46, 1969.
3. **Ewbank, R.,** Social hierarchy in suckling and fattening pigs: a review, *Livestock Prod. Sci.,* 3, 363—372, 1976.
4. **Goodwin, R. F. W.,** Problems of intensive livestock production, *Span,* 12, 45—47, 1969.
5. **Thorpe, W. H.,** Welfare of domestic animals, *Nature (London),* 224, 18—20, 1969.
6. **Bryant, M. J.,** The social environment: behaviour and stress in housed livestock, *Vet. Rec.,* 90, 351—359, 1972.
7. **Bryant, M. J.,** The place of animal behavioural studies in agricultural production, *Agric. Prog.,* 51, 19—26, 1976.
8. **Hughes, B. O.,** Animal welfare and the intensive housing of domestic fowls, *Vet. Rec.,* 92, 658—662, 1973.
9. **Kiley, M.,** The behavioural problems that interfere with production in animals under intensive husbandry, *3rd World Conf. Anim. Prod.,* 4, 16—23, 1973.
10. **Wood-Gush, D. G. M.,** Animal welfare in modern agriculture, *Br. Vet. J.,* 129, 167—174, 1973.
11. **Duncan, I. J. H.,** A scientific assessment of welfare, *Proc. Br. Soc. Anim. Prod.,* 3, 9—19, 1974.
12. **Bareham, J. R.,** Research in farm animal behaviour, *Br. Vet. J.,* 131, 272—283, 1975.

13. **Siegel, P. B. and Gross, W. B.,** Confinement, behavior and performance with examples from poultry, *J. Anim. Sci.,* 37, 612—617, 1973.
14. **Kilgour, R.,** Potential value of animal behaviour studies in animal production, *Aust. Soc. Anim. Prod.,* 10, 286—298, 1974.
15. **Dantzer, R.,** Environment and behaviour in husbandry, *Folia Vet. Lat.,* VI, 76—90, 1976.
16. **Carter, T. C.,** The hen's egg: shell cracking at oviposition in battery cages and its inheritance, *Br. Poult. Sci.,* 12, 259—278, 1971.
17. **Arbi, A., Wodzicka-Tomaszewska, M., and Cumming, R. B.,** Effects of specs (or polypeepers) on egg production, efficiency of feed conversion and behaviour of laying hens in cages and floor pens, *Proc. Aust. Soc. Anim. Prod.,* 12, 226, 1978.
18. **McBride, G.,** Behaviour and the design of the animal husbandry interface, in Intensive Animal Production, as presented at the Proc. 3rd Combined Conf. Aust. Chicken Meats Federation and Aust. Stock Feed Manufacturers Assoc. Aust., Adelaide, 1975, 91—95.
19. Her Majesty's Stationery Office, Welfare of Livestock, Farm Animal Welfare Advisory Committee, Her Majesty's Stationery Office, London, 1970.
20. Her Majesty's Stationery Office, Order of recommendations for the Welfare of Livestock, Pamphlets 1-4, Ministry of Agriculture, Fisheries and Food, London, 1971.
21. **English, P. and Smith, B.,** Save a pig a litter — and you could double your profits, *Pig Farming,* 22, 26—29, 1974.
22. **Titterington, R. W. and Fraser, D.,** The lying behavior of sows and piglets during early lactation in relation to the position of the creep heater, *Appl. Anim. Ethol.,* 2, 47—53, 1975.
23. **Stephens, D. B.,** Studies on the effect of social environment on the behaviour and growth rates of artificially-reared British Friesian male calves, *Anim. Prod.,* 18, 23—34, 1974.
24. **Stephens, D. B. and Baldwin, B. A.,** Observations of the behaviour of groups of artificially reared lambs, *Res. Vet. Sci.,* 12, 219—224, 1971.
25. **Levy, D. M.,** Experiments on the sucking reflex and social behaviour of dogs, *Am. J. Orthopsychiat.,* 4, 203—224, 1934.
26. **Alexander, G.,** Behaviour of newly born lambs, *Proc. Aust. Soc. Anim. Prod.,* 2, 123—125, 1958.
27. **Alexander, G.,** Maternal behaviour in the Merino ewe, *Proc. Aust. Soc. Anim. Prod.,* 3, 105—114, 1960.
28. **Alexander, G. and Williams, D.,** Teat-seeking activity in new born lambs during the first hours of life, *Anim. Behav.,* 14, 166—176, 1966.
29. **Alexander, G. and Williams, D.,** Teat-seeking in new-born lambs: the effects of cold, *J. Agric. Sci. Camb.,* 67, 181—189, 1966.
30. **Lynch, J. J. and Alexander, G.,** The effect of gramineous windbreaks on behaviour and lambing mortality amongst shorn and unshorn Merino sheep during lambing, *App. Anim. Ethol.,* 2, 305—325, 1976.
31. **Lynch, J. J. and Alexander, G.,** Sheltering behaviour of lambing Merino sheep in relation to grass hedges and artificial windbreaks, *Aust. J. Agric. Res.,* 28, 691—701, 1977.
32. **Smith, F. V., van-Toller, C., and Boyes, T.,** The "critical period" in the attachment of lambs and ewes, *Anim. Behav.,* 14, 120—125, 1966.
33. **Hudson, S. J. and Mullord, M. M.,** Investigations of maternal bonding in dairy cattle, *Appl. Anim. Ethol.,* 3, 271—276, 1977.
34. **Hersher, L., Richmond, J. B., and Moore, A. U.,** Modifiability of the critical period for the development of maternal behavior in sheep and goats, *Behaviour,* 20, 310—320, 1963.
35. **Neathery, M. W.,** Acceptance of orphan lambs by tranquilized ewes (*Ovis aries*), *Anim. Behav.,* 19, 75—79, 1971.
36. **Scott, J. P.,** Social behaviour, organization and leadership in a small flock of domestic sheep, *Comp. Psychol. Monogr.,* 18, 1—29, 1945.
37. **Scott, J. P.,** *Early Experience and the Organization of Behaviour,* Wadsworth Publ., Belmont, Calif., 1968, Chaps. 4 and 5.
38. **Kloffer, P. H., Adams, D. K. and Kloffer, M. S.,** Maternal "imprinting" in goats, *Proc. Nat. Acad. Sci. U.S.A.,* 52, 559—608, 1964.
39. **Edey, T. N., Kilgour, R., and Bremner, Kaye,** Sexual behaviour and reproductive performance of ewe lambs at and after puberty, *J. Agric. Sci. Camb.,* 90, 83—91, 1978.
40. **Levine, S.,** Stimulation in infancy, *Sci. Am.,* 202, 81—86, 1960.
41. **Levine, S.,** Infantile experience and resistance to physiological stress. *Science N.Y.* 126, 405, 1957.
42. **Denenberg, V. H. and Bell, R. W.,** Critical periods for the effects of infantile experience on adult learning, *Science N.Y.* 131, 227—228, 1960.
43. **Levine, S.,** Plasma-free corticosteroid response to electric shock in rats stimulated in infancy, *Science N.Y.,* 135, 795, 1962.
44. **Meier, G. W.,** Infantile handling and development in Siamese kittens, *J. Comp. Physiol. Psychol.,* 55, 363—368, 1961.

45. **Fox, M. W. and Stelzner, D.,** Behavioural effects of differential early experience in the dog, *Anim. Behav.,* 14, 273—281, 1966.
46. **Donaldson, S. L., Black, W. C., and Albright, J. L.,** The effects of early feeding and rearing experiences on dominance, aggressive and submissive behavior in young heifer calves, *Am. Zool.,* 6, 559—560, 1966.
47. **Donaldson, S. L.,** The Effects of Early Feeding and Rearing Experiences on Social, Maternal and Milking Parlour Behaviour in Dairy Cattle, Ph.D. thesis Purdue University, Lafayette, Ind., 1970.
48. **von Finger, K. H. and Brummer, H.,** Observations on the sucking habits of calves reared in the absence of dams, *Dtsch. Tieraerztl. Wochenschr.,* 76, 665—667, 1969.
49. **Drori, D., Wallace, M. H., Lewis, J. M. and Hinds, F. C.,** Relation of drinking behaviour to growth in artificially reared lambs, *Ill. Agr. Exp. Stn. Dixon Springs Agric. Center,* 4, 155—156, 1976.
50. **Arnold, G. W. and Maller, R. A.,** Effects of nutritional experience in early and adult life on the performance and dietary habits of sheep, *Appl. Anim. Ethol.,* 3, 5—26, 1977.
51. **Liddell, H. S.,** The behaviour of sheep and goats in learning a simple maze, *Am. J. Psychol.,* 36, 544—552, 1925.
52. **Hemsworth, P. H., Beilharz, R. G., and Galloway, D. B.,** Influence of social conditions during rearing on the sexual behaviour of the domestic boar, *Anim. Prod.,* 24, 245—251, 1977.
53. **Capretta, P. J.,** The establishment of food preferences in chicks *Gallus gallus, Anim. Behav.,* 17, 229—231, 1969.
54. **Arnold, G. W. and Maller, R. A.,** Some aspects of competition between sheep for supplementary feed, *Anim. Prod.,* 19, 309—319, 1974.
55. **Nolan, J. V., Norton, B. W., Murray, R. M., Ball, F. M., Roseby, F. B., Rohan-Jones, W., Hill, M. K., and Leng, R. A.,** Body weight and wool production in grazing sheep given access to a supplement of urea and mollasses: intake of supplement/response relationship, *J. Agric. Sci. Camb.,* 84, 39—48, 1975.
56. **Kilgour, R.,** Social behaviour in the dairy herd, *N.Z. J. Agric.,* 119, 34—37, 1969.
57. **Kilgour, R.,** Animal behaviour in intensive systems and its relationship to disease and production, *Aust. Vet. J.,* 48, 94—98, 1972.
58. **Stokols, D.,** On the differences between density and crowding: some implications for future research, *Psychol. Rev.,* 79, 275—277, 1972.
59. **McBride, G.,** Social adaptations to crowding in animals and man, *The Impact of Civilisation on the Biology of Man,* Boyden, S. V. Ed., Australian National University Press, Canberra, 1970, 142—166.
60. **Donaldson, S. L., Albright, J. L., and Ross, M. A.,** Space and conflict in cattle, *Proc. Ind. Acad. Sci.,* 81, 352—354, 1974.
61. **Stricklin, W. R.,** A theory and model for overcrowding effects on social animals, *Can. J. Anim. Sci.,* 56, 849, 1976.
62. **McBride, G.,** The conflict of crowding, *Discovery,* 27, 16—19, 1966.
63. **Fraser, D., Richie, J. S. D., and Fraser, A. F.,** The term "stress" in a veterinary context, *Br. Vet. J.,* 131, 653—662, 1975.
64. **McBride, G.,** Behavioural measurement of social stress, in *Adaptation of Domestic Animals,* Lea & Febiger, Philadelphia, 1968, 360—366.
65. **Guhl, A. M.,** Social inertia and social stability in chickens, *Anim. Behav.,* 16, 219—232, 1968.
66. **Morris, D.,** The response of animals to restricted environment, *Symp. Zool. Soc. Lond.,* 13, 99—118, 1964.
67. **Wood-Gush, D. G. M., Duncan, I. J. H., and Fraser, D.,** Social stress and welfare problems in agricultural animals, in *Behaviour of Domestic Animals,* 3rd ed., Hafez, E. S. E., Ed., Bailliere Tindall, London, 1975, 182—202.
68. **Done, J. R.,** Ethological Aspects of Sheep in an Unnatural Environment — the Animal House, Thesis, University of New England, Armidale, N.S.W., Australia, 1975.
69. **Hinde, R. A.,** *Animal Behaviour,* McGraw-Hill, London, 1966, 389—390.
70. **McBride, G.,** Behaviour and theory of poultry husbandry, *Proc. Wld. Poult. Congr.,* 12, 102—105, 1962.
71. **Cumming, R. B. and Epps, W. R.,** The Use of Polypeepers or Spectacles on Caged Layers, *Proc. 1st Aust. Poult. Stock Feed Conf.,* Melbourne, 1976, 273—274.
72. **Arbi, A., Wodzicka-Tomaszewska, M., and Cumming, R. B.,** Effects of specs or polypeepers on reporductive efficiency and behaviour of layer hens in cages and floor pens, *Theriogenology,* 8, 147, 1977.
73. **Sanctuary, W. C.,** A Study of Avian Behaviour to Determine the Nature and Persistance of the Order of Dominance in the Domestic Fowl and to Relate These to Certain Physiological Reactions, M.S. thesis, Massachusetts State College, Amherst, 1932.
74. **Guhl, A. M. and Allee, W. C.,** Some measurable effects of social organisation in flocks of hens, *Physiol. Zool.,* 17, 320—347, 1944.

75. **Morgan, W. C. and Bonzer, B. J.**, Stresses associated with moving cage layers to floor pens, *Poult. Sci.*, 38, 603—606, 1959.
76. **Choudary, M. R. and Craig, J. V.**, Effects of early flock assembly on agonistic behavior and egg production in chickens, *Poult. Sci.*, 51, 1928—1937, 1972.
77. **Hughes, B. O.**, Selection of group size by individual laying hens, *Br. Poult. Sci.*, 18, 9—18, 1977.
78. **Connor, J. K. and Burton, H. W.**, Effects of cage population and stocking density of the performance of layers in Queensland, *Aust. J. Exp. Agric. Anim. Husb.*, 15, 619—625, 1975,
79. **McBride, G., James, J. W., and Hodgens, N.**, Social behaviour of domestic animals, *Anim. Prod.*, 6, 129—139, 1964.
80. **Scheel, D. E., Graves, H. B., and Sherritt, G. W.** Nursing order, social dominance and growth in swine, *J. Anim. Sci.*, 45, 219—229, 1977.
81. **Hartsock, T. G., Graves, H. B., and Baumgardt, B. R.**, Agonistic behavior and the nursing order in suckling piglets: relationships with survival growth and body composition, *J. Anim. Sci.*, 44, 320—330, 1977.
82. **Beilharz, R. G. and Cox, D. F.**, Social dominance in swine, *Anim. Behav.*, 15, 117—122, 1967.
83. **Meese, G. B. and Ewbank, R.**, The establishment and nature of the dominance hierarchy in the domesticated pig, *Anim. Behav.*, 21, 326—334, 1973.
84. **Ewbank, R. and Meese, G. B.**, Aggressive behaviour in groups of domesticated pigs on removal and return of individuals, *Anim. Prod.*, 13, 685—693, 1971.
85. **Ewbank, R. and Meese, G. B.**, Individual recognition and the dominance hierarchy in the domesticated pig. The role of sight, *Anim. Behav.*, 22, 473—480, 1974.
86. **Fraser, D.**, The behaviour of growing pigs during experimental social encounters, *J. Agric. Sci. Camb.*, 82, 147—163, 1974.
87. **Meese, G. B. and Baldwin, B. A.**, The effects of ablation of the olfactory bulbs on aggressive behaviour in pigs, *Appl. Anim. Ethol.*, 1, 251—262, 1975.
88. **Bryant, M. J. and Ewbank, R.**, Effects of stocking rate upon the performance general activity and ingestive behaviour of groups of growing pigs, *Br. Vet. J.*, 130, 139, 1974.
89. **Plumlee, M. P., Cline, T. R., Krider, J. L., and Underwood, L.**, Space, protein and feeder type effects on finishing swine, *J. Anim. Sci.*, 42, 1339, 1976.
90. **Ewbank, R.**, Social environment of the pig, in *Pig Production, Proc. 18th Easter School in Agricultural Science, University of Nottingham*, Cole, D. J. A., Ed., Butterworths, London, 1972, 129—139.
91. **Blackshaw, Judith, K.**, Gastric ulcers in pigs, *Pig Farmer*, 12, 525—528, 1978.
92. **Schein, M. W. and Fohrman, M. H.**, Social dominance relationships in a herd of dairy cattle, *Br. J. Anim. Behav.*, 3, 45—55, 1955.
93. **Guhl, A. M. and Atkeson, F. W.**, Social organisation in a herd of dairy cows, *Kansas Acad. Sci.*, 62, 80—87, 1959.
94. **Beilharz, R. G., Butcher, D. F., and Freeman, A. E.**, Social dominance and milk production in Holsteins, *J. Dairy Sci.*, 49, 887—892, 1966.
95. **Dickson, D. P., Barr, G. R., and Wieckert, D. A.**, Social relationship of dairy cows in a feed lot, *Behaviour*, 29, 195—203, 1967.
96. **Friend, T. H. and Polan, C. E.**, Social rank, feeding behavior, and free stall utilization by dairy cattle, *J. Dairy Sci.*, 57, 1214—1220, 1974.
97. **Collis, K. A.**, An investigation of factors related to the dominance order of a herd of dairy cows of similar age and breed, *Appl. Anim. Ethol.*, 2, 167—173, 1976.
98. **Brakel, W. J. and Leis, R. A.**, Intergroup transfers: effects on milk production and behaviour, *Ohio Agric. Res. Develop. Cent. Res. Summ.*, No. 76, 49—50, 1974.
99. **Arave, C. W. and Albright, J. L.**, Social rank and physiological traits of dairy cows as influenced by changing group membership, *J. Dairy Sci.*, 59, 974—981, 1976.
100. **Wagnon, K. A.**, Social dominance in range cows and its effect on supplemental feeding, *Calif. Agric. Exp. Stn. Bull.*, No. 819, 1—32, 1965.
101. **McPhee, C. P., McBride, G., and James, J. W.**, Social behaviour of domestic animals. III. Steers in small yards, *Anim. Prod.*, 6, 9—15, 1964.
102. **Warnick, V. E., Arave, C. W., and Mickelsen, C. H.**, Effects of group, individual, and isolated rearing of calves on weight gain and behavior, *J. Dairy Sci.*, 60, 947—953, 1977.
103. **Borsi, J.**, A comparative study on the behaviour of loose kept growing bulls and its effect on the weight gain, *Allattenyesztes*, 23, 61—70, 1974.
104. **Brown, W. G.**, Some aspects of beef cattle behaviour as related to productivity, Ph.D. thesis, abstracted in *Diss. Abstr. Int. B.*, 34, 1805, 1974.
105. **Friend, T. H., Polan, C. E., and McGilliard, M. L.**, Free stall and feed bunk requirements relative to behavior, production and individual feed intake in dairy cows, *J. Dairy Sci.*, 60, 108—116, 1977.
106. **Schmisseur, W. E., Albright, J. L., Dillon, W. M., Kehrberg, E. W., and Morris, W. H. M.**, Animal behavior responses to loose and free stall housing, *J. Dairy Sci.*, 49, 102—104, 1966.

107. **Kilgour, R. and Scott, T. H.,** Leadership in a herd of dairy cows, *Proc. N.Z. Soc. Anim. Prod.,* 19, 36—43, 1959.
108. **Tulloh, N. M.,** Behaviour of cattle in yards. II. A study of temperament, *Anim. Behav.,* 9, 20—24, 1961.
109. **Beilharz, R. G. and Mylrea, P. J.,** Social position and movement orders of dairy heifers, *Anim. Behav.,* 11, 529—533, 1963.
110. **Gadbury, Jane C.,** Some preliminary field observations of the order of entry of cows into herringbone parlours, *Appl. Anim. Ethol.,* 1, 275—281, 1975.
111. **Ewbank, R.,** Preliminary observations on the apparent lack of dominance and leadership hierarchies in fattening sheep, *Br. Vet. J.,* 129, 501—502, 1973.
112. **Arnold, G. W.,** An analysis of spatial leadership in a small field in a small flock of sheep, *Appl. Anim. Ethol.,* 3, 263—270, 1977.
113. **Squires, V. R. and Dawes, G. T.,** Leadership and dominance relationships in Merino and Border Leicester sheep, *Appl. Anim. Ethol.,* 1, 263—274, 1975.
114. **Fowler, D. G. and Jenkins, L. D.,** The effects of dominance and infertility of rams on reproductive performance, *Appl. Anim. Ethol.,* 2, 327—337, 1976.
115. **Dzuik, P.,** Estimation of optimum time for insemination of gilts and ewes by double-mating at certain times relative to ovulation, *J. Reprod. Fertil.,* 22, 277—282, 1970.
116. **Kilgour, R.,** Animal Handling in Works: Pertinent Behaviour Studies, Proc. 13th N.Z. Meat Ind. Res. Conf., Hamilton, N.Z., July 14 to 15, 1971, 9—12.
117. **Stephens, D. B. and Toner, J. N.,** Husbandry influences on some physiological parameters of emotional responses in calves, *Appl. Anim. Ethol.,* 1, 233—243, 1975.
118. **Pearson, R. A. and Mellor, D. J.,** Some behavioural and physiological changes in pregnant goats and sheep during adaptation to laboratory conditions, *Res. Vet. Sci.,* 20, 215—217, 1976.
119. **Kilgour, R.,** Review of Animal Behaviour in Extensive and Intensive Systems, Proc. Sheep Assembly and Transport Workshop, October 1976, Truscott, G. M. C. and Wroth, R. H, Eds., Western Australian Department of Agriculture, Perth, 1976, 64—84.
120. **Baldwin, B. A. and Stephens, D. B.,** The effects of conditioned behaviour and environmental factors on plasma corcicosteroid levels in pigs, *Physiol. Behav.,* 10, 267—274, 1971.
121. **Arave, C. W., Mickelsen, C. H., Lamb, R. C., Svejda, A. J., and Canfield, R. V.,** Effects of dominance rank changes, age and body weight on plasma corticoids of mature dairy cattle, *J. Dairy Sci.,* 60, 244—248, 1976.
122. **Kilgour, R. and De Langen, H.,** Stress in sheep resulting from management practices, *Proc. N.Z. Soc. Anim. Prod.,* 30, 65—76, 1970.
123. **Pearson, A. J., Kilgour, R., De Langen, H., and Payne, E.,** Hormonal responses of lambs to trucking, handling and electric stunning, *Proc. N.Z. Soc. Anim. Prod.,* 37, 243—248, 1977.
124. **Norris, J.,** Abattoir practice and meat quality, *Meat,* 49, 22—25, 1976.
125. **Obst, J. M. and Deland, M. P.,** Pre-mating plasma corticoid and calving percentage of different breeds of crossbred heifers, *Theriogenology,* 8, 138, 1977.
126. **Ewbank, R. and Mansbridge, R. J.,** The effects of sonic booms on farm livestock, *Appl. Anim. Ethol.,* 3, 292, 1977.
127. **Gross, W. B. and Colmano, G.,** Effect of infectious agents on chickens selected for plasma corticosterone response to social stress, *Poult. Sci.,* 50, 1213—1217, 1971.
128. **Gross, W. B. and Colmano, G.,** Further studies on the effects of social stress on the resistance to injection with *Escherichia coli, Poult. Sci.,* 46, 41—46, 1967.
129. **Thurley, D. C.,** Some Factors Predisposing to Perinatal Lamb Mortality, Proc. 2nd Seminar N.Z. Vet. Assoc. Sheep Soc., Palmerston North, N.Z., June 9 to 11, 1972, 95—102.
130. **Ekesbo, I.,** Animal health, behaviour and disease prevention in different environments in modern Swedish animal husbandry, *Vet. Rec.,* 93, 36—39, 1973.
131. **Ewbank, R.,** Abnormal behaviour and pig nutrition. An unsuccessful attempt to induce tail-biting by feeding a high energy, low fibre vegetable protein ration, *Br. Vet. J.,* 129, 366—369, 1973.
132. **Van Putten, G.,** An investigation into tail-biting among fattening pigs, *Br. Vet. J.,* 125, 511—516, 1969.
133. **England, D. C. and Spurr, D. T.,** Effect of tail-biting on growth rate of swine, *J. Anim. Sci.,* 26, 890—891, 1967.
134. **Hughes, B. O. and Duncan, I. J. H.,** The influence of strain and environment upon feather pecking and cannibalism in fowls, *Br. Poult. Sci.,* 13, 525—547, 1972.
135. **Franklin, M. C.,** The drought feeding of sheep, *Aust. Vet. J.,* 27, 326—333, 1951.
136. **Southcott, W. H. and McClymont, G. L.,** Drought feeding of cattle. I. Comparison of hay-grain and all-grain rations: with observations on vitamin A status, *Aust. J. Agric. Res.,* 11, 439—444, 1960.

137. **Southcott, W. H. and McClymont, G.**, Drought feeding of cattle. II. Comparison of daily and weekly feeding of all-grain rations: with observations on vitamin A status, *Aust. J. Agric. Res.*, 11, 445—456, 1960.
138. **Ryley, J. W., Gartner, R. J. W., and Morris, J. G.**, Drought feeding studies with cattle. V. The use of sorghum grain as a drought fodder for non-pregnant heifers, *Q. J. Agric. Sci.*, 17, 339—359, 1960.
139. **Franklin, M. C.**, Maintenance rations for Merino sheep. I. A comparative study of daily and weekly feeding on rations containing high proportions of wheat and several proportions of roughage to concentrate, *Aust. J. Agric. Res.*, 3, 168—186, 1952.
140. **Arnold, G. W. and Bush, I. G.** Observations on non-feeding in groups of hand-fed sheep, *Field Stn. Rec.*, 7, 47—58, 1968.
141. **Foot, Janet Z. and Russel, A. J. F.**, Some nutritional implications of group-feeding hill sheep, *Anim. Prod.*, 16, 293—302, 1973.
142. **Lynch, J. J. and Alexander, G.**, Animal behaviour and the pastoral industries, in *The Pastoral Industries of Australia*, Alexander, G. and Williams, O. B., Eds., Sydney University Press, Sydney Australia, 1973, 371—400.
143. **Yeates, N. T. M. and Schmidt, P. J.**, *Beef Cattle Production*, Butterworths, London, 1974, 154—156.
144. **Squires, V. R.**, Ecology and behaviour of domestic sheep (*Ovis aries*) a review, *Mammal Rev.*, 5, 35—57, 1975.
145. **Tribe, D. E.**, The behaviour of the grazing animal: a critical review of present knowledge, *J. Br. Grassl. Soc.*, 5, 209—224, 1950.
146. **Hancock, J.**, Grazing habits of dairy cows in New Zealand, *Emp. J. Exp. Agric.*, 18, 249—263, 1950.
147. **Arnold, G. W.**, Some principles in the investigation of selective grazing, *Proc. Aust. Soc. Anim. Prod.*, 5, 258—271, 1964.
148. **McBride, G., Arnold, G. W., Alexander, G., and Lynch, J. J.**, Ecological aspects of behaviour in domestic animals, *Proc. Ecol. Soc. Aust.*, 2, 133—165, 1967.
149. **Lynch, J. J.**, Merino sheep: some factors affecting their distribution in very large paddocks, in *The Behavior of Ungulates and its Relation to Management*, Vol. 2 (No. 24), (New series), Geist, V. and Walther, F., Eds., IUCN Publ., Morges, Switzerland, 1974, 697—707.
150. **Stobbs, T. H.**, Components of grazing behaviour of dairy cows on some tropical and temperate pastures, *Proc. Aust. Soc. Anim. Prod.*, 10, 299—302, 1974.
151. **Jamieson, W. S. and Hodgson, J.**, The grazing behaviour and herbage intake of cattle and sheep, *Br. Vet. J.*, 133, 95, 1977.
152. **Hilder, E. J. and Mottershead, B. E.**, The redistribution of plant nutrients through free-grazing sheep, *Aust. J. Sci.*, 26, 88, 1963.
153. **Geytenbeek, P. E.**, A Survey of Post-Shearing Losses Due to Adverse Weather Conditions. No. 1, Experimental Record, Department of Agriculture, South Australia, 1963, 21—30.
154. **Donnelly, J. B., Lynch, J. J., and Webster, M. E. D.**, Climatic adaptation in recently shorn Merino sheep, *Int. J. Biometeorol.*, 18, 233—247, 1974.
155. **Hopkins, P. S. and Pratt, M. S.**, Some practical considerations for improving the pregnancy rate of tropical Merinos, *Proc. Aust. Soc. Anim. Prod.*, 11, 153—156, 1976.
156. **Smith, I. D. and Alexander, G.**, Perinatal mortality in shorthorn cattle in Northern Queensland, *Proc. Aust. Soc. Anim. Prod.*, 6, 63—65, 1966.
157. **Kilgour, R. and Campin, D. N.**, The behaviour of entire bulls of different ages at pasture, *Proc. N.Z. Soc. Anim. Prod.*, 33, 125—138, 1973.
158. **Dalton, D. C., Pearson, M. E., and Sheard, M.**, The behaviour of dairy bulls kept in groups, *Anim. Prod.*, 9, 1—5, 1967.
159. **Blockey, M. A. and Lade, A. D.**, Social dominance relationships among young bulls in a test of rate of weight gain after weaning, *Aust. Vet. J.*, 50, 435—437, 1974.
160. **Macfarlane, J. S.**, The effect of two post-weaning management systems on the social and sexual behaviour of Zebu bulls, *Appl. Anim. Ethol.*, 1, 31—34, 1974.
161. **Price, M. A. and Yeates, N. T. M.**, Infertile bulls versus steers. I. The influence of level of nutrition on relative growth rate, *J. Agric. Sci. Camb.*, 77, 307—311, 1971.
162. **Hinch, G. N.**, Social behaviour of young partially castrated bulls and steers related to their management, *Proc. Aust. Soc. Anim. Prod.*, 12, 265, 1978.
163. **Hunter, W. K. and Edwards, J.**, The Maintenance of an A.I. Stud in an Inactive State, Proc. 5th Int. Congr. Anim. Reprod. Artif. Insem., Trento, Italy, September 6 to 13, 1964, 341—347.
164. **Kilgour, R.**, Behavioural Problems Associated with Intensifications — Sheep, Proc. NZVA Sheep Section 1st Symp. Massey University, Palmerston North, N.Z., 1971, 18—20.

165. **Lindsay, D. R.,** Mating Behaviour in Sheep, Proc. Int. Cong. on Sheep Breeding, Tomps, G. J., Robertson, D. E., and Lightfoot, R. J., Eds., Muresk and Perth, Western Australia, 1976, 338—344.
166. **Mattner, P. E., Braden, A. W. H., and George, J. M.,** Studies in flock mating of sheep. IV. The relation of libido tests to subsequent service activity of young rams, *Aust. J. Exp. Agric. Anim. Husb.,* 11, 473—477, 1971.
167. **Winfield, C. G. and Kilgour, R.,** The mating behavior of rams in a pedigree pen mating system in relation to breed and fertility, *Anim. Prod.,* 24, 197—201, 1977.
168. **Allison, A. J., and Davis, G. H.,** Studies of mating behaviour and fertility of Merino ewes. I. Effects of number of ewes joined per ram, age of ewe, and paddock size, *N.Z. J. Exp. Agric.,* 4, 259—267, 1976.
169. **Allison, A. J. and Davis, G. H.,** Studies of mating behaviour and fertility of Merino ewes. II. Effects of age of ewe, live weight, and paddock size on duration of oestrus and ram-seeking activity, *N.Z. J. Exp. Agric.,* 4, 268—274, 1976.
170. **Keane, M. G.,** Breeding from ewe lambs, *Farm Food Res.,* 7, 10—12, 1976.
171. **Kilgour, R. and Edey, T. N.,** Courtship and Mating Responses in Mature Ewes and Ewe Lambs at Puberty, Proc. 15th Int. Ethol. Conf., Bielefeld, Germany, August 1977, 90.
172. **Blockey, M. A.,** Studies on the Social and Sexual Behaviour of Bulls, Ph.D. thesis, University of Melbourne, Australia, 1975.
173. **Blockey, M. A.,** Serving capacity — a measure of the serving efficiency of bulls during pasture mating, *Theriogenology,* 6, 393—399, 1976.
174. **Blockey, M. A.,** Mating Management of Beef Bulls, Proc., 54th Annual Conf. Aust. Vet. Assoc., Perth, Australia, May 9 to 13, 1977, 82—83.
175. **Fielden, E. D. and MacMillan, K. L.,** Some aspects of anoestrus in New Zealand Dairy Cattle, *N.Z. Soc. Anim. Prod.,* 33, 87—93, 1973.
176. **MacMillan, K. L. and Watson, J. D.,** Short oestrous cycles in New Zealand dairy cattle, *J. Dairy Sci.,* 54, 15—26, 1971.
177. **Esslemont, R. J.,** Heat detection in large dairy herds, in *The Detection and Control of Breeding Activity in Farm Animals,* Owen, J. B., Ed., University of Aberdeen, Scotland, 1974, 57—70
178. **McBride, G.,** Fitting Farms to Fowls, 16th Ann. N.Z. Poult. Conv., Palmerston North, N.Z., February 4 to 6, 1969.
179. **Hughes, B. O. and Black, A. J.,** The influence of handling on egg production, egg shell quality and avoidance behaviour of hens, *Br. Poult. Sci,* 17, 135—144, 1976.
180. **Hassall, A. C.** Behavioural patterns of beef cattle in relation to production in the dry tropics, *Proc. Aust. Soc. Anim. Prod.* 10, 311—313, 1974.
181. **Kilgour, R.,** The open-field test as an assessment of the temperament of dairy cows, *Anim. Behav.,* 23, 615—624, 1975.
182. **Hamilton, F. J., Manusu, P., Bennett, J. W., and Hutchison, J. C. D.** Observations on the transport of sheep by sea through the tropics, *Aust. Vet. J.,* 37, 297—302, 1961.
183. **Sutton, G. D., Fourie, P. D., and Retief, J. S.,** The behaviour of cattle in transit by rail, *J.S. Afr. Vet. Med. Assoc.* 38, 153—156, 1967.
184. **Sutton, G. D. and van den Heever, L. R.,** The effect of prolonged rail transport on adult Merino sheep. *J. S. Afr. Vet. Med. Assoc.,* 39, 31—34, 1968.
185. **Kilgour, R. and Mullord, M.,** Transport of calves by road, *N.Z. Vet. J.,* 21, 7—10, 1973.
186. **Young, B. A.,** Evaluation of Methods for Transportation of Cattle by Rail, University of Alberta Feeders' Day, Canada, 1973, 49—52.
187. **Truscott, G. M. C.,** Wastage in the Industry, Proc. Sheep Assembly and Transport Workshop, October 1976, Truscott, G. M. C. and Wroth, R. H. Eds., Western Australian Department of Agriculture, Perth, 1976, 7—16.
188. **Biswas, D. K. and Craig, J. V.,** Genotype — environment interactions in chickens selected for high and low social dominance, *Poult. Sci.,* 49, 681—692, 1970.
189. **Freeman, B. M.,** Stress and the domestic fowl: a physiological appraisal, *Wld. Poult. Sci. J.,* 27, 263—272, 1971.
190. **Brown, K. I. and Nestor, K. E.,** Physiological responses of turkeys selected for high and low adrenal response to cold stress, *Poult. Sci.,* 49, 1372, 1970.
191. **Heitman, H., Hahn, LeRoy, Kelly, C. F., and Bond, T. E.,** Space allotment and performance of growing-finishing swine raised in confinement, *J. Anim. Sci.,* 20, 543—546, 1961.
192. **Krider, J. L., Albright, J. L., Plumlee, M. P., Conrad, J. H., Sinclair, C. L., Underwood, L., Jones, R. G., and Harrington, R. S.,** Magnesium supplementation, space and docking effects on swine performance and behavior, *J. Anim. Sci.,* 40, 1027—1033, 1975.
193. **Leng, R. A., Kempton, T. J., and Nolan, J. V.,** Non-protein nitrogen and bypass proteins in ruminant diets, *A.M.R.C. Rev.,* No. 33, 1—22, 1977.
194. **Hilder, E. J.,** The distribution of plant nutrients by sheep at pasture, *Proc. Aust. Soc. Anim. Prod.,* 5, 241—248, 1964.

195. **Alexander, G. and Lynch, J. J.,** unpublished data.
196. **Holder, J. M.,** personal communication.
197. **Blackshaw, J. H.,** personal communication.
198. **Edey, T. N.,** personal communication.
199. **Nolan, J. V.,** personal communication.
200. **Lynch, J. J., Mottershead, B. E. and Alexander, G.,** unpublished data.
201. **Hinch, G. N.,** unpublished data.
202. **Leng, R. A. and Nolan, J. V.,** personal communication.

NUTRITION AND ANIMAL PRODUCTIVITY

A. Bondi

INTRODUCTION

The main purpose of animal production is to supply high-quality food for humans. Although animal products are not essential dietary components for humans other than the very young, meat, milk, cheese, and eggs are very satisfying to the palate and provide satiety. Moreover, animal proteins are of higher nutritional quality than plant proteins because they contain large amounts of essential amino acids required by man. Also, animal products supply vitamins, particularly B_{12}, and valuable minerals. Livestock production is vital to man today and will be equally important in the future. The consumption of animal proteins by the affluent population of the U.S. is very high and provides almost 70% of the protein consumed, whereas the world population obtains only one third of its dietary protein from animal sources. The increasing world population and the rising standard of living will bring about an increased demand for animal proteins.

The advantageous properties of foods of animal origin justify their production in spite of the great superiority of plant production to animal production as regards yield per unit area (Table 1). Considerable losses of energy and protein are involved in the conversion of plant products to animal protein foods owing to the metabolic processes underlying the utilization of the nutrients ingested by animals. The inputs of energy and nutrients supplied by the food provide sources for the total outputs, i.e., animal products, plus the losses which are expended in order to promote the synthesis of animal products from food constituents.

All animals utilize feeds in essentially the same way; foodstuffs, usually mixtures of complex substances, proteins, fats, and carbohydrates ingested in the digestive tract lumen, are decomposed by the process of digestion into simple substances, e.g., amino acids, sugars, etc., which are absorbed into the blood. These nutrients are transported to the organs, where the metabolic processes occur, producing energy or leading to the formation of body tissues or animal products, e.g., milk, eggs, etc.

Dietary strategy of ruminants and monogastric animals differs markedly. Excluding geese, monogastric animals such as pigs and poultry digest very little roughage and consume mainly highly digestible concentrate feedstuffs such as cereal grains or oil seed by-products and compete with man for these foods. Ruminants have in their paunches a complex microbial flora capable of breaking down cellulose into smaller molecules such as volatile fatty acids. In their tissues, these acids (acetic, propionic, and butyric), are main sources of energy, instead of glucose which serves the same purpose in the body of animals with simple stomachs. By breaking down cellulose, the ruminant can make use of foods such as roughages, grasses, straws, and other offals unacceptable to man or monogastric animals. Ruminants exploit the capabilities of the bacteria in the rumen for synthesizing essential amino acids and certain vitamins; these animals are less dependent upon protein quality than monogastric animals and their protein requirements can be covered in part by sources of inorganic nitrogen such as ammonia or urea.

ENERGY EVALUATION

Meeting the energy requirements of animals is the major cost associated with feeding animals, and the efficiency of utilization of energy is, from a quantitative and economic standpoint, the primary consideration. Thus, the ability of the feedstuffs to supply energy to the animal and the efficiency of utilization of energy for body processes will be discussed in the following sections.

Partition of Food Energy

The total content of energy of a food is not available to the animal. Part of it, i.e., that which is nondigested, is voided in the feces and its energy is lost to the animal. The difference between the energy value of the food and that of the associated feces is the digestible energy of the food. The loss by fecal excretion of nondigested food residues is much more important in ruminant than in monogastric animals. Air-dried feeds ingested by ruminants vary in digestibility from about 40% for wheat straw to about 80% for corn. Most of the feedstuffs accepted by monogastric animals are highly digestible (80 to 90%).

Further limiting factors in the utilization of the energy deposited in foods are illustrated in Figure 1. A part of the digested energy is lost from the body in urine, which contains organic waste products such as urea and uric acid, and in the form of combustible gases, mainly methane by ruminants; gaseous products of digestion result from fermentations occurring in the rumen. The difference between the digestible energy in the food and the sum of the methane and urinary energy losses is called the *metabolizable energy* (ME). It represents that portion of the food energy actually capable of transformations in the body. An average of about 80% of digestible energy is metabolizable by ruminants.

The ingestion of food by an animal is followed by losses of energy not only as the chemical energy of its solid, liquid, and gaseous excreta, but also as heat. This increase is known as the *heat increment* (HI). The main causes of HI are the following: First, energy is used in the mastication of food and its propulsion through the alimentary tract and is dissipated from the body as heat, together with the heat loss taking place through the activities of microorganisms (in ruminants). Secondly, there is a heat loss because of the inefficiency of the reactions by which absorbed nutrients are metabolized. For instance, when glucose is oxidized in the muscle in the presence of oxygen, only 44% of the energy of the glucose is efficient as a source of energy, i.e., formation of ATP; 56% is lost as heat. The factors mentioned account for the HI which depends upon the composition of the diet and is larger in ruminants; it amounts to 25% of the total energy content of the food, compared to 10 to 15% in monogastric animals. The deduction of the HI of a food from its ME gives the net energy value of the food (Figure 1). The net energy of a food represents the portion of its energy content available to the animal for useful purposes, i.e., for body maintenance and for various types of production.

Utilization of Food Energy by the Animal

Even in a nonproductive state, animals need energy for sustaining the body, keeping a stable body temperature, and for maintaining muscular activity; the energy requirements for maintenance cover all costs of driving the physiological machinery of the animal which is not growing, working, or yielding any product. Although farm animals are infrequently kept in a nonproductive state, e.g., mature nonlactating and nonpregnant females, some knowledge of maintenance requirements is needed in order to formulate rations for productive animals by adding requirements together that are calculated separately for maintenance and for production.

These allowances for the various farm species are based on the efficiency of energy utilization for maintenance and the various types of animal production. Respective

Table 1
ANNUAL YIELDS FROM ANIMALS AND CROPS

	Energy (Mcal/ha)	Protein (kg/ha)
Dairy cows	2,500	115
Dairy and beef herds	2,400	102
Beef Cattle	750	27
Sheep	500	23
Pigs	1,900	50
Broilers	1,100	92
Eggs	1,150	88
Wheat	14,000	350
Peas	3,000	280
Cabbage	8,000	1,100
Potatoes	24,000	420

From Holmes, W., Animals for food, *Proc. Nutr. Soc.*, 29, 237—243, 1970. With permission.

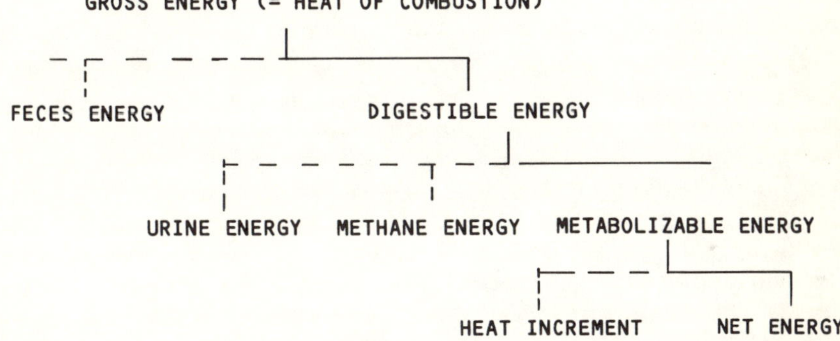

FIGURE 1. Partition of food energy in the animal.

factors expressing the efficiency of utilization of metabolic energy are given in Table 2. The values of these factors are based on average results of metabolic experiments in which the partial efficiency of diets for maintenance and for productive purposes was determined.

The efficiency with which ME is utilized depends upon the interaction of two factors: (1) e.g., the nature of the foods in relation to the nutrients liberated by digestion, e.g., glucose, fatty acids, and amino acids, in which the ME is contained and, (2) the purpose for which these compounds are used by the animal. Thus the variations of coefficients of utilization of metabolic energy for a specific function appearing in Table 2 reflect the influence of the type of rations or nutrients on their utilization.

Efficiency of the utilization of ME for maintenance varies for the different species in relation to their body composition, as will be noted later, and is also influenced by the nature of the diet; this coefficient is higher for single-stomached animals, including very young calves that have not yet begun to ruminate. The range in efficiency for ruminating cattle is from about 60% for very poor roughages high in fiber content to 75% for concentrated foods.

The values of the coefficients of the efficiency of utilization of metabolic energy for body-weight gain in growing animals vary much more than the respective coefficients

Table 2
EFFICIENCY OF UTILIZATION OF METABOLIC ENERGY FOR MAINTENANCE AND PRODUCTION BY CATTLE, SWINE, AND POULTRY[2-7]

Animal	$\frac{\text{Energy retention}}{\text{Metabolic energy intake}} \times 100$	
Cattle		
Maintenance	0.60—0.75	2
Muscular work	0.20—0.30	4
Body-weight gain		
In veal calves	0.68	5
In growing animals	0.25—0.85	
Fat storage in milk cows	0.75	
Fetal tissues in pregnant cows	0.10—0.20	
Milk production		3
From food	0.60—0.75	
From body fat	0.82	
Sheep		
Maintenance	0.54	6
Body-weight gain	0.35—0.48	6
Swine		
Body-weight gain	0.59—0.78	2
Protein gain	0.36—0.77	
Fat gain	0.70—0.75	
Poultry		
Maintenance	0.71—0.92	7
Body-weight gain (growth)	0.60—0.80	
Protein gain	0.51	
Fat gain	0.70—0.84	
Egg production	0.60—0.80	
Egg protein	0.44	
Egg fat	0.74	

for maintenance or other kinds of animal production.[4] This great variability arises mainly from the following reasons: The energy value of the body-weight gain is correlated to the protein to fat ratio in the body-weight gain, since both these components differ considerably in their energy value. The fat to protein ratio in the body-weight gain rises with the age of the animal and also with the increased growth rate, which is caused by level and composition of the diet. Fat-free muscle tissue, e.g., protein, has an average water to protein ratio of 3:1, and 1 g of such tissue means an energy deposition of 1.5 kcal. On the other hand, fat is deposited without water and gives an energy retention of about 10 kcal/g. The energy requirements for body-weight gain can be separated into two components: (1) the energy equivalent deposited in fat and protein and (2) the costs involved in the conversion of nutrients into protein and fat. The energy costs of the gain of protein amount to 15% of the energy value of the protein deposited, whereas a negligible amount of energy is associated with fat deposition.[3] As is obvious from Table 2, protein synthesis is an energetically less efficient process than fat synthesis and applies to swine and chickens as well. Growing and laying chicks convert metabolic energy less efficiently to body and egg protein than to body and egg fat, respectively (see Table 2). This same trend exists in pigs, which shows a less efficient conversion rate of metabolic energy into body protein compared to body fat.

Table 3
NET AVAILABILITY OF METABOLIC ENERGY FOR PRODUCTION OF BODY GAIN AT DIFFERENT LIVE WEIGHTS OF STEERS GIVEN DIFFERENT RATIONS

$$\frac{\text{Energy retention}}{\text{Metabolic energy intake}} \times 100$$

	Live weight (kg)			
	365	450	520	585
Barley diet	77	77	75	84
Dried grass diet	36	30	28	30

Note: Values are calculated from slaughter experiments.

From Kay, M., in *Principles of Cattle Production,* Swan, H., and Browster, W. H., Eds., Butterworths, London, 1976, 255—270. With permission.

The great variations in the efficiency of metabolic energy for production of body-weight gain in growing cattle (see Table 2) may be attributed to the influence of age and growth rate on the composition of body weight gain (i.e., protein:fat ratio); this influence is conspicuous in growing cattle. Furthermore, the efficiency of utilization of ME for growth of ruminant animals varies considerably with the type of diets (Table 3). Increasing the amount of concentrates in the diet is associated with an increase in the relative proportion of propionic acid and a decrease of acetic acid formed in the rumen, while increasing the amount of roughage is associated with an inverse trend in the proportion of both volatile fatty acids. Since propionic acid is used with greater effectiveness than acetic acid, it follows conclusively that increasing the amount of concentrates in the diet increases the efficiency of metabolic energy utilization for production of body-weight gain (Table 3).

The net efficiency of body-weight gain is comparatively high in early life. Young calves such as veal calves in the prerumination stage utilize metabolic energy for body-weight gain with an efficiency of 66 to 69%; in this respect, they are very similar to monogastric animals. Likewise, the net efficiency of lambs on a milk diet is 64% for growth from birth to 1 month of age and 35 to 48% from 2 to 24 months of age[6].

As evidence in Table 2, cattle use metabolic energy for maintenance and milk production with about the same high efficiency, surpassing the respective efficiency for growth in later developmental stages. The efficiency for lactation is thought to be high; the conversion of nutrients ingested by the food into milk constituents such as protein, lactose and lower fatty acids occurs with higher efficiency than their conversion into the higher fatty acids of body fat. A certain physiological condition persisting regularly in high-producing lactating cows associated with depressed efficiency of milk formation, should be mentioned: During the initial stages and peak lactation, when a cow is not able to eat enough to meet the needs of milk secreted, fat reserves stored in the tissues are mobilized and channeled into milk production; fat stores are rebuilt very efficiently during the dry period. This circuitous pathway of milk formation appears to be a normal metabolic adaptation, but the efficiency of milk production via body fat is somewhat depressed. Conversion of the metabolic energy of food to tissue energy and of tissue energy into milk energy gives an overall conversion of only 64% vs. the 75% efficiency of the direct conversion from feed metabolic energy to milk energy. This loss cannot be avoided.

The efficiency of metabolic energy ingested for muscular work is very low; and only one third of the metabolic energy ingested is transformed into mechanical work and two thirds of it is released from the animal as heat and wasted. Likewise, work production by draught horses is the least efficient utilization of metabolic energy among all productive functions of animals.[8]

Charges of Maintenance Needs on the Utilization of Energy for Productive Purposes

With regard to the important types of animal production, the conversion of metabolic energy into animal products is a very efficient process. However, in order to get information about the amount of metabolic energy, generally food energy, that must be invested to produce an energetic unit of an animal product, the energy costs of maintenance and production should be charged against the product obtained. The relative influence of the maintenance requirements on the total input of energy needed for various types of production is illustrated in Table 4. The total energy requirements necessary to produce the unit of weight of an animal product decreases with increasing production level, since high production levels reduce the proportional charge of maintenance on total production costs. Figure 2 uses a milking cow as an example and shows the extent to which the ratio of maintenance requirements to total energy requirements drops as the yield increases.

UTILIZATION OF PROTEIN BY ANIMALS

Apart from the supply of energy, the administration of protein is most important for ensuring satisfactory performance and production of farm animals. Simple-stomached animals must receive the essential amino acids in the correct quantities and mutual proportions and a sufficient amount of the nonessential amino acids to meet their metabolic needs. They obtain the amino acids from the breakdown of protein during digestion and absorption, whereas in ruminant animals this occurs in a different way: digesta, consisting mainly of microbial protein and, to a smaller extent, food protein, reaches the intestine, and, owing to the uniform composition of microbial protein a mixture of amino acids of a quite uniform composition, almost independent upon that of the original diet, is liberated in the intestine and absorbed. Whereas monogastric animals consume only highly digestible feedstuffs, the efficiency of protein-containing feedstuffs for ruminants is limited by the digestibility of the protein. Measures of quality of protein foods for monogastric animals are based on amino acid composition; proteins in ruminant animals are evaluated in terms of digestible protein, i.e., percentage of the protein intake that is not recovered in the resulting fecal excretion.

The efficiency of conversion of digested protein into animal products is reduced by similar charges as those diminishing the utilization of digested energy. Protein is required for maintenance. There is a continuous breakdown and synthesis of individual body proteins; balance between synthesis and destruction represents the maintenance requirement of protein. The efficiency of conversion of ingested protein into animal products varies with the type of production and is also affected by the proportion of protein and energy consumed. Estimates of the efficiency of utilization of digestible protein for milk production vary from 60 to 70%.[11] The biosynthesis of milk proteins occurring in the udder from amino acids arising from the blood has been recognized as a very efficient process. Therefore, for explaining this gap between amounts of protein required and those recovered in milk, it should be taken into account that a certain part of the absorbed amino acid may be used for energy supply.

Considerable variations are evident in the utilization of protein for growth, depending upon the composition of gain, the rates of gain, and the proportions of protein

Table 4
APPROXIMATE PROPORTIONS OF THE TOTAL ENERGY REQUIREMENTS OF ANIMALS WHICH ARE CONTRIBUTED TO BY THEIR REQUIREMENTS FOR MAINTENANCE

	Daily values (kcal net energy) required for:		Maintenance as a percentage of total
	Maintenance	Production	
Dairy cow weighing 500 kg and producing 20 kg milk	8,000	18,400	30
Steer weighing 300 kg and gaining 1 kg	7,000	3,700	65
Pig weighing 50 kg and gaining 0.75 kg	1,730	2,320	43
Fowl weighing 1000 g and gaining 27 g	120	60	66

From McDonald, P., Edwards, R. A., and Greenhalgh, I.F.D., *Animal Nutrition,* 2nd ed., Oliver & Boyd, Edinburgh, 1973, 262. With permission.

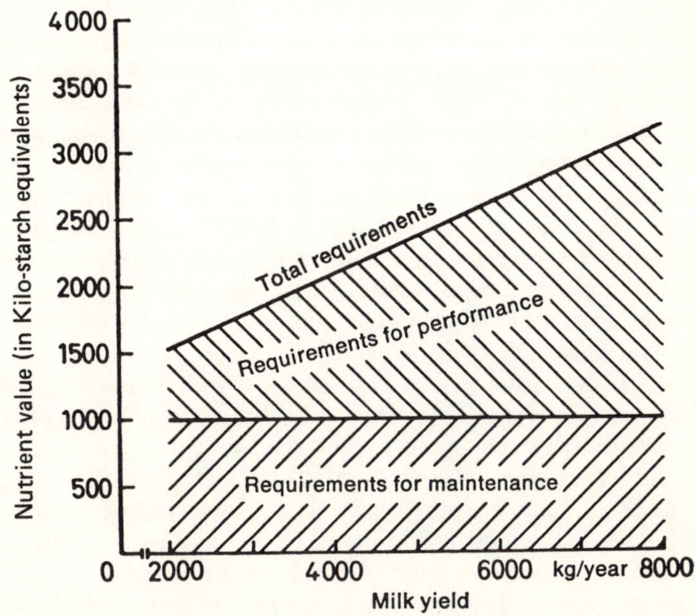

FIGURE 2. Energy requirements of milking cows at different yield levels. (From Oslage, H. J., in *Animal Research and Development,* Vol. 2, Institute for Scientific Cooperation, Tübingen, Germany, 1975, 7 — 19. With permission.)

and energy consumed. The efficiency of utilization of protein by simple-stomached animals is affected if essential amino acids are not fed in the exactly required proportions. Values for the efficiency with which protein is used for production of body-weight gain in growing animals are not given here because they vary considerably, but can be found in related literature.[12-14]

The efficiency of conversion of dietary amino acids into egg protein is very high — close to 100% — when the diet being fed is adequate with respect to the essential amino acids required. However, there is a large gap between the almost total recovery of amino acids supplied in the exactly required proportions to laying hens (in addition to their maintenance needs) and between the gross utilization of dietary protein of only 27% achieved in the U.S. on an annual basis; the reasons for the low gross utilization of egg protein will be outlined later.

It is well known that supplementation of rations with minerals and vitamins is of great importance for ensuring the normal functioning of the animals. Since minerals and vitamins contained in most of the conventional feed additives are highly available, problems dealing with the efficiency of these nutrients will not be considered here.

COMPARATIVE EFFICIENCY OF FARM ANIMALS IN THE CONVERSION OF FEEDSTUFFS TO HUMAN FOODS OF ANIMAL ORIGIN

The values for the efficiencies of utilization of ME by farm animals given in Table 2 were obtained by metabolic experiments of short duration. It was pointed out that the knowledge of these values, apart from their physiological interest, enables the formulation of feed rations. Data for comparing the efficiency of various types of animal production have been obtained by determining the protein-calorie output of animal products vs. respective inputs of feeds on the basis of an individual of each species in terms of productive lifetime performance. Data concerning input-output have also been obtained for whole animal populations in great animal enterprises or even on a country-wide basis. Such data on the overall efficiency of food production take into account the protein-calorie inputs necessary to maintain the breeding-herd population and to cover losses resulting from infertility and mortality. Data on the efficiency of utilization of energy and protein supplied to farm animals, which were calculated in different ways, are presented in Tables 5 through 7 and Figure 3. Different parameters of efficiency were used to express the food protein produced as a function of feed energy and protein consumed. Considerable effort was also devoted to assessing the energy and protein content of the productive output, i.e., body tissue, particularly its edible part, milk and eggs.

A similar relative order of the efficiency of various types of animal production arises from Tables 5 through 7. Highest efficiency of energy and protein conversion to human foods is obtained with milk and egg production, and protein conversion into poultry meat occurs with about the same efficiency. Efficiency of energy utilization by broilers and of protein and energy utilization by swine are intermediate; energy and protein conversion are the lowest in lamb and beef production. In Table 5, amounts of protein and energy contained in edible products are calculated as percentages of their intakes for all classes of livestock consumed during the whole lifetime of the different animal species.[15] These values are based on recent average data obtained in the U.S.

Respective data taken from European average values are presented in Figure 3. This figure includes data referring separately to animals of different production levels. The latter data reveal the increase of efficiency associated with increased production. High production levels reduce the proportional charge of maintenance on total requirements.

Table 6 summarizes data on the comparative efficiency with which farm animals produce food protein relative to the input of digestible energy.[17] Comprehensive data on animal protein production per hectare in the U.S. and the inputs of feed, labor,

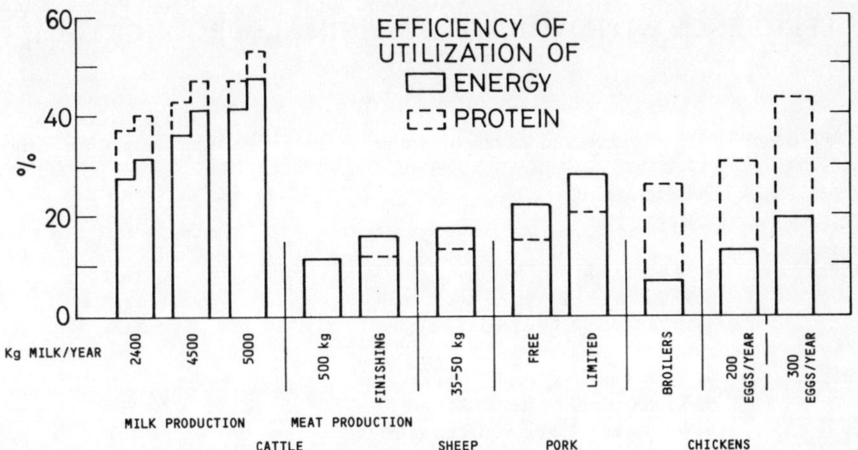

FIGURE 3. Efficiency of utilization of energy and protein by various classes of livestock and for different levels of production. (From Schurch, A., *Mitt. Tierhaltung*, 123, 1, 1969. With permission.)

Table 5
ESTIMATED PERCENTAGE EFFICIENCY OF CONVERTING FEED NUTRIENTS TO EDIBLE PRODUCT

Livestock	Crude protein	Energy
Nonruminants		
Broilers	23	11
Turkeys	22	9
Hens (eggs)	26	18
Swine	14	14
Ruminants		
Dairy cattle	25	17
Beef cattle	4	3
Lambs	4	—

Note: (Total lifetime production/total lifetime input), e.g., for milk protein the calculation is as follows: protein in all milk produced + protein in edible cuts of carcass/total feed crude protein input.

From Wedin, W. F., Hodgson, H. J., and Jacobson, N. L., *J. Anim. Sci.*, 41, 667—685, 1975. With permission.

and fossil energy are presented in Table 7.[18] Fossil energy is the main driving force behind the high yields achieved by modern agriculture. Inputs of fossil energy include energy cost of operation and maintenance of machinery, equipment, building, fertilizers, pesticides, etc., and for some production types, the inputs of fossil energy reach the scope of the input of food energy (Table 7). The data on the kilocalorie ratios of feed energy input to protein output and of fossil energy input to protein output manifest the efficiency of both kinds of energy input for the production of the different kinds of animal proteins (Table 7) and deserve great practical interest.

Table 6
EFFICIENCY WITH WHICH FARM ANIMALS PRODUCE FOOD PROTEIN

Food product	Level and/or rate of output	Protein production (g/Mcal of digestible energy)
Eggs	200 eggs/year	10.1
	250 eggs/year	13.7
Broiler	1.59 kg/12 wk; 3 kg feed/1 kg gain	11.9
	1.59 kg/10 wk; 2.5 kg feed/1 kg gain	13.7
	1.59 kg/8 wk; 2.1 kg feed/1 kg gain	15.9
Pork	91 kg/8.3 mo; 6 kg feed/1 kg gain	5.0
	91 kg/6.0 mo; 4 kg feed/1 kg gain	6.1
	91 kg/4.4 mo; 2.5 kg feed/l kg gain	8.7
	91 kg/3.7 mo; 2.0 kg feed/1 kg gain	
Milk	3,600 kg/yr; No concentrates	10.5
	5,400 kg/yr; 25% of energy as concentrates	12.8
	9,072 kg/yr; 50% of energy as concentrates	16.3
	13,608 kg/yr; 65% of energy as concentrates	20.5
Beef	500 kg/15 mo; 8 kg feed/1 kg gain	2.3
	500 kg/12 mo; 5 kg feed/1 kg gain	3.2
	Highly intensive system; no losses	4.1

From Reid, J. T. and White, O. D., in *New Protein Foods*, Vol. 3, Altschul, A. M. and Wiecke, H. L., Eds., Academic Press, New York, 1978, 117.

The increase of efficiency of milk production associated with increasing milk yield, as manifested in Table 6, is noticeable. The increased efficiency of milk production by higher yielding cows, which produce more than 5400 kg of milk per year, is also a result of the intensification of the energy input. This is accomplished by supplying the portion of the ration that covers the requirements for milk production by concentrate feeds and only the maintenance requirements by forages. Milk production by high-yielding cows (13,500 kg/year, obtaining 65% of the energy supplied as concentrates) is, according to Table 6, the most efficient of all livestock systems in the conversion of digestible energy into edible protein.

On the other hand, cows can produce as much as 5000 kg of milk on an all-forage diet, with an efficiency of 12 g of protein output per megacalorie of digestible energy input, i.e., these cows produce milk with almost the same efficiency as on a ration containing 25% of energy as concentrates (see Table 5). The level of this yield (5000 kg of milk per year) is probably close to the upper limit possible on forage alone.

The high efficiency of protein conversion by milking cows is indicated in Table 7. In 1974, the average yield per cow was 5541 kg in the U.S.; i.e., 59 kg of milk protein was produced from 188 kg feed protein. Of the 188 kg of feed protein, about 98 kg was supplied in concentrates and 90 kg was from forages. The efficiency of the conversion of the protein of concentrates, i.e., the portion of the rations designated to milk production, was 60%; this high figure was obtained because the protein in forages covering the maintenance requirements was not taken into account. The total efficiency of the conversion of food protein into milk protein is 25%, according to average U.S. data (Table 5). When calculated on the basis of the input of digestible protein, the efficiency of the production of milk protein increases to about 30%. The milking goat produces milk protein with about the same efficiency as the milking cow. [18]

Table 7
ANIMAL PROTEIN (kg) PRODUCED PER HECTARE IN THE U.S. WITH VARIOUS INPUTS OF FEED, LABOR, AND ENERGY

				Feed-energy input (10^3 kcal for the production of				Kilocalorie ratio	
Animal product	Animal-protein yield (kg)	Feed-protein input (kg)	Feed-energy input (10^3 kcal)	Feed	Feed and animal	Animal	Labor (man-hours)	Feed input/protein output	Fossil energy input/protein output
Milk	59	188	6,963	2,382	8,561	6,179	23	30	35.9
Eggs	182	672	14,406	6,070	9,560	3,490	174	20	13.1
Broilers	116	651	8,886	6,446	10,233	3,787	38	19	22.1
Catfish	51	484	5,007	2,180	7,068	4,888	55	25	34.6
Pork	65	689	17,021	6,774	9,212	2,438	28	65	35.4
Beef									
Feedlot	51	786	24,952	7,129	15,845	8,716	31	122	77.7
Rangeland	2.2	33	1,420	0	89	89	1	164	10.1
Lamb (rangeland)	0.17	3	128	2	11	9	0.2	188	16.2

From Pimentel, D., Dritschilo, W., Drummel, J., and Kutzman, J., *Science*, 190, 754—761, 1975. With permission. Copyright by the American Association for the Advancement of Science.

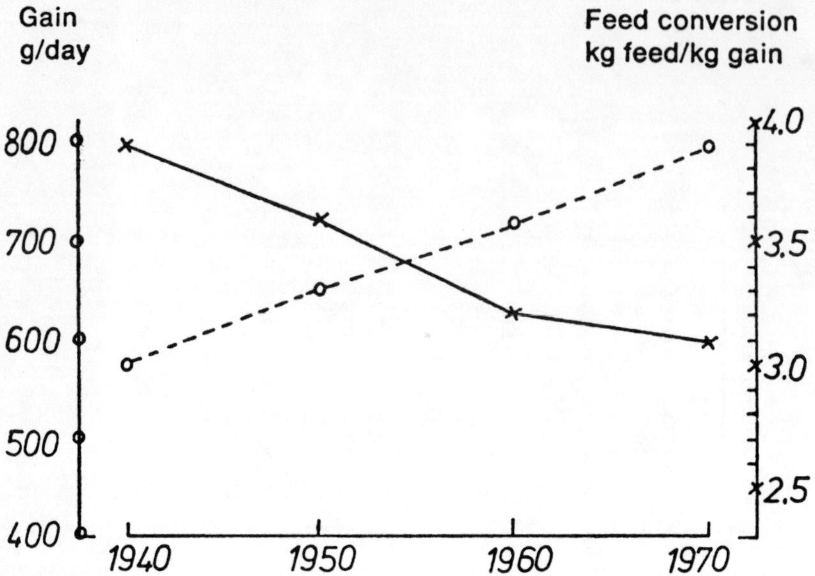

FIGURE 4. Improvement in gains and feed conversion in pigs from 1940 to 1970. (From Oslage, H. J., in *Animal Research and Development,* Vol. 2, Institute for Scientific Cooperation, Tübingen, Germany, 1975, 7 — 19. With permission.)

At 27%, egg production is the next most efficient means of converting feed protein into edible animal protein (Table 5). Due to recent progress in poultry breeding and nutrition, according to data from the U.S.; even less energy is needed for production of egg or broiler protein than for that of milk protein: 30 kcal of feed energy are needed for production of 1 kcal of milk protein, and only 20 kcal of energy are needed for 1 kcal of egg protein (Table 7). Broiler production is very similar to egg production with regard to the feed input in kilocalories to protein output, i.e., 19 kcal energy for 1 kcal protein, whereas the efficiency of protein conversion in broiler production is only 18%, vs. 21% for egg protein production. The data for broiler production given in Table 6 show that as the intensity of production increases the efficiency of protein production increases. This again reflects the effect of diluting the energy cost of maintenance. The same trend arises from recent British data concerning broiler and egg production; the British standards of broiler production, in which birds of 1.6 kg are raised in 56 days with a feed-conversion ratio of 2.5, provide a protein-conversion efficiency of about 20%.[19] By improving the feed-conversion ratio to 2.0 and increasing the live weight of the finished broiler to 2.0 kg, the efficiency of protein conversion is raised to almost 30%. The efficiency of the conversion of food into egg protein is highly correlated to level of egg yield; it is about 20% at yields of 240 eggs per year and rises to about 30% when yields are raised to 320 eggs per year (compare Figure 3).[19] Protein requirements for the maintenance of laying hens and the amino acid composition of practical diets, a composition that is far from being ideally balanced, may account for the great gap between gross and net efficiency of egg protein production.

Pigs produce a relatively low protein product, i.e., ca. 13%, at usual slaughter weight; as outlined on page 197, the efficiency of body growth decreases with increasing fat content of the body gain. For this reason, and because of the great costs of producing the leaner pig, the production of pork products is of comparatively low efficiency.[7] The feed energy input in kilocalories per kilocalories of protein output for pork production is 65 to 1, or about twice that of milk production (Table 7). In recent years, progress has been made in breeding pigs with more lean meat and less fat.[11]

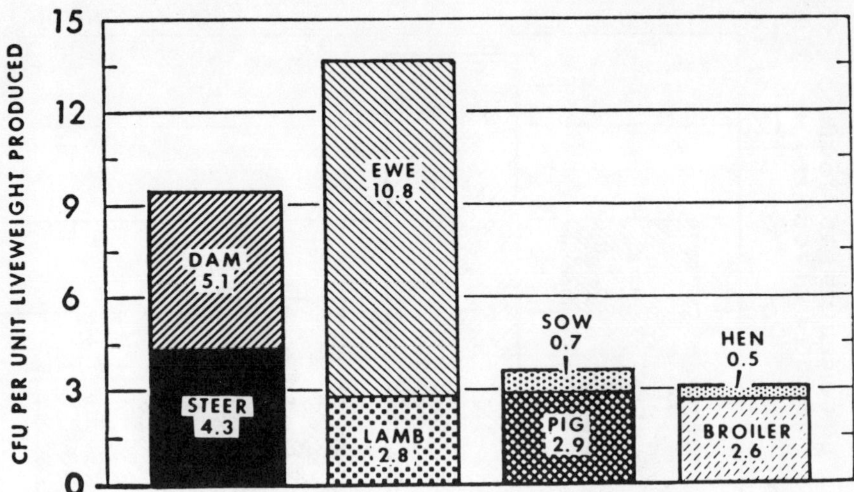

FIGURE 5. Partition of energy requirements of various species of animals between body-weight gain and offspring. CFU = corn equivalent feed units. (From Byerly, T. C., *Science*, 157, 890, 1967. With permission. Copyright 1967 by the American Association for the Advancement of Science.)

Figure 4 shows the improvement in gains and feed conversion in pigs that was achieved in Britain. In growing pigs, as in chicks, the protein-conversion efficiency increases with accelerated growth rate; this efficiency can be raised from 12 to 16% by elevating daily weight gain average from 0.4 to 0.6 kg and by concomitant decreasing of feed-conversion ratios from 2.9 to 2.1.

The production of both protein and energy per unit of energy ingested by meat-producing ruminants is the least efficient production by domesticated animals. The low efficiencies of beef and lamb production (see Tables 5 through 7) is accountable in great part to the high energy ɔst of rearing and maintaining the breeding herd; breeding-herd input of beef cattle represents about one third of the food energy input required for beef production.[18] The normal reproductive rate in ruminant population is low; as a result, an excessive amount of food is used mainly by the mother, for each unit of output in the young. The efficiency of production of lamb meat increases by lambing larger litters; the ewe bearing three lambs needs 60% less feed energy and the ewe with two lambs 40% less than the ewe with a single lamb.[21] It appears from Figures 5 and 6 that the requirements of energy and protein for the dams of cattle and sheep are relatively much higher than those for the dams of pigs and poultry.[22]

The feed efficiency of rangeland beef and lamb production is even lower than that of feedlot beef production, since the feeding value of the plants of natural pasture and rangeland grasses is lower than that of the food for feedlot beef, which in the U.S. consisted of about 42% forage and 58% concentrate foodstuffs in 1975. Of feedlot beef protein produced, 122 kcal of feed energy is consumed per kilocalorie, while 164 or 188 kcal of feed energy is used per kilocalorie of rangeland beef or lamb (Table 7). The difference in the efficiency of protein production of beef between the intensive and extensive systems is a reflection of the longer maintenance period for beef produced extensively. The energy expended in grazing also reduces the efficiency of food conversion. The pastural systems vary in their effectiveness according to climatic conditions. In Texas, with a rainfall of 70 cm/year, 2.2 kg of beef protein is produced per hectare per year; in Utah, with a rainfall of 36 cm/year, only 0.17 kg of protein is produced per hectare (see Table 7). Animal protein yields per hectare of rangeland

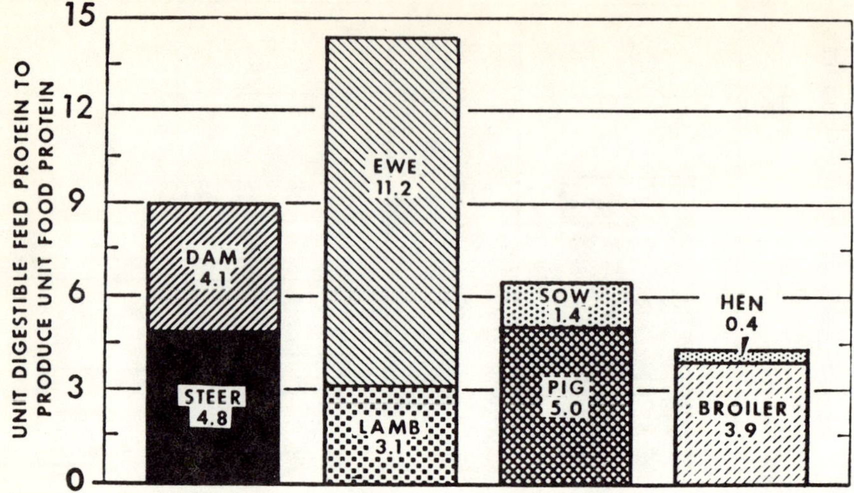

FIGURE 6. Partition of digestible protein requirements between body - weight gain and offspring. (From Byerly, T. C., *Science*, 157, 890, 1967. With permission. Copyright 1967 by the American Association for the Advancement of Science.)

beef and lamb are very low. However, sheep also produce wool; if wool production was included, the calculation of sheep protein production would be higher. Despite the low output of protein per unit of energy consumed (Table 7) by beef and lamb under extensive management conditions, these animals require a minimal supplement of fossil energy.

The 4% efficiency of protein utilization by beef cattle and lambs (see Table 4) can be increased by intensive feeding or rearing systems; intensive beef production with all concentrate, particularly barley rations, results in a 10 to 15% efficiency of protein utilization.[19,20]

A comparison of the efficiencies with which various species of meat-producing animals convert feed into meat are given in Tables 8 and 9.[21] The efficiencies are expressed as a ratio:

$$\frac{\text{total energy in carcass produced}}{\text{gross energy in feed}}$$

These efficiencies are presented separately for individual meat- producing animals (Table 8) and for populations (Table 9). With regard to those species of meat-producing animals dealt with previously, about the same order of feed efficiency arises as is revealed in Tables 5 through 7 and Figure 3. The data given in Tables 8 and 9 reveal clearly the influence of the reproduction rate and number of offspring on feed efficiency.

Efficiency of fish production

On a world-wide basis, fish protein amounts only to 5% of the total protein available to man, whereas total protein produced by livestock amounts to 25% of the total. The data on food efficiency by fish are very scarce. Comparison of food utilization of the carp, a poikilothermic species, with that of poultry showed that the daily maintenance need of energy by carp was one fifth that of the chicken. This probably results from the fact that in fish metabolism is slower at the low body temperature.[23] However, the efficiency with which the total food energy consumed by the carp, which grow from

Table 8
RANGE OF EFFICIENCY VALUES (E) FOR WEANED INDIVIDUALS OF MEAT-PRODUCING ANIMALS

$$E = \frac{\text{Total energy in the carcass}}{\text{Gross energy in feed from independence to slaughter}} \times 100$$

Animal	E
Beef cattle	5.2—7.8
Sheep	11—14.6
Rabbits	12.5—17.5
Pigs	35
Hens	16
Geese	13.4

From Spadding, C. R. W. and Hoxey, A. M., in *Meat,* Cole, D. J. A. and Lawrie, R. A., Eds., Butterworths, London, 1975, 483—506. With permission.

40 to 80 g, was retained in the body was 27%; the broilers' efficiency averaged 30% over the normal growth period. This result did not indicate any advantage of the poikilothermic species with regard to energy utilization. On the contrary, the ratio N retention to N intake was 30% in carp, while it was more than 50% for chickens. Table 7 presents some data concerning the commercial production of catfish; this fish requires the feeding of grains and protein foods suitable for man and monogastric animals. The rate of protein conversion by catfish is about 11%. High inputs of fossil energy are needed for the production of catfish. Large quantities of fossil energy must be expended to produce fish protein. On the coast of England, for instance, about 7920 kcal is required to harvest 1 kg of fish. [18]

TENDENCIES AND TRENDS FOR INCREASING EFFICIENCY OF ANIMAL PRODUCTION[24,25]

The tendency of livestock farmers to raise efficiency of production per head has been implemented during recent years in the U.S., particularly with regard to dairy cattle.[18] From 1960 to 1974, feed consumption per head of dairy cattle rose 40%. This increase was accompanied by large increases in milk production per head and increased efficiency, as evidenced by an 11% reduction in feed units consumed per 100 kg of milk. During this period, the dairy cattle population decreased by 40% and the milk yield only by 4%. A large percentage of the increased amount of feed units consumed by dairy and beef cattle herds in the U.S. derived from concentrate feeds. For beef cattle, the increased rate of feeding decreased efficiency, and there was a 10% increase in feed units per 100 kg of beef produced. The population of beef cattle in the U.S. increased during the above period by 56%, while the production of beef increased only by 36%. This reduction of feed efficiency was accompanied by a desired change in the quality of meat, which became lean and tender. Since 1973, a further improvement of carcass grade and dressing percentage was acquired by increased use of forage instead of grains prior to the finishing period; the improvement in meat quality was at the expense of a further decline in efficiency of feed-conversion.[26] This changed feeding system was installed with regard to the progressing reduction of the grain supply. However, the more the livestock production depends upon concentrates, the easier is the management.

Table 9
RANGE OF EFFICIENCY VALUES (E) FOR POPULATIONS OF MEAT-PRODUCING ANIMALS

$$E = \frac{\text{Total energy in carcass produced}}{\text{Gross energy in feed for the progeny and proportion of parents}} \times 100$$

Animal	E
Suckler cows and calves[a]	3.2
Sheep[b]	
With singles	2.4
With twins	3.4
With triplets	4.2
Rabbits[c]	8.0
Pigs[d]	23—27
Hens[e]	14.6
Geese[f]	10

[a] Feed intake of the cow for 1 year plus feed intake of the calf to slaughter.
[b] Feed intake of the ewe for 1 year plus feed intake of the lamb(s) to slaughter.
[c] One buck to 15 does, each producing 40 progeny per year.
[d] One boar to 20 sows, each producing 20 progeny per year.
[e] One cock to 10 hens, each producing 108 progeny per year.
[f] One gander to 3 geese, each producing 18 progeny per year.

From Spadding, C. R. W. and Hoxey, A. M., in *Meat,* Cole, D. J. A. and Lawrie, R. A., Eds., Butterworths, London, 1975, 483—506. With permission.

Great progress in improving food efficiency has been reached during recent years in the nutrition of pigs and poultry, which are, of course, largely dependent upon concentrates. The goal of producing 1 kg of live gain with about 2 kg of feed has almost been achieved with poultry and swine. A considerably high rate of efficiency in ruminants is reached by the portion of the ration originating from concentrates in comparison to the respective efficiency of roughages. Supplementary feeding with concentrates maintains the milk production and reproductive level of cows kept on forages; such supplementation enables accelerated growth of cattle and more efficient production of meat. However, in the future, grain feeding of ruminants will be restricted in order to avoid competition with grain needs for human and monogastric animals.

In developing countries, ruminants, e.g., beef cattle, sheep, and other meat-producing ruminants, subsist wholly on poor-quality forages produced from rangelands; there is no other possible utilization for these wide areas and they provide man with food that he would not otherwise have. Thus, the relative inefficiency with which food is utilized under such extensive management conditions is not hampering. In other countries, great achievements have been made in developing nutritionally and economically efficient forages and procedures for forage conservation.

Other recent trends in the economical nutrition of farm animals include the adjustment of rations to the use of industrial and agricultural by-products and processed animal wastes without affecting animal productivity and feed efficiency. The efficiency of protein in rations for meat animals and for cows with daily milk yields lower than 20 kg can even be improved by covering a part of the nitrogen requirement (up to 20%) by urea.

Animal productivity has been considerably improved and in the future, will be further raised by two types of genetic means: (1) The continued selection of breeding stock for high performance and conversion rates and (2) the improvment of reproductive efficiencies by crossing widely unrelated genetic stocks.[27,28]

REFERENCES

1. **Holmes, W.**, Animals for food, *Proc. Nutr. Soc.*, 29, 237—243, 1970.
2. **Lenkeit, W. and Breirem, K.**, *Handbook of Animal Nutrition*, Vol. 2, Paul Parey, Hamburg, 1972.
3. **Moe, P. W. and Tyrrell, H. F.**, Observations on the efficiency of metabolizable energy for meat and milk production, in *Nutrition Conference for Feed Manufacturers*, Vol. 7, Swan, H. and Lewis, D., Eds., Butterworths, London, 1974, 27—36.
4. **Millward, D. J., Garlick, P. J., and Reeds, P. T.**, The energy cost of growth, *Proc. Nutr. Soc.*, 35, 339—349, 1976.
5. **Kay, M.**, Meeting the energy and protein requirements of the growing animal, in *Principles of Cattle Production*, Swan, H. and Brewster, W. H., Eds., Butterworths, London, 1976, 255—270.
6. **Graham, N. McC.** Growth in Sheep, in Energy Metabolism of Farm Animals, Schürch, A. and Wenk, C., Eds., European Association for Animal Production, No. 13, Zurich, 1970, 105—108.
7. **De Groote, G.**, Utilization of metabolizable energy, in *Energy Requirements of Poultry*, Morris T. R. and Freeman, B. M., Eds., British Poultry Science, Edinburgh, 1974, 113—134.
8. **Dyrendahl, S.**, Work, in *Handbook of Animal Nutrition*, Vol. 2, Lenkeit, W. and Breirem, K., Eds., Paul Parey, Hamburg, 1972, 674—689.
9. **McDonald, P., Edwards, R. A., and Greenhalgh, I. F. D.**, *Animal Nutrition*, 2nd ed., Oliver and Boyd, Edinburgh, 1973, 262.
10. **Oslage, H. J.**, Modern Animal Nutrition and the Future of Animal Production, in *Animal Research and Development*, Vol. 2, Institute for Scientific Co-operation, Tübingen, Germany, 1975, 7—19.
11. **Van Es, A. T. H. and Boekholt, H. A.**, Protein requirements in relation to lactation cycle, in *Protein Metabolism and Nutrition*, Cole, D. J. A. et al., Eds., Butterworths, London, 1976, 441—456.
12. **Orskov, E. R.**, Factors influencing protein and non-protein nitrogen utilization in young ruminants, in *Protein Metabolism and Nutrition*, Cole, D. J. R., et al., Eds., Butterworths, London, 1976, 457—476.
13. **Chamberlain, A. G.**, Protein requirements of the growing pig, in *Pig Production*, Cole, D. J. A., Ed., Butterworths, London, 1972, 203—224.
14. **Kielanowski, J.**, Protein requirements of growing animals, in *Handbook of Animal Nutrition*, Vol. 2, Lenkeit, W. and Breirem, K., Eds., Paul Parey, Hamburg, 1972, 528—546.
15. **Wedin, W. F., Hodgson, H. J., and Jacobson, N. L.**, Utilizing plant and animal resources in production to human food, *J. Anim. Sci.*, 41, 667—685, 1975.
16. **Schürch, A.**, The future of animal production, *Mitt. Tierhaltung*, 123, 1—10, 1969.
17. **Reid, J. T.**, Comparative efficiency of animals in the conversion of feedstuffs to human foods, Proc. Cornell Nutr. Conf. Feed Manufacturers, Departments of Animal Science and Poultry Science, Cornell University, Ithaca, New York, 1975, 16—24.
18. **Pimentel, D., Dritschilo, W., Drummel, J., and Kutzman, J.**, Energy and land constraints in food protein production, *Science*, 190, 754—761, 1975.
19. **Wilson, P. N.**, The biological efficiency of protein production by animal production enterprises, in *The biological efficiency of protein production*, Jones, J. G. W., Ed., Cambridge University Press, London, 1973, 201—210.
20. **Homb, T. and Joshi, D. C.**, The biological efficiency of protein production by stall-fed ruminants, in *The biological efficiency of protein production*, Jones, J.G.W., Ed., Cambridge University Press, London, 1973, 237—262.
21. **Spadding, C. R. W. and Hoxey, A. M.**, The potential for conventional meat animals, in *Meat*, Cole, D. J. A. and Lawrie, R. A., Eds., Butterworths, London, 1975, 483—506.
22. **Byerly, T. C.**, Efficiency of feed conversion, *Science*, 157, 890—895, 1967.
23. **Blaxter, K. L.**, Conventional and unconventional farmed animals, *Proc. Nutr. Soc.*, 34, 51—56, 1975.

24. **Scrimshaw, N. S., Wang, D. I. C., and Milner, M.,** Protein Resources and Technology: Status and Research Needs, National Science Foundation, NSF Grant AEN 75-13072, Washington, D.C., 1975, 59.
25. **Byerly, T. C.,** Ruminant livestock, research and development, *Science,* 195, 450—456, 1977.
26. **Hodgson, H. J.,** Gaps in knowledge and technology for finishing cattle on forages, *J. Anim. Sci.,* 44, 896—900, 1977.
27. **Frenkle, A. and Willham, R. L.,** Beef production efficiency, *Science,* 198, 1009—1015, 1977.
28. **Cunha, T, J.,** Land animals: opportunities for improved production, in *New Protein Foods,* Vol. 3, Altschul, A. M. and Wiecke, H. L., Eds., Academic Press, New York, 1978, 198—225.

CASTRATION AND ANIMAL PRODUCTIVITY*

J. D. Turton

The history of castration is probably almost as old as the history of the domestication of animals to fulfill man's requirements for meat, animal products, and draft power. From prehistoric bones found at Skara Brae in Orkney, Scotland the existence of castrated male cattle was postulated on the basis of the shape of the horn core.[1] The adoption of castration was probably originally related to the greater tractability of the castrate and the greater ease with which it was husbanded in the presence of the mature female. Later, the idea of limiting indiscriminate breeding occurred, and the first indication of a market demand was a preference for the fatter and more tender carcass of the mature ox and wether.

In general terms, the effect of castration is to modify the secondary sex characteristics of an animal. Sexual drive and aggressiveness are reduced or abolished, thus simplifying husbandry practices. Body form and composition are modified, resulting in differing carcass characteristics. The balance between fore- and hindquarters is changed; the uncastrated animal having a relatively greater development of forequarter musculature. Also, the amount and distribution of fat in the carcass are altered by castration. The meat of entire males is traditionally described as tougher and darker in color than that of castrates and thus is less acceptable to the consumer. A sexual odor or taint has been ascribed to boar meat, and a strong taste to the meat of the bull and ram. This resulted in a resistance in some parts of the world in accepting bull, ram, or boar carcasses.

The age at which an animal is castrated and slaughtered, relative to its age at sexual maturity, influences the effects of castration. The age at slaughter, in turn, depends upon market demands, methods of husbandry, and species and breed of the animal. Twenty years ago, although castration had long been an almost universal practice, precise experimental evidence of its effects on the performance of farm livestock was very limited.[2] Even in 1962, not many investigations had been carried out on the subject, and furthermore, many of the studies were of little scientific value.[3] Subsequently, many reports on the effects of castration appeared in the literature, including a number of reviews.[4-10]

Much of the detailed data on the experimental work will be presented in the form of tables referred to as data set 1, and the text will summarize conclusions that can be reached on the effects of castration. By this means, it is hoped that the general reader can obtain a picture of the main effects of castration, while those who may wish to obtain more detail can trace this via the tables. A good proportion of the work has been published in languages other than English, and the tables contain additional data to those which have already appeared in English abstracts. It is hoped that this will be of assistance to those who cannot read the papers in their original language. Experimental work for which no statistical analysis of the data is reported in the source scrutinized has not been included in the tables, but is summarized in the text referred to as data set 2. Comparisons between entire and castrated animals will, whenever possible, be given as the difference between the two means. This difference will be expressed as a percentage of the lower mean in the case of traits that are not themselves expressed as percentages. For traits expressed as percentages, the difference between the means will be given. Sometimes an experiment has included several groups of animals; in these cases, more than one entire versus castrate comparison will result. In other experiments, only a single value may be available. Comparison values generally

* Tables follow text, beginning on page 224.

varied considerably from experiment to experiment or even within the same experiment. Standard errors of the overall (unweighted) means for traits will be given. The coefficients of variation (CV) for the traits were not related to the number of comparison values (n) used in computing each mean, with the regression of CV on n being nonsignificant.

Taken as a whole, carcass studies embrace a large number of individual traits, and experiments often cannot be compared because they deal with different traits or apparently similar traits that are measured in different ways in different countries. For example, the cuts into which carcasses are separated differ between countries and even between regions within the same country, and dressing percentages are often not strictly comparable. Therefore, in order to allow comparisons with some validity, the carcass traits chosen for scrutiny are those which are for the most part independent of cutting method and are most likely to have a common interpretation in different countries.

The discussion here will be limited to the main species in which castration is of importance, namely, sheep, cattle, and pigs. Where only a single average figure is given for a trait, this will refer to data set 1 unless otherwise indicated.

SHEEP

The classic studies on castration were carried out in sheep and reported as long ago as 1932.[11] The general findings can be summarized as follows: At 5 months of age, sex differences between the ram and wether are noticeable. The musculature and bone of the ram are better developed, but the wether exhibits greater fat development. Castration alters the muscle:bone proportion. Muscular development in the ram is greater than in the ewe, but the proportion of muscle to bone is not higher because of the greater thickening of bones in the former. Castration prevents this thickening, thus raising the proportion of muscle to bone in younger animals. Subsequently, a greater prolongation of bone development occurs, so that after approximately 11 months of age, the proportion of muscle to bone in castrates again approaches that of rams. Data on sheep experiments are given in Table 1.

The average daily gain of rams in these experiments exceeded that of wethers by 13.14 ± 1.92%, and the superiority of rams for body weight was 9.72 ± 1.86%.

For data set 2, the superiority of rams for body weight was 7.36%; no data were available on average daily gain.[57-64] The superiority of rams increased with age, and for rams above 1 year was very marked. The higher percentage values for average daily gain, as compared with body weight, are a statistical artifact. This is illustrated in the following example:

	Initial weight (kg)	Final weight (after 100 days of fattening)	Average daily gain (kg)
Rams	20	42	0.22
Wethers	20	40	0.20

The superiority of the rams as compared to the wethers in their average daily gain was

$$\frac{0.02}{0.20} \times 100 = 10\%$$

In final weight, the superiority of the rams was

$$\frac{2}{40} \times 100 = 5\%$$

In the efficient utilization of food, rams were superior to wethers by 16.96±6.96%. Ram carcasses were higher in lean meat content than wether carcasses by 4.43 ± 1.36 percentage units and had appreciably less fat, as evidenced by less fat cover or fat trim. Loin-eye area, unadjusted for carcass weight, was 4.78 ± 2.60% higher in rams, but this superiority was mainly due to a higher carcass weight. Differences in meat characteristics were also evident, although there is very little data to suppor this. Shear values for ram meat were 12.11 ± .32% higher in rams than wethers, but taste panel evaluations did not indicate any noticeable differences. Castration significantly affected the proportions of some classes of fatty acid in sheep fat, but this does not seem to be of commercial significance. Dressing percentage is not given in the tables, for reasons given earlier. It tended to be slightly higher in wethers than in rams in about two thirds of the cases. In some cases, testes weight was included in ram carcass weight, which biased the comparisons.

The adverse effect of castration on growth rate and food conversion in sheep is well established, although the magnitude of the effect varies considerably with age and with other factors not yet adequately studied. Castration has been found to interact significantly with breed, but not with nutrition, although more evidence on these points is required before any firm conclusion can be drawn.[31,43] The ram is marginally superior in its production of lean meat, but the greater fat cover of the wether is advantageous in the case of fore- and hindlimb roasts. As yet, rising production costs have not resulted in mobilization of opinion toward the abandonment of castration of entire male lambs in countries where castration is traditionally and widely practiced, although the advantages of such a course of action were pointed out more than 25 years ago[6,11]

For lambs, the inhibiting effect of castration on wool growth is barely noticeable. However, at approximately 12 months of age or older, fleece weight may be as much as 18% greater in rams than in wethers.[30,67,70] The effects on wool fineness and crimp have not been found to be significant.[26,30.]

CATTLE

Most of the interest in whether or not to castrate animals has centered on cattle. There are three main reaons for this. Whereas in some countries (e.g., the U.S., Canada, and Great Britain) castration has been the predominant and frequently the exclusive practice, in continental western and eastern Europe, production of bull beef has been and still is the dominant practice. This inevitably suggests that there are good reasons for looking into the justification for castration. Secondly, rising costs of production have led agricultural scientists and farmers to look for ways of increasing production efficiency, and it has long been known that bulls tend to grow more rapidly than steers. Thirdly, feedlot methods of management lend themselves better to the production of bull beef than to the extensive methods of husbandry, or to the methods whereby cattle are slaughtered at a somewhat older age than they are at present. The use of feedlot methods has increased over the past 20 years.

Data on cattle experiments are given in Table 2. Cattle results for data set 2 are also available.[146-187] In addition, there is a substantial body of data recorded on bull — steer comparisons by the Meat and Livestock Commission (MLC) in Great Britain.[188,189] Details of MLC data are given separately in Table 3, but the comparisons have been included in the overall means for data set 2. In data sets 1 and 2, the overall mean superiority of bulls over steers was 12.77 ± 1.32 and 14.78%, respectively, for average daily gain, and 9.11 ± 1.63 and 7.75% for body weight at various slaughter ages. Food utilization efficiency of bulls was better than that of steers by 13.86 ± 1.63 and 9.24%. The standard errors conceal to some extent the variable results obtained over a wide range of countries and management systems. The coefficients of variation of the group means in the experiments cited for data set 1 range from 70 to 100%. Nevertheless, under reasonably good feeding and management, the advantage of the bull over the steer is marked. The advantage is much less variable when results are examined over a wide range of environmental conditions, as in the complete data sets.

Before dealing with carcass traits, it is necessary to summarize the effects of castration on the muscle weight distribution of the bovine carcass. Confusion is possible because muscle weights may be considered both in absolute terms and as percentages of total carcass muscle.[190] Muscles may be grouped according to their growth characteristics. Specifically, a growth coefficient (*b*) can be defined that represents the ratio of the percentage of postnatal growth of a muscle or muscle group to the growth of total muscle. These coefficients can then be used to define high impetus muscles (*b* significantly > 1), average impetus muscles (*b* not significantly different from 1), and low impetus muscles (*b* significantly < 1). Combinations can occur, such as high-average, with significant differences in *b* between growth phases which are separate in time. The effects of castration are most easily seen by plotting groups of *b* values for specific muscles or muscle groups against total carcass muscle weight.[190]

The *b*-value differences between bulls and steers are negligible in several muscle groups, e.g., distal pelvic limb muscles, muscles of spinal column and abdominal wall, and distal thoracic limb muscles. For proximal muscles of the pelvic limb, *b* values are higher in steers than in bulls, and the opposite relationship occurs for the muscles of the neck and thorax. The proportion of total muscle, accounted for by muscles that form the most expensive cuts of meat, (muscles of the proximal hindlimb, loin, and proximal forelimb) is about 1% higher in steers than in bulls. Results have also been presented on the effect of castration on the absolute weights of individual muscles.[191] The percentage weight reduction of muscles in steers relative to their entire monozygotic twins was highest for the muscles attaching the scapula to the thorax and neck: 50% for the splenius, 30% for the semispinalis capitis, and 23% for the rhomboideus. Other shoulder muscles showed the second largest decrease: approximately 12 to 15% for the deltoid, teres minor, and teres major muscles. The reduction in total muscle weight in the steers relative to the bulls was about 7%. Some muscles showed less than this 7% decrease, mainly those of the lower thorax and forearm: the longissimus dorsi and psoas muscles, the abdominal musculature, and the quadriceps and gastrocnemius muscles. However, they fell below the 7% level only by 2 or 3%.

In bull and steer carcasses of equal weight, the weight of the hindquarter muscle is the same, the weight of the forequarter muscle is greater in bulls, the bulls have less fat, and there is no difference in bone. Experiments were performed which assessed carcass composition in terms of lean, fat, bone, and measures of meatiness, e.g., rib eye area. In the two data sets, the lean percentage of bulls exceeded that of steers by 4.18 ± .25 and 5.09 percentage units and the fat percentage of the bulls was lower by 5.73 ± 0.49 and 3.27 percentage units. These figures refer to a large number of studies in which slaughter endpoint and many other experimental features varied considerably. Nevertheless, bulls had a higher lean and a lower fat content than steers virtually without exception. Bone percentage was about 1.7% higher in bulls than in steers (based on only six comparisons). The greater meatiness of bulls was reflected in higher area of the rib or loin eye, both adjusted and unadjusted for carcass weight. In the two cases, the superiority was 5.92 ± 1.94 and 12.76 ± 1.33%. Proximate analyses indicated that the protein percentage of meat was higher in bulls than in steers by 0.47 ± 0.18 in data set 1, but lower by 0.13 in data set 2. Thus, castration does not seem to affect this trait to any marked degree. Fat percentage of meat was higher in steers in the two data sets, by 1.94 ± 0.45 and 3.06, respectively.

Tenderness of bull meat, as assessed by shear value, was consistently higher than that of steer meat by 18.71 ± 4.44%. However, not much consideration should be given to this result because not only do taste panel assessments frequently fail to indicate a significant difference, but the average consumer is unable to detect this difference with any degree of reliability.

Some significant interactions of the castration effect with genotype and other factors have been reported. Genotype for meat production, as assessed by a progeny test, interacted significantly with castration. The effect was greater as genotypic rating for meat production increased (higher daily gain, etc.).[103] Similarly, the castration effect increased in successive growth stages and with increasing muscle mass in bulls.[123,191] Such relationships do not always occur, as evidenced by the lack of an interaction between castration and genotype in a study involving Hereford and Aberdeen Angus cattle.[194]

The castration effect appears to interact significantly with plane of nutrition, provided that nutritional differences have large enough effects on growth.[104] There is some evidence to suggest that, on pasture, the superiority of bulls over steers with respect to daily gain may be minimal or disappear.[68,91,192,193] However, this is probably a function of an overall level of daily gain, so that at the same levels of gain, the bull — steer comparison would be similar on pasture and feedlot.

Some bull — steer comparisons have been assessed at the economic level.[70,87,188,189] Earlier results were somewhat inconclusive, but recent MLC results have indicated appreciably better gross margins for bulls. Of course, costs and income are notoriously unstable factors, so that economic evaluations are valid only at the time they are made or so long as there is no marked change in them. They are, nevertheless, useful if expressed as relative profitability.

The general conclusion from the studies reviewed and from farming experience is that, under suitable management systems, castration of bulls is unjustified. Keeping of bulls has been shown to be free of managemental problems under grass/cereal and grass finishing systems provided proper attention is paid to safety. Feed costs are now so high that it is no longer justifiable to deliberately foster a practice that reduces growth rate and feed-conversion efficiency. The objections of the meat trade are based on prejudice, but the cost of maintaining this prejudice has now become excessive.

PIG

Over the past few years, there has been increased interest, particularly in Great Britain, in the possibility of using boars for pork and bacon production. More recent research has provided answers to some, but not all, of the key questions relevant to the matter. Data on pig experiments (data set 1) are given in Table 4. For average daily gain, boars had a superiority over barrows of 1.51 ± 0.12%. For data set 2, the corresponding mean was 1.18%.[223-231] Boars had higher gains than barrows in about 55% of the comparisons, barrows were superior in about 36%, and there was little or no difference in the remaining 8%. In studies reviewed in 1969, boars were superior in 45% of the cases and barrows in 35%.[4] Results of such comparisons are affected by management and nutrition, and it seems likely that the highest levels of feeding and management must be employed if the growth potential of boars is to be exploited to the fullest. The boar — barrow difference in growth rate, in itself, is not sufficient to support the case of either the supporters or the opposers of castration.

For food conversion efficiency, boars had a superiority of 5.74 ± 1.30 and 3.49% in the two data sets. In about three fourths of the comparisons, boars had an advantage, and barrows had a slight superiority in the remainder. In the 1969 review, boars were found to be superior in about 66% of cases.[4] The advantage of boars is more marked and more consistent than was the case for daily gain, and again, the advantage is best expressed under proper feeding and management.

Considering carcass traits, boars produce a higher lean content and less fat than barrows. In the two data sets, lean percentage for boars was higher by 6.37 ± 1.74 and 4.33 percentage units. With the exception of one comparison, boars always had the higher lean content. For fat percentage, boars had a lower value by 4.77 ± 0.94 percentage units for data set 1; only four comparisons were available for data set 2, and these showed a lower boar average by 22.8 percentage units. In no comparison were boars fatter than barrows. The greater fatness of barrows was also indicated by backfat thickness. Boars had thinner backfat by 23.16 ± 2.45 and 14.38% in the two data sets. The increased leanness and reduced fatness of the boar is arguably its greatest advantage over the barrow. Fat is expensive and inefficient to produce, and generally the consumer does not want it. The greatest disadvantage of the pig as a converter of feed to meat is that it wraps its protein in three or more centimeters of unwanted adipose tissue. The increased meatiness is reflected in greater loin eye area, boars exceeding barrows by 11.36 ± 2.22% in data set 1.

More evidence is required about the interaction of castration and nutritional factors. Existing evidence suggests that, within limits, protein level of the ration and castration do not interact significantly. Therefore, it is not worth feeding boars a higher level of protein than that normally given to barrows.[207,235] Thus, experimental evidence indicates that boars, under the right management, have some advantage in food utilization efficiency and a marked carcass advantage, as shown by a higher lean and a lower fat content.

Boar Taint

An unpleasant odor, referred to as boar taint, boar odor, or sex odor, has long been associated with cooked boar meat. The meat trade in most developed countries has shown a profound unwillingness to accept boar carcasses and, upon accepting any, subjects them to a financial penalty compared with barrow or gilt carcasses. Some of the prejudice against boar meat is probably related to the fact that service boars, particularly older ones, have a strong odor derived partly from secretions originating in the preputial sac and also from the slightly pungent, musty odor of the animal's breath and saliva.[232] It has become the general practice to equate such smells with a characteristic odor sometimes detected when frying or grilling boar pork or bacon.[232] It is not, perhaps, an unreasonable attitude to adopt in the absence of any knowledge about the precise origin of the odor.

However, the whole basis for assessing the presence and importance of boar taint was changed with the discovery that the source of the odor was the steroid 5α-androst-16-en-3-one, more conveniently referred to as androstenone.[233] This steroid accumulates in the fat of boars of about 3 months of age and older, but is absent from the fat of comparable gilts and barrows. Androstenone can be estimated by chromatography or by human testers trained to recognize its odor in heated boar fat. The term boar taint is implicitly pejorative, and where applicable, androstenone odor would seem to be a better term. Shortly after the discovery regarding androstenone, it was found that a human sex difference exists in the ability to detect its smell; 44.3% of men tested were unable to detect the odor, but only 7.6% of women.[234] The latter also found the odor significantly more unpleasant that did the former. This finding is of importance both for the meat industry and for the design of experiments based on taste panel assessment of pig meat. Future testing programs on boar meat should request the opinion of those consumers most likely to be involved in the preparation and cooking of pork and bacon.[234]

Subsequent to the initial work on androstenone, which was carried out in Great Britain at the Agricultural Research Council's Meat Research Institute, Langford, Bristol, more research on the subject has been carried out at this Institute and elsewhere. A dialog has been conducted with the meat trade in Great Britain in an attempt to influence it to accept boar carcasses without any financial penalty vis-a-vis barrow or gilt carcasses. Two reviews on boar taint appeared shortly after the work on androstenone.[10,235] Many of the studies reviewed were carried out prior to the attribution of taint to androstenone. Nevertheless, it is of interest to summarize some of the conclusions in these reviews in order to ascertain how they compare with the most recent work. Both reviews indicate considerable variation in the literature as to the presence of taint in boar meat. This is not surprising considering the fact that confusion existed as to the precise nature of the taint. Some workers were probably evaluating a broad spectrum of pig odors rather than the specific odor attributable to androstenone. The age and the breed type of the pig also varied among studies. Some studies found odors of varying degree but others did not.

American work suggested that the meat of about 30% of the boars killed at 90 kg live weight or above had a medium or strong taint.[235] Work carried out in Denmark indicated that the androgen-stimulated increased meatiness of boars, compared with barrows, is not necessarily accompanied by taint. This conclusion was based on a very low correlation (0.05) between odor score and loin eye area.[235] Both reviews indicated that the factors affecting the incidence and intensity of taint were not clearly identified, and there was no evidence on the relative importance of those factors that seemed to be operating. Two questions were posed: (1) Are androstenone level and odor intensity inherited: and (2) do nutrition and environment interact with androstenone level[235] Also, attention was drawn to the necessity for carrying out work on the effects of breed, weight, maturity, and nutrition. One reviewer[10] considered the stage of maturity to be an important factor, while another[235] believed that the available evidence did not indicate, with any certainty, the existence of a relationship between taint and age at puberty.

Since these reviews were published, some additional evidence has been reported. In an interesting study, androstenone and other abnormal odors, e.g., skatole odor, were scored separately (the only study at the time of this writing to have done this).[242] The study involved 945 boar, barrow, and gilt carcasses evaluated by two trained panels. The tests were carried out over a period of 10 to 12 weeks and involved carcasses at three factories. The results are particularly instructive in two ways. In the first place, while boars rated significantly higher than barrows and gilts for androstenone odor, as would be expected, there was no significant difference for abnormal (nonandrostenone) odor, except at one factory, where boars scored significantly higher (more abnormal odor) than gilts. Secondly, there were highly significant differences between judges in about one half of the weekly test periods, and the mean score of one panel was higher than that of the other panel, although panel and factory were confounded. Nevertheless, this illustrated the need for caution in interpreting results obtained by different panels. The sex × time (morning and evening) and the sex × time × judges interactions were not significant, but the sex × judges interaction was often significant.

One would expect the incidence and/or level of taint to increase as age and weight increased. In general, this is illustrated by experimental results, although in one report, no significant differences were found between boars slaughtered at 55, 70, 85, or 100 kg.[236,244-247,249] Also, when a correlation exists it can be low, as evidenced by a value of 0.2 for weight and taint of boars killed at 54 to 77 kg.[236] Age and weight have been almost invariably confounded in experiments, with notable exceptions in two studies.[243,246] In the first of these reports, Large White boars were killed at various live weights, and fat samples were scored by a trained panel extremely sensitive to taint.[246] The proportion of boars whose fat was free of taint was 76% at 43 kg, 58% at 55 kg 58% at 78 kg, 48% at 92 kg, and 41% at 118 kg ($p<0.05$). Intensity of taint tended to increase with increasing slaughter weight. There was some variation in age at slaughter within each of the slaughter-age groups, but multiple regression analysis indicated that, apart from the 118-kg group, there was no significant relationship between age at slaughter within weight groups and the incidence of taint, although histograms indicated a trend in three of the groups. For the heaviest group, the age varied from 185 to 365 days, and the incidence of taint increased with age.

In the second study, a trained panel was used to evaluate androstenone and other abnormal odors in Large White, Landrace, and Large White × Landrace carcasses weighing 56.7 to 72.6 kg from 96 boars, 96 barrows, and 96 gilts.[243] Although the usual differences were found between boars and the other two classes of pig, the most interesting feature of this report relates to the examination of breed and growth-rate differences as they affect odor. For boars killed at the same age, faster growing animals had significantly more androstenone odor than slower growing boars and boars killed at lower weights. There was a similar growth effect for nonandrostenone odor.

Although there is some conflict between the two sets of results with regards to the relationship between growth rate and taint, they are not totally incompatible bearing in mind that there was a significant relationship in one of the groups and a nonsignificant one in the others.[246] It is not unreasonable to conclude that the incidence and, probably, the severity of taint increase within certain slaughter-age limits; when conditions are such that weight-age correlations are very high, a similar relationship with age will apply. However, within the range 50 to 100 kg, taint probably does not greatly increase as weight increases.[236] Because of differences in the way in which taint has been assessed, estimates of its incidence vary greatly between experiments. For instance, in an experiment with Large Whites in France, only 9.5% of the boars killed at 80 kg exhibited taint, compared with 42% in another experiment.[246,247] In the French experiment, the incidence increased to 13.6% at 100 kg.

There is, as yet, little evidence on breed or nutrition effects. In an experiment which involved Large Whites and Landraces, no significant breed difference was found for the level of taint in fat; however, there is unpublished evidence that Large Whites have lower androstenone levels than Landraces.[237,243] The incidence of taint was not found to be related significantly to the level of feeding, although there was a tendency for strength of taint to increase as intensity of feeding decreased from high through medium to low.[246]

Heritability of taint, based on the results of odor tests on 1907 Danish Landrace boars culled from service stations, was 0.13 ± 0.08.[248] A larger value, 0.54 ± 0.32, was obtained from data on 72 paternal half-sib families from 30 state breeding centers. Both values have large standard errors ($0.05< p <0.10$); therefore, more precise estimates are required.

The present position may be summarized as follows:

1. The cause of taint (androstenone) is known, and it seems that other unpleasant odors in meat are as often associated with barrows or gilts as with boars, although experimental corroboration of this is desirable.
2. The incidence and degree of taint increase as slaughter weight increases; although the correlation between the two traits can be small, the interrelated effects of age, weight, and degree of maturity on taint have not been clearly separated.
3. Evidence on breed and nutrition effects is sparse, but neither effect seems to be of major importance.
4. There is some additive genetic variance for the breeder to manipulate, but whether or not selection against taint is necessary or would be cost-effective is arguable in light of the latest studies on consumer acceptance of boar meat. It is also not yet known whether there are any sizeable genetic correlations between taint and traits of major economic importance.

Consumer Reactions to Meat and Meat Products from Boars

In recent years, several studies have been carried out in Great Britain on consumer reaction to boar meat and meat products compared with meat or meat products from barrows and/or gilts.[236,238-241]

In one study, pork joints from boars and gilts killed at 24 weeks of age were distributed to 1560 consumers in 419 households.[239] Odor during roasting of the meat was judged by the cook and family members. Judgements showed no overall significant differences between the acceptability of boar and gilt meat. Two consumer panels were involved, the first chosen by taking every 65th entry in an electoral register, and the second comprising households which had returned adverse comments on the odor of boar bacon in an earlier test. The results given by the two types of panels were in close agreement.

In a marketing trial, pork carcasses from ten Large White boars raised to 54 to 77 kg were supplied weekly to a shop in sufficiently quantity to supply the total amount of pork sold there.[236] The customers were not told that boar pork was being sold, nor that any test was being carried out. For the first 4 weeks of the test, only gilt or barrow pork was sold from the shop, followed by boar pork for the next 10 weeks. Boar, gilt, and barrow carcasses were assessed for taint by a trained panel by heating fat slivers on a soldering iron. Boar taint was not recorded in any of the gilt or barrow carcasses, 76 boar carcasses showed weak taint, 14 emitted zero or negligible taint, and 10 showed taint a little below the medium level. No complaints about the boar pork were received from customers, and in follow-up interviews with 41 customers, no adverse reactions to it were recorded. Of the 41 customers interviewed, 22 preferred pork sold during the "boar period" to that sold prior to it, 18 made no distinction, and 1 person found it inferior. A number of criticisms of the design of this test might be raised, and indeed the authors of the report do this themselves, but one must agree with their assessment that the results indicate a high level of customer satisfaction with boar pork. It seems clear that, although sensitive, trained testers are able to detect low or moderate levels of androstenone in the fat of boars of pork weight, such levels have not aroused any antagonism in consumer populations thus far sampled.

Three other trials investigated the acceptability of products derived from boar meat.[238,240,241] In one of these, sausages prepared from the meat of boars killed at 100 kg live weight and a control product prepared from barrow or gilt meat were submitted to consumer panels comprised of 47 cooks and 156 family members.[240] There was no evidence that the sausages made from boar meat were less acceptable than the control sausages. The two types of sausage were also tested by a trained panel. Seven of its eight members were unable to detect an androstenone odor in the boar sausages and one member recorded a weak odor. The judgements of the trained panel were made more difficult because of the spices in the sausage (which are absent in pork fat).

In another study, unsmoked, Wiltshire-cured bacon from 109-kg boar carcasses and 90.9-kg gilt carcasses was distributed to 387 persons in 125 households.[238] The carcasses were mainly from Large Whites and Landraces. Based on heated backfat tests by a trained panel, the boar carcasses with the most intense androstenone odor were selected for processing, and the gilt carcasses were selected for their freedom from any foreign odor. There was a correlation of 0.83 ($p < 0.01$) between the trained panel results and the androstenone level in the kidney fat determined by chromatography; the correlation would probably have been higher if the same fat sample had been used for both tests. Less than 1% of the consumers differentiated unambiguously against boar bacon while accepting that from gilts. About 90% of the consumers regarded boar bacon as perfectly normal, and most of the other 10% were dissatisfied with both boar and gilt bacon. It is worth stressing that the experiment was set up so as to maximize the odor difference between boar and gilt bacon; this should be kept in mind when the results are interpreted. It was suggested that carcasses with androstenone content above 1μg/g of fat should not be processed into bacon, although chemical assessment is too complicated for a factory floor test; a rapid subjective test would be required.

A study to assess consumer reaction to boar bacon was set up jointly by the Pigs Marketing Board of Northern Ireland and the Ulster Curer's Association. This development reflected the interest of the meat trade in determining whether or not boar meat should be accepted as a normal part of the pig meat trade.[241] Bacon was distributed to 524 households, boar bacon first, then barrow bacon. The boars to be processed were selected by a trained panel using the heated fat test; there were 13 boars rated as having a slight taint, 13 medium, and 13 strong. Carcass weight of boars was

61.4 to 73.2 kg, and that of barrows was 63.6 to 70.5 kg. The sides were cured by the usual Wiltshire process. Consumers rated the bacon on a seven-point scale for each of six quality traits, including aroma. Results are presented in the form of boar-barrow comparisons, and a least squares analysis was made of factors likely to affect scores; many correlations and regressions for pairs of traits were also calculated. The overall conclusion from the study was that no marked preference for either boar or castrate bacon was shown by cooks, purchasers, or eaters, although for most traits boar bacon scored slightly better. About 13% (69 persons) marked boar bacon as having a "much stronger" or a "very much stronger" aroma than their usual bacon, but 12% marked barrow bacon in the same categories. Of the 69, 55 found the strong aroma "much more appetizing" or "very much more appetizing" than usual, and only 3 marked it less appetizing. The final recommendation of the report was that producers should cease to castrate and that boar bacon should be sold under the same label as barrow bacon, without any distinction between the two being noted.

These tests indicate that, for sizeable consumer populations in three widely separated areas of Great Britain, boar products can be marketed without adverse consumer reaction. The overall conclusions in regard to pigs is that the use of boars rather than barrows offers substantial advantages in terms of a greater production of lean meat for the same input costs. Evidence is accumulating which indicates that boar meat and products derived from it are acceptable to consumers. The way is open for the financial benefits accruing from greater production efficiency to be shared between producer and consumer.

CONCLUSION

As this review indicates, there is a large body of data on the effects of castration. However, a number of areas require more investigation. The first involves the interactions between castration and other factors, especially breed and nutrition. In general, the most productive genotypes seem to benefit most from the avoidance of castration. More information is needed on feeding and management regimes that permit optimum exploitation of the greater growth potential and lean meat production of entire animals. Secondly, an economic evaluation must also take place. In the final analysis, everything in a farming operation is reduced to economic terms, taking into consideration both short- and long-term objectives. Efficiency of production must take into account not only growth, feed efficiency, and the carcass, but also the cost of castration and any mortality attributable to it. In a national context, one must also consider how many superior breeding males are lost through castration and what loss of genetic gain this entails, the loss being translated into financial terms.

Experimenters have chosen to work in terms of carcass composition and measurements rather than, for example, total protein in the carcass (see discussion to reference 4), which could be regarded as a more objective end point, particularly in evaluating feed efficiency. However, because the consumer buys kilograms or pounds of meat and not protein, the traditional carcass traits used by experimenters are arguably more realistic. The gross effects of castration are now fairly well quantified, although more work on the aspects mentioned immediately above is still needed. In this more critical work, there may well be an advantage in using total protein production as the end point.

NOTE ADDED IN PROOF STAGE

Since preparation of the manuscript, a certain amount of additional material on the effects of castration has been published. Most of this material adds nothing new to the results and conclusions of the work published earlier. Some studies, however, merit specific mention, as they throw additional light on areas requiring more investigation, or, in one instance, deal with a new facet of the subject. In the latter case, an analysis of data on 3822 calves in 11 herds in Victoria, Australia, suggested that the superiority of bulls over steers for preweaning growth rate was due, at least partly, to the early castration of poorly growing male calves.[250] Such a selection bias is likely to occur in studies not set up as controlled experimental comparisons, with sex treatments being allocated at random to the experimental animals.

Two consumer studies on bull vs. steer beef gave somewhat conflicting results. The first, which involved a trained taste panel, found no significant difference in palatability of semimembranosus muscle between bulls and steers, although bull meat was significantly tougher by the Warner-Bratzler shear test.[251] In the other study, 166 households made 603 judgements on the eating quality of bull and steer beef.[252] In 236 comparisons, bull beef was considered tougher than steer beef, in 184 it was considered more tender, and in 183 no difference was detected.

Two reports in pigs have provided information on the interaction of nutritional factors with castration. In the first of these, which comprised two experiments with Dutch Landraces, 40 boars and 40 barrows in experiment 1 and 110 boars, 110 barrows and 132 gilts in experiment 2 were either fed *ad lib.* or on a restricted ration.[253] On *ad lib.* feeding, barrows had higher feed consumption than boars by 18.6 and 15.7% in the two experiments, and a higher rate of weight gain by 5.5 and 9.9%. On restricted feeding, however, boars had a higher rate of gain than barrows by 4.2 and 2.6%. On both feeding regimes, feed conversion efficiency was better in boars by 6.2 to 13.8%. Boars had significantly less fat and more lean in the carcass than barrows and meat quality was not significantly affected by castration.

In the other report, which covered a factorial experiment with 192 British Landraces, boars, barrows, and gilts were fed diets containing 20 or 23.5% crude protein and 1.00, 1.34, or 1.68% lysine, at four levels of maximum daily feed intake.[254] Boars had significantly higher average daily gain and feed conversion efficiency than barrows and gilts. In the case of boars and gilts, average daily gain was best at a maximum daily feed intake of 2.66 kg, whereas for barrows, it continued to increase for intakes up to 2.99 kg. There was a significant feed intake × sex interaction for backfat thickness. Increasing the maximum daily feed intake did not significantly affect backfat thickness in boars, but increased it in barrows and gilts. The average daily muscle weight gain of boars was higher on the ration with 20% protein than on that with 23.5%, whereas it was similar on the two levels in gilts (for this trait, no data were given for barrows). The addition of extra lysine to the rations of boars and barrows worsened their growth rate and feed conversion efficiency.

The results of these studies suggest that the boar performs best, vis-a-vis the barrow, when feed intake is kept below the maximum the animals will consume, and support the conclusions of previous studies to the effect that boars should not be fed higher protein levels than barrows.

As a postscript to the studies on consumer reaction to boar bacon in Northern Ireland, it appears that processors are still somewhat reluctant to handle meat from boars, although there have been no complaints about taint.[255] The processors complain of thin, soft backfat, and bellies unsuitable for slicing. In addition, the extra trimming loss with boars (about 1 kg, including testes) is unpopular. Several of the major supermarket chain stores have shown no interest in purchasing boar bacon.

Table 1
SHEEP EXPERIMENTS ON THE EFFECTS OF CASTRATION

Experimental groups	Number of animals	Body weight or growth rate (kg)[a]		Food utilization efficiency	Carcass and/or meat characters	Ref.
		Final weight				
Hampshire wethers	17	35.0 (20 weeks)				12
Hampshire rams	14	36.7 (20 weeks)				12
Shropshire wethers	13	46.1 (52 weeks)				12
Shropshire rams	20	46.5 (52 weeks)				12
		21-month weight				
Castrates	22	47.1[a]				13
Castrates	19	46.8[a]				13
Rams	19	57.3[b]				13
		Final weight (11 months)				
Ausimi wethers	7	37.6				14
Ausimi rams	34	40.6				14
Rahmani wethers	5	35.8				14
Rahmani rams	10	37.4				14
		Live weight (8—10 weeks)				
Rams	31	26.7[a]				15, 55
Wethers (castrated at 2 weeks)	33	25.7[b]				15, 55
Tsigai breed		Final weight				
Castrated surgically	6	31.2				16
Uncastrated	6	31.7				16
		7 month weight				
Castrated surgically at 4 months	10	45.7				17
Uncastrated	10	45.6				17
		Weaning weight	17-month weight			
Poll wethers	35	21.6	47.7			
	29	23.2	45.9			18
Horned wethers	41	21.6	48.0			
	24	23.1	46.4			18
Poll Rams	34	23.8	62.8			
	29	24.4	55.9			
Horned rams	38	23.5	62.7			
	29	25.6	56.9			18
		Rams vs. wethers $P < 0.005$ at both ages				

Growth data on 251 lambs at weaning and 144 yearlings		Average daily gain (ADG) to weaning: rams > wethers by 0.014 kg($P<0.01$)	Rib eye area of yearlings adjusted for carcass weight rams 16.9 and 17.1 cm^2 vs. 14.6 and 16.6 cm^2 in wethers ($P<0.01$)				19
			Adjusted fat thickness in yearlings: 9.9 and 8.5 mm in rams vs. 15.9 and 11.0 mm in wethers ($P<0.01$)				
Carcass data on 64 lambs and 77 yearlings		ADG to 450 days: rams > wethers by 0.023 and 0.041 kg ($P<0.05$)	Eating quality up to 7 months: no significant difference (NSD) between rams and wethers				19
Crossbreds		Average weekly gain (3—4 months to 10—11 months)		% neck			
Rams	6	0.75[a]		6.23			20
Wethers (castrated at 1 month)	6	0.62[b]		4.94			20
Dohne Merinos		ADG to 32 kg		Fat thickness (mm)			
Castrated by 7 days of age	30	0.17		2.74			21
Castrated at about 18 kg	31	0.17		2.34			21
Uncastrated	32	0.18		1.99			21
Age at slaughter (weeks) castrated at 4 weeks		Final live weight		Adjusted carcass weight[b]		Rib-eye area (adjusted) (cm^2)	
8	5	16.7		7.0			22, 22(a)
12	5	19.7		8.9			22, 22(a)
16	5	26.9		12.4		15.1	22, 22(a)
28	5	29.4		14.0		15.5	22, 22(a)
Rams							
8	5	17.5		7.6			22, 22(a)
12	5	20.1		9.2			22, 22(a)
16	5	28.7		14.5		12.3	22, 22(a)
28	5	32.7		16.9		14.7	22, 22(a)
Experiment also included groups of ♀♀ and spayed ♀♀		Statistical analysis did not separate effects of castration and spaying					
Four-breed types		Slaughter Weight		Retail trimmed meat (kg)	Fat trim (kg)	Shear value in kg/cm^2	
Rams	203	43.2	Rams[c]	15.5	2.1	2.05	23
Wethers	186	45.4	Wethers[c]	10.9	2.7	1.74	23
Merinos and crossbreds							
Rams	20		NSD in muscle, fat, or bone components of joints between rams and wethers; data corrected for side weight and age				24
Wethers (Slaughtered at 13.5, 19.0, 24.5, 30.0, or 35.5 kg)	20						24
				Shear value of chop meat ($P<0.05$)	Cooking loss% ($P<0.05$)		
Wether carcasses	90	39.2	Wether	4.06	26.3		25
Ram lamb carcasses	112	42.2[a]	Ram	4.74	24.9		25

Table 1 (Continued)
SHEEP EXPERIMENTS ON THE EFFECTS OF CASTRATION

Experimental groups	Number of animals	Body weight or growth rate (kg)[a]		Food utilization efficiency		Carcass and/or meat characters			Ref.
Ram, wether, and ewe carcasses for study of meat quality (Ages at slaughter 119—304 days)	259								25
Wethers and rams; wool examined annually over 6 years	5					Percentage of paracortex, fiber, and crimp frequency: NSD between rams and wethers			26
Southdown × western lambs	40	Age at slaughter (days)							
Castrated bilaterally		192 (a)							27
Castrated unilaterally		170 and 173							27
Left entire (Slaughter at 37—38 kg)		172 (b)							27
East Friesian × native and Chios × native lambs: 3 groups castrated and 1 entire	35	NSD in growth from 2 to 4 months							28
Polish Merino and Blackheaded rams and wethers (killed at 150 days)	48					NSD between rams and wethers for muscle dry matter, crude protein, and fat %			29
Merino lambs (castration at 3 weeks)	56	ADG to weaning		kg feed/kg gain		Character	Rams	Wethers	
		Rams	0.22	Rams	2.9[a]	Eye-muscle width (cm)	5.01	4.93	30
		Wethers	0.21	Wethers	4.2[b]	Eye-muscle depth (cm)	2.29	2.60	
		ADG, weaning to slaughter at 36 kg							
		Rams	0.20				0.38		
		Wethers	0.15			Backfat (cm)		0.49	
Restricted feed	32	ADG		Mcal metabolizable energy per kg gain					31
Ram lambs		0.336 (a)		13.66(a)		47.38(a)% rib-cut lean; 33.63(a), % fat			
Wether lambs		0.295 (b)		15.27(b)		38.61(b), % rib-cut lean; 43.06(b), % fat			
Unrestricted feeds									
Ram lambs		0.336		13.29					
Wether lambs		0.340		13.16					
Polish Merinos									
Slaughtered at 100 days	66	ADG				NSD for meat composition and organoleptic traits			32
Rams		0.236(a)							
Wethers		0.215(b)							
Slaughtered at 181 days									
Rams		0.194(a)							
Wethers		0.192(b)							
German Mutton Merinos	40								
Fattened to 35 kg									33
Rams		0.197(a)							
Wethers		0.220(b)							

Fattened to 40 kg						
Rams		0.212(a)				
Wethers		0.221(b)				
Fattened to 45 kg						
Rams		0.193(a)				
Wethers		0.164(b)				
Fattened to 50 kg						
Rams		0.210(a)				
Wethers		0.194(b)				
Hampshire × crossbred lambs	60	Live weight at slaughter				34
Rams		45				
Wethers		45.2				
(self-fed and slaughtered at 36, 45, or 54 kg)		Carcass weight per day of age				
		0.168				
		0.160				
Hampshire × blackface lambs (slaughtered at 36, 45, or 54 kg)	30 rams 30 wethers		NSD overall between rams and wethers in muscle fiber or fat cell diameter			35
Sudan Desert Sheep	30	Slaughter weight		Longissimo dorsi (l.d.) (cm^2)	Percentage of meat	36
Rams		38.11		8.6	76.9	
Wethers		37.76		8.3	78.7	
(slaughtered at 14 months, after a 2-month feeding trial)						
Crossbreds castrated at:	59	ADG				37
10 days		0.277 (a)				
18 kg		0.267 (b)				
Left entire		0.327 (b)				
Crossbreds castrated at	31					37
10 days		0.228 (a)				
Left entire		0.272 (b)				
Hampshire × blackface lambs (slaughtered at 36, 45, or 54 kg)	60			Fatty Acids in Fat (%)		38
			Perinephric	Rams	Wethers	
			C18	26.85 (a)	29.07 (b)	
			C18:2	8.84 (a)	7.27 (b)	
			C18:3	2.87	2.47	
			Subcutaneous			
			C16	23.18 (a)	24.34 (b)	
			C18	16.22 (a)	17.92 (b)	
			C18:1	42.71 (a)	41.37 (b)	
			C18:2	9.17 (a)	7.94 (b)	

Table 1 (Continued)
SHEEP EXPERIMENTS ON THE EFFECTS OF CASTRATION

Experimental groups	Number of animals	Body weight or growth rate (kg)[a]		Food utilization efficiency	Carcass and/or meat characters				Ref.
Hampshire lambs	43	Wt/day of age		Live weight gain (g)/ Mcal digestible energy	Fat thickness (cm)	Cutability percentage			39
Entire		0.308 (a)		56.7	0.61 (a)	67.2 (a)			
Made cryptorchid		0.289 (b)		51.5	0.62 (a)	66.3 (a)			
Castrated at 35 days		0.265 (b)		43.9	0.94 (b)	62.8 (b)			
(Slaughtered at approximately 46—49 kg)					NSD in organoleptic traits, marbling, lean texture, color, and firmness				
German Blackheaded									
Mutton sheep	65	ADG			Carcass length (cm)				40
Rams		0.275			70.55 (a)				
Wethers		0.275			69.25 (b)				
(Fattened to 40 kg wethers Castrated at 1 week)									
Suffolk, Cheviot, and crossbred sheep	57	ADG (g)[c]		kcal/kg gain[c]	Protein % of carcass[c]	Shear values[c]			41
Castrated by four methods at various ages		−14 to +20		−2.10 to +8.68	−2.4 to +10.4	−1.15			
Entire (part of larger experiment)		+20		−4.59	7.4	−0.69 to +1.62			
		Treatment effects significant)		(Treatment effects significant)	(Treatment effects significant)				
Vasectomized	43	Weight gain							42
Castrated		9.2 (a)							
Entire males		7.7 (b)							
(fattened for 179 days)		9.3 (a)							
Sheep of 7 genetic groups	441 (At weaning) 400 (At slaughter)	Weight per day of age							43
		At weaning	At approximately 44 kg						
Rams		0.28 (a)	0.279 (a)						
Rams implanted with stilbestrol		0.27 (a)	0.278 (a)						
Short-scrotum males		0.27 (a)	0.279 (a)						
Wethers castrated at birth		0.25 (a)	0.252 (b)						
Rambouillet type range feeder lambs	54	Final Weight			Retail meat (%)	Fat thickness (cm)	Loin eye (cm^2)	Shear value (kg/cm^2)	44
Ram		34.3 (a)			74.7 (a)	0.73 (a)	10.71	3.35	
Wether					71.6 (b)		10.97		
(Fed for 30, 60, or 90 days from 150, 180, or 210 days of age)		32.0 (b)				1.03 (b)		2.93	

Hampshire-sired lambs Castrated at 1 week Left entire (Slaughtered at 45 kg)	20		Specific fatty acids in back and subcutaneous fat (%) C14:0 — C18:2 7.5 (a) — 9.9 (a) 4.5 (b) — 7.9 (b)	45
Light wethers (50 kg at slaughter) Heavy wethers (65 kg) Heavy rams (68 kg)	140	ADG 0.23 (a)[f] 0.26 (b)[f] 0.30 (c)[f]	l. d. (cm^2) — Fat (cm) — Primal cuts (%) — Taste panel (overall) 13.05 (a) — 0.83 (a) — 58.48 (a) — 5.60 14.24 (b) — 1.09 (b) — 54.25 (b) — 5.80 14.95 (c) — 0.72 (c) — 55.67 (c) — 5.59 Some significant differences in the fatty acid composition of fat	46
Hampshire-sired wethers and rams (slaughtered at 36, 45, and 54 kg)	60		Superiority of meat traits at 36, 45, or 54 kg Flavor 0—4 Tenderness 5.3—22.5 Overall satisfaction 1.3—11.8 Shear value 43—45 Wethers better than rams ($P < 0.05$ and 0.01) Wethers > rams (fat trim %) by 3.1—13.3 % depending on slaughter weight ($P < 0.01$)	47
Tsigai wethers and rams (slaughtered at 153 or 174 days)	40		NSD for carcass and meat characters	48
Rambouillet crossbreds Rams Wethers (Slaughtered at 36—64 kg)	102	ADG — Food conversion ratio 0.292 (a) — 5.8 0.235 (b) — 6.4	Boneless cuts (%) — Fat trim (kg) 44.68 (a) — 5.05 (a) 43.36 (b) — 6.49 (b) Shear value (kg) — l. d. area (cm^2) 4.91 — 14.49 (a) 5.02 — 13.57 (b)	49
Ausimi and Rahmani males (half castrated at birth)	40	Preslaughtered weight NSD		50
Rambouillet, Suffolk, or S × R lambs Entire Cryptorchid Castrated (Slaughtered at approximately 45 kg)	101	Weaning weight 26.2 26.8 26.6 Feedlot ADG 0.32 0.32 0.28	Carcass weight 22.3 22.4 22.3 NSD in fatty acid composition of fat	51
Market lambs of five breeds and three crosses	209		NSD in organoleptic traits	52
Fat-tailed males Half left entire Half castrated at 4 weeks	38	ADG during fattening 0.209 (a) 0.169 (b)	Forequarter weight — Saddle weight — l.d.(cm^2) 11.5 (a) — 3.9 (a) — 17.0 (a) 9.9 (b) — 31.1 (b) — 15.0 (b)	53

Table 1 (Continued)
SHEEP EXPERIMENTS ON THE EFFECTS OF CASTRATION

Experimental groups	Number of animals	Body weight or growth rate (kg)[a]	Food utilization efficiency	Carcass and/or meat characters						Ref.
(all slaughtered at 29 weeks after fattening)										
2 × 3 factorial experiment	30	Weight gain over last 84 days of trial		Fat measurement points			Energy storage (Mcal)			54
				C	Z	J	Fat	Fat-free	l.d.(cm^2)	
Entire males		13.54 (a)		3.7(a)	8.8(a)	16.4(a)	43.19(a)	6.40(a)	11.35(a)	
Castrated males on 3 diets for 92 days; (slaughtered at approximately 42 kg)		11.15 (b)		5.6(b)	13.5(b)	20.2(b)	56.32(b)	2.33(b)	10.35(b)	
Hampshire, Suffolk, and Hampshire × Suffolk rams killed at				L. S.[c] means						
				Flavor*	Tenderness*	Aroma	Shear value			55
183 days				5.8 (a)	6.8 (a)	6.4 (a)	6.4 (a)			
237 days				5.3 (b)	5.7 (b)	5.3 (b)	8.0 (b)			
295 days				5.6 (ab)	5.3 (b)	6.1 (a)	8.2 (b)			
Whiteface wethers killed at 300 days				6.4 (c)	6.9 (a)	4.4 (c)	7.2 (ab)			
				(1 = no aroma)						
				*high = best						

[a] Where means for a given trait have alphabetically different letters within parenthesis, they are different at the 5% or higher level of significance.
[b] Adjusted for initial weight.
[c] Least squares (means).

Table 2
CATTLE EXPERIMENTS ON THE EFFECTS OF CASTRATION

Experimental groups	Number of animals	Body weight or growth rate (kg)[a]	Food utilization efficiency	Carcass and/or meat characters			Ref.
Herefords		Average daily gain (ADG) (over 210-252 days) on feed		Significant differences for steer values minus bull values			65
Bulls	10	1.06 (a)		hindquarter (%) 1.9—2.3			65
Steers (castrated at 1 month)	10	0.91 (b)		kidney knob (%) 0.47—1.07			65
Steers (castrated at weaning)	10	0.91 (b)					
Bulls	12	1.10 (a)		Tenderness score in second group bulls < steers (significant)			65
Steers (castrated at 1 month)	12	0.89 (b)					65
Steers (castrated at weaning)	12	0.87 (b)					65
Herefords	252—day feeding test	ADG (to 13-15 months)		Hindquarter (%)		Edible (%)	
Bulls	10	1.0 (a)		46.2		77.7	66
Steers	10	0.91 (b)		47.8		73.7	66
Steers	10	0.91 (b)		48.5		74.1	66
	210—247 days on test						
Bulls	12	1.1 (a)		46.6		77.5	66
Steers	12	0.89 (b)		48.5		74.1	66
Steers	12	0.88 (b)		48.5		74.4	66
	8—196 days on test						
Bulls	20	1.1 (a)		47.2		77.5	66
Steers	8	0.94 (b)		49.0		73.2	66
Steers	5	0.84 (b)		49.0		73.9	66
				Tenderness (highest = best)	Intramuscular fat (%)	Hydroproline (%) (Measure of connective tissue)	
			Bull	7.25 ± 0.11	2.38 ± 0.11	0.046 ± 0.0019	
			Steer	7.78 ± 0.08	5.24 ± 0.30	0.046 ± 0.0013	
		ADG (over 411 days)	Starch unit per kg gain				
Bulls	3	1.14 (a)	3.73				67
Steers (castrated at 36 days)	4	0.88 (b)	4.71				67
Steers (castrated at 437 days)	4	0.95 (b)	4.36				67

Table 2 (Continued)
CATTLE EXPERIMENTS ON THE EFFECTS OF CASTRATION

Experimental groups	Number of animals	Body weight or growth rate (kg)[a]	Food utilization efficiency	Carcass and/or meat characters	Ref.
Czech Pieds		ADG: Pasture (91 days)	ADG: Fattening period (142 days)		
Bulls	26	0.51 (a)	0.94 (a)	No significant difference (NSD) in meat composition	68
Steers (castrated at start of fattening	20	0.66 (b)	0.81 (b)		68
Steers (castrated during fattening)	26	0.49 (c)	0.71 (c)		68
Swedish (Red-and-White)				Subcutaneous fat (%); I/M fat (%)	
Bulls	10(MZ twins)			3.21 (a); 1.45 (a)	69
Steers (castrated at 1, 6, or 12 months)	10(MZ twins)			4.70 (b); 2.87 (b)	
69				Mesenteric fat (%); Perinephric fat (%)	
				1.21 (a); 2.19 (a)	
				1.56 (b); 3.48 (b)	
		ADG (1) (2) (3) (4)	Food unit per kg gain (1) (3)		
Bulls	47	0.82 0.35 0.94	3.16 5.42		70
Steers (castrated at 5½ months)	40	0.81 0.37 0.60 0.43	3.27 6.34		
		(1) = first winter (2) = first summer (3) = second winter (4) = second summer			
Swedish Red-and-White		Final live weight (25 months)	Food unit per kg of gain		
Bulls	12 (MZ twins)	483	5.5		71
Steers	12 (MZ twins)	451	5.9		71
Criollos		ADG (over 65 days)	kg of TDN[b] per kg of gain		
Bulls	16	1.12 (from 231 kg)	4.64		72
Steers (castrated at 230 kg)	10	1.18 (from 304 kg)	4.38		72
Holsteins		ADG (34—200 kg)			
Bulls	10	0.70			72
Steers (castrated at 15-105 days)	9	0.67			72
Yugoslavian Simmentals		ADG (to about 400 kg)	Food unit per kg of gain		
Bulls	30	1.09 (a)	8.03		73
Steers	30	0.97 (b)	907		73

		ADG (during fattening)		Oat units per kg of gain	Fat in meat (%)		Protein in meat (%)	
Bulls	12	1.01 (a)		5.58	14.68 (a)		18.89	74
Steers (fattened 5-15 months)	12	0.87 (b)		6.75	17.80 (b)		18.32	74
Kula breed		ADG (over 85 days of fattening)						
Bulls	46	0.66 (a)						75
Steers	46	0.81 (b)						75
Holstein-Friesians		ADG	kg of TDN[b] per 50 kg of gain		Rib eye (cm²)		Hindquarter (%)	
Bulls (killed at 360 kg)	15	1.07 (a)	381	173	58.4 (a)		48.4 (a)	76
Steers (killed at 360 kg)	15	0.96 (b)	411	186	51.2 (b)		49.3 (b)	76
Bulls (killed at 450 kg)	15	1.05 (a)	431	196	63.4 (a)		47.1 (a)	76
Steers (killed at 450 kg)	15	0.99 (b)	473	215	59.0 (b)		49.0 (b)	76
					Meat (%)			
					Lean	Fat	Bone	
					64.0	18.0	18.0	
					60.1	21.2	17.9	
					63.0	18.8	18.1	
					60.0	23.9	16.1	
Friesian or Friesian × Hereford		ADG (to 55 weeks)			Fat cover (mm)	Muscle (%)	Fat (%)	
Bulls	6	1.04			5.8 (a)	64.2 (a)	16.8 (a)	20
Steers (castrated at 7 months)	5	0.91			19.6 (b)	61.8 (b)	29.2 (b)	20
Black Pied Lowland		Final weight			Carcass bone (%)			
Bulls	8	261			21.13 (a)			77
Steers (castrated at 4 wk)	9	255			19.88 (b)			77
Least squares analysis of 7971 records of Angus, Hereford, and Shorthorn cattle		ADG (birth to weaning) Least squares constants bull 0.108; steer 0.000						78
Butana zebus		Final weight			Meat and fat in cuts (%)			
Bulls	9	195 (at 9 months)			79.9			79
Steers (On feed for 156 days)	9	191 (at 12 months)			79.3			79
Friesians		ADG (to 17 months)	kg of feed per kg of gain		Lean (%)	Fat trim (%)	Rib eye area per 45 kg (cm²)	
Bulls	8	0.69	6.29 (a)		73.2	4.6 (a)	13.43	80
Steers	8	0.62	7.08 (b)		71.7	7.2 (b)	12.14	80
Bulls	8	0.71			74.1	5.4 (a)	13.47	80
Steers	8	0.63			70.8	7.2 (b)	11.76	80
Bulls	10	Final weight	Starch units per kg of gain					
Steers (castrated at 6 month)	10	469 (a)	3562 (a)		In 3-rib cut, lean content of bulls			81

Table 2 (Continued)
CATTLE EXPERIMENTS ON THE EFFECTS OF CASTRATION

Experimental groups	Number of animals	Body weight or growth rate (kg)[a]		Food utilization efficiency	Carcass and/or meat characters			Ref.
(MZ twins fattened for 18 month)		419 (b)		4215 (b)	17.6 % > that of steers ($P < 0.001$); fat content of steers 33.3 % > that of bulls ($P < 0.01$)			81
Bulls	11				Rib steaks evaluated by a tenderometer;			82
Steers (castrated at 10—13 weeks) (killed at 22—23 months)	11				bull meat less tender than steer meat ($P <$ 0-10); NSD in cooking loss			82
Herefords (grade)		14-month weight	ADG (in 7 months)		Rib cut composition over 7-month period (%)			
					Fat	Lean	Bone	
Bulls	19	414 (a)	1.19 (a)		30.8 (a)	51.8 (a)	17.4 (a)	83
Steers (castrated at 3.2 months)	19	407 (b)	1.06 (b)		40.1 (b)	44.1 (b)	15.8 (b)	83
Bulls	9				NSD between LS[b] means for bulls			84
Steers	9				and steers with respect to shear values, tenderness, and flavor.			84
Swedish Red-and-White		ADG (at 19—23 months)			Fat thickness (mm)	Kidney and (%) visceral fat	Hindquarter (%)	
Bulls	24	0.73 (a)			2.05 (a)	2.72 (a)	48.0 (a)	85
Steers	24	0.62 (b)			2.62 (b)	3.70 (b)	49.7 (b)	85
Swedish Friesian								
Bulls	24	0.79 (a)			1.57 (a)	2.09 (a)	49.4 (a)	85
Steers	24	0.68 (b)			2.49 (b)	3.29 (b)	50.5 (b)	85
Yugoslavian Simmentals		ADG	Final weight	Food units per kg gain				
Bulls	9	1.17 (a)	473	7.49				86
Vasectomized males	9	1.18 (a)	483	7.47				86
Steers	9	0.99 (b)	429	8.66				86
Bulls Steers Some animals implanted with stilbestrol	Numbers not stated	ADG on feed (176 days) 1.20		kg of feed per kg of gain 7.7	Difference bulls minus steers in cost of producing 45 kg boneless beef varied in 4 experiments between \$11.51 and \$7.88			87
Bulls	134				Significant differences between bulls			88
Steers + heifers (assumed to be the same tenderness, flavor, etc.)	84				and steers + heifers for following traits of rib roasts: at 500—599 days of age, marbling, shear values, tenderness; at 600—699 days, marbling, shear values, tenderness, flavor, juiciness. All differences in favor of steers + heifers. No significant differences for ages 300—499 days.			88

		ADG (from 12 weeks to slaughter)					
Bulls	12	1.21 (a)					89
Steers	12	1.03 (b) slaughtered at approximately 400 kg					89
Zebu							
Bulls	20	NSD in ADG up to 4 years on range					90
Steers (castrated at 24 weeks)	20						90
Zebu (in Brazil)							
Entirely on pasture		ADG (8—9 months to 18—19 months)		Kidney fat (%)	Fat thickness (mm)	Rib eye area (cm^2)	
Bulls	11	0.49		2.4	1.5	30.0	91
Steers	10	0.41		4.0	3.3	28.8	91
Pasture + postweaning feed supplement (high protein)							
Bulls	11	0.63		2.0	1.5	34.4	91
Steers	10	0.54	Overall castration effect significant	4.8	3.8	28.1	91
Pasture + pre- and postweaning supplements (low protein)							
Bulls	13	0.57		2.2	1.8	33.8	91
Steers	11	0.47		4.0	3.0	30.0	91
Pasture + pre- and postweaning supplements (low protein)							
Bulls	11	0.61		2.2	1.3	35.6	91
Steers	10	0.49		4.4	3.0	29.4	91
				$P < 0.001$	$P < 0.001$	$0.025 < P < 0.05$	
				Significance of effects tested overall			
		ADG preweaning					
Bulls	19	0.75					92
Steers	19	0.72					92
Herefords (on range)							
Bulls	9	0.68					92
Steers	10	0.65					92
Bulls	14	0.83 (a)					92
Steers	10	0.75 (b)					92
Bulls	16	0.65 (a)					92
Steers	11	0.59 (b)					92
Bulls	19	0.74					92
Steers	11	0.74					92
Friesians		ADG (lifetime)	kg of TDN[b] per kg of meat produced				
Indoor rearing (to 13 months)							
Bulls	8	0.92 (a)	7.72 (a)				93
Steers	8	0.84 (b)	9.12				93
Grazing + indoor rearing (to 16 months)							
Bulls	8	0.77					93
Steers	8	0.73					93

Table 2 (Continued)
CATTLE EXPERIMENTS ON THE EFFECTS OF CASTRATION

Experimental groups	Number of animals	Body weight or growth rate (kg)[a]		Food utilization efficiency		Carcass and/or meat characters			Ref.
						Rib cut (standardized carcass weight)			
						Muscle (%)	Fat (%)	Bone (%)	
Friesians		ADG (150—300 kg)							
Bulls	5					61.6 (a)	21.9 (a)	16.5 (a)	94
Steers	6	bulls 1.35				57.8 (b)	28.6 (b)	13.6 (b)	94
Herefords × Friesians									
Bulls	10	steers 1.24				60.5 (a)	22.8 (a)	16.8 (a)	94
Steers	12					55.8 (b)	30.2 (b)	14.0 (b)	94
Sudanese cattle		ADG over 1 year period (160 to 200-250 kg)							
Supplemented for 58 days									
Bulls	9	0.25							95
Steers	9	0.21							95
Not supplemented									
Bulls	9	0.18							95
Steers	9	0.11							95
High-plane feeding		ADG (to about 470 kg)		Starch unit per kg of gain					
Bulls	9	0.89 (a)		4.22					96
Steers	10	0.83 (b)		4.76					96
Moderate feeding									
Bulls	10	0.82		4.22					96
Steers	9	0.80		4.36					96
MZ Swedish Red-and-White twins	28	ADG		kg of feed per kg of gain		Muscle (%)			97
castrated at		Bulls	Steers	Bulls	Steers	Bulls		Steers	
1 month		0.607 (a)	0.549 (b)	5.51	6.01	69.4 (a)		63.9 (b)	
6 months		0.644 (a)	0.590 (b)	5.38	5.85	72.0 (a)		64.7 (b)	
12 months		0.647 (a)	0.599 (b)	5.43	5.89	68.1 (a)		63.5 (b)	
Plus entire controls for each castration group (slaughtered at 25 months						Fat (%)			
						Bulls		Steers	
						9.7 (a)		15.4 (b)	
						10.1 (a)		17.1 (b)	
						12.1 (a)		16.9 (b)	
Initial weight (kg)	48			kg of feed per kg of gain (over 18-week period)		Intramuscular fat (%)			98
Friesland 113				Bulls	Steers	Bulls		Steers	
Jersey 159				2.12 (a)	2.32 (b)	1.09 (a)		1.86 (b)	
Brown Swiss 205									

Hereford bulls and steers on 50% or 70% concentrates half the bulls and half the steers implanted with stilbestrol	60			WB shear values / Panel tenderness / Overall palatability Bulls 10.2 / 4.65 / 4.91 Steers 8.8 / 6.14* / 5.80* *High = best	99
Holstein-Friesian calves Some bulls and steers implanted with stilbestrol	40	312-day ADG (nonimplanted animals) Bulls 0.995 Steers 0.841			100
Hereford-type (killed at 448 days) Bulls Steers	39	ADG 1.03 0.96		Rib eye (cm^2) 60.9 (a) 54.2 (b)	101
Jersey (J), Simmental × Jersey (S×J), and Brown Swiss × Jersey (BS×J)	6 bulls and 6 steers per breed group	ADG (to 15 months) Bulls > steers by 15% ($P < 0.01$)	Bulls > steers by 11%	Lean (%): J bulls 66.2 (a); J Steers 63.6 (b); S×J bulls 64.4; S×J steers 63.3; BS×J bulls 62.6; BS×J steers 63.2 Fat (%): J bulls 8.8 (a); J steers 15.8 (b); S×J bulls 11.9 (a); S×J steers 17.4 (b); BS×J bulls 12.4 (a); BS×J steers 16.6 (b)	102
26 Swedish Friesian (SF) groups 26 Swedish Red-and-White (SRW) groups	12—13 males per group	Net ADG SF bulls 0.385 SF steers 0.321 SRW bulls 0.335 SRW steers 0.294		Fat (mm) SF bulls 1.4 SF steers 2.1 SRW bulls 1.5 SRW steers 2.6	103
Yugoslavian Simmental bulls and steers on high plane (HP) and moderate plane (MP) feeding (slaughtered at approximately 470 kg)	38	ADG HP bulls 0.894 (a) HP steers 0.832 (b) MP bulls 0.824 MP steers 0.80	kg of starch equivalent per kg of gain HP bulls 4.22 HP steers 4.76 MP bulls 4.22 MP steers 4.34		104
Conventional castrates	15	ADG 0.742 (a)		Meat + fat (%) 81.03 Protein (% of meat) 21.33 Fat (% of meat) 7.12	105

Table 2 (Continued)
CATTLE EXPERIMENTS ON THE EFFECTS OF CASTRATION

Experimental groups	Number of animals	Body weight or growth rate (kg)[a]	Food utilization efficiency	Carcass and/or meat characters			Ref.
Partial castrates	15	0.821 (b)		8.02	20.96	7.28	
Bulls	15	0.841 (b)		82.04	21.46	6.59	
(Slaughtered at approximately 365—410 kg)							
				Rib cut composition			
Friesian DZ twin pairs in individual stalls and killed at same age (SA) or same weight (SW)	30	ADG	Mcal ME/kg gain	Fat (%)		Protein (%)	106
SA bulls		1.06 (a)	14.3 (a)	22.7 (a)		17.6 (a)	
SA steers		0.97 (b)	15.5 (b)	31.7 (b)		15.8 (b)	
SW bulls		0.98 (a)	14.2 (a)	20.6 (a)		17.5 (a)	
SW steers		0.88 (b)	16.1 (b)	32.7 (b)		16.1 (b)	
		ADG	kg of feed per kg of gain	Forequarter (%)		Kidney fat (%)	106
Bulls	7—8 per group	1.26 (a)	5.36 (a)	30.7 (a)		1.93 (a)	
Steers	7—8 per group	1.07 (b)	6.06 (b)	35.7 (b)		2.93 (b)	
Both on five commercial farms							
Aberdeen-Angus	157		Steers consumed 141 kg TDN[b] more than bulls	Longissimus dorsi (l.d.) (cm^2)	Fat over l.d. (cm)	Total retail product (kg)	107
Bulls				71.0 (a)	0.9 (a)	156.1 (a)	
Steers				66.1 (b)	1.4 (b)	142.9 (b)	
(killed at 445 or 480 days in a 3-year period				(adjusted carcass weight of 235 kg)			
				Fat (%) 12th rib	Protein (%) 12th rib	Shear value	
				46 (a)	47 (a)	63 (a)	
				57 (b)	36 (b)	50 (b)	
				Organoleptic traits: bulls slightly inferior to steers			
Grade Herefords	72	Postweaning ADG on range	kg of feed per kg of gain (first 105 days of fattening)	l.d. area (cm^2)	Fat (cm)	Separable muscle (%)	108
Conventionally castrated at 8 weeks		0.01	6.92 (a)	63.0	2.45 (a)	57.3 (a)	
Partially castrated at 8 weeks		0	7.03 (b)	62.8	2.38 (a)	56.6 (a)	
Conventionally castrated at 8 weeks		0	6.71 (c)	63.3	2.28 (a)	56.7 (a)	

Left entire (kept on range for first year of life, then fattened in yards		0		6.38 (d)	66.8	1.68 (b)		59.8 (b)	
		ADG during fattening		From approximately 320 to 440 kg					
		1.21 (a)		8.26					
		1.61 (b)		8.96					
		1.31 (c)		7.95					
		1.45 (d)		8.02					
			ADG	kg of feed per kg gain	l.d.[c] area (cm^2)			l.d.[c] area (cm^2) per 100 kg carcass	109
Herefords	60								
Castrated at birth		Bulls	1.23 (a)	6.75	82.17 (a)			32.08 (a)	
Castrated at 2 months		Steers castrated at birth	1.04 (b)	7.80	68.97—69.42 (b)			30.04-31.43 (b)	
Castrated at 7 months		2 months	1.05 (b)	7.80	68.97—69.42 (b)			30.04—31.43 (b)	
Castrated at 9 months		7 months	1.01 (b)	8.15	68.97—69.42 (b)			30.04—31.43 (b)	
Left entire (Slaughtered at approximately 370—420 kg)		9 months	0.98 (b)	8.15	68.97—69.42 (b)			30.04—31.43 (b)	
					Fat (cm)			Edible (%)	
					0.64 (a)			74.32 (a)	
					0.84—1.14 (b)			69.10—70.08 (b)	
					0.84—1.14 (b)			69.10—70.08 (b)	
					0.84—1.14 (b)			69.10—70.08 (b)	
					0.84—1.14 (b)			69.10—70.08 (b)	
					NSD for tenderness, flavor, juiciness, or shear value				
Friesians killed at	40	ADG			Meat (%)	Fat (%)		Eye muscle (cm^2)	110
17 months									
Bulls		0.72 (a)			69.0 (a)	9.3 (a)		73.1 (a)	
Steers		0.63 (b)			66.2 (b)	12.0 (b)		65.9 (b)	
23 months									
Bulls		0.77 (a)			71.8 (a)	10.7 (a)		84.1 (a)	
Steers		0.68 (b)			64.1 (b)	18.6 (b)		70.6 (b)	
Yugoslavian Simmentals	40	ADG		l.d. (cm^2)	Meat (%)	Fat (%)	Protein (%) of meat	Fat (%) of meat	111
Bulls on high-high feeding		0.894 (a)		88.9	74.7 (a)	8.97 (a)	23.17	2.12	
Steers on high-high feeding		0.832 (b)		73.3	70.4 (b)	13.57 (b)	22.52	3.22	
Bulls on medium-high feeding		0.824 (c)		82.4	73.4 (c)	9.17 (c)	23.72	1.90	
Steers on medium-high feeding (Slaughtered at approximately 470 kg)		0.800 (d)		75.8	68.5 (d)	15.18 (d)	22.98	2.91	
Holstein-Friesian × zebu	30	ADG (during fattening)							112

Table 2 (Continued)
CATTLE EXPERIMENTS ON THE EFFECTS OF CASTRATION

Experimental groups	Number of animals	Body weight or growth rate (kg)[a]		Food utilization efficiency	Carcass and/or meat characters				Ref.
Bulls		0.78 (a)							
Steers (Fattened on pasture plus concentrates to 444 kg)		0.73 (b)							
Grade Herefords (Slaughtered at 400—570 kg)	42	Total gain		kg TDN[b] per kg of gain (during finishing)	l.d.[c] area (cm^2)				113, 114
First experiment									
Bulls		251.9		5.40	73.9 (a)				
Steers		228.6		6.08	62.8 (b)				
Second experiment					Retail yield (%)				
Bulls		282.1 (a)		5.96	74.89 (a)				
Steers		244.3 (b)		6.35	67.04 (b)				
					Steers significantly better than bulls for tenderness. NSD for flavor, juiciness, or shear values				
Nellore cattle (fattened for 29 months)	55	31 month live-weight							115
Bulls			425						
Steers castrated at									
2 months			360						
12 months			345						
24 months			390						
Five trials in different Australian environments, using Hereford, zebu × dairy, Beef Shorthorn, and Hereford × Shorthorn cattle: steers vs. hemicastrates (slaughtered at 364 kg)	82	ADG of hemicastrates as (%) of steer value 2% in low growth rate conditions to 25.5% in high-growth rate conditions $P<0.05$ or <0.01 in 4 of the 5 trials							116
Hereford and Shorthorn × Hereford cattle on grass (slaughtered at 10 months)	30	Live weight gain							117
		Days 58—86	Days 58—170		Muscle (%)	Fat (%)	Shear value	Taste panel tenderness	
Entire		29.5 (a)	117.3 (a)		61.6 (a)	14.4	7.36 (a)	25.1 (a)	
Unilateral castrates		32.3 (b)	117.7 (a)		62.1 (a)	13.6	9.5 (b)	24.6 (a)	
Bilateral castrates		28.2 (a)	106.8 (b)		57.6 (b)	20.5	6.4 (a)	28.2 (b)	
				Bulls significantly better than steers					

Half-sib Japanese Blacks	12	ADG		Lean (%)		Fat (%)		118
Bulls		1.03 (a)		66.9 (a)		19.7 (a)		
Steers		0.85 (b)		61.2 (b)		26.1 (b)		
(Fattened for 308 days)								
Aberdeen-Angus	218	Live weight (at slaughter)	Digestible energy (Mcal) consumed per kg of edible product	Edible product (kg/day of age)				119
Bulls		333.6 (a)	6.0 (a)	0.379 (a)				
Steers		306.3 (b)	12.8 (b)	0.267 (b)				
(Slaughtered at 13—15 months of age)			(Maintenance requirement similar)					
Ad lib feeding	20	ADG	Food consumption per kg of gain	Muscle (%)	Fat (%)	Meat protein (%)	Meat fat	120
Bulls (MZ twins)		0.888 (a)	4.73	70.7 (a)	12.7 (a)	21.78	3.91	
Steers (MZ twins)		0.735 (b)	5.04	67.3 (b)	15.0 (b)	21.58	5.12	
Restricted feeding								
Bulls (MZ twins)		0.863 (a)	4.46 (a)	69.1 (a)	13.6 (a)	21.54	4.73 (a)	
Steers (MZ twins)		0.721 (b)	5.64 (b)	62.7 (b)	20.7 (b)	21.04	7.17 (b)	
(Slaughtered at 455 kg)								
Friesians	18	ADG	kg of feed per kg of gain	Fat thickness (cm)	l.d. area (cm²)	Shear value (kg) 9th rib	Shear value (kg) 11th rib	121
Bulls		1.14 (a)	4.46 (a)	1.89 (a)	48.7	2.56	1.95	
Induced cryptorchids		0.99 (a)	4.94 (a)	1.35 (b)	50.6	2.20	1.85	
Steers		0.80 (b)	6.18 (b)	2.14 (a)	42.9	2.13	1.99	
(Slaughtered at 350—400 kg)								
Aberdeen-Angus and Hereford calves 210 days on feedlot	60	ADG		Fat (cm)	Rib eye (cm²)	Cutability (%)		122
Left entire		1.20 (a)		0.93 (a)	80.3 (a)	52.2 (a)		
Castrated at birth		1.13 (b)		1.35 (b)	63.6 (b)	49.0 (b)		
Castrated at weaning		1.17 (c)		1.40 (b)	65.4 (c)	49.2 (b)		

Hereford × Friesian cattle (slaughtered at approximately 420 kg) on	36	ADG		kg concentrate dry matter per kg of gain		Fat (%) of side		Lean (%) of side		123
		Bulls	Steers	Bulls	Steers	Bulls	Steers	Bulls	Steers	
High protein diet		1.23 (a)	1.03 (b)	4.21 (a)	5.02 (b)	21.9 (a)	27.0 (b)	60.4 (a)	56.8 (b)	
Medium protein diet		1.20 (a)	1.09 (b)	4.27 (a)	4.79 (b)	22.9 (a)	29.5 (b)	60.2 (a)	53.5 (b)	
Low protein diet		1.14 (a)	0.97 (b)	4.37 (a)	4.90 (b)	22.3 (a)	27.3 (b)	60.7 (a)	56.4 (b)	

Table 2 (Continued)
CATTLE EXPERIMENTS ON THE EFFECTS OF CASTRATION

Experimental groups	Number of animals	Body weight or growth rate (kg)[a]	Food utilization efficiency	Carcass and/or meat characters		Ref.
Aberdeen-Angus, Hereford, and Brown Swiss				Shear value	Overall satisfaction*	124
Bulls				4.18 (a)	5.40 (a)	
Steers (Slaughtered at 384 kg)				3.0 (b)	6.74 (b)	
Santa Gertrudis and Charolais cattle	90			Shear value	Overall satisfaction*	124
Bulls				4.18 (a)	4.0 (a)	
Steers				3.0 (b)	5.2 (b)	
(Slaughtered at 438 kg)				*High = best		
Salers cattle	40	ADG (for 107 days preslaughter)	kg of feed per kg of gain	Composition of 11th rib cut		125
				Muscle (%)	Fat (%)	
Bulls		1.181 (a)	9.8 (a)	67 (a)	14.8 (a)	
Steers		0.916 (b)	12.1 (b)	62 (b)	20.4 (b)	
(Slaughtered at 24 months)						
Friesian bulls	36	ADG on grass				126
Cryptorchids		0.76 (a)				
Steers		0.80 (a)				
Each group subdivided on low,		0.63 (c)				
medium, and high planes of nu-		ADG in feedlot				
trition, then switched to feedlot		1.66				
(Killed at 360 kg live weight)		1.56				
		1.47				
		Sex × nutrition not significant				
Polled Sinú, zebu, and zebu × Polled Sinú cattle on grass	30	ADG		l.d.[c] area per 100 kg of carcass (cm^2)		127
Bulls		0.371 (a)		33.2		
Steers		0.313 (b)		32.85		
Polish Red-and-White Lowland	24	ADG	Oat units per kg gain	l.d.[c] (cm^2)		128
Slaughtered at 350 kg						
Bulls		0.79	5.5	65.9		
Steers		0.78	5.6	67.9		
Slaughtered at 450 kg						
Bulls		0.73	7.8	76.0 (a)		
Steers		0.67	8.8	66.8 (b)		

San Martin and Holstein-Friesian group, Half implanted with stilbestrol	32	Total gain per head (over 259 days)							129
Bulls		146 (a)							
Steers		124 (b)							
Half not implanted									
Bulls		131 (a)							
Steers		108 (b)							
Aberdeen-Angus, Hereford, and Brown Swiss	90				Shear value (kg)				130
Bulls					4.20 (a)				
Steers					3.00 (b)				
Averaging 385 days at slaughter)									
Santa Gertrudis and Charolais (averaging 484 days at slaughter)					NSD				
Holstein-Friesian	45				Cutability (%)	Shear value	Tenderness rating*	Total acceptability	131
Bulls					51.7 (a)	6.5	4.3 (a)	4.6 (a)	
Steers					49.4 (b)	6.0	6.4 (b)	6.1 (b)	
					*High = good				
Italian Friesian	24	ADG (from initial weight of approximately 315 kg)	Food unit consumed per kg of gain		Rib cut				132
					Lean (%)			Fat (%)	
Bulls		1.04 (a)	7.33 (a)		62.5 (a)			18.1 (a)	
Steers		0.74 (b)	5.84 (b)		58.3 (b)			22.3 (b)	
(Fattened for 129—164 days									
Zebus on grazing	24	Final body weight			Backfat (mm)			Eye-muscle depth (mm)	133
Half on good veld plus final fattening period									
Bulls		378.9			2.4			99	
Steers		377.4			1.0			95	
Half on poor veld plus final fattening period									
Bulls		314.3			3.0			90	
Steers		320.7			0.9			94	
Zebu (2 × 2 factorial experiment)			kg of food per kg of gain						
High plane	12	Final body weight	First period	Second period	Backfat (mm)			Eye-muscle depth (mm)	
Bulls		371.5 (a)	6.22	8.24	2			98	
Steers		344.3 (b)	7.15	9.44	9			95	
Low plane									
Bulls		348.1 (a)	4.36	5.32	4			97	
Steers		329.2 (b)	6.55	5.65	7			93	

Table 2 (Continued)
CATTLE EXPERIMENTS ON THE EFFECTS OF CASTRATION

Experimental groups	Number of animals	Body weight or growth rate (kg)[a]		Food utilization efficiency		Carcass and/or meat characters				Ref.
Friesian										
Half implanted with hexestrol	40	ADG		kg of TDN[b] per kg of gain	TDN[b] per kg of lean meat	Meat (%)	Fat (%)		Eye muscle per 45 kg carcass (cm^2)	135
Bulls		0.72 (a)		3.72	4.03	70.0 (a)	12.1 (a)		13.6	
Steers		0.78 (a)		3.37	4.35	66.6 (b)	15.2 (b)		13.3	
Half not implanted										
Bulls		0.80 (a)		3.31	4.13	68.7 (a)	13.4 (a)		13.6	
Steers		0.67 (a)		4.0	4.48	65.2 (b)	17.2 (b)		13.4	
Twin pairs of cattle, one member castrated and the other entire (slaughtered at 45-445 kg)	20					No significant effect of castration on muscle fiber diameter, DNA, or total protein				136
Holstein × Brahman and Holstein × Santa Gertrudis on molasses diets	176	ADG		Mcal of metabolizable energy per kg of gain		Edible product (%)				137
Bulls		0.86 (a)		16.17 (a)		70.99				
Steers (Slaughtered at 395 kg)		0.76 (b)		18.95 (b)		69.29				
						Meat:bone ratio				
						3.56 (a)				
						3.38 (b)				
Hereford and Friesian bulls and steers killed at 16, 22, 24, or 25 months	87					Bull meat significantly tougher than steer meat by Volodkevich bite tenderometer, Warner-Bratzler shear, and taste panel				138
Holstein-Friesians	30	ADG		kg of feed per kg of gain		Fat (cm)	l.d. (cm^2)	Cutability (%)	Meat acceptability	139
		63—190 days	190—402 days							
Entire		1.136	1.208	7.8		0.66 (a)	74.2 (a)	52.0	6.3 (a)	
Castrated		1.000	1.042	8.8		0.99 (b)	63.2 (b)	51.5 (a)	6.0 (b)	
Short scrotum (Slaughtered at 402 days)		0.991	1.113	8.0		0.58 (a)	72.9 (a)	52.7 (b)	5.8 (b)	
						(High = good)				
Russian Black Pieds	30	15-month body weight		Food units per kg of gain			Fat in meat (%)			140
							12 months	15 months		
Castrated		458.0 (a)		6.4			12.16 (a)	18.26 (a)		
Entire and implanted with stilbestrol		514.0		5.8			12.72 (a)	15.08 (b)		
Entire (Slaughtered at 12 or 15 months)		495.0 (b)		6.0			9.48 (b)	13.41 (c)		

				Carcass fat content bulls < steers by 12.3% ($P < 0.001$)			
Holstein-Friesians, half castrated at 136 kg	36			Rib roast data			141
Bulls					Bulls	Steers	
Steers				% drip	8.81 (a)	5.14 (b)	
(Slaughtered at 475 kg)				Tenderness	5.36 (a)	4.34 (b)	
				Juiciness	5.09 (a)	4.53 (b)	
				Flavor			
				Fat	4.88 (a)	4.69 (b)	
				Lean	5.31 (a)	4.91 (b)	101
				Overall score	5.33 (a)	4.40 (b)	
				l. dorsi fat%	4.60 (a)	2.14 (b)	
				(Low = good for organoleptic traits)			
Five breed/crossbred groups of bulls and five similar groups of steers in progeny tests	2311	Bulls vs. steers (net daily gain)					142
		0.610 (a) vs. 0.491 (b)					
		0.664 (a) vs. 0.565 (b)					
		0.634 (a) vs. 0.579					
		0.694 (a) vs 0.586 (b)					
		0.670 (a) vs. 0.576 (b)					
Nellore cattle in feedlot for 112 days	32	ADG					144
Bulls		0.96					
Steers		0.94					
Holstein-Friesians in feedlot for 112 days	48	ADG	kg of dry matter per kg of gain	Internal fat (%)		Eye-muscle area (cm^2)	143
Bulls		1.29 (a)	6.61	1.70 (a)		49.35 (a)	
Steers		1.13 (b)	6.92	2.32 (b)		43.82 (b)	
	40	ADG	Meat (%)	Fat (mm)	Eye muscle (cm^2)	Saleable meat (kg)	145
Bulls on grass		0.50	74.7 (a)	0	54.9 (a)	167.1 (a)	
Steers on grass (Killed at 427 kg)		0.49	69.2 (b)	0.4	50.0 (b)	143.0 (b)	

[a] Where means for a given trait have alphabetically different letters within parentheses, they are different at the 5% or higher level of significance.

[b] Total digestible nutrients.

[c] Longissimus dorsi.

Table 3
CATTLE (MLC DATA)

Groups recorded	Body weight or growth rate (kg)			Carcass traits		Profitability (in pounds sterling)
Cereal beef production	Average daily gain (ADG) in kg			Carcass weight per day of age		Gross margin per head
Approximately 450 Friesian bulls (slaughtered at 333 days) in 8 units	1.32			0.693		32
Steers at equivalent units (slaughtered at 328 days)	1.18			0.642		20
	ADG (kg)			Carcass weight per day of age		Gross margin per head
	Grazing	Finishing	Overall			
Approximately 400 Friesian bulls in seven units using the 18-month beef system	0.86	0.91	0.86	0.503		54
Friesian steers on equivalent units	0.77	0.82	0.77	0.455		44
	Sale weight (kg)		ADG			Gross margin per head
Finishing of approximately 100 suckled bull calves	458		0.863			Bulls > steers by 85%
Equivalent steers	415		0.772			
Friesians in cereal beef production				Lean (%)	Fat (%)	
Bulls				66.3	16.6	
Steers				61.0	22.5	
Friesians in 18-month beef production						
Bulls				69.0	13.4	
Steers				62.4	19.6	
Hereford × Friesian in 18-month beef production						
Bulls				67.5	14.9	
Steers				63.8	18.9	

[a] Data from References 188 and 189.

Table 4
PIG EXPERIMENTS ON EFFECTS OF CASTRATION

Experimental groups	Number of animals	Body weight or growth rate (kg)	Food utilization efficiency	Carcass and/or meat characters				Ref.
Barrows castrated at		Average daily gain (ADG) (18—100 kg)	kg of feed per kg of gain	Significant comparisons, boar vs. barrow				195
18 kg	4	0.64	1.74	Carcass length (cm)	77.0 vs. 71.5—74.0			195
45 kg	4	0.66	1.80	Backfat (cm)	2.7 vs. 3.6—4.4			195
64 kg	4	0.71	1.63	Preferred cuts (%)	72.8 vs. 64.9—68.8			195
82 kg	4	0.65	1.67	Lean in loin plus backfat (%)	61.7 vs. 40.9—51.2			195
Boars	4	0.60	1.75	Palatability score	3.3 vs. 4.5—4.8			195
(Crossbreds fattened to approximately 100 kg)								
Barrows castrated at		ADG (weaning to 93 kg)		Significant differences among groups, boars vs. barrows				
Birth	16	0.80	1.61	Backfat	1.9 vs. 2.1—2.5			196
6 weeks	15	0.79	1.64	Shoulder (%)	28.2 vs. 27.0—27.9			196
12 weeks	15	0.79	1.61	Middle (%)	47.9 vs. 48.1—49.9			196
16 weeks	15	0.79	1.61	Fat firmness				196
20 weeks	20	0.80	1.49	(Iodine no.) (softer fat in boars)	59.0 vs. 55.6—58.0			196
Boars	14	0.79	1.45					196
Gilts	16	0.78	Differences among groups significant Barrow vs. boar not tested statistically					196
Large Whites	Killed at 152 days			Significant average boar-barrow differences				197
				Proximate analysis of meat				
Boars	3			Fat (%)	−4.82			197
Barrows	3			Moisture (%)	2.72			197
	Killed at 220—227 days			Protein (%)	0.66			197
				Bone (%)	0.64			
	4			Shoulder (%)	1.01			
	4			Fat in back (%)	−1.54			
				Muscle in leg (%)	−1.17			
				Bone in shoulder (%)	1.08			
Dutch Landrace		ADG (40—80 kg)		Carcass length (cm)	Backfat (cm)	Fat (%)	Meat (%)	198
Boars	7	0.78		81.1	2.4	27.4	61.8	
Barrows	8	0.70		79.3	2.6	28.8	61.4	
Large Whites								
Boars	8	0.78 (a)		78.1	2.6	28.2	61.9	
Barrows	8	0.72 (b)		76.5	2.8	29.3	61.5	

Table 4 (Continued)
PIG EXPERIMENTS ON EFFECTS OF CASTRATION

Experimental groups	Number of animals	Body weight or growth rate (kg)	Food utilization efficiency	Carcass and/or meat characters					Ref.
Dutch Landrace		ADG (17—92 kg)							
Boars	38	0.57	3.18	82.7 (a)	2.8 (a)	28.8 (a)	63.8 (a)		
Barrows	32	0.60	3.18	81.6 (b)	3.4 (b)	31.2 (b)	62.3 (b)		
		ADG (22—95 kg)							
Boars	28	0.64 (a)	3.16	77.8 (a)	3.0 (a)	27.9 (a)	62.6 (a)		
Barrows	28	0.62 (b)	3.27	76.4 (b)	3.6 (b)	30.6 (b)	61.0 (b)		
		ADG (23—90 kg)							
Boars	34	0.66 (a)		79.5	3.1 (a)	29.3 (a)	60.9 (a)		
Barrows	18	0.70 (b)		78.5	3.8 (b)	32.2 (b)	59.2 (b)		
Large Whites		ADG (to 110 kg)			Boars	Barrows			
Boars	7	0.78		% Shoulder	35.7 (a)	32.9 (b)			
Barrows (castrated at 5 weeks)	7	0.82		% Middle	29.4 (a)	32.8 (b)			
				% Lean	41.0 (a)	35.9 (b)			
				% Fat	31.0 (a)	40.0 (b)			
				% Bone	9.3 (a)	7.8 (b)			
		ADG (to 93—98 kg)		Significant comparisons boars vs. barrows					
Boars	57	0.87	1.55	Carcass length (cm)		76.0 vs. 73.4			
Barrows	30	0.83	1.69	Backfat (cm)		3.2 vs. 3.8			199
(Mainly Durocs)				Fat (%)		17.1 vs. 20.9			199
Included in larger experiment in which other boars were implanted with stilbestrol				Shoulder (%)		18.8 vs. 17.3			
Large Whites		ADG (to 89 kg)	kg of feed per kg of gain	Carcass length (cm)		Backfat (cm)			
Boars	24	0.66 (a)	1.39 (a)	80.6		3.9 (a)			
Barrows (castrated at 8 weeks)	24	0.60 (b)	1.57 (b)	80.0		4.3 (b)			200
				Forecut (%)		Loin eye (cm^2)			200
				54.6		24.8 (a)			
				54.5		21.7 (b)			
Large White × Landrace		ADG (23—110 kg)	Food units per kg of gain	Lean cuts (%)	Fat cuts (%)	Backfat (cm)			
Boars	4	0.66	4.1	66.9 (a)	17.9 (a)	2.8 (a)			201
Barrows	4	0.64	4.2	60.9 (b)	24.3 (b)	3.8 (b)			201
Large Whites	32			Backfat (cm)	Lean (%)	Fat (%)	Bone (%)		202
Standard level of protein		ADG (29—111 kg)						Loin eye (cm^2)	
Boars		0.79		1.26 (a)	42.6 (a)	27.9 (a)	8.6 (a)	26.2 (a)	
Barrows		0.79		1.54 (b)	37.9 (b)	35.9 (b)	7.6 (b)	22.2 (b)	

High level of protein								
Boars		0.85						
Barrows		0.78						
Norwegian Landraces		ADG			Backfat (mm)		Longissimus dorsi (cm²)	203
Boars	20	0.646			25.3 (a)		30.6	
Barrows	40	0.655			29.1 (b)		30.1	
(Slaughtered at 88—92 kg)								
		ADG		Meat (%)	Fat (%)	Loin eye (cm²)	Protein in meat (%)	204
Bulgarian White boars		0.597		53.8	33.8	30.1	22.07	
Barrows (castrated at 4 months)		0.672		47.1	39.6	26.5	22.9	
Bulgarian White boars		0.701 (a)		43.0	34.4	23.2	21.56	
Barrows (castrated at 40 days)		0.760 (b)		41.9	42.2	24.4	21.55	
Barrows (castrated at 6 months)		0.751		44.8	38.7	25.5	21.95	
Large Whites (half castrated at 80 days	22	ADG	Food conversion index	Carcass length (cm)		Backfat (mm)	Meat:fat	205, 206
Boars		0.783	3.23	98.37 (a)		35 (a)	1.04 (a)	
Barrows		0.782	3.12	96.0 (b)		40 (b)	0.91 (b)	
Pigs fed from 22.5 kg to 88.6 kg on (1) growing ration (17% protein) or (2) growing ration to 50 kg then finishing ration (13% protein)	56	Overall ADG	kg of feed per kg of gain			Boars	Barrows	207
Boars		0.73 (a)	3.20 (a)	Backfat (mm)		31.0 (a)	35.3 (b)	
Barrows		0.68 (b)	3.70 (b)	Lean in ham face (%)		50.68 (a)	45.24 (b)	
				Loin (%)		24.77	25.32	
				Ham (%)		28.39	28.42	
				Loin-eye (cm²)		26.39	24.77	
Dutch Landraces (fattened from 20—90 kg)	32	ADG	kg of food per kg of gain	Carcass length (cm)		Fat (cm)	Eye muscle (cm²)	208
Boars		0.643	3.1	97.5		3.1	29.9	
Barrows		0.633	3.3	95.8		3.4	28.2	
Large Whites (fattened from 20—90 kg)								
Boars		0.651	3.1	93.3		3.0	28.5	
Barrows		0.624	3.4	92.4		3.5	23.7	

		ADG		kg of feed per kg of gain		
Saddlebacks left entire or castrated at 7, 21 or 56 days (2 replicates R_1 and R_2)	32	R_1	R_2	R_1	R_2	209
Boars		0.658	0.609	3.69	3.86	
Barrows		0.604—0.652	0.505—0.601	3.41—3.85	3.74—4.0	
		Significant differences among groups				

Table 4 (Continued)
PIG EXPERIMENTS ON EFFECTS OF CASTRATION

Experimental groups	Number of animals	Body weight or growth rate (kg)	Food utilization efficiency	Carcass and/or meat characters		Ref.
	110	ADG	kg of feed per kg of gain	Backfat (cm)		210
Boars (fattened to 110 kg)		0.808 (a)	3.05 (a)	3.51 (a)		
Barrows (fattened to 110 kg)		0.727 (b)	3.51 (b)	3.94 (b)		
Durocs (half castrated at 21 days; slaughtered at 100—114 kg)	14	ADG		Fat (cm)	Boar odor (%)	211
Boars		0.747	No significant difference (NSD)	4.6	75	
Barrows		0.719		5.5	0	
Norwegian Landraces (fattened to 90 kg)	52			Lean (%)	Fat (%)	212
Boars				50.53 (a)	22.57 (a)	
Barrows				45.58 (b)	29.73 (b)	
				Weights of 24 muscles significantly greater in boars than in barrows by 5.9% (adductor) to 17.5% (Extensor carpi radialis)		
British Landrace × Large White pigs (slaughtered at 100 kg)	24	ADG	kg of feed per kg of gain	Lean (%)	Intermuscular fat (%)	213
Partially castrated		0.73	2.41	52.3	6.4	
Testes but not epididymides removed		0.70	2.41	49.2	7.0	
Completely castrated		0.70	2.40	50.0	7.6	
Left entire		0.72	2.23	60.3	5.5	
				Significant difference NSD for cooked meat evaluation		
		ADG	Food units per kg of gain	Backfat (cm)	Fat:lean (%)	214
Boars	56	0.743 (a)	2.80 (a)	2.66 (a)	81 (a)	
Complete castrates		0.692 (b)	3.09 (b)	3.17 (b)	115 (b)	
Partial castrates		0.735	2.86	2.82	84	
Testes but not epididymides removed		0.688	3.03	3.07	104	
				Boar odor:boars significantly > barrows		
Large White pigs (slaughtered at 102 kg) castrated at	84	ADG (30—100 kg)		Lean cuts (%)	Backfat (%)	215
20 kg		0.634		42.9	35.1 (b)	
70 kg		0.661		43.6	33.3 (b)	
90 kg		0.616		47.3	26.8 (a)	
Left entire		0.627		48.4	25.2 (a)	

Landrace × Large White pigs (slaughtered at 102 kg) castrated at							
20 kg		0.624		43.5 (c)		33.9 (b)	
70 kg		0.657		44.8 (c)		31.0 (b)	
90 kg		0.631		48.2 (b)		25.3 (a)	
Left entire		0.628		50.1 (a)		24.1 (a)	
				Backfat (mm)	Meat protein (%)	Meat fat (%)	
Boars fed to 100 kg on	24	ADG	kg of feed per kg of gain				216
An *ad lib.* diet		0.682	3.26 (a)	23.0 (a)	14.3 (a)	33.5	
A restricted diet		0.555	3.18 (a)	20.5 (a)	14.7 (a)	31.5	
Barrows fed to 100 kg on							
An *ad lib.* diet		0.627	3.69 (b)	32.0 (b)	12.3 (b)	41.3	
A restricted diet		0.470 (b)	3.84 (b)	30.5 (b)	12.3 (b)	41.9	
	32		NSD in nitrogen retention or nitrogen and energy digestibility	Fat thickness (sum of three measurements) (cm)		Loin eye (cm²)	217
Boars castrated at 70 kg				9.78 (a)		31.4 (a)	
Entire boars				9.47 (a)		33.2 (a)	
Barrows				11.96 (b)		27.3 (b)	
				NSD in proximate analysis of longissimus dorsi muscle			
				Panel scores for taint at 90 kg live weight (0 = no taint)			
		ADG (after 70 kg)	kg of feed per kg of gain	Panel 1 (score range of 1—3)		Panel 2 (score range of 1—5)	218, 219
Boars castrated at 70 kg	32	0.93	3.56 (a)	0.25		0.41	
Entire boars		0.90	3.32 (b)	0.78		1.68	
Barrows		0.87	4.07 (c)	0.42		0.47	
		NSD in ADG to 70 kg		Correlation of taint score with weight (70—84 kg) 0.06 or not significant			
Large Whites (fattened to 97 kg)	12	ADG Similar in boars and barrows	kg of feed per kg of gain Boars better than barrows by 14% $P < 0.05$	Lean weight:boars > barrows by 10% Fat weight:boars < barrows by 20% Skin weight:boars > barrows by 20% $P < 0.05$ for all 3 traits			220
		ADG	kg of feed per kg of gain	Fat (mm)		Eye muscle (cm²)	221
Boars	72	0.78	2.84 (a)	35.6 (a)		35.1 (a)	
Barrows		0.79	3.03 (b)	44.7 (b)		32.5 (b)	
Fed on rations containing 16, 18, or 20% protein and slaughtered at 90 kg							
Yorkshires fattened in Spring	69	ADG	kg of feed per kg of gain	Backfat (cm)		Loin eye (cm²)	222
Boars		0.940	2.63	2.97		32.7	
Barrows		0.958	2.77	3.31		28.4	

Table 4 (Continued)
PIG EXPERIMENTS ON EFFECTS OF CASTRATION

Experimental groups	Number of animals	Body weight or growth rate (kg)	Food utilization efficiency	Carcass and/or meat characters		Ref.
Autumn						
Boars		0.894	3.07	3.10	33.5	
Barrows		0.826	3.42	3.56	28.8	
		Sex differences (including gilt) significant	Sex differences in spring (including gilt) significant	Sex differences (including gilts) significant		

[a] Where means for a given trait have alphabetically different letters within parenthesis, they are different at the 5% or higher level of significance.

REFERENCES

1. **Trow-Smith, R.**, *A History of British Livestock Husbandry to 1700,* Routledge & Kegan, London, 1957.
2. **Pálsson, H.**, Conformation and body composition, in *Progress in the Physiology of Farm Animals,* Vol. 2, Hammond, J., Ed., Butterworths, London, 1955, 430—542.
3. **Turton, J. D.**, The effect of castration on meat production and quality in cattle, sheep and pigs, *Anim. Breeding Abstr.,* 30, 447—456, 1962.
4. **Turton, J. D.**, The effect of castration on meat production from cattle, sheep, and pigs, in *Meat Production from Entire Male Animals,* Rhodes, D. N., Ed., J & A Churchill, London, 1969, 1—50.
5. **Brännäng, E.**, *Effects of Castration and Ovariectomy on Growing Cattle,* Kvalitetstryck AB, Stockholm, 1971, 1—16.
6. **Field, R. A.**, Effect of castration on meat quality and quantity, *J. Anim. Sci.,* 32, 849—858, 1971.
7. **Lougnon, J.**, Influence de la castration sur les performances et les besoins alimentaires des porcs charcutiers, *Ind. Aliment. Anim.,* 216, 28—33, and 36, 1970.
8. **Anastasijević, V.**, Problem of castration and its effect on fattening capacity and carcass characters in pigs, (in Serbo-croation) *Stocarstvo,* 23, 363—374, 1969.
9. **Walstra, P. and Kroeske, D.**, The effect of castration on meat production in male pigs, *World Rev. Anim. Prod.,* 4 (19-20), 59—64, 1968.
10. **Martin, A. H.**, The problem of sex taint in pork in relation to the growth and carcass characteristics of boars and barrows: a review, *Can. J. Anim. Sci.,* 49(1), 1—10, 1969.
11. **Hammond, J.**, *A Survey of the Problems Involved in Meat Production,* Oliver & Boyd, Edinburgh, 1932.
12. **Hunt, W. E., Meade, D., and Carmichael, B. E.**, Effect of castration of lambs on the development and quality of meat, *Md. Agric. Exp. Stn. Bull.,* 417, 259—278, 1938.
13. **Riches, J. H. and Johnstone, I. L.**, An experiment to determine the relative growth and productivity of rams and wethers under identical field conditions, *Aust. Vet. J.,* 25, 270—272, 1949.
14. **Badreldin, A. L.**, Growth and carcase percentage in Ossimi and Rahmani sheep, *Bull. Fac. Agric. Fouad I Univ., Cairo,* 3, 1—16, 1951.
15. **Pattie, W. A., Armstrong, F. J., and Godlee, A. C.**, The influence of the poll gene and castration on lamb growth, *Proc. Aust. Soc. Anim. Prod.,* 4, 175—177, 1962.
16. **Gligor, V., Nedelniuc, V., Tacu, A., Florescu, U. S., Bica, M., Raicu, E., Rosca, N., Popescu, C., and Harsian, A.**, The physiological basis for the use of stimulators in fat lamb production (in Rumanian), *Lucr. Stiint. Inst. Cercet. Zooteh.,* 20, 395—421, 1962.
17. **Gligor, V., Nedelniuc, V., Timariu, S., Tascenco, V., Popescu, C., Rosca, N., Tacu, A., Florescu, S., Jurencova, G., Raicu, E., and Bica, M.**, The physiological basis for the use of stimulators to fatten Merinos, (in Rumanian) *Lucr. Stiint. Inst. Cercet. Zooteh.,* 21, 5—32, 1963.
18. **Dun, R. B.**, The influence of the poll gene and of castration on production characters of male Merino sheep, *Aust. J. Exp. Agric. Anim. Husb.,* 3, 262—265, 1963.
19. **Bradford, G. E. and Spurlock, G. M.**, Effects of castrating lambs on growth and body composition, *Anim. Prod.,* 6, 291—299, 1964.
20. **Prescott, J. H. D. and Lamming, G. E.**, The effects of castration on meat production in cattle, sheep and pigs, *J. Agric. Sci.,* 63, 341—357, 1964.
21. **Coetzee, C. G.**, Effect of castration on growth rate and carcass composition of lambs, *Proc. S. Afr. Soc. Anim. Prod.,* 4, 165—167, 1965.
22. **Everitt, G. C. and Jury, K. E.**, Effects of sex and gonadectomy on the growth and development of Southdown × Romney cross lambs. I. Effects on liveweight growth and components of live weight. *J. Agric. Sci.,* 66, 1—14, 1966.

22a. **Everitt, G. C. and Jury, K. E.**, Effects of sex and gonadectomy on the growth and development of Southdown × Romney cross lambs. II. Effects on carcass grades, measurements and chemical composition, *J. Agric. Sci.,* 66, 15—27, 1966.

23. **Ray, E. E. and Mandigo, R. W.**, Genetic and environmental factors affecting carcass traits of lambs, *J. Anim. Sci.,* 25, 449—453, 1966.
24. **Seebeck, R. M.**, Composition of dressed carcasses of lambs, *Proc. Aust. Soc. Anim. Prod.,* 6, 291—297, 1966.
25. **Oliver, W. M., Carpenter, Z. L., King, G. T., and Shelton, J. M.**, Qualitative and quantitative characteristics of ram, wether, and ewe lamb carcasses, *J. Anim. Sci.,* 26, 307—310, 1967.
26. **Scheepers, G. E.**, The influence of age and sex of sheep on the cortical segmentation of Merino wool, *S. Afr. J. Agric. Sci.,* 10, 551—554, 1967.
27. **Dutt, R. H., Dame, P. R., and Renfro, R. E.**, Effects of unilateral castration on body weight and accessory gland development in ram lambs, *Ky. Agric. Exp. Stn. Prog. Rep.,* 176, 37—38, 1968.

28. **Vlachos, K., Karagiannidis, A., and Koutsoutis, Ch. D.**, Investigations on growth capacity in male lambs castrated according to different methods, (in Greek), *Bull. Physiol. Pathol. Reprod. Artif. Insemination Thessaloniki, Univ.*, 4(1), 55—61, 1968.
29. **Załuska, K., Mielnik, J. and Groth, I.**, Porównanie zawartości suchej masy, białka ogólnego i tłuszczu surowego w mięsie jagniąt rasy merynos polski i czarnogłówka w zależności od rasy i badanego mięśnia, *Rocz. Nauk Roln. Ser. B.*, 90, 311—324, 1968.
30. **Cloete, J. G., Dreyer, J. H., Mulder, A. M., and Rossouw, J. W.**, Influence of endogenous testicular androgens on the utilization of dietary components, endocrine activity and productivity of male Merino hoggets, *Agroanimalia*, 1, 5—12, 1969.
31. **Prescott, J. H. D.**, The influence of castration on the growth of lambs in relation to plane of nutrition, in *Meat Production from Entire Male Animals*, Rhodes, D. N., Ed., J & A Churchill, London, 1969, 109—128.
32. **Doroszewski, B., Osikowski, M., Doroszewska, Z., and Janasz, M.**, Jakość miesa tryczków i skopków rasy merynos ubijanych w różnym wieku, *Rocz. Nauk Roln. Ser. B.*, 92, 223—237, 1970.
33. **Göhler, H.**, Zum Problem der Lämmermast unter besonderer Berücksichtigung der Schlachtwertbestimmung, *Arch. Tierz.*, 13, 69—83, 1970.
34. **Kemp. J. D., Crouse, J. D., Deweese, W., and Moody, W. G.**, Effect of slaughter weight and castration on carcass characteristics of lambs, *J. Anim. Sci.*, 30, 348—354, 1970.
35. **Moody, W. G., Tichenor, D. A., Kemp, J. D., and Fox, J. D.**, Effects of weight, castration and rate of gain on muscle fiber and fat cell diameter in two ovine muscles, *J. Anim. Sci.*, 31, 676—680. 1970.
36. **Osman, A. H., El Shafie, S. A., and Khattab, A. G. H.**, Carcass composition of fattened rams and wethers of Sudan Desert sheep, *J. Agric. Sci.*, 75, 257—263, 1970.
37. **Simms, R. H., Perry, T. W., and Andrews, F. N.**, Influence of delayed castration and of diethylstilbestrol implantation on the performance of suckling lambs, *J. Anim. Sci.*, 30, 970—973, 1970.
38. **Tichenor, D. A., Kemp. J. D., Fox, J. D., Moody, W. G., and Deweese, W.**, Effect of slaughter weight and castration on ovine adipose fatty acids, *J. Anim. Sci.*, 31, 671—675, 1970.
39. **Wilson, L. L., Ziegler, J. H., Rugh, M. C., Watkins, J. L., Merrutt, T. L., Simpson, H. J., and Kreuzherger, F. L.**, Comparison of live, slaughter and carcass characteristics of rams, induced cryptorchids and wethers, *J. Anim. Sci.*, 31, 455—458, 1970.
40. **Witt, M. and Kallweit, E.**, Der Einfluss der Kastration auf Mast- and Schlachtleistung bei männlichen Lämmern, *Zuchtungskunde*, 42, 391—398, 1970.
41. **Baillargeon, J. M., Lemay, J. P., Holtmann, W. B., and Charette, L. A.**, Comparison de diverses methodes de castration et de sterilisation des agneaux. I. Influence de ces méthodes sur la croissance, l'efficiencé alimentaire, le rendement a l'abattage et la rentabilité. II. Influence sur la carcasse, *Can. J. Anim. Sci.*, 51, 579—599, 1971.
42. **González, J. and Cardozo, A.**, Deferencetomia y orquidectomia en la producción ovina, in 3rd Reunion Latinoamericana Producción Animal, Bogotá, 1971, 109.
43. **Glimp, H. A.**, Effects of sex alteration, breed, type of rearing and creep feeding on lamb growth, *J. Anim. Sci.*, 32, 859—862, 1971.
44. **Ray, E. E. and Kromann, R. P.**, Effects of sex, age of lamb and length of feeding upon energy metabolism and carcass traits of lambs, *J. Anim. Sci.*, 32, 721—726, 1971.
45. **Crouse, J. D., Kemp. J. D., Fox, J. D., Ely, D. G., and Moody, W. G.**, Effect of castration, testosterone and slaughter weight on fatty acid content of ovine adipose tissue, *J. Anim. Sci.*, 34, 384—387, 1972.
46. **Jacobs, J. A., Field, R. A., Botkin, M. P., Riley, M. L., and Roehrkrasse, G. P.**, Effects of weight and castration on lamb carcass composition and quality, *J. Anim. Sci.*, 35(5), 926—930, 1972.
47. **Kemp, J. D., Shelley, J. M., Jr, Ely, D. G., and Moody, W. G.**, Effects of castration and slaughter weight on fatness, cooking losses and palatability of lamb, *J. Anim. Sci.*, 34, 560—562, 1972.
48. **Pinkas, A., Solomonov, Kh., and Petrov, N.**, Effect of castration on meat production and characters in male lambs (in Bulgarian), *Zhivotnovud. Nauki*, 9(5), 87—93, 1972.
49. **Shelton, M. and Carpenter, Z. L.**, Influence of sex, stilboestrol treatment and slaughter weight on performance and carcass traits of slaughter lambs, *J. Anim. Sci.*, 34, 203—207, 1972.
50. **Younis, A. A., Kotby, S., and Kamar, G. A. R.**, Effect of castration on live body weight and certain carcass traits in Ossimi and Rahmani lambs, *Egypt. J. Anim. Prod.*, 12(2), 91—97, 1973.
51. **Veseley, J. A.**, Growth rates, carcass grades, and fat composition in ram lambs, wether lambs, and induced cryptorchids, *Can. J. Anim. Sci.*, 53(2), 187—192, 1973.
52. **Bell, T. D., Orme, L. E., Everson, D. O., and Hodgson, C. W.**, Carcass characteristics of lambs of different breeding and sex, *Idaho Agric. Exp. Stn. Res. Bull.*, 546, 1974, 1—12.
53. **Assadi-Moghaddam, R. and Nik-Khah, A.**, Untersuchungen zum Einfluss der Kastration auf Gewichtszunahme und Schlachtkörpermerkmale der männlichen Lämmer des Fettschwanzschafes. *Züechtungskunde*, 47(5), 351—356, 1975.

54. **Price, M. A.**, The effects of added dietary lipid on the body composition of rams and wethers, *J. Agric. Sci.*, 84(2), 201—208, 1975.
55. **Misock, J. P., Campion, D. R., Field, R. A., and Riley, M. L.**, Palatability of heavy ram lambs, *J. Anim. Sci.*, 42(6), 1440—1444, 1976.
56. **Pattie, W. A., Godlee, A. C., and Bouton, P. E.**, The effects of castration and of the poll gene on prime lamb production, *Aust. J. Exp. Agric. Anim. Husb.*, 4, 386—391, 1964.
57. Ministry of Agriculture, United Kingdom, Report, Transcoed Experimental Husbandry Farm, Her Majesty's Stationery Office, London, 1963, 4—6.
58. **Erokhin, A. I.**, Is it necessary to castrate ram lambs for meat production (in Russian), *Ovtsevodstvo*, 11(7), 13—15, 1965.
59. **Grebenjuk, A. Z. and Kazanchev, S. C.**, Castrating ram lambs for meat production, (in Russian), *Ovtsevodstvo*, 14(6), 14—15, 1968.
60. **Korotkov, V. I.**, Is it more advantageous to fatten wethers or ram lambs? (in Russian), *Ovtsevodstvo*, 12(5), 27—29, 1966.
61. **Mihálka, T.**, Növendék kos vagy ürü hizlalása megfelelöbb-e pecsenye célra? *Kiserletugyi Kozl. B.*, 1960(2), 69—79, 1961.
62. **Dobrev, D.**, The choice of suitable rations and the time for fattening wethers (in Bulgarian), *Izv. Inst. Zhivotnovud. Sofia*, 17, 137—148, 1963.
63. **Walker, D. E.**, The influence of sex upon carcass quality of New Zealand fat lamb, *N.Z. J. Sci. Technol. Sect. A*, 32(1), 30—38, 1951.
64. **Mochalovskiǐ, A. N.**, New methods of sterilising rams and the effect on physiological and production characters (in Russian), *Sb. Nauchno. Tr. Leningr. Nauchno. Issled. Vet. Inst.*, 10, 280—284, 1963.
65. **Klostermann, E. W., Kunkle, L. E., Gerlaugh, P., and Cahill, V. R.**, The effect of age of castration upon rate and economy of gain and carcass quality of beef calves, *J. Anim. Sci.*, 13, 817—825, 1954.
66. **Wierbicki, E., Cahill, V. R., Kunkle, L. E., Klosterman, E. W., and Deatherage, F. E.**, Meat quality. Effect of castration on biochemistry and quality of beef, *J. Agric. Food Chem.*, 3, 244—249, 1955.
67. **Tyleček, J.**, The effect of castrating at different times on meat production during fattening and on the quality of carcass characters (in Czechoslovakian), *Sb. Cesk. Akad. Zemed. Ved. Zivocisna Vyroba*, 2(30), 633—656, 1957.
68. **Tyleček, J.**, The advantage of castrating bulls in fattening young stock at pasture (in Czechoslovakian), *Sb. Vys. Sk. Zemed. Brne Rada A*, 2, 129—142, 1958.
69. **Danl, O.**, Effect of castration on composition of the depot fats of monozygous twin cattle, *J. Sci. Food Agric.*, 13, 520—524, 1962.
70. **Skjervold, H., Gravir, K., and Tandberg, O. V.**, Kjøttproduksjonsforsøk med storfe. Sammenligning mellom okser og kastrater av norske raser og krysninger med engelske kjøttferaser. *Meld. Nor. Landrukshoegsk.*, 39(3), 39, 1960.
71. **Brännäng, E.**, Kastrationsförsok pa SRB-tvillingar, *Lantmannen*, 71, 46, 1960.
72. **Baca, A. S. F., González, G. E., Madariegue, M. F., and Nolte, M. M.**, Effects of castration in fattening young and adult cattle, (in Spanish), *Rev. Fac. Med. Vet. Univ. Nac. San Marcos Lima*, 16/17, 231—239, 1961—62.
73. **Čobić, T., Bačvanski, S., Vučetić, S., Stojanović, N., and Filipović, V.**, The effect of castration and method of housing of young bulls during fattening on weight gains and food conversion (in Serbocroatian), *Vet. Glas.*, 16, 715—723, 1962.
74. **Prés, J.**, Different methods of feeding and fattening young cattle of the Black Pied Lowland breed from the physiological-nutritional and economic angle (in Polish), *Rocz. Nauk Roln. Ser. B*, 81, 1—21, 1962.
75. **Kadiǐski, E. G. and Petkov, P.**, Comparative fattening trials with steers and bull calves at pasture and in byres (in Bulgarian), *Nauchni Tr. Vissh. Selskostop. Inst. Sofia Zootekh. Fak.*, 14, 47—60, 1964.
76. **Nichols, J. R., Ziegler, J. H., White, J. M., Kesler, E. M., and Watkins, J. L.**, Production and carcass characteristics of Holstein-Friesian bulls and steers slaughtered at 800 or 1,000 pounds, *J. Dairy Sci.*, 47, 179—185, 1964.
77. **Bielińska, K., Bieliński, K., Borzuta, K., Góźdź, H., Chrząszcz, T. and Słaboń, W.**, The effect of castrating young bulls of the Black Pied Lowland breed on their fattening and slaughter value when fattened to 250 kg live weight (in Polish), *Rocz. Nauk. Roln. Ser. B*, 86, 91—101, 1965.
78. **Cunningham, E. P. and Henderson, C. R.**, Estimation of genetic and phenotypic parameters of weaning traits in beef cattle, *J. Anim. Sci.*, 24, 182—187, 1965.
79. **El Shafie, S. A.**, Fattening of Sudan zebu cattle. I. Weight gain and carcass analysis of castrated and non-castrated Butana calves, *Sudan, J. Vet. Sci. Anim. Husb.*, 6, 33—40, 1965.
80. **Harte, F. J., Curran, S., and Vial, V. E.**, The production of beef from young bulls. I., *Ir. J. Agric. Res.*, 4, 189—204, 1965.

81. **Witt, M. and Andreae, U.,** Kastrationseffekte bei männlichen eineiigen Rinderzwillingen, *Z. Tierz. Züechtungsbiol.*, 81, 1—45, 1965.
82. **Woodhams, P. R. and Trower, S. J.,** Palatability characteristics of rib-steaks from Aberdeen Angus steers and bulls, *N.Z. J. Agric. Res.*, 8, 921—926, 1965.
83. **Bailey, C. M., Probert, C. L., and Bohman, V. R.,** Growth rate, feed utilization and body composition of young bulls and steers, *J. Anim. Sci.*, 25, 132—137, 1966.
84. **Bailey, C. M., Probert, C. L., Richardson, P., Bohman, V. R., and Chancerelle, J.,** Quality factors of the longissimus dorsi of young bulls and steers, *J. Anim. Sci.*, 25, 504—508, 1966.
85. **Brännäng, E.,** Studies on the effect of breed and castration on food consumption, growth and carcass characters under alternate pasture and indoor feeding, (in Swedish), *Lantbrukshoegsk. Medd. Ser. A*, No. 52, 1—24, 19 66.
86. **Čobić, T., Maslarović, B., Bačvanski, S., Ognjanovič, A. and Vučetić, S.,** A comparison of vasectomy and castration for the fattening of bull calves (in Serbo-croatian), *Arh. Poljopr. Nauke*, 19(65), 14—22, 1966.
87. **Conrad, B. E., Marion, P. T., Neal, E. M., King, G. T., Allen, J. H., and Riggs, J. K.,** Young bulls, steers and heifers for slaughter beef production, *Beef Cattle Res. Texas*, 28—29, 1966.
88. **Field, R. A., Nelms, G. E., and Schoonover, C. O.,** Effects of age, marbling and sex on palatability of beef, *J. Anim. Sci.*, 25, 360—366, 1966.
89. **Forbes, T. J. and Irwin, J. H. D.,** A comparison of five breeds and crosses for intensive beef production, *Rec. Agric. Res.*, (Belfast), 15(2), 39—50, 1966.
90. **Macfarlane, J. S.,** Castration in farm animals, *Vet. Rec.*, 78, 436, 1966.
91. **Quinn, L., Mott, G. O., Bisschoff, W. V. A., and Da Rocha G. L.,** Response of male zebu calves to creep feeding, castration, diethylstilbestrol and supplementary feeding on pasture (in Portugese), *Pesqui Agropecu. Bras.*, 1, 303—317, 1966.
92. **Thurber, S. W., Dunbar, J. R., and Smith, D. P.,** Effects of castration age and diethylstilbestrol on weight gains in male calves, *Calif. Agric.*, 20(10), 12—14, 1966.
93. **Harte, F. J. and Curran, S.,** The production of beef from young bulls. II., *Ir. J. Agric. Res.*, 6, 101—118, 1967.
94. **McDonald, I. and Kay, M.,** A note on the composition of live weight gains estimated by regression analysis, *Anim. Prod.*, 9, 553—556, 1967.
95. **Mukhtar, A. M. S.,** Effect of castration and feed supplementation on liveweight gains of western Sudan range cattle, *Indian Vet. J.*, 44, 496—500, 1967.
96. **Čobić, T.,** Castration experiments with Yugoslav Simmental cattle. I. The effect of castration on growth and live-weight gains, *Anim. Prod.*, 10, 103—107, 1968.
97. **Brännäng, E.,** Studies on monozygous cattle twins. XVIII. The effect of castration and age of castration on the growth rate, feed conversion and carcase traits of Swedish Red and White cattle, *Lantbrukshoegsk. Ann.*, 32, 329—415, 1966.
98. **Armstrong, C. W. B. and Naudé, R. T.,** The effect of rhythmic changes in the feeding level on the feed utilization and intramuscular fat of young bulls and steers of the milking breeds, *Proc. S. Afr. Soc. Anim. Prod.*, 6, 105—107, 1967.
99. **Carpenter, Z. L., King, G. T., Legg, W. E., and Riggs, J. K.,** Palatability characteristics of young bull, steer and heifer carcasses, *Beef Cattle Res. Texas*, 41—42, 1967.
100. **Jadhav, D. S.,** Studies on raising Holstein males for meat and an associated study regarding their feedlot activities, *Diss. Abstr. B*, 27, 4188-B, 1967.
101. **King, G. T. and Carpenter, Z. L.,** Cutability of bull, steer and heifer carcasses, *Beef Cattle Res. Texas*, 38—41, 1967.
102. **Naudé, R. T. and Armstrong, C. W. B.,** Beef production from Jersey and Jersey crossbred steers and bulls, *Proc. S. Afr. Soc. Anim. Prod.*, 6, 156—161, 1967.
103. **Brännäng, E.,** In studie i avkommebedömningsteknik för tillväxt-och slaktegenskaper hos kombinerade mjölk-köttraser, *Lantbrukshoegsk. Medd. Ser. A*, 101, 48, 1968.
104. **Čobić, T.,** Castration experiments with Yugoslav Simmental cattle. I. The effect of castration on growth and live-weight gains, *Anim. Prod.*, 10, 103—107, 1968.
105. **Ivanov, P., Ivanova, S., and Aleksandrov, S.,** Comparative fattening of partial castrates, steers and bulls, (in Bulgarian), *Zhivotnovud. Nauki.*, 4(7), 9—16, 1967.
106. **Preston, T. R., MacDearmid, A., Aitken, J. N., MacLeod, N. A., and Philip, E. B.,** The effect of castration on growth, feed conversion and carcass quality of Friesian cattle given all-concentrate diets, *Rev. Cubana Ciencia Agric.*, (English Edition) 2, 183—190, 1968.
107. **Arthaud, V. H., Adams, C. H., Jacobs, D. R., and Koch, R. M.,** Comparison of carcass traits of bulls and steers, *J. Anim. Sci.*, 28, 742—745, 1969.
108. **Bailey, C. B. and Hironaka, R.,** Growth and carcass characteristics of bulls, steers, and partial castrates kept on range for the first year of life and then fattened, *Can. J. Anim. Sci.*, 49, 37—44, 1969.

109. **Champagne, J. R., Carpenter, J. W., Hentges, J. F., Jr., Palmer, A. Z., and Koger, M.**, Feedlot performance and carcass characteristics of young bulls and steers castrated at four ages, *J. Anim. Sci.*, 29, 887—890, 1969.
110. **Harte, F. J.**, The production of beef from young bulls. III., *Ir. J. Agric. Res.*, 8, 293—305, 1969.
111. **Čobić, T.**, Effect of time of castration on fattening performance and carcass characters in Yugoslav Pied bulls, (in Serbo-croation), *Zb. Rad. Inst. Stočar.*, (Novi Sad), 2, 3—56, 1969.
112. **Kaspar, A. and Willis, M. B.**, Apuntes sobre las tases relativas de crecimiento de toros y novillos con pasto suplementado en los trópicos, *Rev. Cubana Ciencia Agric.*, 3, 17—18, 1969.
113. **Hedrick, H. B., Thompson, G. B., and Krause, G. F.**, Comparisons of feedlot performance and carcass characteristics of half-sib bulls, steers and heifers, *J. Anim. Sci.*, 29, 687—694, 1969.
114. **Hedrick, H. B. and Thompson, G. B.**, Quantitative and qualitative characteristics of beef as influenced by sex and length of time on feed, in *Proc. 2nd World Conf. Anim. Prod., College Park, Md., 1968*, American Dairy Science Association and American Society of Animal Sciences, printed by Bruce Publ., St. Paul, Minn., 1969, 343—344.
115. **Roverso, E. A., Imai, A., Tundishi, A. G. A., and da Finseca, J. C.**, Efeito da idade e método de castracão no desenvolvimento de bovinos da raça Nelore, *Bol. Ind. Anim.*, 26, 67—72, 1969.
116. **Price, M. A. and Yeates, N. T. M.**, Growth rates and carcass characteristics in steers and partial castrates, in *Meat Production from Entire Male Animals*, Rhodes, D. N., Ed., J & A Churchill, London, 1969, 69—77.
117. **Watson, M. J.**, The effects of castration on the growth and meat quality of grazing cattle, *Aust. J. Exp. Agric. Anim. Husb.*, 9, 164—171, 1969.
118. **Yoshida, S., Ueda, K., Terada, T., Tanaka, S., and Ozawa, S.**, Comparative studies on meat production in young growing fattening bulls and steers (in Japanese), *Bull. Chugoku Agric. Exp. Stn. Ser. B. Livest. Div.*, 16, 73—102, 1969.
119. **Bidart, J. B., Koch, R. M., and Arthaud, V. H.**, Comparative energy use in bulls and steers, *J. Anim. Sci.*, 30, 1019—1022, 1970.
120. **Brännäng, E., Henningsson, T., Liljedahl, L. -E. and Lindhé, B.**, Studies on monozygous cattle twins. XXI. The effect of castration and intensity of feeding on the growth rate, feed conversion and carcase traits of Swedish Red and White cattle, *Lantbrukshoegsk. Ann.*, 36, 91—113, 1970.
121. **Kellaway, R. C. and Gaden, E. R.**, Methods of sterilisation in relation to growth and carcass characteristics of male Friesian cattle, *Proc. Aust. Soc. Anim. Prod.*, 8, 231—236, 1970.
122. **Glimp, H. A. and Tuma, H. J.**, The effect of method of sex alteration on growth and carcass traits of cattle, Beef Cattle Field Day, Clay Center, Report, US Meat Animal Research Center, Clay Center, Neb., 1970, 52—57.
123. **Robertson, I. S., Paver, H., and Wilson, J. C.**, Effect of castration and dietary protein level on growth and carcass composition in beef cattle, *J. Agric. Sci.* 74, 299—310, 1970.
124. **Reagan, J. O., Carpenter, Z. L., Smith, G. C., and King, G. T.**, A comparison of palatability traits for beef produced by bulls versus steers, *Beef Cattle Res. Texas*, 66—69, 1970.
125. **Geay, Y. and Malterre, C.**, Influence de la castration et de la nature des glucides de la ration sur la croissance et la qualité des carcasses de bovins abattus à 24 mois. *Ann. Zootech.*, 20, 251—257, 1971.
126. **Kellaway, R. C.**, Growth, fertility and carcase studies with bulls, induced cryptorchids and steers, *Aust. J. Exp. Agric. Anim. Husb.*, 11, 599—603, 1971.
127. **La Hoz, E., Patiño, O., Castro, A., and Reyes, L.**, Efecto de raza y castración en ceba de bovinos Cebu, Romosinuano y Cebu × Romosinuano, en sistema rotacional de pasto para (Brachiaria mutica). in 3rd Reunión Latinoamericano Producción Animal, Bogotá, 1971, 35.
128. **Zieminski, R.**, Badania nad zdolnością opasowa i wartością rzeźna młodego bydła rasy nizinnej czerwono-białej, *Rocz. Nauk Roln. Ser. B*, 93(1), 47—64, 1971.
129. **Ramirez Maya, L. F. and Patiño, H. O.**, Efecto del implante con estilbestrol y la castración en la ceba de ganado Sanmartinero y Holstein en praderas de clima frió, in 3rd Reunión Latinoamericano Producción Animal, Bogotá, 1971, 33.
130. **Reagan, J. O., Carpenter, Z. L., Smith, G. C., and King, G. T.**, Comparison of palatability traits of beef produced by young bulls and steers, *J. Anim. Sci.*, 32, 641—646, 1971.
131. **Ziegler, J. H., Wilson, L. L., and Coble, D. S.**, Comparisons of certain carcass traits of several breeds and crosses of cattle, *J. Anim. Sci.*, 32, 446—450, 1971.
132. **Giannotti, D., Trimarchi, G., and Turriani, G.**, Riflessi della castrazione e della sterilizzazione mediante schiacciamento della coda dell'epididimo in vitelloni di razza Frisona allevati per la produzione della carne, *Riv. Zootec. Agric. Vet.*, 10(2), 43—63, 1972.
133. **Hale, D. H. and Oliver, J.**, The effect of castration and vasectomy on male zebus which grazed veld under two systems of management, *S. Afr. J. Anim. Sci.*, 2(1), 27—31, 1972.
134. **Hale, D. H. and Oliver, J.**, Effect of castration and plane of nutrition on growth of male zebus, *S. Afr. J. Anim. Sci.*, 2(1), 33—34, 1972.

135. **Harte, F. J. and Curran, S.**, Production of beef from young bulls. IV. *Ir. J. Agric. Res.*, 11(3), 251—259, 1972.
136. **LaFlamme, L. F., Trenkle, A., and Topel, D. G.**, Effect of castration or breed type on growth of the longissimus muscle in male cattle, *Growth*, 37(3), 249—256, 1973.
137. **Losada, H., Martin, J. L., Willis, M. B., and Preston, T. R.**, Effect of castration and housing system on growth and carcass composition of F_1 Holstein × Brahman and F_1 Holstein × Santa Gertrudis bulls fed on molasses based diets, *Cuban J. Agric. Sci.*, 7(2), 179—183, 1973.
138. **Joseph, R. L. and Connolly, J.**, Tenderness of bull and steer beef, *Ir. J. Agric. Res.*, 13(3), 307—322, 1974.
139. **Wilson, L. L., Rugh, M. C., Ziegler, J. H., and McAllister, T. J.**, Live and carcass characteristics of Holstein castrated, short scrotum and intact males, *J. Anim. Sci.*, 39(3), 448—492, 1974.
140. **Arzumanyan, E. A. and Ertuev, M. M.**, Comparison of the meat production of bulls and steers, (in Russian), *Izv. Timiryazevskh. Akad.*, 2, 164—175, 1975.
141. **Forrest, R. J.**, Effects of castration, sire and hormone treatments on the quality of rib roasts from Holstein—Friesian males, *Can. J. Anim. Sci.*, 55(3), 287—290, 1975.
142. **Gaillard, C.**, Nachzuchtprüfungsergebnisse der Fleischleistungsprüfung 1972/73, *Mitt. Schweiz. Verb. Kunstl. Besamung Schweiz. Arbgemeinsch. Kunstl. Besamung*, 13(2), 40—43, 1975.
143. **Velloso, L., Silva, L. R. M. da, Boin, C., and Rocha, G. L. da**, Desenvolvimento de bovinos mestiços Holandeses inteiros e castrados, em regime de confinamento e as caracteristicas das carcaças, *Bol. Ind. Anim.*, 32, 37—45, 1975.
144. **Velloso, L., Boin, C., and da Rocha, G. L.**, Bovinos da raca Nelore, inteiros e castrados, em confinamento, *Bol. Ind. Anim.*, 32(1), 9—14, 1975.
145. **Mickan, F. J., Thomas, G. W., and Spiker, S. A.**, A comparison between Friesian bulls and steers on pasture for lean meat production, *Aust. J. Exp. Agric. Anim. Husb.*, 16(80), 297—301, 1976.
146. **Bocsor, G., Bárczy, G., Czakó, J. and Kállay, L.**, Adatok a növendék bikák és tinok hizlalásához, *Allattenyesztes*, 4, 121—130, 1955.
147. **Danilevskiĭ, P. and Maseljuk, V.**, Rearing and fattening entire bulls (in Russian), *Molochnoe Myasn. Skotovod* 6(3), 27—30, 1961.
148. **Migda, I. and Mochalovski, A.**, It is advantageous to fatten uncastrated bulls (in Russian), *Molochnoe Miyash Skotovod.*, 4(8), 47, 1959.
149. **Vezzani, V. and Raimondi, R.**, L'influenza della castrazione sullo sviluppo somatico e sui caratteri delle carni di vitelli piemontesi all'ingrasso, *Riv. Zootec.*, 27, 341—347, 1954.
150. **Boyarskiĭ, L. G.**, The effectiveness of fattening entire bull calves, (in Russian), *Zhivotnovodstvo*, 26(1), 27—30, 1964.
151. **Dikiĭ, N. and Astakhova, M.**, Comparative fattening of bulls and steers (in Russian), *Molochno Myasn. Skotovod. (Kiev)*, 7(10), 24—25, 1962.
152. **Ivanov, P. and Michev, M.**, Comparative fattening trials with Red bulls and steers, (in Bulgarian), *Izv. Inst. Zhivotovud. Sofia*, 18, 5—22, 1963.
153. **Ivanov, P., Vankov, K., and Aleksiev, A.**, Comparative experiment to establish the optimum live weight for intensively fattened bulls and steers (in Bulgarian), *Zhivotnovud. Nauki*, 3, 93—102, 1966.
154. **Ivanov, P., Vankov, K., and Aleksiev, A.**, The optimum live weight for first generation Red Danish crossbred bulls and steers (in Bulgarian), *Zhivotnovdstvo*, 21(3), 24—27, 1967.
155. **Kochenov, D. A.**, The effect of castration at various ages on growth and beef characters of young cattle (in Russian), *Tr. Vses. Nauchno Issled. Inst. Zhivotnovod.*, 24, 49—56, 1962.
156. **Kr"stanov, Kh.**, The fattening of Montafon crossbred bull calves and steers (in Bulgarian), *Izv. Nauchno Issled. Inst. Zhivotnovud. Sofia*, 15, 113—125, 1962.
157. **Miletić, D., Kulaš, C. and Dimitrijević, L.**, The effect of vasectomy in the fattening of cattle (in Serbo-croatian), *Vet. Glas.*, 17, 695—697, 1963.
158. **Peregoncuk, S. T.**, Intensive fattening of entire bulls (in Russian), *Zhivotnovodstvo*, 24(10), 58—63, 1962.
159. Anon., La production des taurillons de boucherie, *Rev. Elev.*, 20(11), 21—33, 1965.
160. **Richter, K., Cranz, K. L., and Schmidt, K. -H.**, Mastversuche mit Jungbullen und Jungochsen. I. Mitteilung. Untersuchungen über den Einfluss einer frühzeitigen Kastration auf die Mastleistung, Schlachttier-und Schlachtkörpergüte. II. Mitteilung. Untersuchungen über den Einfluss einer späten Kastration auf die Mastleistung, Schlachttier- und Schlachtkörpergute, *Zuchtungskunde*, 32, 217—230; 560—574, 1960.
161. **Richter, K., Cranz, K. L., and Schmidt, K. -H.**, Mastversuche mit Jungbullen und Jungochsen. III. Mitteilung: Weitere Untersuchungen über den Einfluss einer späten Kastration auf die Mastleistung, Schlachttier- und Schlachkorperqualitat, *Zuchtungskunde*, 33, 493—510, 1961.
162. **Rostovcev, N. F. and Cherkashchenko, I. I.**, Comparative studies in rearing bulls and steers for meat (in Russian), *Zhivotnovodstvo*, 28(12), 33—37, 1966.
163. **Spivak, M. G.**, The meat production of Simmental bulls and steers (in Russian), *Tr. Vses. Nauchno Issled. Inst. Zhivotnovod*, 28, 109—116, 1966.

164. **Rostovcev, N. F. and Cherkashchenko, I. I.**, The rearing for meat of young cattle of the basic breeds in the USSR (in Russian), *Dokl. Vses. Akad. Skh. Nauk.*, 2, 28—34, 1966.
165. **Rostovcev, N. F. and Shvarts, V. E.**, The effect of castration on growth, hormonal activity of the thyroid and digestion in young cattle (in Russian), *Dokl. Vses. Akad. Skh. Nauk.*, 5, 23—25, 1966.
166. **Watson, W. P.**, Sire testing in Ontario. Beef bulls rated on the performance of progeny, *Scott. Agric.*, 35, 195—196, 1956.
167. **Ivanov, P. and Zahariev, Z.**, Intensive fattening of Kula bull calves and steers (in Bulgarian), *Nauchni Tr. Vissh. Selskostop. Inst. Sofia Zootekh. Fak.*, 14, 9—21, 1964.
168. **Bonini, P.**, Aspetti tecnici ed economici della produzione del baby-beef nelle comuni condizioni delle aziende agrarie dell'alto milanese, *Progresso Vet.*, 21, 384—396, 1966.
169. **Mglinets, A. I.**, The meat quality of bulls and steers (in Russian), *Sb. Nauchn. Rab. Vses. Nauchno Issled. Inst. Zhivotnovod.*, 5, 54—57, 1967.
170. **Berezovoĭ, A. S., Berezovaya, L. P., and Zaritskaya, A. F.**, The effect of crossbreeding and castration on meat quality of young cattle (in Russian), *Tr. Opyt. Sta. Myasn. Skotovod. Kiev*, 2, 107—114, 1968.
171. **Epifanov, G. V.**, Meat production and meat quality of young Simmentals (in Russian), *Tr. Vses. Nauchno Issled. Inst. Zhivotnovod.*, 1, 122—133, 1968.
172. **Gaĭko, A. A.**, Increasing meat production of cattle (in Russian), in *Plemen. Delo i Zhivotnovodstve*, Urozhaĭ, Minsk, 1968, 74—78.
173. **Kadiĭski, E.**, Effect of method of castration on fattening ability in bulls (in Bulgarian), *Nauchni Tr. Vissh. Selskostop. Inst. Sofia Zootekh. Fak.*, 19, 97—110, 1968.
174. **Logunova, R. D. and Shuvalov, P. T.**, Physiological maturity of uncastrated and castrated bulls reared for meat (in Russian), *Sb. Nauchn. Rab. Kurgan. Obl. Gos. Selkh. Opyt. Sta.*, 2, 94—104, 1968.
175. **Mieth, K. and Berg, F.**, Die Jungbullen-Weidemast nach verschiedenen Kastrations- und Sterilisationsverfahren, *Monatshefte VetMed.*, 24, 168—171, 1969.
176. **Mirzaev, Z. K.**, The effect of castration on the morphological composition of meat (in Russian), in *Sb. Statei Molodyth Uchenykh Dagestanskogo Filiala Akad. Nauk SSSR*, 1969, 153—154.
177. **Paisnev, S. G.**, Conformation type and meat production of young Russian Black Pied cattle in relation to sex (in Russian), *Sb. Nauchn. Rab. Vses. Nauchno Issled. Inst. Zhivotnovod.*, 15, 34—36, 1969.
178. **Paishev, S. G.**, Development of young bulls, steers and heifers to 18 month of age under intensive conditions (in Russian), *Sb. Nauchn. Rab. Vses. Nauchno Issled. Inst. Zhivotnovod*, 15, 52—54, 1969.
179. **Paton, A. F.**, A commercial study of bulls and steers reared in individual pens on slats, in *Meat Production from Entire Male Animals*, Rhodes, D. N., Ed., J & A Churchill, London, 1969, 97—102.
180. **Spedding, A. W.**, Some data on commercial bull beef production in the United Kingdom, in *Meat Production from Entire Male Animals*, Rhodes, D. N., Ed., J & A Churchill, London, 1969, 91—95.
181. **Cherekaev, A., Stepanenko, Ya., and Cherekaeva, I.**, Effect of castration on fattening in cattle (in Russian), *Molochnoe Myasn. Skotovod.* 15(12), 9—10, 1970.
182. **Khrapkovskiĭ, A. I. and Mglinets, A. I.**, Meat production and quality of Hereford × Simmental bulls and steers (in Russian), *Dokl. Vses. Akad. Skh. Nauk.*, 7, 29—30, 1970.
183. **Pegov, V. I.**, Meat production of young bulls castrated by the bloodless method (in Russian), *Uch. Zap. Kazan. Vet. Inst.*, 106, 189—194, 1970.
184. **Sharandina, G. I.**, Meat quality and physiological indices of young Simmental cattle in relation to hormonal state (in Russian), *Tr. Vses. Nauchno Issled. Inst. Myasn Skotoved.*, 15(1), 88—95, 1970.
185. **Tugaĭ, L. N.**, Skeletal growth of young Black Pied bulls on moderate feeding as affected by castration (in Russian), *Korma Korml. Skh. Zhivotn. Resp. Mezhved. Temat. Nauch. Sb.*, 10, 97—100, 1967.
186. **Danilevskaya, N. T.**, Post-embryonal growth of the skeleton of young cattle castrated at various ages (in Russian), *Korma Korml. Skh. Zhivotn Resp. Mezhved. Temat. Nauch. Sb.*, 10, 101—110, 1967.
187. **Fomina, A. A.**, Results of histological studies of muscle tissues of steers and bulls (in Russian), *Uch. Zap. Mord. Gos. Univ.*, 59, 97—102, 1967.
188. Anon., Data Sheets on Beef Production and Breeding, Meat and Livestock Commission, Milton Keyner, U.K., 1976, 45—47.
189. Anon., Bull Beef, Meat and Livestock Commission, Milton Keynes, U.K., 1976, 1—12.
190. **Berg, R. T. and Butterfield, R. M.**, *New Concepts of Cattle Growth*, Sydney University Press, Sydney, Australia, 1976, 65—142.
191. **Brännäng, E.**, Studies on monozygous cattle twins. XXIII. The effect of castration and age of castration on the development of single muscles, bones and special sex characters. II. *Swed. J. Agric. Res.*, 1, 69—78, 1971.

192. **Homb, T.**, Sammenligning av okser ok kastrater i kjottproduksjonen, *Beretn. Foringst. Norges Landbruksh.* No. 87, 1958, 70 pp.
193. **Homb, T.**, The use of bulls and steers for fattening, *8th Int. Congr. Anim. Prod.*, Verlag Eugen Ulmer, Stuttgart, Germany, 1961, 18—19.
194. **Glimp, H. A., Dikeman, M. E., Tuma, H. J., Gregory, K. E., and Cundiff, L. V.**, Effect of sex condition on growth and carcass traits of male Hereford and Angus cattle, *J. Anim. Sci.*, 33, 1242—1247, 1971.
195. **Bratzler, L. J., Soule, R. P., Jr., Reineke, E. P., and Paul, P.**, The effect of testosterone and castration on the growth and carcass characteristics of swine, *J. Anim. Sci.*, 13, 171—176, 1954.
196. **Charette, L. A.**, The effects of sex and age of male at castration on growth and carcass quality of Yorkshire swine, *Can. J. Anim. Sci.*, 41, 301—39, 1961.
197. **Carroll, M. A., Hill, F., and O'Donovan, P. B.**, Some effects of castration on pig carcases of pork and bacon weights, *Ir. J. Agric. Res.*, 2, 177—194, 1963.
198. **Kroeske, D.**, Het kastreren van beerbiggen. Een schadelijke gewoonte of een noodzakelijk kwaad? *Veeteelt Zuivelber*, 6, 254—260, 1963.
199. **Teague, H. S., Plimpton, R. F., Jr, Cahill, V. R., Grifo, A. P., Jr, and Kunkle, L. E.**, Influence of diethylstilbestrol implantation on growth and carcass characteristics of boars, *J. Anim. Sci.*, 23, 332—338, 1964.
200. **Blair, R. and English, P. R.**, The effect of sex on growth and carcass quality in the bacon pig, *J. Agric. Sci.*, 64, 169—176, 1965.
201. **Matassino, D., Bordi, A., and Gargiulo, V.**, Alcuni confronti fra maschi interi e castrati nei suini. Nota preliminare, *Prod. Anim.*, 4, 193—215, 1965.
202. **Prescott, J. H. D. and Lamming G. E.**, The influence of castration on the growth of male pigs in relation to high levels of dietary protein, *Anim. Prod.*, 9, 535—545, 1967.
203. **Vold, E.**, Fleischproduktionseigenschaften bei Ebern und Kastraten. II. Untersuchungen des Rückenspeckes von Ebern und Kastraten, *Meld. Nor. Landbrukshoegsk.*, 46(20), 15, 1967.
204. **Angelov, A., Georgiev, I., and Pinkas, A.**, Influence of sex and functional status of sexual glands on fattening capacity of Bulgarian White pigs (in Bulgarian), *Zhivotnovud. Nauki*, 5(7), 13—22, 1968.
205. **Monetti, P. G., Mordenti, A., Manfredini, M., and Santoro, P.**, Effetti della castrazione in suini maschi macellata al p.v. di 95 kg. I. Incrementi ed indici di conversione, *Atti Soc. Ital. Sci. Vet.*, 21, 455—458, 1968.
206. **Mordenti, A., Manfredini, M., Monetti, P. G., and Barbieri, L.**, Effetti della castrazione in suini maschi macellati al p.v. 95 kg. II. Qualità delle carcasse, *Atti Soc. Ital. Sci. Vet.*, 21, 458—464, 1968.
207. **Wong, W. C., and Boylan, W. J., and Stothers, S. C.**, Effects of dietary protein level and sex on swine performance and carcass traits, *Can. J. Anim. Sci.*, 48, 383—388, 1968.
208. **Anastasijević, V.**, Effect of partial castration on fattening capacity and production of meat in Dutch Landrace and Large White pigs (in Serbo-croatian), *Arh. Poljopr. Nauke*, 22(79), 25—62, 1969.
209. **Rodrigues, A. J., Gorni, M., De Almeida, M. A. C., Leitão, P. J. P., and Kalil, E. B.**, Efeito de idade de castracão no desenvolvimento e producão dos suínos, *Bol. Ind. Anim.*, 26, 83—91, 1969.
210. **Witt, M. and Schröder, J.**, Verlauf der Mastleistung bei Ebern, Börgen und Sauen im Mastabschnitt von 40 bis 110 kg Lebendgewicht, *Fleischwirtschaft*, 49, 353—356, 1969.
211. **Spers, A., Rodrigues, A. J., and Neto, L. P.**, Efeito de castracão parcial e total no desempenho, qualidade de carcaca e comportamento sexual dos suínos, *Bol. Ind. Anim.*, 26, 131—145, 1969.
212. **Vold, E.**, Fleischproduktionseigenschaften bei Ebern und Kastraten. III. Untersuchungen der Schlachtkörperzusammensetzung, sowie der Fleisch- und Speckqualität bei Ebern und Kastraten, *Meld. Nor. Landbrukshoegsk.*, 48(23), 50, 1969.
213. **Rhodes, D. N. and Patterson, R. S. L.**, Effects of partial castration on growth and the incidence of boar taint in the pig, *J. Sci. Food Agric.*, 22, 320—324, 1971.
214. **Staun, H.**, Experiments with boars and different methods of castration, *Arsskr. K. Vet. Landbohojsk.*, 1971, 60—71, 1971.
215. **Texier, C., Desmoulin, B., and Dumont, B. L.**, Influence de la castration tardive du porc mâle sur la qualité des carcasses et l'utilisation de la viande, in *Journées de la Recherche Porcine en France*, Institut Technique du Porc, Paris, 1970, 209—216.
216. **Desmoulin, B.**, Qualité de carcasses de porcs Large-White: aptitudes aux rationnements suivant le sexe et après la castration, in *Journées de la Recherche Porcine en France*, Institut Technique du Porc, Paris, 1973, 189—199.
217. **Newell, J. A. and Bowland, J. P.**, Comparison of intact, late-castrated, and diethylstilbestrol (DES)-implanted boars with barrows and gilts: nitrogen and energy digestibility, nitrogen retention, carcass measurements, muscle analyses, and residual DES in muscle tissue, *Can. J. Anim. Sci.*, 53(3), 579—585, 1973.

218. **Newell, J. A. and Bowland, J. P.**, Comparison of boars, barrows and gilts for meat production, in *Proc. 3rd World Conf. Anim. Prod.*, Sydney University Press, Australia, 1973, 555—539.
219. **Newell, J. A., Tucker, L. H., Stinson, G. C., and Bowland, J. P.**, Influence of late castration and diethylstilbestrol implantation on performance of boars and on incidence of boar taint, *Can. J. Anim. Sci.*, 53(2), 205—210, 1973.
220. **Desmoulin, B., Bonneau, M., and Bourdon, D.**, Étude en bilan azoté et composition corporelle des porcs mâles entiers ou castrés de race Large White, in *Journées de la recherche porcine en France*, Institut Technique du Porc, Paris, 1974, 30.
221. **Pay, M. G. and Davies, T. E.**, Growth, food conversion and carcass characteristics in castrated and entire male pigs fed three different dietary protein levels, *J. Agric. Sci.*, 81(1), 65—68, 1973.
222. **Siers, D. G.**, Live and carcass traits in individually fed Yorkshire boars, barrows and gilts, *J. Anim. Sci.*, 41(2), 522—526, 1975.
223. **Calder, A.**, Producing pork from pigs, *Rhod. Agric. J.*, 60, 102—104, 1963.
224. **Nilsson, N. E.**, Kastrationens inflytande på fläskkvaliteten *Svenska Svinavelsfor. Tidskr.*, 10, 185—189, 1961.
225. Anon., Beretning om de af Landøkonomisk Forsøgslaboratorium og De samvirkende danske Andels-Svineslagterier invaerksatte avls-og fodringsforsøg med svin, 1961. Bilag til De samvirkende danske Andels-Svineslagteriers delegeretmøde den 16. og 17. marts 1961. Frederiksberg Bogtrykkeri, Copenhagen, 1961, 1—99.
226. **Sybesma, I.**, De invloed van het tijdstip van castreren op de slachtkwaliteit van de varkens, *Tijdschr. Diergeneeskd.*, 87, 788—789, 1962.
227. **Snovl'anski, B. and Malkin, I.**, The effect of castrating piglings on growth during the suckling period (in Russian), *Vet. Glas.*, 15, 481—484, 1961.
228. **Ushkalov, E. N.**, Castrating pigs for fattening (in Russian), *Zhivotnovodstvo*, 11, 100—101, 1955.
229. **Wallace, L. R.**, The influence of sex upon carcass quality and efficiency of food utilisation, *Proc. N.Z. Soc. Anim. Prod.*, 4, 64—70, 1944.
230. **Grosse, F.**, Der Einfluss des Kastrationsalters auf die Ansatzleistung beim Schwein, *Arch. Tierz.*, 6, 210—230, 1963.
231. **Żebrowski, Z.**, Carcass characters of meat and meat-lard breeds of pig and their crosses (in Russian), *Mezhdunar. Skh. Zh.*, 5(3), 98—107, 1961.
232. **Patterson, R. L. S.**, Boar taint, in *Veterinary Annual.* Vol. 13, 1972, 37—41.
233. **Patterson, R. L. S.**, 5α-androst-16-ene-3-one: —compound responsible for taint in boar fat, *J. Sci. Food Agric.*, 19, 31—38, 1968.
234. **Griffiths, N. M. and Patterson, R. L. S.**, Human olfactory responses to 5α-androst-16-en-3-one — principal component of boar taint, *J. Sci. Food Agric.*, 21, 4—6, 1970.
235. **Wismer-Pedersen, J.**, Boars as meat producers, *World Rev. Anim. Prod.* 4 (19-20), 100—109, 1968.
236. **Rhodes, D. N. and Krylow, A.**, A marketing trial of pork from boars, *Inst. Meat Bull.*, 89, 2—4, 1975.
237. **Rhodes, D. N. and Patterson, R. L. S.**, Effects of partial castration on growth and the incidence of boar taint in the pig, *J. Sci. Food Agric.*, 22, 320—324, 1971.
238. **Rhodes, D. N.**, Consumer testing of bacon from boar and gilt pigs, *J. Sci. Food Agric.*, 22, 485—490, 1971.
239. **Rhodes, D. N.**, Consumer testing of pork from boar and gilt pigs, *J. Sci. Food Agric.*, 23, 1483—1491, 1972.
240. **Rhodes, D. N. and Krylow, A.**, A consumer trial of sausages made from boar pork, *Inst. Meat Bull.*, 92, 13—14, 1976.
241. **Lesser, D., Baron, P. J., and Robb, J. D.**, *Boar bacon — A Consumer Survey*, Pigs Marketing Board (Northern Ireland)and Ulster Curers' Association, 1976, 1—97.
242. **Robb, J. D., Patton, J., and Weatherup, S. T. C.**, The occurrence of abnormal odour in pig carcase fat, in 21st European Meeting of Meat Research Workers, Berne, Switzerland, 1975, 135—137.
243. **Robb, J. D., Patton, J., and Weatherup, S. T. C.**, The effects of breed, age and carcase weight on the occurrence of abnormal odour in boar carcase fat, in 21st European Meeting of Meat Research Workers, Berne, Switzerland, 1975, 138—139.
244. **Jonsson, P.**, Relationship between age of boars and intensity of their odour, *Forsogslab. Arb., Kbh.*, 145—147, 1968.
245. **Jonsson, P., Wismer-Pedersen, J., Jensen, P., and Banyai, A.**, Sex odour in Danish Landrace boars, *Forsogslab. Arb., Kbh.*, 107—115, 1969.
246. **Elsley, F. W. H. and Livingstone, R. M.**, Effect of slaughter weight and feeding level on the incidence of boar taint, in *Meat Production from Entire Male Animals*, Rhodes, D. N., Ed., J & A Churchill, London, 1969, 273—284.
247. **Desmoulin, B., Dumont, B. -L., and Jacquet, B.**, Suitability of Large White boars for meat production, in *Journées de la Recherche Porcine en France*, 1971, Institut Technique du Porc, Paris, 187—195.

248. **Wismer-Pedersen, J., Jonsson, P., Jensen, P., and Banyai, A.,** The occurrence of sex odour in Danish Landrace boars, in *Meat Production from Entire Male Animals,* Rhodes, D. N., Ed., J & A Churchill, London, 1969, 285—295.
249. **Staun, H.,** Experiments with boars and different methods of castration, *Arsskr. K. Vet. Landbohojsk.,* 1971, 60—71, 1971.
250. **Hopkins, I. R.,** The effects of selection on sex differences in pre-weaning growth in beef cattle, *Anim. Prod.,* 25(1), 39—45, 1977.
251. **Jacobs, J. A., Miller, J. C., Sauter, E. A., Howes, A. D., Araji, A. A., Gregory, T. L., and Hurst, C. E.,** Bulls versus steers. II. Palatability and retail acceptance, *J. Anim. Sci.,* 45(4), 699—702, 1977.
252. Meat Research Institute, UK, Biennial report 1975—77, Agricultural Research Council, 1977, 127 pp.
253. **Walstra, P., Buiting, G. A. J., and Mateman, G.,** Fattening of boars. I. Influence of castration and feeding method on growth, food conversion and carcass quality, *Rep., Inst. Veeteelkundig Onderzoek "Schoonoord",* No. B-128, 1977, 78 pp.
254. **Trapnell, M. G., Cooke, B. C., and Curran, M. K.,** The growth response of boars, gilts and castrates to different feed and protein levels, *Paper Summ., Brit. Soc. Anim. Prod., Winter Meeting,* No. 31, 1978, 2 pp.
255. **Patton, J.,** Personal Communication, 1979.

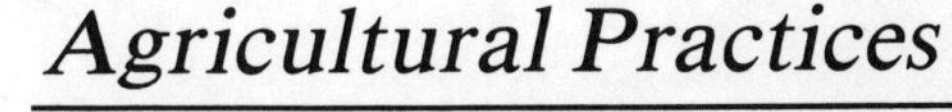

Agricultural Practices

AGRICULTURAL PRODUCTIVITY: POTENTIAL AND CONSTRAINTS *

Theodore C. Byerly

PRODUCTION RESOURCES: SOIL, WATER, AND ENERGY

Agricultural productivity may be measured in terms of total production and yield per hectare or animal unit. Productivity so defined is determined by quantity and quality of resources used, the technology applied in their use, and the impact of weather, pests, and diseases.

The principal resources used are soil, water, nutrients (both plant and animal), seed and livestock breeding animals, crop, machine, and livestock inventories, and energy and pesticides. The productive use of these resources is limited by the availability and use of capital credit and management skills.

Soil, water, and human resources available in 1977 and potentially available for use in the year 2000 are shown in Table 1.

The estimates of energy available for agricultural production in relation to arable land are of particular interest. While these estimates are very crude approximations, the differences among the developing countries and more developed market and centrally planned economies are larger than any probable error in these estimates. The estimated hp/ha in the developed market economies (DME) is about 1.3, for centrally planned economies (CPE) about 0.52, for less developed countries (LDC) about 0.38, and for the U. S. about 1.17. Human and animal labor comprise more than 80% of the total hp equivalent available in the LDC compared to less than 5% in DME. Availability of untiring, mechanical power enables cultivators in DME to plow, plant, and reap during brief periods of favorable weather while LDC cultivators are much more constrained by weather. Scarcity of fossil fuel may continue to make human and animal power more cost effective than mechanical power on the millions of small holdings in LDCs.[52]

Crop Production and Yield

Average production and yields of major crops are summarized for 1977 (Table 2). Drought in Australia reduced yield and production in Oceania.

Cereals are harvested from almost half the arable area. Oil seed crops, including cotton, occupy about 9% of the area and pulses about 5%.

Yield variation among crops is due in part to differences in water content, e.g., cereals contain about 11% water, root crops about 80%. Important inherent differences in yield capacity measured as dry matter, metabolizable energy, protein or other desired trait do exist. These will be discussed in this chapter.

Yield differences among country categories and within crop categories reflect differences in climate, weather, resource quality and inputs of fertilizer, pesticides, and technology. We have noted the apparent gross difference in energy available among country categories.

Yields for the U.S. exceed the world average in each category in which it is represented in Table 2. DME countries, of which the U.S. is one, in aggregate, also exceed world average in these categories.

CPE countries in aggregate exceed world average in several crop categories. LDC countries have aggregate average yields below world average in every crop category except coffee and cocoa.

* Tables follow text, beginning on page 288.

In addition to the crops included in Table 2, there are others for which production data are available but no data for area harvested. Production of these crops is listed in Table 3.

In total, they occupy at least 15 million hectares. These crops added to those in Table 2 thus account for about 1142 million hectares of the 1488 listed in Table 1. The area unaccounted for includes areas used to produce forage for livestock, subsistence gardens and orchards, fallow, idle land, and crop failure.

Forage produced from arable land has been estimated to produce more than 10^{12}Mcal of metabolizable energy in forage for livestock. This is equivalent to about 800 million metric tons of dry matter. Cereal crop residues amount to about the same tonnages as the harvested cereals, in sum, more than a billion metric tons of dry matter, of which much is used as livestock feed.[29]

Inventory numbers of principal livestock species for 1977 are shown in Table 4. The production of carcass meat and the yield per inventory head are shown in Table 5.

Table 6 gives the 1977 production and yield figures for cow's milk and hens' eggs. The average milk production for the same period for buffalo, sheep, and goats is shown in Table 7. Data on the numbers milked of the species in Table 7 are not available.

Cereals vs. Grain Legumes

Average maize yields in the world for 1977 were about 2950 kg/ha, and for soybeans about 1570 kg/ha. In the U. S. average yields for maize were about 5700 kg/ha, for soybeans about 1995 kg/ha, the maize average being almost three times that of soybeans in the U.S.; for the world the maize average was almost twice that of soybeans.

For peanuts the world average production was 942 kg/ha, and for U.S. peanuts, averaged 2725 kg/ha. It is seen that for the world maize averaged three times the yield of peanuts; for the U.S. the maize yield is twice that of peanuts.

The yield of "pulses" (beans, peas, chickpeas, lentils) was lower than those for soybeans and peanuts. The world average for pulses for 1977 was about 683 kg/ha; the yield of all cereals for the world was about 1957 kg/ha (Table 2).

Cereal area harvested increased from the 1961 — 65 average of about 676 million hectares to about 745 million hectares in 1977, an increase of about 10%. The area of pulses harvested was about 68 million hectares in the 1961 — 65 period, and about 70 million hectares in 1977. During the same period, world soybean acreage increased by about 80%, from 27.7 million hectares in 1963 to 49.4 million hectares in 1977; and peanut acreage increased from 17.9 million hectares to 18.5 million hectares. The U.S. and Brazil, respectively, were responsible for about 12.5 and 7.5 million hectares of the increase in soybean acreage. The Brazilian increase was dramatic — from 0.3 million hectares in 1963 to 7.8 million hectares in 1977. Brazil is now a substantial factor in world trade in soybeans.*

In countries depending chiefly on vegetable rather than animal protein, there is some apprehension that high-yielding cereals may displace food legumes which have lower yields but better protein quality than do cereals.

Legume roots are generally nodulated by symbiotic bacteria (*Rhizobium* spp.) which fix atmospheric N_2. About 4 kg of carbohydrate photosynthate is metabolized for each kg/N_2 fixed. Millington and Callaghan[106] stated:

* World production of sunflower oil is second to soybean oil; in 1980, 14.62 million metric tons of soybean oil were produced and 5.56 million metric tons of sunflower oil.[107] Oil varieties were introduced into the U.S. from the U.S.S.R. in 1967.[107,108] About 40,000 ha of oil varieties were harvested in the U.S. in 1967; the total had increased to about 1.62 million ha in 1980.[109,110]

Just as the free living *Azotobacter* require energy foods, so the *Rhizobia* derive sugars parasitically from the host plant. This represents a loss to the plant of 15 to 20% of the sugars produced by photosynthesis, but in return the plant receives 80 to 90% of the nitrogen fixed by the *Rhizobia*.

Amount of photosynthate may be increased by CO_2, an enrichment practicable only in controlled environments. Nodulated legumes show little direct response to nitrogen fertilizer. Addition of fertilizer nitrogen to nitrogen fixing legumes decreases N_2 fixation and does not increase total nitrogen input. Under good field conditions, nodulated grain legumes fix about 75 kg/ha N. Forage legumes with a longer growing season, e.g., alfalfa, may average about 150 kg/ha N. (See in-text table, page 278.)

The five countries included in Table 8 produced about 60% of the world cereal crop in 1977. Relative amounts of the major cereals vary widely. The U.S. produces about 18% of all cereals, 70% of the world maize crop. The U.S.S.R. produces a fourth of the wheat, China a third of the rice, and the U.S.S.R. about 30% of the barley. In wheat production in 1977 no other country exceeded the five listed in the table, but several exceeded the U.S., U.S.S.R., and France in rice production — Indonesia, Bangladesh, Thailand, Japan, and Burma among them. Canada exceeded the U.S. in barley production, and Canada and several European countries exceeded India in barley production.

Figure 1 shows yield of all cereals plotted against N fertilizer consumption as kg/ha of cereals harvested in the world and in the U.S. More than half the N fertilizer is used on cereal crops. The slope of the two lines in the figure indicates that for each increase of 1 kg N/ha an increase of 16 to 17 kg cereals occurred. Since only a portion of the N fertilizer was used on cereals the actual ratio was higher.

The intercept values, 1060 kg cereal/ha for the world and 1500 kg cereal/ha for the U.S. indicate yields likely without the use of any N fertilizer or alternate source of N. The higher base yield for the U.S. reflects its generally fertile soils and generally favorable climate for cereal production.

Assuming that the 16:1 ratio of cereal/N fertilizer continues, increasing the 1973 yield 60% to match projected population increase by the year 2000 would require an additional 35 million metric tons of N fertilizer above 1977 use. Ewell projected an increase of 75 million tons above 1974 consumption of fertilizer by the year 2000 to meet projected demand for cereals in the developing countries.[27]

Efficiency of Resource Use

Area of cropland harvested in the U.S. increased until about 1930 and then declined to 1970 in response to crop adjustment programs. The area harvested increased after 1970 in response to increased export demand (Figure 2). Production in 1977 is in excess of probable demand. Continuing abundance may be used for "gasohol" production.

Total inputs, farm produced and purchased, measured in 1976 dollars, increased to about 1930 and have been relatively constant since that time. Farm output and the output/input ratio in 1975 were two and a half times greater than in 1910 (Figure 2).

Horse, mule, and human labor have been largely replaced by tractor, truck, and electrically delivered fossil fuel energy. Tractor fuel constitutes only a fraction of the energy used directly and indirectly in agricultural production.[64,81] Farm output in relation to available tractor hp has decreased steadily (Figure 3).

The Law of Diminishing Returns

Increases in agricultural productivity must finally reach an asymptote. Yield asymptotes are specific for site, crop, time, and technology. Corn, sorghum, soy, broilers, turkeys, beef cattle, and hogs — these are the crops for which the U.S. excels. Yield asymptotes for average cornbelt corn yields 25 years ago were assumed to be about 5

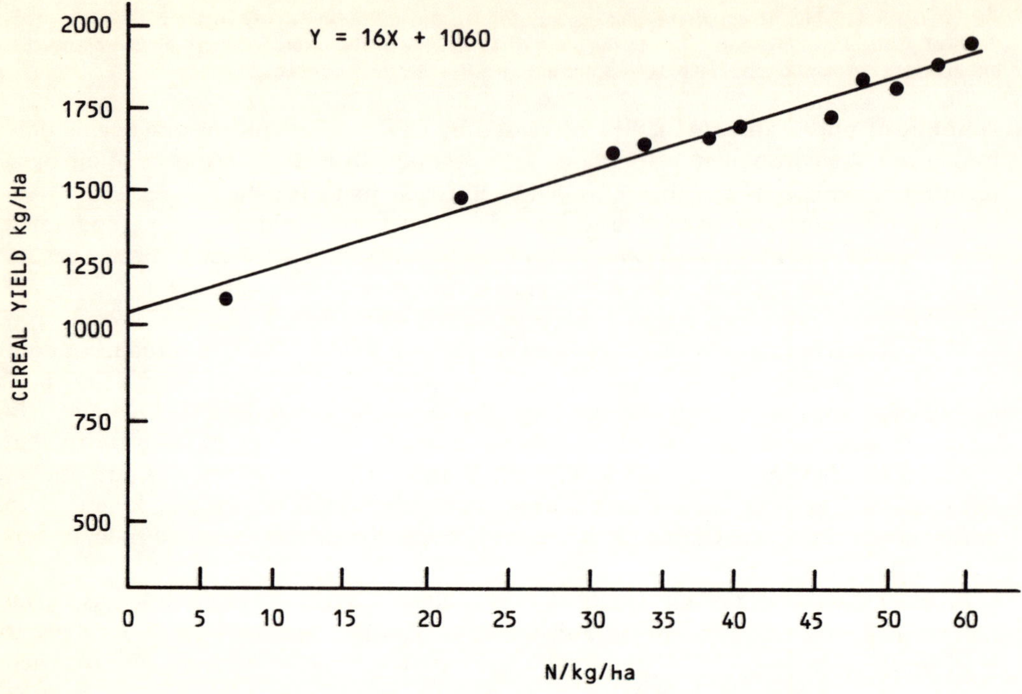

FIGURE 1. World cereal yield and N fertilizer consumption 1950—1977.

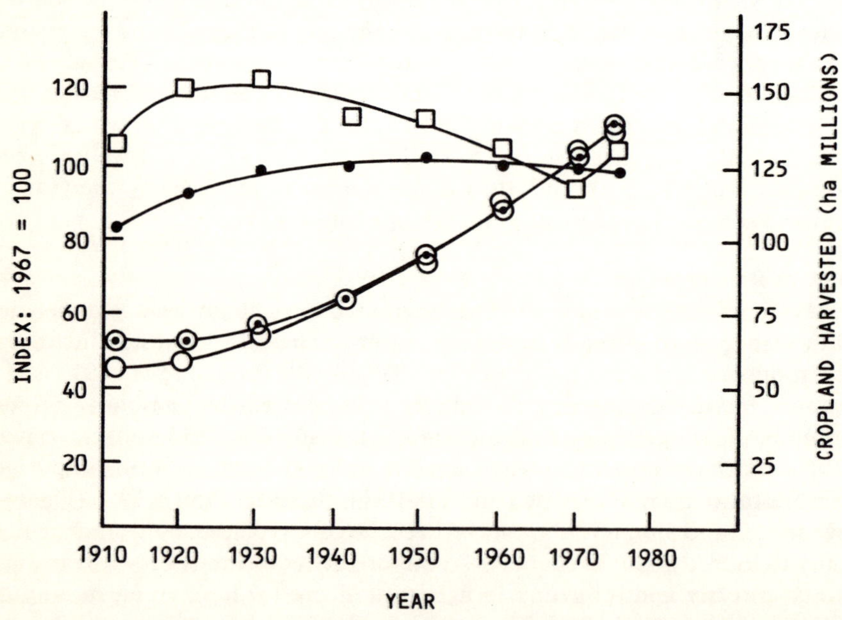

FIGURE 2. 1910—1975 U.S. harvested cropland: land □, farm input ●, farm production ○, output/input ⊙. (Data from Durost, D. D. and Black, E., Stat. Bull. 561, U.S. Department of Agriculture, Washington, D.C. 1976.)

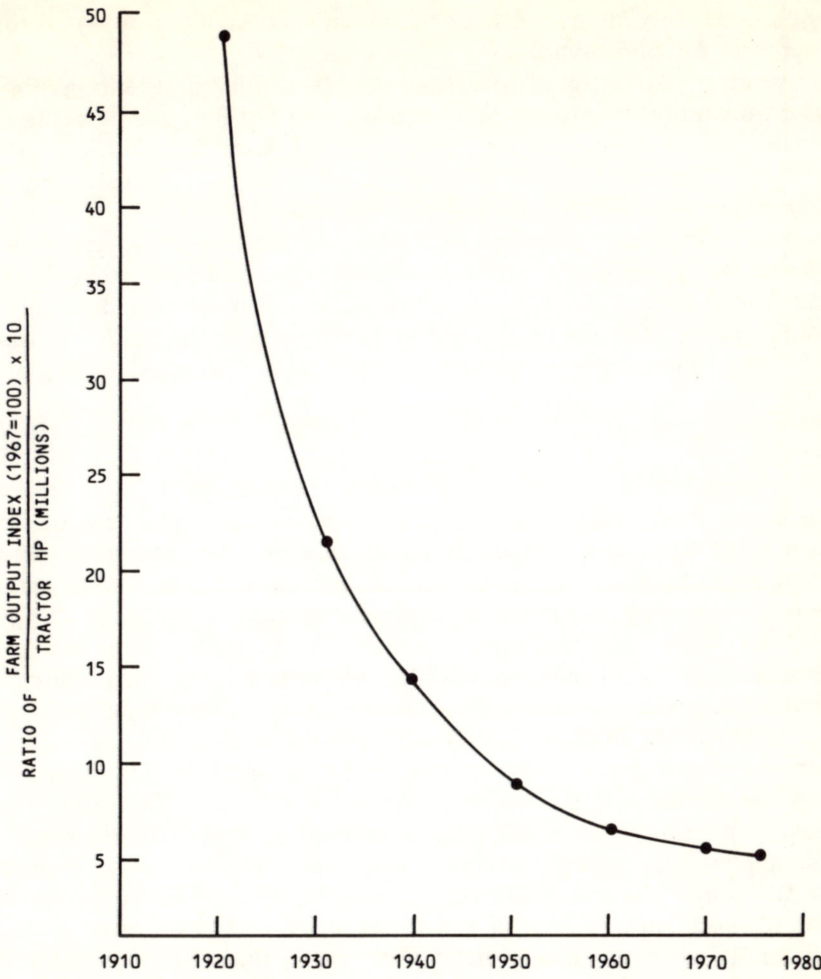

FIGURE 3. Diminishing ratio of Farm-output/tractor-horsepower, 1910—1975, U.S.

metric tons/ha. That yield is now below expected average. A new asymptote of 10 metric tons/ha is reasonable. It is approachable only within the limits of the law of diminishing returns.

Justus von Liebig recognized[98] that adding mineral nutrients or nitrogen to soils already rich in these elements would not increase crop yields. The Spillman[75] equation is $Y = M - AR^x$, in which Y is yield when x units of fertilizer nutrient are applied; M is the maximum yield as x increases indefinitely; and R is the ratio of a decreasing geometric series of the increments in yield in response to successive increments in x.

The operation of the law of diminishing returns is demonstrated by the ratio of farm output to tractor horsepower shown in Figure 3. As tractor horsepower increased from 10 million in 1920 to 230 million in 1973, the ratio decreased from about 48 index points per 10 million tractor hp to less than 5.

PRODUCTION SYSTEMS

In the world generally, agricultural technology is adapted to widely varying production systems. Grazing systems and dryland-rainfed cereal, cotton, and oil seed production require relatively large land areas with relatively small energy inputs (other than solar energy used in photosynthesis) per unit area.

Intensive crop systems, e.g., irrigation, double cropping, genetically high-yielding seeds and animal breeding stocks, and high levels of fertilizer and pesticide chemicals, may be labor intensive (as are most vegetable and fruit crops) or fuel energy intensive, e.g., cereal production in industrial countries, or both. Such systems limit harvested area, conserving land for environmental and other uses.

All technologies involve management based on experience, discovery, research, and development though in widely varying mixes. In every case productivity is determined by interaction of genetic capacity, nutrition, and environment, and depends on protection from diseases, pests and other hazards. In crop production, with soil, water, seeds adapted to site, timely culture and pest management are principal interacting parameters.[18]

Small Holders

Small holdings and labor intensive agriculture are generally, but not necessarily, less efficient economically than larger holdings. Economically, unit cost of inputs purchased in small quantities is generally higher than for the same input purchased in larger quantities. Machines, e.g., tractors, of small capacity are generally more expensive per unit of capacity than machines of larger capacity.

Production per physical unit input of energy, for example, of chemicals, of water, of improved seeds, or of managerial skill, need not be lower than returns on larger units. Indeed, proprietor-operated small holdings often achieve higher yields than large holdings whether individually or collectively operated.

Wortman[103] stated that "Farmers, even those who have tiny land holdings, are willing to change to new, more productive systems if they can." Opportunity to change includes information and demonstration of technology adapted to their needs, availability of supplies of necessary purchased inputs and credit to procure them, and markets for their products which will assure equitable return for their effort. He cited examples of mixed culture of corn and wheat which he had observed in the People's Republic of China with unit area yields 40% greater than that obtained by monoculture. Nonetheless, China, too, is mechanizing her agriculture. The Food and Agricultural Organization[28c] reported 200,000 tractors in the People's Republic of China in 1977, 50% more than in 1970. Planting labor and harvesting labor are often critically important to yield and quality of product. Availability of machines and the fuel to operate them facilitate timely planting and harvest.

Small holders in many tropical developing countries continue to use the ancient practice of slash-and-burn, girdling trees to kill them, burning when dry, planting in the ash-covered soil. Slash-and-burn is not a destructive system when the carrying capacity of the ecosystems where it is practiced is not exceeded. In many tropical areas this may mean a 25-year rotation, 20 years or longer in trees, 2 or 3 years in food crops.

Deep-rooted trees lift mineral nutrients from their root zones and deposit them in stem and leaf. Slash-and-burn leaves these nutrients in ash on the soil surface where they may be utilized by crop plants. Nutrients exhausted, a new area must be slashed, burned, and cultivated. Where human population needs more than about 5% of the arable land under cultivation at one time, slash-and-burn must fail.

We now harvest crops from about 35% of the world's potentially arable land. Carrying capacity of cropland, in terms of people supplied with food, in the U.S. has increased from 1.25 people/ha in 1952 to more than 2 people/ha in 1977.[39] Greenland[32] has suggested that small holders can modify their traditional methods of shifting cultivators and double carrying capacity with minimal monetary cost. They would need high-yielding, pest-resistant crop plants, adapted legumes, and some phosphorus.

Monoculture vs. Mixed Cropping

It is often argued that plant and animal ecosystems consisting of two or more species, cultivars, or genotypes may utilize resources of the system more efficiently than monocultures. Grazing land mixtures of grasses, legumes, and browse species often exceed monocultures in biomass and quality of forage produced. Legumes in the mixture may provide some nitrogen for use by nonleguminous plants in the mixture. Information on binary crop plant mixtures indicates that total biomass production of such mixtures is often no greater than that of monocultures. Trenbath[87] cited, as conditions under which mixtures may out-yield monocultures, differing maturity dates of the components, differing rooting depths, nutritional complementarity, and enhanced light-use efficiency. Factors cited as responsible for underyielding of mixtures include allelopathy and infection of susceptible components by pathogens carried by infected resistant components.

Increases in total annual yields per unit area may be achieved by planting successive crops. Such systems may involve interplanting of succeeding crops prior to maturity of the preceding crop. Such successions may be of the same or different plant species. Examples of such successions include use of cereal grains as "nurse" crops for establishment of forage grasses and legumes, successive rice crops in much of Southeast Asia, soybeans following fall-sown cereals in the southern half of the U.S.

Successions include "cover crops" which may reduce erosion during the winter and contribute improved tilth and some nitrogen to the succeeding crop when "plowed down" rather than harvested.

Winter cereals and cool weather legumes provide grazing for livestock in many countries, including the U.S., in areas roughly bounded by 30°N and 30°S. Wheat, rye, oats, and clovers are grazed on millions of acres. *Trifolium alexandrinum* (berseem) is a clover widely used for winter grazing in Egypt and other Middle Eastern countries. Potential area of this grazing resource in the countries between 30°N and 30°S is roughly that of the wheat and barley areas sown. Grass, legume, and weedy species provide some grazing on other croplands between growing seasons.

Winter cereal grazing is highly variable in productivity. Fall rains may stimulate lush fall growth providing abundant grazing throughout a mild winter. Drought may delay germination and fall growth, limiting grazing to a brief spring period. In many areas use of chemical fertilizers, especially nitrogen, greatly increases forage production. Fertilization with nitrogen at the close of the winter grazing system may be necessary in order to assure acceptable grain yields of winter grazed cereals. In the U.S. gulf coast states rye and winter oats are often sown for winter pasture only. Economic returns from such winter cereal grazing has been greatly constrained by recent increases in fertilizer nitrogen prices.

Organic Farming

Organic farming may be defined as use of manure, composts, crop residues and grass-legume rotations in lieu of synthetic fertilizers and pesticides.

Klepper et al.[48] reported data for 16 matched pairs of cornbelt farms for 1974. One set (organic) used no synthetic fertilizer or pesticides; the other set (conventional) did. Basic data are shown in Table 9.

The two sets of farms had beef, dairy, or hog enterprises, with an average population of 137 (organic farms) and 128 (conventional farms) animal units. Both sets of farms used animal manures. The organic farms spread 3.8 t/ha on 26 ha of cropland, and the conventional farms spread 2.8 t/ha on 30 ha. Crop yields per hectare on the two sets of farms did not vary significantly. Aggregate production of corn, wheat, oats, and soybeans on the organic farms was 209 t vs. 382 t on the conventional farms.

Livestock wastes produced in large scale confined feedlot cattle and pigs and in egg, turkey, and broiler operations are a potential source of some additional N as fertilizer. Storage and transportation problems deter such use.[83]

CLIMATE AND WEATHER

Weather is the major cause of annual fluctuations in crop yields. Fluctuations from trend line may confound long term estimates of yield increases attributable to technology. Thompson[84] calculated Great Plains wheat yield increases from 1935 to 1961 as about equally due to technology and to favorable weather following the very unfavorable weather of the 1930s. Yields of corn, sorghum, and soybeans in the rainfed areas of the Midwest show similar fluctuations due to weather.[19] Long time climatic changes may change fertile areas to barren ones — or vice versa.[8]

Time trends for corn, wheat, sorghum, barley, and even soy, for the period 1930 to date reflect increasing inputs of technology. Deviations may be more than half due to weather — periods of excessive heat, cold, drought, or excessive moisture during the growing season, modulated by soil moisture reservers and, for fall sown wheat, temperature during the preceding winter. Other occasionally overwhelming causes of variation from time trend line may be caused by pests and disease, e.g., wheat rust.[36,84]

Apparent leveling off of time trend yield curves during the 70s has generated speculation that technology response is declining.

Solar Energy and Photosynthesis

Solar energy reaching the earth's surface may be converted or conducted into the air as sensible heat, conducted into soil or water, used to evaporate water, or used in photosynthesis.

The maximum thermal efficiency of transfer of sunlight energy to photosynthate by plants is about 14%.[104] About 10% is lost by reflection from the leaf surface; about 46% is in the photosynthetically effective spectrum wavelengths of 0.4 μ to 0.7 μ. Of this portion, about 33% may be stored in photosynthate.

Lemon[50] observed photosynthesis in a New York cornfield in August with efficiencies of about 4%. Efficiency for the growing season was 2% or less. Mutual shading by the leaves of a plant reduces the sunlight energy absorbed. Lemon observed that the leaves of a corn plant may have an aggregate surface four to five times that of the earth surface under them. Plant breeders have changed corn leaves from the former drooping posture to an upright one to provide maximum effective exposure to sunlight and they have thus increased corn yield.

Genetic and Environmental Factors Affecting Photosynthesis

In C_3 plants the 3 carbon phosphoglyceric acid is the first stable carbon compound formed in photosynthesis.[14] In C_4 plants, the first stable carbon may be malic or another 4-carbon acid.[49] Plants with the C_4 pathway use less water per unit dry matter produced than C_3 plants. C_3 plants lose photosynthate through photorespiration, which increases as ambient temperature increases. Photorespiration may consume 25% or more of photosynthate formed by C_3 plants.[89] Some plants with C_4 pathway give highest yields of dry matter. Sugar cane (*Saccharum sativa*) and Napier grass (*Pennesetum purpureum*) are examples. In temperate climates, among crop plants with determinate growth, C_4 species such as maize (*Zea mays*) and sorghum (*Sorghum*) which thrive in warm weather may outyield C_3 species, e.g., wheat (*Triticum*) or barley (*Hordeum*) which grow best in cool weather. In cool climates C_4 species may be replaced by C_3 species in natural plant communities used for grazing.

Alfalfa, a C_3 species with indeterminate growth, may equal C_4 species in dry matter

(DM) production in warm, dry, irrigated areas but at a water cost per unit; DM produced is twice that of corn or sorghum.[9,73,105]

A third photosynthetic pathway (CAM) is used by many crassulaceous species which can fix carbon dioxide in the dark. In such plants phosphoenopyruvate (PEP) and atmospheric CO_2 react to form malate.[96] PEP is formed from stored carbohydrate.

Water

Average annual precipitation in the U.S. is about 750 mm, a total of 4.75×10^9 acre feet. Of this amount, about 250 mm runs off the land. The remaining 500 mm is used in evapotranspiration or percolates to ground water.[42,100] About 345 million acre feet are diverted for household (8%), industrial (46%), or irrigation (46%) use. Most of the household and industrial water is recycled while most of that used for irrigation is "consumptively" used, returned to the air by evapotranspiration.

In the 17 western states with an average precipitation of 520 mm, average evapotranspiration exceeds precipitation in most of the area, while in the eastern 31 contiguous states (average precipitation 1200 mm) precipitation may exceed evapotranspiration. Seasonal differences are large, so that drainage is necessary for cropland and summer droughts limit productivity.[69]

In most agricultural areas of the world water availability is a limiting factor in agricultural productivity. Genetically high-yielding crop plants must have ample but not excessive supplies of water throughout the growing season in order to reach that potential.

Water is not only necessary for plant growth and metabolism, but evaporation from leaf surface modulates excessive heat through evaporative cooling and maintains moist surfaces in stomates and areas where O_2 — CO_2 exchange takes place.

Crop plants vary genetically in their water requirements. Length of growing season, ambient humidity, insolation temperature, and air movement all affect consumptive use. Annual plants use little water when small, but require larger amounts as vegetative growth and photosynthesis increase.

Troughton[88] remarked, "The results of Shantz and Piemeisel[73] provide, in retrospect, evidence that C_4 type plants use half as much water as C_3 type plants, in producing the same amount of dry matter." Crassulaceous plants, for example *Bryophyllum calycinum,* assimilate CO_2 in the dark.[17]

The data in Table 10 for irrigation water use are from observations made at Mesa, Arizona where annual precipitation is about 200 mm. The water required for wheat, 1380 mt water per ton of grain DM, shows higher efficiency of water use than the 1000 t/1000 lb grain cited by Callaghan and Millington for dry land production in Australia.[13] The Arizona yields on which estimates are shown in Table 10 are based on the state yields for 1974 from the U.S. Department of Agriculture.[93] Wheat yields in Arizona for that year averaged 66 bushels/acre compared to 13.1 bushels/acre in Australia. The higher Arizona yield probably accounts for the more efficient water use.

Yield data in Table 10 are calculated on a DM basis. For barley, sorghum, and wheat only grain is included, while for alfalfa the entire aerial part of the plant is harvested. Assuming that grain and straw or stover are equal in DM, the cereals required for each metric ton of DM: barley — 920 t; sorghum — 695 t; wheat — 690 t. These are compared to 1500 t for alfalfa. Briggs and Shantz[6] established the fact that alfalfa requires about twice as much water to produce a pound of DM as sorghum does.

Halvorson[34] showed that in the state of Washington 100 mm of soil moisture is needed for vegetative growth of the wheat plant. He reported that each additional 25 mm (ca. 100 t/ha) produced 400 kg of grain with stiff strawed semidwarf wheat but only 380 kg with tall cultivars.

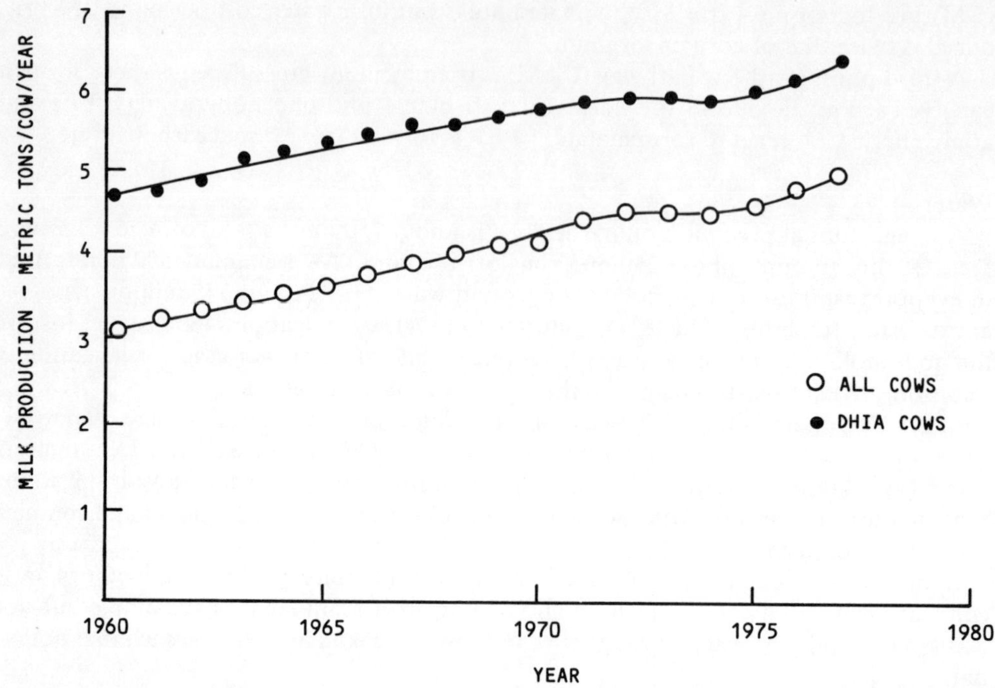

FIGURE 4. U.S. milk production per cow, 1960—1977.

About 16 million hectares were irrigated in the U.S. during 1976. About 10 million hectares were irrigated with pumped water, the remainder by gravity flow from streams and reservoirs. About 81 × 10^9 t of irrigation water were pumped; about 100 × 10^9 t were obtained from surface water. Total energy requirement for irrigation is about one fifth of all energy used directly in agricultural production.[64]

In Arizona about 10,000 t of irrigation water are used per hectare of irrigated land at a cost of about 17.6 Mcal of energy for pumping and distribution. This is about the amount used to produce cotton. The energy expended in irrigating the cotton is about equal to the gross energy of the seed cotton harvested.[70]

Selective Breeding to Enhance Productivity

Selective breeding for a highly heritable trait is one method of increasing yield. This method has been highly effective in increasing milk yield of cows in the U.S. Artificial insemination (AI) of superior sires has accounted for about one third of the increase in yield per cow shown in Figure 4.

Milk production per cow in the U.S. increased from about 3190 kg/cow/year in 1960 to about 5000 kg/cow/year in 1977. At least a third of the increase was due to the use of improved sires, largely through AI. Herds participating in the Dairy Herd Improvement Association increased from about 4100 kg/cow/year to 6550 kg/cow/year during the same period (Figure 4).[47,94]

Selective breeding for short, stiff straw in wheat (semidwarf) and rice have major potential for increased yield because such genetic stocks are fertilizer responsive, while tall stocks fall to the ground, plants shade one another, and photosynthetic surface is so limited that high rates of nitrogen fertilization may result in reduced yields. Selection for photoperiod has produced genetic stocks of maize and soybeans adapted to day lengths both further from and nearer to the equator. Similarly, wheat stocks have been selected which are insensitive to day length and thus are adapted to tropical latitudes. Other examples of such selection include resistance to plant diseases, the method of choice for protection against cereal rusts, and of fungal and bacterial diseases of many vegetable, fruit, and sugar crops.

Hybrid breeding has been a major factor in increasing yield of such crops as maize, sorghum, hogs, and eggs. Probably 20% of current U.S. yields of these crops are due to vigor resulting from hybrid breeding.

The vulnerability implicit in selective breeding may be illustrated by the 1970 experience in the U.S. with "Southern Corn Blight". This disease has long been a minor problem in the Southern states. In 1970, its virulence increased, weather conditions were favorable to its development, and large areas in the cornbelt states were affected.

Most of the commercial maize then carried the "Texas cytoplasmic male sterile" gene used in production of hybrid seed corn without de-tasseling. That gene also made the maize carrying it vulnerable to Southern Corn Blight. Losses measured in terms of reduction in anticipated yield have been estimated at 20 million metric tons of grain.

Breeders replaced the vulnerable gene with others not so vulnerable within a year.[30,35]

FERTILIZATION

From the time man became a cultivator until the synthesis of organic chemicals by Wohler in 1840, he sowed, scratched, planted, harvested a crop or two, and started over again. "Swidden agriculture" they called it in Europe. "Slash-and-burn" we call it now in the extensive tropical and subtropical areas where the practice continues. Ash from the trees provided essential mineral nutrients. Unburned humus on the forest floor provided a little nitrogen.

Fallow periods provided time for mineralization of soil nitrogen and accumulation of some that fell in rain and some contributed by free living nitrogen fixing bacteria and blue green algae.

The practice of manuring with animal and human wastes, composted plant wastes, and green manuring helped. The plow killed plants, and part of their nitrogen was released for crop use.

But not until World War I did fixed atmospheric nitrogen become available for extensive fertilizer use and not until the post World War II era did abundant natural gas for manufacture of fixed N fertilizer make it cheap and abundant. The price of N fertilizer in the U.S. was as high in 1949 as in 1974 when the energy shortage drove N fertilizer prices up threefold. The price has since dropped.

N fertilizer used on maize in 1976 in the U.S. was about 145 kg/ha, on wheat 40kg/ha, and on cotton 70 kg/ha.

Figure 5 shows average U.S. maize yield in relation to rate of commercial N fertilizer use in its production from 1950 to 1954 to 1977. The rate of N use for maize production increased about tenfold during the period. Maize yield doubled. Favorable weather was probably responsible for part of the increased yield. See section on Climate and Weather.

Attributing all N fertilizer to cereals, as in Figure 1, gives a minimal estimate of efficiency of use of fertilizer N use by cereals. The apparent value of 16 kg cereal for each kg N fertilizer used is probably about half the true value. Assuming a harvest index of 0.5 and a nitrogen contents of whole plant cereal as 1%, this would yield a 64% conversion, which is reasonable for recent levels of N fertilizer use.

Figure 1 indicates that without synthetic N fertilizer or added N from other sources, world cereal yields would fall to 1060 g/ha, slightly below the 1950 yield. This residual, intercept yield would be achieved by N recycled through rain, N fixed by legume symbiotic bacteria, by N fixed by free living bacteria (e.g., *Azotobacter*), by symbiotic bacteria (e.g., *Spirillum*), and by blue green algae, and from soil reserves. These latter are still large in many grassland and peat areas.

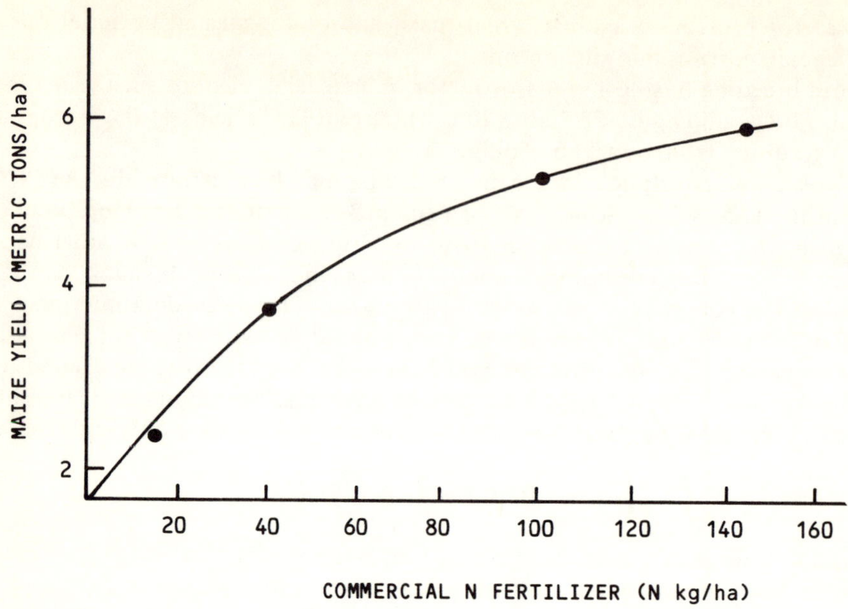

FIGURE 5. U.S. maize yield and commercial N fertilizer — N kg/ha. (Maize yield and the estimated use of commercial N fertilizer on maize were calculated from data in the U.S. Department of Agriculture Agricultural Statistics for the years 1972, 1973, 1974, 1975, and 1976.)

Crops harvested remove plant nutrients from the soil which must be replaced in order to maintain productivity. Recycling of plant residues, animal and human wastes, and nitrogen and sulfur compounds deposited by rain contributes to the replacement process. With due regard for use of animal manure as a fuel, its wide dispersion on pasture and range, and its wastage in storage and feedlots, perhaps 10 million metric tons of nitrogen from manure are applied by cultivators to the fields of the world.[82]

Chemical fertilizers are used in increasing amounts. In addition to those listed in Table 11, several mineral nutrients are necessary in small amounts. Large quantities of lime are applied to correct soil acidity.

Legumes

Results of legume-wheat succession in Australia indicate accumulation of about 56 kg N/ha/year in "Subclover" pastures.[13] This may be compared with the gain of about 900 kg N/ha in 7 years of continuous crested wheat grass-alfalfa unharvested. Yields of wheat in successive years following several years of subclover averaged about 2.6 t/ha/year. Nitrogen in the grain amounted to about 55 kg/year. Total loss of N from the soil was about 130 kg/ha/year, of which 42% was harvested in the grain. Thus about 13 years of subclover were required to supply the N used and lost by six successive wheat crops.

Callaghan and Millington[13] noted that on some "red-brown earth" soils with 400 to 625 cm in annual precipitation, continuous cropping of alfalfa had dropped the water table, originally within 3 ft below the surface to 10 m below the surface. In Australia the marginal precipitation limit for wheat is about 250 mm/year. In such areas, drought defined as 5 successive months in which evaporation is more than three times precipitation, may be expected in 2 years out of 3.[65,85,90]

Maize and Nitrogen

In the cornbelt, 63 years of continuous corn resulted in decrease in soil nitrogen

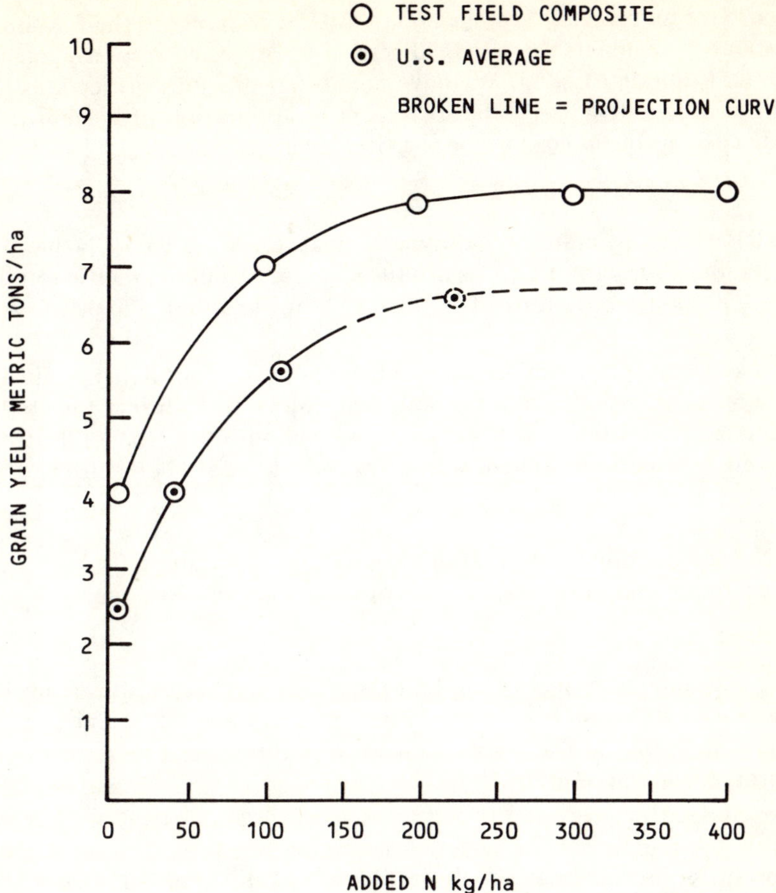

FIGURE 6. Maize yield response to nitrogen.

from initial 3.8 t/ha to a final 0.9 t/ha. Corn yields during the last 4 years reported were about 1.1 t/ha. Under a 4-year rotation of corn, wheat, oats and red clover, soil N after 63 years was about 2.2 t/ha and corn yield about 2.6 t/ha. Smith[74] stated:

Although legumes can have marked benefits both in adding nitrogen, and improving soil structures, a legume crop removed for hay depletes soil minerals and leaves little nitrogen. When a hay crop is removed, the nitrogen carried away in the forage frequently represents that fixed from the atmosphere by the bacteria while that remaining in the roots represents little beyond the amount absorbed from the soil.

Smith concluded that yields of 6 metric tons of maize per hectare could be obtained by use of sufficient N fertilizer. His report was published at about the time that use of synthetic N became general on cornbelt maize. Such use now averages about 145 kg/ha. Average corn yield for the U.S. was about 2.5 t/ha in 1952, compared to current yields of about 5.0 t/ha.

Ten states produced more than 80% of the U.S. 1977 maize crop. These states used about half of all the synthetic N fertilizer.[94] Such use has increased about tenfold since 1950. Maize yields increased from about 2.5 t/ha during 1950 to 1954 to about 5.7 t/ha in 1977 (Figure 5).

The composite N fertilizer-cornyield response curve in Figure 6 indicates that test field yields of maize increased by about 30 quintals/ha in response to the first 100 kg N/ha. Response to the second 100 kg was only about 8 quintals/ha, half the projected world response for all cereals. Average apparent U.S. response to the first hundred kg N/ha was about the same as the test field response. Projected response to the second hundred kg/ha is about 10 q/ha. We have noted that previous projections have generally been exceeded.[24,77,80,92,93,101] Improvement in application of current technology might raise the asymptote at least to the test field level.

Soybeans

Evans and Barber[26] estimated that soybeans may fix 57 to 94 kg N/ha. The 1975 U.S. crop of about 21 million hectaves produced about 38 million metric tons of beans containing 1.9 million metric tons of N, of which not less than 300,000 t came from the soil.

Nodulated soybeans grown in fertile cornbelt soils fix about half the nitrogen they use and obtain the other half from the soil. Johnson et al.,[44] during the 1971 to 1973 period, estimated that Illinois soybeans removed about 70 kg/ha of N from fields where they were grown. Soybeans show little response to added N fertilizer.

Cotton

Rates of N fertilizer applied to cotton vary widely, from about 70 kg/ha in Texas to about twice that rate in the irrigated fields of California and Arizona.

Wheat

N fertilizer was applied to more than half the wheat acreage at rates from 10 kg/ha in dryland wheat to 70 kg/ha on irrigated wheat and to wheat in humid areas. Winter wheat responds to spring fertilization by foliar application with increase in yield and increase in protein content of grain.[40]

Rice

Stiff-strawed rice is responsive to N fertilizer.[113] Tall, weak-strained *indica* types lodge under heavy N fertilization and show little yield response to N. Doyle[20] summarized 38 N-fertilizer rice yield tests in 20 countries. He reported that yield of paddy rice as 12.67 kg/ha (y) per kg N applied. (Equation: $y = 12.67 \times x - 5.67$.) A yield response curve for Arkansas rice (Figure 7) shows the usual diminishing response to added increments of N. The Arkansas data show a yield response of about 32 kg/kg N for the first 100 kg and about 12 kg for the second 100 kg.

Brady,[4] director of International Rice Research Institute, reported that high-yielding rice varieties introduced into several Asian countries about 1965 had increased by 1973 crop year to more than 35% of the harvested rice area in Pakistan, Malaysia, and the Philippines. Examination of data[28a,28b] on rice production indicates an increase from 1967 to 1974 of about 5% in area and 25% in yield. Exports and imports of rice for the three countries approximately balanced.

Per capita supply-production and export-import were unchanged, about 85 kg per capita in 1969 and in 1974. Thus high-yielding rice and the package of practices necessary to its success kept pace with population increase.

Brady also reported that the IRRI yields, where water, fertilizer, weeds, insects, and diseases are controlled, when compared to yields obtained by Philippine farmers without such control, indicated that these factors increased yield by 2 to 3 t/ha.[18]

Evans and Barber[26] estimated that biological nitrogen fixation by legumes and some other organisms was as follows:

Organism	N_2/kg/ha/year
Clover	104—160
Alfalfa	128—600

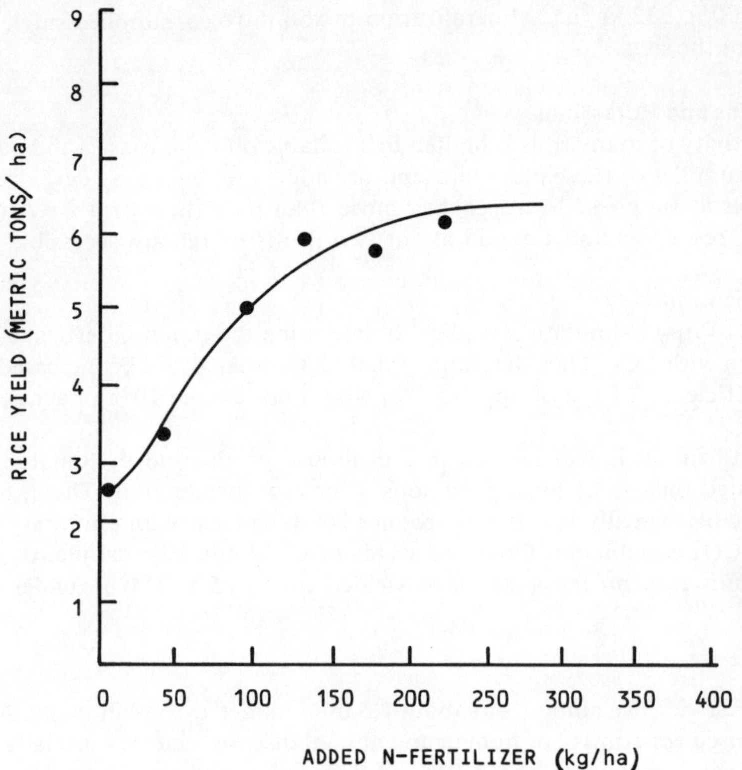

FIGURE 7. Rice yield response to N fertilizer. (From Doyle, J. J., Agric. Studies No. 70, Food and Agriculture Organization, Rome, 1966. With permission.)

Lichens	39—84
Bluegreen algae	25
Azotobacter	0.3

Using the mean value for alfalfa, the alfalfa hay area harvested in 1974 may have fixed 1.32 million t nitrogen, of which most was harvested in the hay crop (*vide supra*)

Evans and Barber further stated,[26] "There is no doubt that nitrogen fixation occurs in root environments of non nodulated species, but this type of fixation in well-aerated environments is sporadic, difficult or impossible to reproduce and for the most part fails to occur at rates sufficient to meet the requirements of intensive crops." Compare this view with von Bulow and Dobereiner.[97]

Sugar Crops

Some varieties of sugar cane have a higher nitrogen requirement for maximum yield of DM than for maximum sugar yield, while other varieties may have about the same requirements for both. Sugar beets appear to have a higher requirement for maximum DM than for maximum sucrose.

For sugar cane, Stanford and Ayers[78] found a requirement for near maximum yield of about 2 kg/ton of DM produced.

Stanford et al.[79] reported that residual NO_3 N in the root zone and N mineralized during the growing season are utilized by sugar beets with an efficiency of about 73% under optimal fertilization. They concluded that N use for sugarbeets in southern Idaho is excessive in many fields. In 1976 they reported that soils at 30 sites in southern Idaho varied in requirements for added N necessary for maximum sugar beet sucrose yield from 0 to 332 kg/ha. Mineralization of soil nitrogen supplied sufficient nitrogen to twelve of the sites.[15]

Phosphorus and Potassium

Productivity of many soils is limited by available phosphorus (P) and potassium (K). World supplies of these plant nutrients are adequate, but many developing countries lack domestic supplies. Morocco has more than half the world's readily accessible phosphate resources and Canada about two thirds of readily accessible potassium.[71]

CO_2 Fertilization

Allen et al[2] used simulation studies to determine the potential efficacy of cornfield fertilization with CO_2. They determined that CO_2 intake could be increased up to 45%, but that efficiency of use of applied CO_2 would not exceed 10% under cornfield conditions.

CO_2 fertilization is widely used in greenhouse production of tomatoes. Bassham[3] has suggested the use of huge greenhouses for crop production. There, he estimates, it would be biologically feasible to produce 200 t/ha/year with photorespiration eliminated by CO_2 enrichment. Observed yields of C_4 humid tropical plants, e.g., Napier grass (*Pennisetum purpureum*), have yielded up to 85 t DM/ha under field conditions.[17]

Pesticides

World pesticide use amounts to about 1.5 million metric tons annually. A substantial portion is used for control of human and animal disease vectors, especially in countries where malaria is endemic. About 60% of the pesticide chemicals used in the U.S. are used in agricultural production.[46] The remainder is used by households, industry, institutions, and public agencies (Table 12).

Pesticides are an essential adjunct to crop production. Insects, fungi, nematodes, weeds, birds, and rodents inflict substantial losses to unprotected crops.

Genetic, other biological, and cultural methods of pest control may be used with chemicals in "integrated pest management systems". Such systems may minimize development of pest populations resistant to chemical and biological control agents, and hazards to nontarget organisms and the environment. Adoption of "integrated pest management" systems is deterred by the necessity for judgment as to the point where probable pest damage requires intervention with chemical control. When, on occasion, the decision is too long delayed, substantial crop loss may occur.

Use of many pesticides in the U.S. has been restricted of eliminated by regulatory action by the Environmental Protection Agency that administers the Federal Insecticide, Fungicide, and Rodenticide Act (FIFRA).[111] Atlernate pesticides have replaced some of those eliminated. Integrated pest management (IPM) is increasing.[112]

LIVESTOCK AND POULTRY PRODUCTION IN U.S.

Livestock and poultry use much of the energy they consume to support activity, obtain food, and maintain body temperature. In industrialized countries intensive livestock and poultry producers confine livestock and bring feed to them. In poultry production, temperature of animal quarters is partially controlled. These processes substitute fossil fuel energy for feed energy.

Growth of animals and their productivity is constrained by the law of diminishing returns just as are crop production processes.

Feed used by livestock and poultry in the U.S. is shown in Table 13.

Beef

Liveweight production by cattle and calves increased from about 11 million metric tons in 1952 to about 19 million metric tons in 1972. During this period liveweight produced by feedlot cattle increased from 1.5 million t to about 6 million t, accounting for about three fourths of the total increase (Figure 8). Of the 1.5 million t increase in production form nonfeedlot cattle, about half was due to increase in numbers. The other half was due to an increase of about 2 kg in production per capita. This increase may be attributed to an industry shift to the production of larger, faster-growing cattle.

Grain and other concentrates used in feedlot beef production increased from about 14 million metric tons in 1952 to about 40 million t in 1972. During 1973—75, export demand for grain and a poor crop year in 1974 increased grain prices sharply. Feedlot cattle in 1974 used only about 25 million metric tons of grain and concentrates compared to the 40 million used in 1972. Roughage used was about the same in the 2 years.

Concentrate/roughage ratio, calculated on a corn-equivalent basis, grain and other concentrates supplied about 70% of the nutrients consumed by feedlot cattle during the 1952—72 period compared to about 8% for other beef cattle.

Current abundant grain supplies have resulted in return to high concentrate/roughage ratios for feedlot cattle. As Arne Paulsen[62] stated, "When converting grain and feed to livestock becomes a profitable venture, it is probably not competitive with feeding people." Among major food producing livestock species, curtailment of grain use in 1974 varied widely. Concentrates used for milk cows declined very little. Use by swine and poultry dropped about 10% below 1972 usage.[62]

The various species of livestock and poultry vary widely in the proportion and amounts of different feed resources they consume (Table 13). Feedlot cattle consumed one fifth as much feed as "other cattle" and produced two fifths as much beef (Table 14).

Table 15 shows that in terms of grain used by food-producing livestock, and of all feed used, milk gives the largest output per unit input. This is also true on a DM, energy, or protein basis of calculation.

Feedlot cattle and pigs are about equally productive in terms of liveweight produced per unit of grain used; broilers and turkeys are much more productive.

Sheep are relatively productive in terms of liveweight per unit of grain used; in terms of all feed their productivity is relatively low. Sheep are better adapted to many range areas than cattle are. Ewe/lamb enterprises can make more efficient use of semiarid range, where herbage production is low, than cow/calf units can.[16]

Table 16 shows the "cattle equivalent" numbers of livestock and poultry and the energy and protein content of their edible products for the U.S. in 1977. Cattle comprised about two thirds of the product-edible energy and edible protein.

Milk Production

Measured in corn equivalent feed units (CFU), milk cows of the U.S. consume about a sixth of the feed consumed by all livestock and about one seventh of the grain and by-product feeds. Production of milk per cow increased from about 3190 kg in 1960 to about 5000 kg in 1977. A substantial portion of the increase was due to use of superior sires in artificial insemination (Figure 4). The increase was accompanied by an increase in CFU consumed per cow from about 3625 kg in 1960 to about 5400 kg in 1976. Feed required to produce a kg of milk decreased from about 1.23 kg CFU to 1.08 kg CFU.

Milk cows in the U.S. consumed about 421 g of grain and other concentrates per kilogram of milk produced in 1977, which provided about 40% of CFU consumed by milk cows in the country.

The values shown in Table 17 reflect an efficiency of about 60% in conversion of

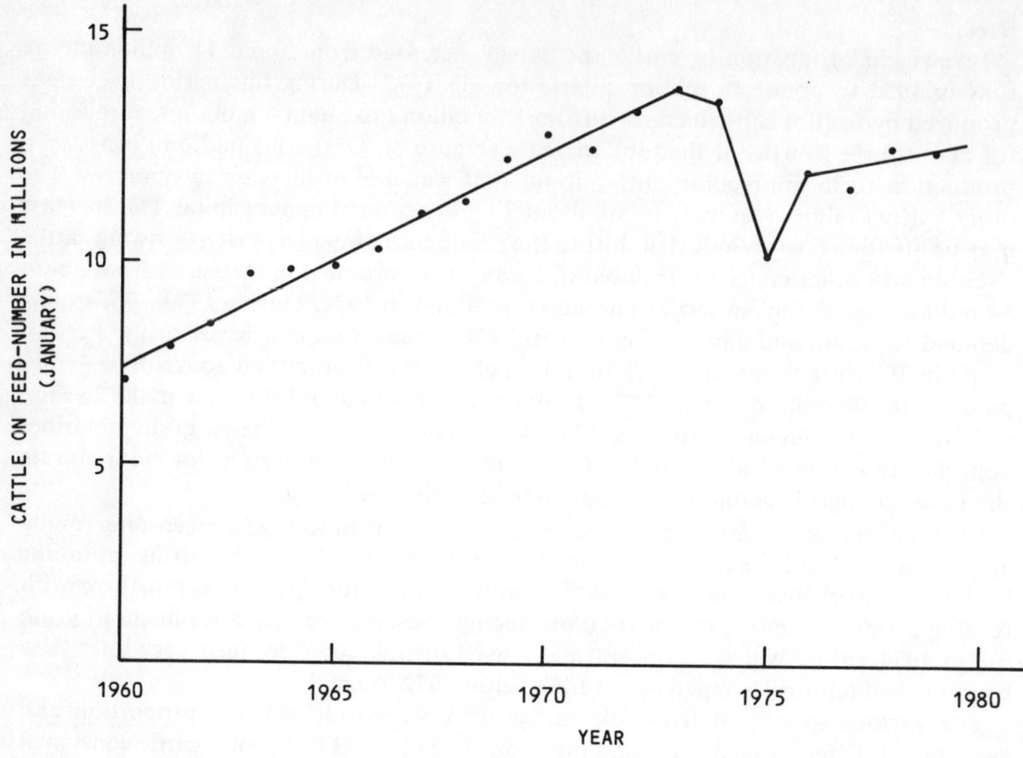

FIGURE 8. Cattle on feed January 1st (in millions).

metabolizable energy (ME) and digestible protein in feed above maintenance requirement to edible energy and protein in milk.

Digestibility of gross energy and crude protein in feeds used for lactating cows producing at the higher levels indicated in the table must exceed 60% in order to sustain such rates of milk production. About 25 to 30% ME and crude protein (CP) in feed is produced in milk at these higher levels of production.

Sheep

Ewes producing a single lamb per year are relatively inefficient in conversion of feed ME to edible meat. When wool is included apparent efficiency is substantially increased. Since adult wethers have only maintenance and wool production energy and protein cost, they can subsist in areas with vegetation too sparse to support high rates of reproduction.

In countries where sheep are milked, efficiency in terms of edible product is higher than in countries where, as in the U.S., only meat and wool are produced. Data in Table 18 show that in France, where both meat and milk are produced, edible protein per capita for sheep is three times that in the U.S. where only meat is produced.

Pigs

Data in Table 19 indicate wide differences among the countries included in turnoff and edible product per capita in the 1977 inventory. Turnoff (number slaughtered/inventory number) in the U.S. was about 145%, in the LDC less than 50%. Yield of pork per inventory head in the U.S. was about 110 kg per capita in inventory while in China it was only about 43 kg per capita in inventory.

Productivity of the U.S. pig population increased in terms of pork per inventory

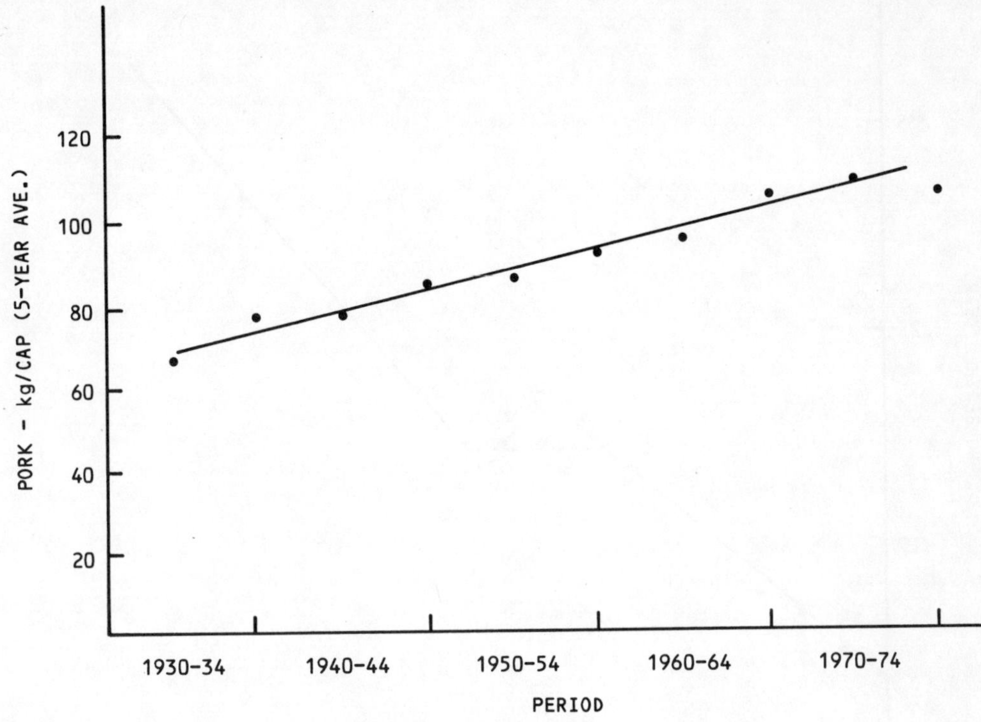

FIGURE 9. Pigs in inventory (5-year averages) and pork production per pig.

head as shown in Figure 9. Production has increased from about 82 kg/head in 1950 to about 105 kg/head in 1974. Lard, on the other hand, peaked at about 25kg/head in 1955, and declined to about 11 kg/head in 1974. These changes reflect more effective disease control as well as breeding improvement. Pigs saved per sow farrowing increased from 6.6 in 1950 to 7.1 in 1974.

Change in ratio of pork to lard increased from 3.3:1 in 1950 to 9.5:1 in 1974. This change resulted chiefly from selective breeding for meat type.[10,92,93]

Egg Production

Egg production per hen in the U.S. increased from 174 in 1950 to 231 in 1974. The period was one of almost complete transition from standardbred stock to crossbred and hybrid matings. While hybrid egg-laying stock produced more eggs per hen than the older standardbred stock, it was equally vulnerable to Marek's disease, a neoplastic disease of viral origin. Morbidity and mortality from Marek's contributed to a plateau in egg production per hen from about 1965 to 1970. An effective vaccine which protected layers from the disease was developed by research workers in the Regional Poultry Laboratory.[66,67] It was applied in 1971 and subsequent years, and the response in egg production per hen was prompt and sustained as indicated in Figure 10.

Broilers

Broiler production in the U.S. has increased from about 70,000 t in 1935 to more than 5 million metric tons liveweight in the 'seventies. Metabolizable energy and protein consumed by broilers has decreased from about 12 Mcal ME/kg liveweight and 720 g CP/kg in 1935 to about 6.5 Mcal ME and 400 g protein/kg currently. Time from hatching to market weight of 1.7 kg has decreased from about 12 weeks in 1935 to 7 weeks currently (Figure 11).

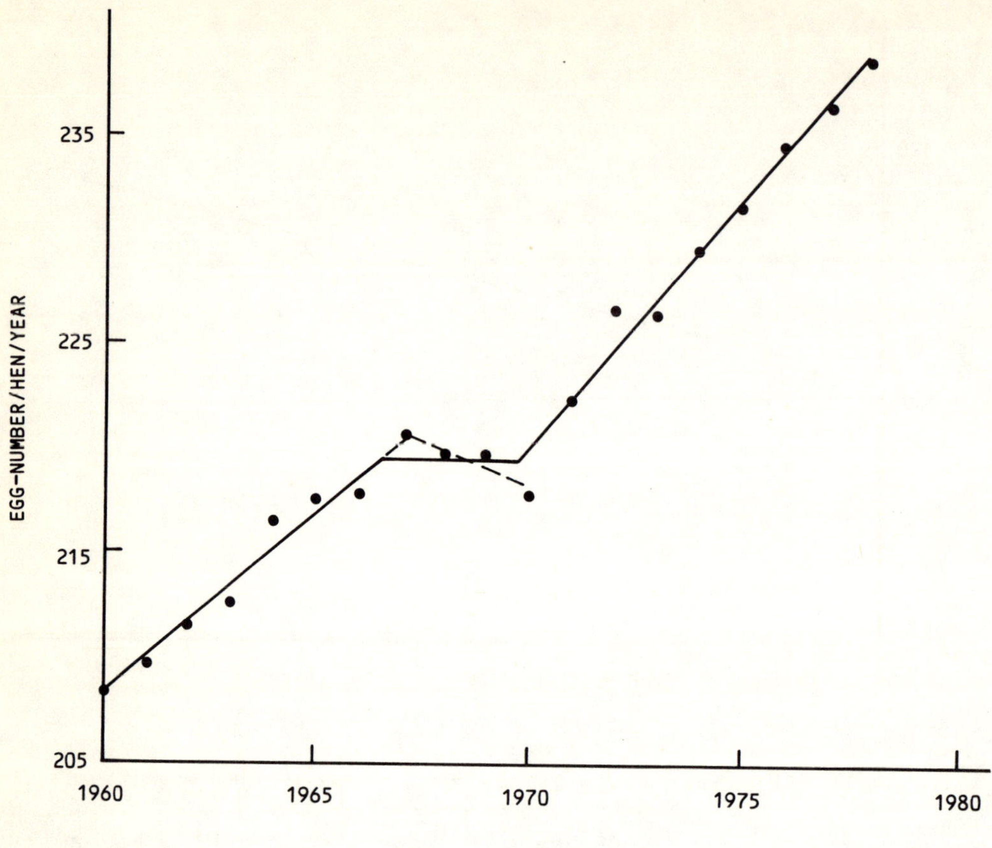

FIGURE 10. Egg production.

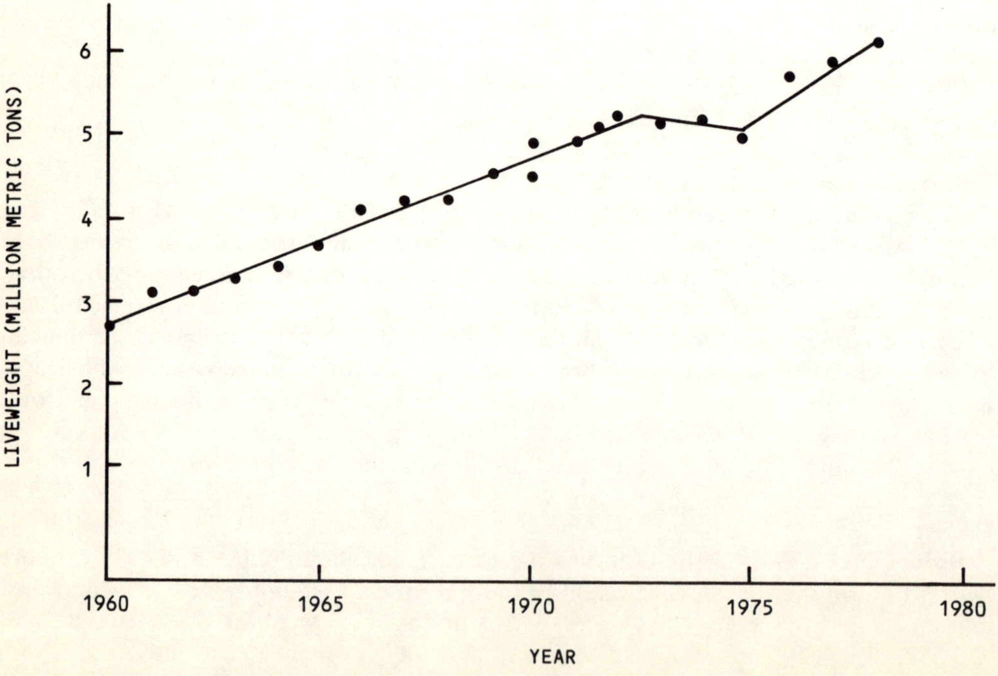

FIGURE 11. Broiler production, U.S.

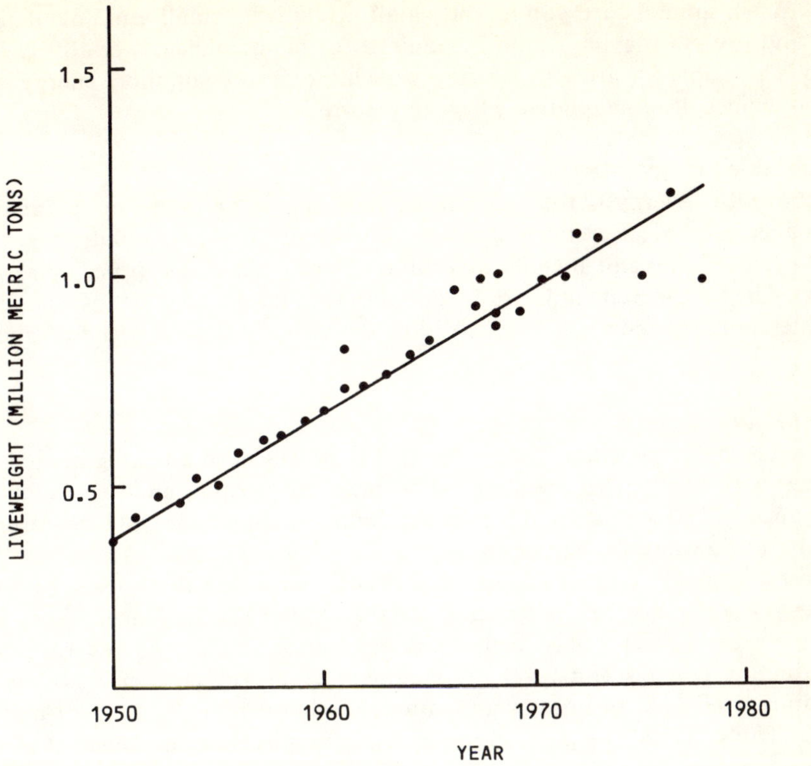

FIGURE 12. Turkey production, U.S.

Turkeys

Turkeys are relatively efficient as converters of feed to lean meat.[43,113,114] Annual U.S. production has increased from about 375 thousand metric tons in 1950 to more than a million recently, as shown in Figure 12. Small-turkey numbers have been static in recent years, while large turkeys for institutional use and further processing have continued to increase. Rather large, price-related variations in annual production have occurred.

GROWTH

Minot[53] demonstrated that, in guinea pigs, percent rate of growth "diminishes, almost uninterruptedly from the time onwards, when the animal recovers from the postnatal loss of weight."

Moderated by interaction with myriad environmental parameters — e.g., photoperiod, temperature, nutrition, spatial relations — Minot's discovery is true for all living things, both individuals and populations. Growth may be interrupted or continuous, determinate or indeterminate. Even for organisms and populations with indeterminate growth, senescence may be correlative with accumulated nonproductive components. In mobile animals, energy cost of movement of ever-increasing mass is associated with decreased movement. Activity cost must be proportional to body weight albeit large animals may be less active than smaller ones.

The Minot dictum is, in fact, a statement of the law of diminishing returns. Gross efficiency of feed use in livestock and poultry production is bound by this rule. Hendricks[38] developed a simple method for relating cumulative feed consumption and body weight. When animals are young and small a relatively small amount of the *ad lib.* energy and protein they consume is required for maintenance, a relatively large proportion is available for growth. As they grow larger, more and more energy is required for maintenance, leaving relatively less for growth.

Metabolizable Energy (ME)

Metabolizable energy is that portion of feed energy or tissue energy available for maintenance, storage, secretions, activity (other than "work"), and the heat increment of feeding. ME does not include digestible energy voided, as urine, or as gas, e.g., methane. The heat increment is proportional to feed intake, and is thus a larger portion of the metabolizable energy of feeds of low digestibility than for feed of high digestibility.

ME for Maintenance

Maintenance energy is the energy cost of life processes in a resting animal. Activity associated with feeding, reproduction, and play is generally, and here, included with maintenance ME. The National Research Council maintenance ME requirements include a 10% allowance for activity.

Because the energy cost of activity is proportional to the first power of liveweight, a smaller proportion of ME is required for the smaller species (sheep, pigs, and poultry) than for cattle. Activity is further reduced by confinement, a general practice for the production of eggs and broilers. Maintenance energy cost increases as ambient temperature decreases for poultry and animals generally.[12] The data for maintenance energy in Table 21 and the portion required for maintenance in Table 22 assume ambient temperature of 15° C.

Apparent energy requirements for individually growing pigs decrease about 1% for each degree C in ambient temperature. Stahly et. al.[76] reported data for feed intake, gain, and carcass traits for such pigs reared at ambient temperatures of 10°C, 12.5°C, and 35°C. Intake of a 3.2 Mcal ME/kg diet was 10% greater at 10°C than at 12.5°C, and 15% greater at 12.5°C than at 35°C. Gain at 35°C was reduced in comparison with the lower temperatures.

Metabolizable Energy Required for Production and Reproduction

Use of metabolizable energy (ME) for gain in weight may be less efficient than for milk and eggs production. Net energy for gain (NEG) for beef cattle in *Nutrient Requirements of Beef Cattle,*[58] based on the work of Lofgreen and Garrett,[51] are about 55% of ME. Higher efficiencies are probably achievable. For example, Robison's[72] values for pigs from 30 to 100 kg liveweight, indicate that 70 to 80% of ME is available for production. We have assumed about 55% NEG of ME for all young meat animals.

The efficiencies in Table 20 show the large relative cost of maternal feed in producing ruminants for meat. Opportunities for increasing ruminant fecundity are limited. The increased efficiency of twin lamb production is large. It is possible that three successive reproductive cycles in 2 years can be used. However, it is notable that energy efficiency of two litters of pigs from the same dams in 1 year changes energetic efficiency very little.

Opportunities for utilizing a larger portion of ruminant milk as human food are substantial in countries which accept milk, butter, and cheeses as desirable. Specialization of dairy and meat production industries may, however, result in greater net efficiency of energy and protein from meat and milk.

This is generally assumed to be the case for poultry meat and eggs. Nonetheless, feed cost for broiler breeders constitutes about 8% of the feed cost of broiler production. It may be possible to reduce it by use of recessive dwarf breeder hens carrying genes for rapid growth and heavy adult weight.[33]

Data in Table 21 do not include costs of replacing breeding stock and of maintaining barren females and breeding males. These costs would be balanced partially by the liveweight of breeding stock sold for slaughter. Death losses of breeding stock may be estimated as about 5% for cattle and 10% for the other species.

Protein Requirements

Protein requirements are best expressed in relation to energy requirements. Protein deficiency depresses energy intake. Protein excess is wastefully metabolized for energy. Intensively managed livestock and poultry receive fixed ratios. Range and pastured animals may receive protein supplements during winter or dry season.

Protein requirements vary with age, gain, and reproduction phases. Forages on which ruminants largely feed vary seasonally in protein content. During periods of rapid growth, grasses such as crested wheat grass (*Agropyron cristatum*) may contain 80 g of total protein (CP) — 65 g digestible protein (DP) for each Mcal/ME. Dry and weathered, it may contain only 12 g CP (2 DP) for each Mcal/ME. Fresh, immature, crested wheat grass consumed by ruminants contains luxus amounts of protein, much of which is metabolized for energy. Animals subsisting on dry and weathered crested wheat grass are sure to lose weight and condition.

Grams of protein/Mcal ME are shown in Table 22 for several species and life stages of livestock and poultry. Only mature, dry, nonpregnant females, and castrates can subsist on less than 20 g DP/Mcal ME. (See References 57-59.) Requirements for late pregnancy, lactation, and egg production are much higher.

SUMMARY AND PROJECTION

Current agricultural productivity would need to increase about 50% in order to provide supplies needed to maintain current levels of use by the projected 6.3 billion people in the year 2000. This result can be achieved by increasing yields on presently arable land or by increasing arable area. For either course, water, nitrogen, mineral plant nutrients, supplies, and favorable weather are necessary. Technology applied in effective use of these resources, pest management, genetically productive plant seed, and livestock and poultry breeding stock are critical requirements everywhere.

Doubling arable area would make it possible to derive more of the nitrogen required for food crop production from legumes and animal manure. Total dependence on biologically fixed N would be likely to result in reduced yields per hectare in many DME countries, including the U.S. In many developing countries, increased use of legumes and manures could lead to increased quantitative and qualitative agricultural productivity.

Nichiporovich[61] has estimated the photosynthetically active radiation (PAR) reaching the earth's surface each year as about 280×10^{18} kcal. He estimated the annual production of biomass by autotrophic plants as about 100×10^{9} t, containing gross energy of about 450×10^{15} kcal. Thus no more than 0.16% of PAR energy is stored as photosynthate.

Nichiporovich estimated mean influx of PAR to cultivated areas during the growing season as about 3×10^{9} kcal/ha. He projected a possible future efficiency of use of PAR in crop production at 2%. This could result in a sevenfold increase over total 1969 production if realized on 3×10^{9} potentially arable hectares.

In order to achieve this result Nichiporovich estimated that 2 to 3×10^{12} t water, 15 $\times 10^{9}$ t C, 2 to 3×10^{9} t mineral plant nutrients and 0.5×10^{9} t of nitrogen would need to enter the biological cycle.

Nichiporovich's estimates of potential agricultural productivity are tenfold greater than those needed to supply the projected 6.3 billion people in the year 2000 with food

Table 1
AGRICULTURAL LAND AND ENERGY RESOURCES

Area	Total land (ha × 10^6)	Arable land 1977	Arable land 2000[b]	Grazing land 1977	Grazing land 2000	Irrigated land 1977	Irrigated land 2000[c]	Energy[a] (estimated millions hp) Human	Animal	Tractor[d]	Total
DME	3,158	394	715	889	1450	31	68	4.0	7.5	512	523.5
CPE	3,476	420	595	733	600	106[e]	120	39.5	42.0	145	221.5
LDC	6,444	674	2,000	1,435	1,840	98	180	55.5	131.5	70	255.0
World	13,078	1,488	3,200	3,057	3,890	225	385	99.0	181.0	720	1,000.0
US	913	191	250	244	310	16	20	0.3	4.5	219	223.8

[a] Human labor estimated @ 1/8 hp; animal horsepower @ 0.5 horse, mule, ass, and camel populations; @ 0.1 the cattle and buffalo population in LDC and CPE. There is some use of cattle for draft in some DME countries. Data are from the FAO Production Yearbook 1977,[28c] except as noted.

[b] Rounded.

[c] Estimated at 1977 % of arable.

[d] Tractors estimated at 40 hp, except for the U.S. for which 50 hp is estimated.[95]

[e] Includes estimate of 10 million ha for U.S.S.R.

at current rates. Our projected increase of 50 × 10^6 t of nitrogen above current use seems modest by comparison with his 500 million metric tons projection.

Past projections of agricultural productivity have been exceeded by production.[39] Past and recent evaluations of future productivity have generally been limited to crop productivity. Recommendations of research priorities, too, have emphasized genetic engineering, nitrogen fixation, and photosynthesis.[7,91]

Increased productivity may indeed be limited by technology for increasing efficiency of these basic processes. Increased efficiency of livestock and poultry productivity is feasible and compatible with increase in crop productivity.[29]

Duckham[21] declared that agricultural productivity could be increased by 50% by applying what we now know. Increased yields through application of existing technology on existing arable land could accomplish such an increase.

Alternately, area of land under cultivation and grazing can be increased, albeit at great expense. Increase of food supply to meet population growth and economic demand projected to the year 2000 is biologically feasible. As Timmer[86] pointed out in his review of Duckham, Jones, and Roberts' book, *Food Production and Consumption,* it may be "impossible to minimize economic cost, social upheaval, support energy, and number of decision makers simultaneously."

Among the costs of increasing agricultural production is the reduction of forests, especially tropical forests. This issue, the paradox of conversion of tropical forest lands to agriculture was stated by Nelson[60] as follows:

Who is to say that the destruction of a hectare of tropical forest in order to produce corn to feed a campesino and his family is a low-priority present use and that harvesting of the same hectare for ten years hence is a high-priority future use? Or conversely, who decides that clearing forests for farm lands in the head waters of a river is a high-priority present use and that external diseconomies in the form of destruction wrought by floods downstream in twenty years time constitute a low-priority sequence?

Table 2
1977 AVERAGES OF CROP AREA YIELD AND PRODUCTION[a]

	DME			CPE			LDC			World			U.S.		
	Area (ha × 10^6)	Yield (kg/ha)	Production (t × 10^6)	Area (ha × 10^6)	Yield (kg/ha)	Production (t × 10^6)	Area (ha × 10^6)	Yield (kg/ha)	Production (t × 10^6)	Area (ha × 10^6)	Yield (kg/ha)	Production (t × 10^6)	Area (ha × 10^6)	Yield (kg/ha)	Production (t × 10^6)
Cereals	160.6	3,127	502.3	277.9	1,906	529.8	307.2	1,390	426.9	745.1	1,957	1,459.0	71.9	3,667	261.7
Roots	3.6	22,204	80.6	26.8	11,470	309.9	21.4	8,480	181.6	51.8	10,987	570.2	0.6	27,945	16.5
Pulses	3.2	962	3.1	18.8	1,080	2.04	48.2	507	24.4	70.1	683	48.0	0.7	1,425	10.6
Oilseeds	36.3	1,725	62.6	38.1	1,005	38.3	61.1	765	46.8	135.5	1,089	147.6	31.0	1,784	55.3
Sugar	2.9	44,030	127.9	5.5	26,095	143.7	0.6	30,333	8.6	9.0	32,155	290.1	0.5	46,232	22.8
Sugar cane	0.9	79,184	70.5	0.7	65,124	47.7	11.6	53,464	619.3	13.2	55,845	737.5	0.3	81,769	25.1
Coffee	—	—	—	—	—	—	9.1	478	4.3	9.1	478	4.3	—	—	—
Cocoa	—	—	—	—	—	—	4.7	300	1.4	4.7	300	1.4	—	—	—
Tea	0.1	1,734	0.1	0.4	1,017	0.4	1.1	1,129	1.2	1.6	1,121	1.8	—	—	—
Tobacco	0.8	1,903	1.6	1.3	1,385	1.7	2.3	985	2.3	4.4	1,272	5.6	0.4	2,245	0.9
Cotton[b]	5.8	60.3	3.5	7.9	646	5.1	19.4	294	5.7	33.2	431	14.3	5.4	593	3.2
Other fibers	—	600	3.2	0.7	2,285	1.6	4.5	889	4.0	5.3	1,075	5.7	—	—	—
15 vegetables	3.2	17,635	56.4	3.0	11,610	34.8	3.6	9,916	35.6	9.7	13,290	128.9	0.6	23,230	14.3
Melons	0.4	16,210	7.1	0.9	9,445	8.7	1.0	12,710	12.4	2.3	11,975	28.2	0.1	13,850	1.8
Grapes	5.9	6,550	38.4	2.0	4,850	9.7	2.3	5,455	12.6	10.2	5,607	57.0	0.3	12,850	3.9

[a] DME: Developed Market Economies; CPE: Centrally Planned Economies; LDC: Developing Market Economies. All are listed in the FAO Production Yearbook 1977, p. 273.[28c] DME includes U.S., Canada, Japan, Israel, South Africa, Australia, New Zealand, and Western Europe. CPE includes the countries of Eastern Europe, U.S.S.R., Peoples Republic of China, Mongolia, North Korea, Vietnam, Kampuchea, LDC includes all other countries. Crops include — cereals: wheat, rice, rye, barley, oats, maize, sorghum and millet; roots: potatoes, sweet potatoes, cassava, and yams; pulses: beans, peas, chick peas, lentils, and pigeon peas; oil seeds: soy, flax, peanut, sunflower, rape, cottonseed, sesame, safflower; fiber: flax, jute, hemp, and cotton lint. Relevant minor crops are also included in each category.

[b] Cotton area is included with oilseeds also.

Table 3
PRODUCTION FROM TREE CROPS AND SMALL FRUITS[a]

	DME	CPE	LDC	World	U.S.
Tree fruits	52.5	10.6	43.5	106.6	19.9
Tree nuts	1.1	0.6	1.3	3.0	0.4
Small fruits	1.2	0.5	0.1	1.8	0.4
Coconuts	—	0.2	32.2	32.4	—
Olives	6.0	—	2.1	8.1	—
Palm kernels	—	—	1.5	1.5	—
Pineapples	1.0	0.9	4.2	6.1	0.6
Bananas and plantains	0.6	1.0	54.8	56.4	—
Totals	62.4	13.8	139.7	215.9	21.3

[a] Production in metric tons × 10^6.

Table 4
NUMBERS OF PRINCIPAL LIVESTOCK SPECIES, 1977[28c]

	DME[a]	CPE[a]	LDC[a]	World[a]	U.S.[a]
Cattle	295.3	214.8	702.8	1212.9	122.8
Buffalo	0.1	33.8	96.9	130.8	—
Sheep	330.4	294.2	433.3	1027.9	12.8
Goats	16.8	74.2	319.4	410.7	1.4
Poultry[b]	1773.8	2745.5	2107.7	6597.0	397.5
Pigs	173.9	377.6	114.8	66.3	54.9
Horses, mules and asses	15.1	32.1	67.9	115.1	0.1
Camels	—	1.9	11.9	13.8	—

[a] Millions.
[b] Chickens, ducks, and turkeys.

Table 5
1977 MEAT PRODUCTION AND YIELD FROM INDIGENOUS ANIMALS

	DME		CPE		LDC		World		U.S.	
	Production	Yield	Production	Yield	Production	Yield	Production	Yield	Production	Yield
Cattle and buffalo	24.1	81.7	11.1	44.3	12.3	15.4	47.5	30.1	11.6	93.6
Sheep and goats	2.4	7.0	2.0	5.9	3.0	4.0	7.4	5.1	0.2	11.0
Pigs	19.2	110.2	21.2	56.1	3.5	23.8	43.9	65.9	6.0	109.3
Poultry	13.9	0.8	6.6	0.2	3.8	0.2	24.3	0.4	7.2	1.8

Calculated from data in Reference 28c. Production in metric tons × 10^6; yield in kg per capita.

Table 6
PRODUCTION AND YIELD OF EGGS AND COWS' MILK — 1977 AVERAGE

	DME	CPE	LDC	WORLD	USA
Cows					
Production (metric tons × 10^6	212.8	138.8	57.5	409.0	55.8
Milk yield[a] (kg per capita)	3738.0	2197.0	689.0	2010.0	5078.0
Eggs					
Production (metric tons × 10^6	11.6	9.1	4.2	24.9	3.8
Yield[b] (kg per capita)	6.7	3.3	1.9	3.8	9.5

[a] Yield per cow milked.
[b] Yield per inventory head.
[c] Data calculated from Reference 28c.

Table 7
MILK PRODUCTION OF BUFFALO, SHEEP AND GOATS: 1977[a]

	DME	CPE	LDC	World	U.S.
Buffalo	0.1	1.2	26.2	27.5	—
Sheep	2.5	1.6	3.2	7.3	—
Goats	1.4	0.8	4.3	6.5	—

[a] Production in metric tons × 10^6. Calculated from Reference 28c.

Table 8
WORLD CEREAL CROP IN 1977[28c]

	Wheat		Rice		Maize		Barley		Other[a]		Total	
	metric tons × 10^6	kg/ha	metric tons × 10^6	kg/ha	metric tons × 10^6	kg/ha	metric tons × 10^6	kg/ha	metric tons × 10^6	kg/ha	metric tons × 10^6	kg/ha
U.S.	55.1	2058	4.5	4955	161.5	5700	9.1	2357	31.5	2715.5	261.7	3667
U.S.S.R.	92.0	1484	2.2	4029	11.0	3270	52.7	1526	30.0	1220.8	187.9	1502
China	40.0	1270	131.5	3546	33.6	2962	15.4	1495	21.9	802.1	242.4	2061
India	29.1	1394	74.0	1873	6.8	1133	1.6	1035	21.1	611.6	132.6	1286
France	17.5	4230	—	—	8.6	5294	10.3	3536	3.1	2809.1	39.5	4069
World	386.6	1664	366.5	2566	349.9	2952	173.1	1894	183.1	1140.1	1459.0	1957
Subtotals	233.7		212.2		221.5		89.1		107.6		864.1	

[a] Principally millet, sorgo, and rye.

Table 9
ORGANIC AND CONVENTIONAL CORNBELT FARMS: A COMPARISON OF PRODUCTION BY 16 PAIRED FARMS

Farms	Area (ha)	Cropland (ha)	Cereals[a] (ha)	Cereals[a] (mt)	Soybeans (ha)	Soybeans (mt)	Other crops (ha)	Pasture and other (ha)
Organic (16)	191	108	48	166	22	43	37	83
Conventional (16)	185	145	76	303	40	79	26	40

[a] Cereals included corn, wheat, and oats.

Calculated from data in Klepper, et al., *Am. J. Agric. Econ.*, 59, 1-24, 1977. With permission.

Table 10
IRRIGATION WATER USED AND CROP PRODUCTIVITY[25,88]

Crop	Days irrigated (number)	Water used (t/ha)	Dry matter produced (t/ha)	Water / Dry matter
Alfalfa	300	20,000	13.3	1,500
Barley	150	6,250	3.4	1,800
Cotton	240	10,175	3.2	3,170
Potatoes	120	7,000	7.8	900
Sorghum	90	6,275	4.5	1,395
Sugar beet	300	10,570	13.3	720
Wheat	150	5,655	4.1	1,380
Cantaloupe	210	4,715	1.7	2,770
Lettuce	105	2,100	2.1	1,000
Carrots	210	4,100	2.1	1,950

Table 11
FERTILIZER CONSUMPTION — 1977 (METRIC TONS × 10^6)

Area	Nitrogen	P_2O_5	K_2O
DME	20.5	13.1	11.5
CPE	16.6	9.8	9.4
LDC	7.7	4.6	2.3
World	44.8	27.5	23.2
U.S.	9.6	5.1	5.3

Data from *Nitrogen,* Suppl. No. 18, Nov./Dec. 1978.

Table 12
PESTICIDE CONSUMPTION 1973 (THOUSANDS OF METRIC TONS)

Area	Insecticides	Fungicides	Fumigants	Herbicides	Rodenticides	Total
DME	376.7	271.0	32.8	130.2	1.0	811.7
CPE[a]	108.0	95.0	1.8	94.8	1.5	301.1
LDC	133.7	37.7	2.4	15.8	0.1	189.7
World	618.4	403.7	37.0	240.8	2.6	1302.5
USA	332.8	72.6	13.0	29.2	0.1	447.7

[a] Data for PRC is not included; for U.S.S.R. data is apportioned as in reporting countries in Eastern Europe.

Data from FAO Production Yearbook 1974, Food and Agriculture Organization, Rome. With permission.

Table 13
FEED CONSUMED BY LIVESTOCK & POULTRY — U.S. 1978 (MILLIONS OF METRIC TONS)

	Cereals		Byproducts[a]		Harvested roughage[a]		Pasture and range[b]		CFU[c]
	Amt.	All feed (%)	Amt.	All feed (%)	Amt.	All feed (%)	Amt.	All feed (%)	Totals
Dairy cattle	20.0	28.2	6.0	8.4	30.0	42.3	15.0	21.1	71.0
Feedlot cattle	30.0	68.9	5.0	11.5	7.0	16.1	1.5	3.5	43.5
Other beef cattle	7.0	3.6	3.0	1.5	40.0	20.5	145.0	74.4	195.0
Sheep	0.2	3.3	0.3	4.9	0.6	10.0	5.0	81.8	6.1
Pigs	42.0	63.4	17.0	25.7	—	—	7.2	10.9	66.2
Layers	13.7	60.4	8.0	35.2	—	—	1.0	4.4	22.7
Broilers	9.1	47.6	10.0	52.4	—	—	—	—	19.1
Turkeys	2.6	44.1	3.0	50.9	—	—	0.3	5.0	5.9
Horses	4.0	22.6	0.2	1.2	4.5	25.4	9.0	50.8	17.7
Other livestock	3.3	53.2	0.3	4.8	1.6	25.9	1.0	16.1	6.2
Totals and averages	131.9	29.1	52.8	11.6	83.7	18.4	185.	40.9	453.4

[a] Calculated from data in Economics, Statistics, and Cooperative Service Bulletin.[23]

[b] Estimated from data in USDA 1977.

[c] CFU = Corn-equivalent feed units, the amount of feed equivalent to the feeding value of corn containing 78.6% total digestible nutrients (TDN). (See Reference 42a.)

Table 14
U.S. INVENTORY AND PRODUCTIVITY OF CATTLE, SHEEP, CHICKENS AND TURKEYS — 1977 (IN MILLIONS)

		Production		Live or Product Wt.	
	January 1 Inventory	No. Total[a]	Inventory (%)	Metric tons	Inventory (%)
All Cattle	122.8	40.0	33	18.5	150.0
All Sheep	12.8	6.6	312	0.32	25.0
Hogs	54.9	79.4	145	8.7	158.0
Chickens[b]	930.0	3645.0	392	6.1	6.5
Turkeys[b]	25.0	135.6	542	1.2	48.0
Laying Hens[c]	275.0	—	—	3.7	13.5
Milk Cows[c]	11.0	—	—	55.6	5012.0

[a] Calf, lamb and pig crop minus death loss.

[b] January 1 estimated inventory includes 0.167 of broilers and turkeys produced during 1976.

[c] Included in "chickens" and "cattle", respectively.

From Economics, Statistics, and Cooperative Service, Bull. No. 522, U.S. Department of Agriculture, Washington, D.C., 1979.

Table 15
LIVEWEIGHT, MILK, AND EGGS PRODUCED IN U.S. IN 1977 IN RELATION TO FEED RESOURCES USED (IN METRIC TONS × 10^6)[93]

	Livewt. produced	Livewt./cereals	Livewt./all feed
Dairy cattle	53.6[a]	2.7[a]	0.78[a]
Feedlot cattle	5.0[b]	0.17	0.12
Other cattle	13.5	1.93	0.07
Sheep	0.32	1.6	0.05
Pigs	8.7	0.25	0.16
Hens	4.2[c]	0.33[c]	0.17[c]
Broilers	5.9	0.77	0.38
Turkeys	1.2	0.43	0.18

[a] Milk.

[b] Estimated.

[c] Eggs and chickens other than broilers.

Table 16
CATTLE UNITS OF CATTLE, SHEEP, HOGS, CHICKENS AND TURKEYS AND THEIR PRODUCTION OF EDIBLE ENERGY AND PROTEIN — JANUARY 1, 1977

	Cattle units (millions)	Edible energy (EE) produced (Mcal × 10^9)				Edible protein produced[a] (kg × 10^6)			
		Meat[b]	Milk or eggs	Total	Mcal/CU	Meat[b]	Milk or eggs	Total	Kg/CU
Cattle	122.8	37.0	36.1	73.1	59.5	1504	1831	3335	27.2
Sheep	3.0	0.38	—	0.38	126.7	26	—	26	8.7
Hogs	18.4	27.8	—	27.8	1511.0	522	—	522	28.4
Chickens	11.1	6.1	5.3	11.4	1027.0	549	403	952	85.6
Turkeys	1.3	1.4	—	1.4	1077.0	132	—	132	109.2
Total	156.6	72.68	41.4	114.08	720.5	2733	2234	4967	36.9

Note: Factors: estimated metabolic weight of inventory numbers in Table 14 — cattle 82.6; hogs 27.7; sheep 18.8; chickens 1.0; turkeys 4.3. Calories: cattle 2 Mcal/kg liveweight produced — sheep 1.2; hogs 3.2; chickens 1.0 and turkeys 1.2. Edible protein: cattle 8% of liveweight — sheep, 8; hogs, 6; chickens, 9 and turkeys, 11%. Milk has 0.65 Mcal/kg and 3.5% edible protein — eggs have 1.5 Mcal/kg and 11.5% edible protein. One cattle unit (CU) is the equivalent in metabolic weight of one head of cattle in inventory. Metabolic weight is the three fourths power of liveweight, in kg.

[a] About 6% of harvested milk protein is fed calves or other livestock or wasted in unused cheese whey. About 6% of chicken eggs laid are used for hatching; these amounts have been deducted.

[b] Edible offal is included in meat.

Table 17
COW'S MILK PRODUCTION IN 1977: METABOLIZABLE ENERGY (ME) AND CRUDE PROTEIN (CP) REQUIREMENT AND EFFICIENCY

	Cows milked (millions)	Yield (kg)	Feed per cow		Production			
			MEI (mcal/g)	CPI (year)	(Mcal/cow)	(CP/kg/cow)	ME/MEI	EP/CPI
DME	57.0	3,738	10,217	512.5	2,430	130.8	0.238	0.255
CPE	63.2	2,197·	8,432	386.1	1,435	77.0	0.17	0.199
LDC	83.4	689	5,540	225.5	448	24.1	0.08	0.107
World	203.6	2,010	8,050	365.2	1,307	70.4	0.162	0.193
U.S.	11.0	5,078	11,772	622.4	3,300	177.7	0.28	0.285
U.S.S.R.	42.0	2,246	8,487	390.9	1,460	78.6	0.142	0.201
Oceania	2.9	2,905	9,254	444.1	1,888	101.8	0.203	0.229
France	10.2	2,942	9,297	447.1	1,912	102.8	0.026	0.229
China	6.5	590	6,567	264.1	384	20.7	0.059	0.079
India	17.4	486	5,305	214.0	316	17.0	0.059	0.079

Note: Milk estimated at 3.5% fat. MEI and CP calculated from NRC 1977 for 600 kg/liveweight cows for DME and CPE; 450 for LDC and India; 538 for World. MEI = 365 (0.133W3/4 kg) + 1.16 milk/kg. CP = 359/mcal MEI maintenance + 829 kg milk. ME and CP for rearing, replacement and for bull are not included.

Table 18
SHEEP PRODUCTIVITY — MEAT, MILK, WOOL, EDIBLE PROTEIN AND ENERGY

Area	Inventory (millions)	Slaughter (millions)	Carcass (10^6 metric tons)	Milk (10^6 metric tons)	Wool[a] (10^6 metric tons)	Production edible pro.[b] kg/cap meat	kg/cap	Energy[c] Mcal/cap
DME	330.4	136.4	2196	2466	805	6.7	1.4	22.8
CPE	264.2	99.9	1600	1649	372	6.1	1.2	20.2
LDC	433.3	128.5	1790	3153	334	4.1	1.0	17.1
World	1027.9	364.7	5586	7268	1521	5.4	1.2	19.7
U.S.	12.8	6.5	161	—	24	12.6	1.8	28.2
U.S.S.R.	139.8	60.0	960	100	275	6.9	1.0	16.0
Oceania	194.2	64.0	1061	—	636	5.5	0.8	12.1
France	10.9	8.1	142	892	11	8.2	6.1	27.0
China	76.0	23.5	353	472	37	4.7	1.0	15.4
India	40.3	12.9	117	—	20	2.4	0.3	5.3

[a] Scoured wool.
[b] Calculated at 14% of carcass weight and 6% of milk. Edible offals not included.
[c] Calculated at 2.2 Mcal/kg carcass weight[94] and 1.1 Mcal/kg milk.[44,45]

Table 19
PIGS

Area	Inventory (millions)	Slaughter (millions)	Carcass meat (10^6 metric tons)	Meat (kg/cap)	Edible pro. (kg/cap)	Energy (Mcal/ME/cap)
DME	173.9	261.7	19,164	110.2	8.8	440.8
CPE	377.5	312.9	21,219	56.1	4.5	224.8
LDC	114.8	64.9	3,482	30.3	2.4	121.2
World	666.2	639.5	43,865	65.9	5.3	263.6
U.S.	54.9	81.2	6,010	109.5	8.8	438.0
U.S.S.R.	63.1	59.0	4,900	77.7	6.2	310.8
Oceania	4.3	5.2	255	59.3	4.7	237.2
France	11.6	19.2	1,515	130.6	10.4	522.4
China	243.3	182.5	10,448	42.9	3.8	171.6

[a] Edible offals not included. *U.S. Dep. Agric. Agric. Handb. 8,* 1964.

Calculated from Watt and Merrill, Table 2, medium fat class, 8% protein, 4 mcal/kg.

Table 20
DAILY METABOLIZABLE ENERGY REQUIRED FOR MAINTENANCE OF LIVESTOCK AND POULTRY

Animal	Liveweight (kg)	A $W^{3/4}$[a] (kg)	Estimate published	Ref.
Cow	350	10.76	10.76	57, Table 2
Cow	450	12.99	13	58, Table 1
Cow	600	16.09	16.12	57, Table 2
Cow	700	18.09	17.10	57, Table 2
Bull	600	16.09	18.29	57, Table 1
Bull	800	20.00	21.00	58, Table 10
Bull	1000	23.67	26.83	57, Table 1
Calf	150	5.69	5.60	58, Table 1
Calf	200	7.08	7.00	58, Table 1
Calf	300	9.80	9.50	58, Table 1
Ewe	60	2.59	2.60	59, Table 3
Sow	200	6.38	6.34	56, Table 4
Hen	1.75	0.182	0.18[b]	55, Table 14
Hen	2.5	0.242	0.252[b]	55, Table 13
Hen	4.0	0.34	0.307[b]	55, Table 14
Turkey hen	5.0	0.401		
Turkey hen	8.0	0.571		

[a] "A" is 0.133 for cattle, 0.12 for sheep, pigs, chickens and turkeys. See text.

[b] Calculated for diet containing 2.9 Mcal/ME/kg.

Table 21
METABOLIZABLE ENERGY REQUIRED BY DAM AND PROGENY MEAT ANIMALS AND POULTRY

	Dam					Progeny[a]				Total Mcal ME	
				ME — Mcal			Livewt.				
	Livewt. (kg)	Time (days)	Progeny (number)	total	per capita	Age/market (days)	initial[b]	market	ME	per capita	kg/live-weight
Beef cow[c]	500	365	1	5900	500	600	150	500	7020	12920	25.8
Ewe	60	365	1	1188	1188	180	25	50	274	1458	29.1
Ewe	60	365	2	1278	639	200	20	45	320	959	21.3
Sow	135	200	7[d]	1649	235	180	12	100	1141	1376	13.8
Sow	170	365	14[e]	2963	212	180	12	100	1141	1353	13.53
Hen[f]	4	300	100	102	1.02	50	0.04	1.75	11.7	12.79	73.2
Turkey	5	240	80	117	1.44	90	0.045	5	39.27	40.71	8.0
Turkey	8	240	60	157	2.62	150	0.05	10	92.85	95.47	9.5

[a] We have assumed 55% ME available for deposit in gain, 60% above maintenance in milk and wool, and 70% for eggs. The equation for cattle is MEI = T ($0.133W^{75}$). For other species, MEI = T ($0.120W^{75}$ = ME for maintenance. For gain, ME content for cattle and pigs is assumed to be 5 Mcal/kg; wool 5 Mcal/kg; lamb 4 Mcal/kg; broilers 2 Mcal/kg; turkeys 3 Mcal/kg. For cows' milk 0.65 Mcal/kg; ewe's milk 1.1 Mcal/kg; sow's milk 1.2 Mcal/kg. For eggs 1.5 Mcal/kg.[5,12,31,45,57,99]

[b] "Initial" weight produced by milk or egg.

[c] Beef example assumes steer calf 150 days suckling, 300 days grass and harvested roughage, 150 days in feedlot; finished at choice.

[d] One litter.

[e] Two litters.

[f] Broiler breeder.

Table 22
PROTEIN REQUIREMENT — GRAMS PROTEIN (CP) PER MCAL ME[a]

Required for:	Beef cattle	Milk cows	Pigs	Sheep	Chickens	Turkeys
Growth	50	40	50	45	60	70
Finishing[b]	30	—	40	45	50	43
Late pregnancy	30	44	45	45	—	—
Lactation	50	50[c]	45	45	—	—
Egg production	—	—	—	—	46[d]	46
Adult males	40	—	45	40	42	42

[a] CP = crude protein.
[b] Castrates: steers, wethers, barrows. Young males: cocks and toms.
[c] 20 kg 3.5% fat milk from 600 kg cow. Calculated from data in *Nutrient Requirements of Domestic Animals,* No. 3, 5th rev. ed., National Academy of Sciences, Washington, D.C., 1978.
[d] 60% egg production.

REFERENCES

1. **Allen, G. C. and Devers, M.,** Livestock-Feed Relationships, National and State, Suppl. to Stat. Bull. 530, U.S. Department of Agriculture, Washington, D.C., 1974.
2. **Allen, L. H., Jensen, S. E., and Lemon, E. R.,** Plant response to carbon dioxide under field conditions: a simulation, *Science,* 173, 256—258, 1971.
3. **Bassham, J. A.,** Increasing crop production through more controlled photosynthesis, *Science,* 197, 630—638, 1977.
4. **Brady, N. C.,** Rice responds to science, in *Crop Productivity: Research Imperatives,* Brown, A.W.A., Byerly, T. C., Gibbs, M., and San Pietro, A., Michigan Agricultural Experiment Station, East Lansing, 1975, 62—96.
5. **Brande, R., Coates, M. E., Henry, K. M., Kon, S. K., Rowland, S. J., Thompson, S. Y., and Henry, D. M.,** A study of the compostion of sow's milk, *Br. J. Nutr.* 1, 64—77, 1947.
6. **Briggs, L. J. and Shantz, H. L.,** The Water Requirements of Plants, Bur. Plant Ind. Bull. 285, U.S. Department of Agriculture, Washington, D.C., 1913.
7. **Brown, H. S.,** *World Food and Nutrition Study,* National Academy of Sciences, Washington, D.C., 1977.
8. **Bryson, R. A.,** Shooting at a moving target, in *Crop Productivity: Research Imperatives,* Brown, A. W. A., Byerly, T. C., Gibbs, M., and San Pietro, A., Eds., Michigan Agricultural Experiment Station, East Lansing, 1975, 109—132.
9. **Bukovac, M. J., Moss, D. N., and Zelitch, I.,** Carbon input, in *Crop Productivity: Research Imperatives,* Brown, A.W.A., Byerly, T. C., Gibbs, M., and San Pietro, A., Eds., Michigan Agricultural Experiment Station, East Lansing, 1975, 177—200.
10. **Byerly, T. C., Gous, R. M., Kessler, J. W., and Thomas, O. P.,** Bodyweight and Maintenance Feed Requirements of Laying Hens, Maryland Nutr. Conf. Feed Manufacturers, Baltimore, University of Maryland, College Park, 1977, 36—40.
11. **Byerly, T. C.,** Contributions of the USDA in production research, in *Agricultural and Food Chemistry,* AVI Publishing, Westport, Conn. 1978, 10—24.
12. **Byerly, T. C.,** Prediction of the food intake of laying hens, *Br. Poult. Sci.,* 327—363, 1979.
13. **Callaghan, A. and Millington, A. J.,** *The Wheat Industry in Australia,* Angus and Robertson, Sydney, Australia, 1956.
14. **Calvin, M. and Benson, A. A.,** The path of carbon in photosynthesis, *Science,* 107, 476—480, 1948.
15. **Carter, J. R., Westerman, D. T., and Jensen, M. E.,** Sugarbeet yield and quality as affected by nitrogen level, *Agron. J.,* 68, 49—55, 1976.
16. **Cook , C. W.,** Energy budget of the range and range livestock, *Colo. State Univ. Exp. Sta. Bull.* TB, 109, 1970.

17. **Cooper, J. P., Ed.,** *Photosynthesis and Productivity in Different Environments,* Cambridge University Press, London, 1975.
18. **Dalrymple, D. G.,** The adoption of high yielding grain varieties in developing nations, *Agric. Hist.,* 53, 704—720, 1979.
19. National Research Council, *Climate and Food: Report of the Committee on Climate and Weather Fluctuations and Agricultural Production,* National Academy of Sciences, Washington, D.C., 1976.
20. **Doyle, J. J.,** The Response of Rice to Fertilizer, FAO Agric. Studies No. 70., Food and Agriculture Organization, Rome, 1966.
21. **Duckham, A. N.,** Biological efficiency of food producing systems in AD 2000, *Chem. Ind. London,* 6 July, 903—906, 1968.
22. **Durost, D. D. and Black, E.,** Changes in Farm Production and Efficiency, Stat. Bull. 561. U.S. Department of Agriculture, Washington, D.C., 1976, 1—68.
23. Economics, Statistics and Cooperative Service, Livestock and Meat Statistics, Stat. Bull. No. 522., U.S. Department of Agriculture, Washington, D.C., 1979.
24. **Englestad, O. P. and Parks, W. L.,** Variation in optimum nitrogen rates for corn, *Agron. J.,* 63, 21—23, 1971.
25. **Erie, L. J., French, O. F., and Harris, K.,** Consumptive use of water by crops in Arizona, *Ariz. Agric. Exp. Sta. Bull.,* No. 169, 1948.
26. **Evans, H. J. and Barber, L. E.,** Biological nitrogen fixation for food and fiber production, *Science,* 197, 332—339, 1977.
27. **Ewell, R.,** Food and fertilizer in the developing countries, 1975—2000, *Bioscience,* 25 (12), 771, 1975.

28a. FAO Production Yearbook 1972 (No. 26), Food and Agriculture Organization, Rome.

28b. FAO Production Yearbook 1974 (No. 28), Food and Agricuture Organization, Rome.

28c. FAO Production Yearbook 1977 (No. 31), Food and Agriculture Organization, Rome, 1978.

29. **Fitzhugh, H. A., Hodgson, H. J., Scoville, O. J., Nguyen, Thanh D., and Byerly, T. C.,** Role of Ruminants in Support of Man, Winrock Livestock Research and Training Center, Morrilton, Ark., 1978.
30. **Frankel, O. N., Ed.,** Crop Genetic Resources in their Centers of Diversity, Food and Agriculture Organization, Rome, 1973.
31. **Fuller, H. L. and Mora, G.,** Energetic efficiency of different dietary fats for growth of young chicks, *Poult. Sci.,* 56, 549—557, 1977.
32. **Greenland, D. J.,** Bringing the green revolution to the shifting cultivator, *Science,* 190, 841—844, 1975.
33. **Guillaume, J.,** The dwarfing gene dw, *World Poult. Sci. J.,* 32, 285-304, 1976.
34. **Halvorson, A. R.,** The basis of nitrogen and phosphorus recommendations when soil tests are used, in Proc. of the Walla Walla-Pendleton Fertilizer Ind. Conf., Washington State University, Pullman, 1965, as cited in Decker, W. L., *Climate and Food, Report of the Committee on Climate and Weather Fluctuations and Agricultural Production,* National Academy of Science, Washington, D.C., 1976.
35. **Harpstead, D. D.,** Man-molded cereal — hybrid corn's story, in The 1975 Yearbook of Agriculture, U.S. Government Printing Office, Washington, 1975.
36. **Hayes, P. R. and Schaefer, M. J.,** *Probablistic Climate and Yield Forecasting,* C. F. Kettering Foundation, Yellow Springs, Ohio, 1977.
37. **Hayes, P. R. and Schaefer, M. J.,** A Case Study for the Northern Plains, Systems Research Center, Case Western Reserve University, Cleveland, Ohio, 1977.
38. **Hendricks, W. A.,** Fitting the curve of the diminishing increment to feed consumption liveweight growth curves, *Science,* 74, 290—291, 1931,
39. National Research Council, *Agricultural Production Efficiency,* National Academy of Sciences, Washington, D.C., 1975.
40. **Hucklesby, D. P., Brown, C. M., Howell, S. E., and Hageman, R. H.,** Late spring applications of nitrogen for efficient utilization and enhanced production of grain and grain protein of wheat, *Agron. J.,* 63, 274—283, 1971.
41. **Ibach, D. E.,** A graphic method of interpreting response to fertilizer, in *U.S. Dep. Agric. Handb. No. 93,* 1956.
42. **Jackson, W. A., Knexek, B. D., and van Schilfgaarde, J., Water, soil and mineral input, in** Crop Productivity: Research Imperatives, Brown, A.W.A., Byerly, T. C., Gibbs, M., and San Pietro, A., Eds., Michigan Agricultural Experiment Station, East Lansing, 1975, 201—274.

42a. **Jennings, R. D.,** Consumption of feed by livestock, 1909-1956, Product Res. Rep. No. 21, Agricultural Research Service, U.S. Department of Agriculture, Washington, D.C., 1958, 1—128.

43. **Jensen, L. S.,** Standards show faster growth, improved feed efficiency, *Turkey World,* 52, 10—14, 1977.
44. **Johnson, J. W., Welch, L. F., and Kurtz, L. T.,** Soybeans' role in nitrogen balance, *Ill. Res.,* 16 (3), 6—7, 1974.

45. **Kammlade, W. G.** *Sheep Science,* Lippincott, Philadelphia, 1947.
46. **Kennedy, D.,** *Pest Control, Contemporary Pest Control Practices and Prospects,* Vol. 1, National Academy of Sciences, Washington, D.C., 1975.
47. **King, G. J., Randall, L. F., and Keenast, A. A.,** *Dairy Herd Improvement Association Letter,* 50 (3) 27, 1974.
48. **Klepper, R., Lockerets, W., Commoner, B., Geitler, M., Fast, S., O'Leary, D., and Blobaum, R.,** Economic performance and energy intensiveness on organic and conventional farms in the Cornbelt: a preliminary comparison, *Am. J. Agric. Econ.,* 59, 1—24, 1977.
49. **Kortschak, H. P., Hartt, C. E., and Burr, G. O.,** Carbon dioxide fixation in sugar cane leaves, *Plant Physiol.,* 40, 209—213, 1965.
50. **Lemon, E. R.,** The Energy Budget at the Earth's surface, in Parts I and II, Product Res. Rep. No. 71., Agriculture Research Service, U.S. Department of Agriculture, Washington, D.C., 1963.
51. **Lofgreen, G. P. and Garrett, W. N.,** A system for expressing net energy requirements and feed values for growing and finishing beef cattle, *J. Anim. Sci.,* 27, 793—806, 1968.
52. **McDowell, R. E.,** Ruminant Products More than Meat and Milk, Winrock Rep., Winrock Int. Livestock Res. and Training Center, Morrilton, Ark., 1978.
53. **Minot, C. S.,** Senescence and rejuvenation, *J. Physiol.,* 12, 97—159, 1891.
54. **Morrison, F. B.,** *Feeds and Feeding.* 21st ed., Morrison Publishing, Ithaca, New York, 1948.
55. National Research Council, *Nutrient Requirements of Domestic Animals, Poultry,* 7th rev. ed., No. 1, National Academy of Sciences, Washington, D.C., 1977.
56. National Research Council, *Nutrient Requirements of Domestic Animals, Swine,* 7th rev. ed., No. 2, National Academy of Sciences, Washington, D.C., 1973.
57. National Research Council, *Nutrient Requirements of Domestic Animals, Dariy Cattle,* 5th rev. ed., No. 3, National Academy of Sciences, Washington, D.C., 1978.
58. National Research Council, *Nutrient Requirements of Domestic Animals, Beef Cattle,* 5th rev. ed., No. 4, National Academy of Sciences, Washington, D.C., 1976.
59. National Research Council, *Nutrient Requirements of Domestic Animals, Sheep,* 5th rev. ed., No. 5, National Academy of Sciences, Washington, D.C., 1975.
60. **Nelson, M.,** *The Development of Tropical Lands: Policy Issues in Latin America,* Johns Hopkins University Press, Baltimore, 1974.
61. **Nichiporovich, A. A.,** The role of plants in bioregeneration systems, *Annu. Rev. Plant Physiol.,* 20, 185—208, 1969.
62. **Paulsen, A.,** Feeding Animals versus Feeding People, Midwestern Conf. Food and Social Policy, Sioux City, Iowa, Oct. 22, 1976.
63. **Pierre, W. H., Dumeriel, L., Jolley, V. D., Webb, J. R., and Shrader, W. D.,** Relationship between corn yield, expressed as a percentage of maximum and the N percentage in the grain, *Agron. J.,* 69, 215—220, 1977.
64. **Pimentel, O.,** Energy and land constraints in food protein production, *Science,* 1190, 754—761, 1975.
65. **Prescott, J. A.,** Climatic Expressions and Generalized Climatic Zones in Relation to Soils and Vegetation, Proc., Spec. Conf. Agri., 1949, 27—33, Adelaide and Canberra, as cited by Callaghan, A. and Millington, A. J., *The Wheat Industry in Australia,* Angus and Robertson, Sydney, Australia, 1956.
66. **Purchase, H. G.,** An Evaluation of Research on Lymphoid Leukosis and Marek's Disease, Agriculture Research Service, U.S. Department of Agriculture, Washington, D.C., 1975.
67. **Purchase, H. G., Okazaki, W., and Burmester, B. R.,** Long term field trials with the herpes virus of turkeys vaccine against Marek's disease, *Avian Dis.,* 16, 34—44, 1972.
68. **Ranson, S. L. and Thomas, M.,** Crassulacean acid metabolism, *Annu. Rev. Plant Physiol,* 11, 81—110, 1960.
69. **Raney, W. A.,** Water research and agriculture in humid areas, in *Research on Water,* Hamilton, H. L. and Stelly, M., Eds., ASA Spec. Publ. Ser., No. 4, Soil Science Society of America, Madison, Wis., 1964, 31—41.
70. **Reeve, R. C.,** Potential for Saving Energy in Irrigation, Agriculture Research Service, U.S. Department of Agriculture, Washington, D.C., 1977.
71. **Reidinger, R. B.,** World Fertilizer Review and Prospects to 1980—81, Foreign Agriculture Economic Report, No. 110, U.S. Department of Agriculture, Washington, D.C., 1976.
72. **Robison, O. W.,** Growth patterns in swine, *J. Anim. Sci.,* 42, 1024—1035, 1976.
73. **Shantz, H. L. and Piemeisel, L. N.,** The water requirements of plants in Akron, Colorado, *J. Agric. Res.,* 34, 1093, 1927.
74. **Smith, G. E.,** Soil fertility and corn production, *Mo. Agric. Exp. Sta. Bull.,* No. 583, 1952.
75. **Spillman, W. J.,** Use of the Exponential Yield Curve in Fertilizer Experiments, *U.S. Dep. Agric. Tech. Bull.,* No. 348, 1933.

76. **Stahly, T. S., Cromwell, G. L., and Aviotti, M. P.,** Effect of environmental temperature and dietary lysine source and level on the performance and carcass characteristics of growing swine, *J. Anim. Sci.,* 49, 1242—1251, 1979.
77. **Stanford, G.,** Rationale for optimum nitrogen fertilizer in corn production, *J. Environ. Qual.,* 2 (2), 159—165, 1973.
78. **Stanford, G. and Ayres, A. S.,** The internal nitrogen requirements of sugar cane, *Soil Sci.,* 98, 338—344, 1964.
79. **Stanford G., Carter, J. N., Westerman, D. T., and Meisenger, J. J.,** Residual nitrate and mineralizable soil nitrogen in relation to soil uptake by irrigated sugar beets, *Agron. J.,* 69, 303—307, 1977.
80. **Statistical Research Service,** Cropping Practices, SRS-17, U.S. Department of Agriculture, Washington, D.C., 1971.
81. **Steinhart, J. S. and Steinhart, C. E.,** Energy use in the U.S. food system, *Science,* 184, 305—316, 1974.
82. **Stewart, B. A., Woolhiser, D. A., Wischmeier, W. M., Caro, J. H., and Fyere, M. H.,** Control of Water Pollution from Cropland, Vol. 1, Agricultural Research Service, U.S. Department of Agriculture, and Environmental Protection Agency, Washington, D.C., 1975.
83. **Stucker, T. and Erickson, L., 1975.** Livestock wastes as a substitute for commercial nitrogen fertilizer, *Ill. Res.,* 17 (5), 10—11, 1975.
84. **Thompson, L. M.,** Weather and production of corn in the U.S. cornbelt, *Agron. J.,* 61, 435—456, 1969.
85. **Thornthwaite, C. W.,** An approach toward a rational classification of climate, *Geogr. Rev.,* 38, 55—94, 1948.
86. **Timmer, C. P.,** Energy and the food system, a review of *The Efficiency of Human Food Chains and Nutrient Cycles,* by Duckham, A. N., Jones, J. G. W., and Roberts, E. H., Eds., *Science,* 197, 1354, 1977.
87. **Trenbath, B. R.,** Biomass productivity of mixtures, *Adv. Agron.,* 26, 177-—210, 1974.
88. **Troughton, J. H.** Photosynthetic mechanisms in higher plants, in *Photosynthesis and Productivity in Different Environments,* Cooper, J. P., Ed., Cambridge University Press, London, 1975, 351—391.
89. **Troughton, J. H. and Slatyer, O.,** Plant water status leaf temperature and the calculated mesophyll resistance to carbon dioxide of cotton leaves, *Aust. J. Biol. Sci.,* 22, 815—827, 1969.
90. **Trumble, H. C.,** Rainfall, evaporation and drought frequency in South Australia, *J. Dep. Agric. S. Aust.,* 52, 55—64, 1948.
91. United States Congress, Office of Technology Assessment, Organizing and Financing Basic Research to Increase Food Production, U.S. Government Printing Office, Washington, D.C., 1977.
92. United States Department of Agriculture, Agricultural Statistics, Washington, D.C., 1972.
93. U.S. Department of Agriculture, Agricultural Statistics, Washington, D.C., 1975.
94. U.S. Department of Agriculture, Agricultural Statistics, Washington, D.C., 1978.
95. Balance Sheet of the Farming Sector, Suppl. No. 1, AIB, Economics, Statistics and Cooperative Service, U.S. Department of Agriculture, Washington, D.C., 1978.
96. **Vickery, H. B.,** The formation of starch in the leaves of *Bryophyllum calcinum* cultured in darkness, *Plant Physiol.,* 27, 231—239, 1952.
97. **von Bulow, J. F. W. and Dobereiner, S.,** *Proc. Nat. Acad. Sci. U.S.A.,* 72, 2389, 1975.
98. **von Liebig, J.,** *Die Grundsatze der Agrikultur-Chemie,* Bieweg & Cohn, Braunschweig, 1855.
99. **Watt, B. K. and Merrill, A. L.,** Composition of Foods, in *U.S. Dep. Agric. Handb. 8,* 1964.
100. **Wadleigh, C. A.,** Fitting modern agriculture to water supply, in *Research on Water,* ASA Spec. Publ. Ser. No. 4., Soil Science of America, Madison, Wis., 1964, 8—14.
101. **Welch, L. F., Mulvaney, D. L., Oldham, M. G., Boone, L. V., and Pendleton, J. W.,** Corn yields with fall, spring and side dress nitrogen, *Agron. J.,* 63, 21—23, 1971.
102. **Wells, F. J.,** *The Long-Run Availability of Phosphorus,* Resources of the Future, Inc., Johns Hopkins University Press, Baltimore, 1975.
103. **Wortman, S.,** World crop productivity: challenge to science, in *Crop Productivity: Research Imperatives,* Brown, A. W. A., Byerly, T. C., Gibbs, M., and San Pietro, A., Eds., Michigan Agricultural Experiment Station, East Lansing, 1975, 43—61.
104. **Yocum, C. S.,** Photosynthesis, in The Energy Budget at the Earth's Surface, Part I, Production Research Rep. No. 71, Agricultural Research Service, U.S. Department of Agriculture, Washington, D.C., 1963, 28—33,
105. **Zelitch, I.,** *Photosynthesis, Photorespiration and Plant Productivity,* Academic Press, New York, 1971.
106. **Millington, A. J. and Callaghan, A.,** *The Wheat Industry in Australia,* Angus and Robertson, Sydney, Australia, 1956, 80—81.

107. Fats and Oils Situation, FOS-301, Economics and Statistics Service, U.S. Department of Agriculture, October 1980, Washington, D.C.
108. **Piestevoit, G. V.,** Current work in sunflower breeding at Uniimk (USSR), Proc. 3rd Intl. Sunflower Conf., Crookston, Minn., 1978, 46—52.
109. **Doty, H. O.,** Competitive position of new oil seed sunflower with soybeans, *Sunflower,* 5(5), 1979, 16—19.
110. Agricultural Statistics, U.S. Department of Agriculture, Washington, D.C., 1979.
111. Status Report on Rebuttable Presumption Against Registration (RPAR), TS-791, Office of Pesticide Programs, U.S. Environmental Protection Agency, Washington, C.C., 1980.
112. **Eichers, T. B.,** Evaluation of pesticide supplies and demand for 1980, AER Report No. 454, Economics, Statistical Cooperatives Service, Agriculture, Washington, D.C., 1980.
113. **Hargrove, T. R. and Cabanilla, V. L.,** The impact of semidwarf varieties on Asian rice-breeding programs, *Bioscience,* 29, 731—735, 1979.

CHEMICALS FOR CROP AND LIVESTOCK PROTECTION

Keith C. Barrons

One has only to visit the poorer parts of the world to recognize the quantitative aspects of good nutrition. Without abundant food production at home or the monetary means to pay for imports, hunger is inevitable, at least for the poorer segments of a population. Stroll down the side streets of Port-au-Prince, Lima, or Calcutta and you will see the stark reality of calorie as well as protein deficiency. Go into the heavily populated countryside of many "third world" countries and you will see walking reminders that living on the land is no guarantee of good nutrition.

Of course, abundance does not assure well-balanced nutrition; however, without abundance, there can be no hope that the masses will have a healthful diet. Even though a country's available food, if evenly divided, would provide a reasonable diet for all, malnutrition of many is inevitable. No one has yet found a way to equitably divide an adequate total amount of food; a shortage would intensify the problem. The abundance that has blessed the technically advanced and agriculturally productive countries in recent decades reduces the chances of hunger by keeping prices lower than they otherwise would be. Lest one questions the importance of food abundance to food prices, think back to the sugar at $0.60/lb in late 1974 when there was a temporary, though hardly acute, shortage of this commodity. Food subsidies for the poor, such as the U.S. food stamp program and the various domestic and foreign relief activities, have little chance of proving meaningful or even existing if there are shortages.

REQUIREMENTS FOR ABUNDANCE

What gives us abundance in the more fortunate parts of the world? Conversely, why are so many countries perennially short of the food needed for good nutrition of their masses of people? There is no one simple answer, but some important factors contributing to abundance are understood. Nutritionists, concerned with the quality of diets, should also have a grasp of the following quantitative aspects of food supply, for without quantity our concern for good nutrition can become an exercise in futility.

People — Our infinite capacity to reproduce, in contrast to finite food production resources, has resulted in rapid population growth rates in many countries, often exceeding expansion in the food supply. Recent public health programs and improved medical services, assuring that more people survive to reproduce, have resulted in births far exceeding deaths. This is in sharp contrast to former days when a large family was needed to assure survival of a few. Lower birth rates in the technically advanced countries have tended to compensate for reduced mortality, but this has not been true in vast regions of Africa, Asia, and Latin America. No matter what progress is made in food production efficiency, a slowing-down in birth rates is essential if the presently food-short peoples are to ever be better nourished.

Natural resources — Most food must come from the land. Only about 3% is derived from aquatic sources, and much of this is concentrated in a few parts of the world, e.g., Japan and Northern Europe. Land adaptability for food production is essential from the standpoint of topography, climate, rainfall distribution, and fertility.

Infrastructure — The infrastructure of finance, roads, and other transportation facilities, and storage, processing, marketing, and distribution is essential to an effective food system, even in a country with abundant labor and little dependence on mechanization. Storage facilities are needed to provide abundance not only between harvests but also to provide a reserve in the event of a poor crop. Food reserves are vital to continuing good nutrition.

Production — The production factor is dependent on the farmer who raises the food. What enables and encourages him to produce abundantly? He must have certain mined or manufactured supplies. In a high-labor, low-capital economy such as those in most developing countries, growers still need fertilizer and crop and livestock protection chemicals if high yields are to be achieved. Where a small labor force must feed the populace, mechanical equipment and the energy to run it are also imperative.

Incentive for the farmer is also vital; a food system that assures him of a market for his produce beyond that needed for home consumption encourages investment and hard work. Conversely, nothing discourages productivity as much as the specter of market gluts and ruinous prices at harvest time.

Given land, a favorable climate, available supplies, incentive, and the infrastructure necessary to support the producer, many technical factors become important to abundant production. Vast improvements in technology have enabled farmers in the agriculturally advanced world to double yields per unit area of many crops. U.S. corn, for example, now averages nearly three times as many bushels per acre as it did only 40 years ago (Figure 1). This "yield revolution" has resulted from many decades of research and development, and the continuing support of these activities is essential to future abundance.

The technical influences involved in food abundance may be considered in five categories:

Genetically improved varieties and breeds — The importance of breeding has been emphasized in recent news about increased yields obtained from dwarf Mexican wheat, hybrid corn, and "miracle" rice. Actually, there is no successful agricultural enterprise today that has not benefited from advances in genetics and the scientific breeding of the last century.

Superior nutrition — More than a century of research on the mineral nutrition of plants, together with developments in the large-scale production of fertilizers by the chemical industry, made possible today's vastly better-nourished crops. Improved nutrition has also had a major impact on the efficiency of animal agriculture, particularly poultry.

Better management — Improved crop husbandry practices made possible through increased knowledge of soils, irrigation, and plant responses to their environment have contributed significantly to increased yields. Both livestock and poultry are being produced more efficiently because of advanced management practices, e.g., caged layers in the poultry industry.

Farm mechanization — Mechanization is vital to total production in the labor-short developed countries, but not as critical to productivity per unit area as other factors. The evidence: high yields in a number of labor-rich countries where relatively little farm equipment is employed. Nonetheless, equipment that makes it possible to irrigate extensively and to more adequately perform planting, harvesting, and crop protection operations at just the right time can have a beneficial impact on yields everywhere.

Control of damaging pests — The plant breeder has given us genetic resistance to many diseases, and research on sanitation, cultural, and management practices have pointed the way to mitigation of a number of pests. Nature's ways of keeping populations in check through predators and parasites have been encouraged and some important biological control methods are now available.

After the above methods of controlling insects, fungi, nematodes, weeds and other pests have all been put to work, however, there is still a wide gap that must be filled with crop and livestock protection chemicals, often called pesticides. Unfilled, this gap in protecting our food supply would result in lower general productivity and higher costs. At times it would result in severe losses and human suffering such as has occurred in the past, e.g., the great Irish potato famine of the mid-19th century when fungicides to control potato blight were unknown. Much progress has been made in recent years in devising integrated pest management programs involving various methods of control, but in most integration systems chemicals remain as one important "tool". Indeed, chemicals are still often the first line of defense.

We must defend ourselves against the ravages of pests if food abundance and good nutrition are to be a continuing reality. This chapter is about crop and livestock protection chemicals and their relationship to the consistent high level of food production so essential to good nutrition for the populace.

CLASSES OF PESTS AND CHEMICALS FOR THEIR CONTROL

A wide range of organisms can, if their populations get out of hand, be damaging to the productivity of crops and livestock. The major groups include fungi, bacteria, insects, mites, viruses, snails and slugs, weeds, nematodes, birds, and rodents and other mammals.

When these organisms affect plants in the U.S., they are legally classified as pests and chemicals used for their control are regulated under the pesticide laws. Insects affecting animals are also considered as pests and fall under these same regulations. Synthetic chemicals or biologically produced substances used for the control of diseases or various parasites of animals (other than insects) are legally considered as drugs and are regulated under the drug laws. In the U.S. and most other countries, both pesticides and drugs must have governmental approval before they can be sold.

Let us look at some representative pests of food plants and animals and the crop and livestock protection chemicals that are essential to a high level of year-in and year-out productivity.

Fungi

Over the last century, genetic resistance to specific diseases has been identified in many crop plants, and breeders have often succeeded in combining such resistance with other desirable traits to form useful varieties and hybrids. Notable among these are rust-resistant wheats used in important grain-growing countries throughout the world. Breeding for disease resistance is a never-ending job; fungi often mutate to form new physiological races to which the old resistant varieties may be susceptible. Sanitation, rotation, and other cultural practices are widely employed methods of mitigating the severity of fungal infection of plants. However, there are many fungi attacking foliage or the below-ground portion of plants that can only be successfully controlled by the use of fungicides.

The old saying when planting corn seed: "One for the cutworm, one for the crow, one to damp off and one to grow" is reflective of the uncertainties of obtaining a good stand of seedlings that beset growers before the availability of fungicidal seed treatment. If the soil became cold and wet, seed might rot and replanting would be necessary. Modern fungicidal corn seed treatment minimizes such losses and permits earlier planting and thus the use of higher yielding hybrids that require a long season for their development. These yield at least 10 bushels more per acre than the early hybrids that would have to be grown, usually with later planting, if seed-treatment fungicides were not available. For the U.S., with more than 70 million acres of corn, this means an increase in production of at least 700 million bushels, a tremendous contribution to the world's food supply.

The fungus which causes scab of apples is an almost universal problem of this important fruit crop. It is true that you can get a lot of apples from a backyard tree, good for sauce or pie, even though scab lesions are present of the surface of the fruit. However, with appreciable scab infection, apples do not keep well in storage. Fungicides have long been used for the control of this disease, and few consumers know what it looks like.

Potato late blight, mentioned earlier as the cause of the disastrous famine in Ireland in the 1840s, and other fungus diseases of this crop would make potato growing extremely risky under many climatic conditions. Fungicides, first used on this important food plant nearly a century ago, now protect it throughout Europe, eastern North America, and other areas where a damp climate is conducive to development of disease. Nearly 300 million metric tons of potatoes are produced in the world annually. The per capita consumption is particularly high in Europe, where it has long been a staple of people with low incomes. Disruptions of the potato crop such as those occurring occasionally before protection with fungicides could have a disastrous effect on the nutrition of tens of millions. Fortunately, the fungicidal properties of copper sulfate were discovered during the latter part of the 19th century; the presently used organic fungicides of the dithiocarbamate type were discovered more recently. Today the potato crop is relatively well protected from both insects and fungi; variations in amounts produced now related primarily to rainfall differences.

The history of potato yields in the U.S. makes an interesting case study of the importance of all the technical advances of the last 60 years (Table 1). The marked increases in yield are, of course, the result of many factors, but improved fungicides played an important role. Better insecticides are also important. Not many years ago, growers hardly knew what healthy potato foliage looked like because of the effect of ever-present leaf hoppers. Now, without hopper damage, foliage remains active longer resulting in more and larger potatoes. Improved varieties and better plant nutrition are also important factors in higher potato yields and in several areas where rainfall is undependable, supplemental irrigation has contributed to more dependable crops.

Insects

Some plants grown under favorable conditions have relatively few insect problems, but when potentially damaging insect species increase to unusual levels, crop protection chemicals can assure productivity, benefiting not only the farmer, but also the public, who require food every day until the next crop is harvested. In the case of the green bug, an aphid of wheat, years may pass without an insecticidal spray or dust. Similar occasional outbreaks of aphids may occur on sorghum and peas. With many species, natural controls usually keep insect numbers in check, but for reasons not well understood, a population explosion is occasionally experienced. Armyworms and grasshoppers are other insects that occasionally occur in vast numbers and have the capacity to cause sharp yield depressions.

There are many crop insects, on the other hand, that occur in damaging numbers almost every year, and the grower must be prepared with control measures. For example, the corn rootworm is so prevalent in some areas that an insecticidal treatment at planting time is necessary. The larvae feeding on the roots may reduce plant vigor to the extent that yield are reduced, stalks are weakened, and machine harvesting becomes inefficient. Later in the season, the adult beetles of this species feed on corn silks, preventing complete pollination.

Many factors have contributed to the tremendous increase in corn productivity in recent decades (Figure 1), including better fertilization, high-yielding hybrids, and the seed treatments already mentioned; corn rootworm control with insecticides has also

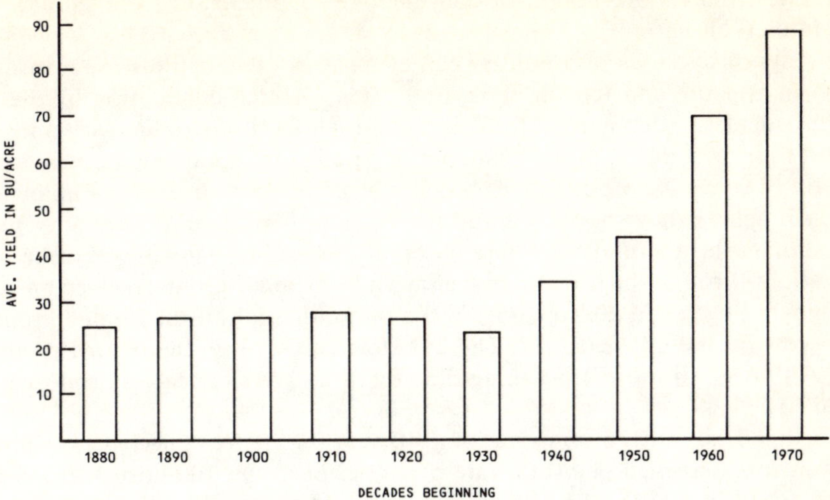

FIGURE 1. A century of corn in the U.S.

TABLE 1
AVERAGE PER-ACRE-YIELD OF POTATOES IN THE U.S.[a]

Decade beginning	Yield in cwt
1920	56
1930	67
1940	82
1950	165
1960	208
1970	247

[a] Data from U.S. Department of Agriculture.

played an important role. It is true that increased acreage with corn following corn has encouraged high worm populations, but root damage was not well recognized until practical controls were developed. Weak stalks were less detrimental in the days of hand harvesting. The nearly 6 billion bushels of corn raised in the average year of the 1970s had to be harvested mechanically; straight stalks are therefore imperative if losses are to be avoided. These huge crops have been vital factors in our abundance of eggs, poultry, red meat, and dairy products as well as foods derived directly from corn. At yields per acre of the 1930s we would have had less than 2 billion bushels available each year, and every food to which corn contributes would be scarce and far more expensive than it is today.

Many fruits and vegetables that provide us with so much enjoyment, as well as protective vitamins and minerals, are particularly vulnerable to insect attack. The so-called Kohl crops — cabbage, cauliflower, broccoli, and related species — are usually beset by leaf-eating worms and sometimes by aphids. A good insecticide program chosen among those approved by pesticide control officials is just as important to the grower as procuring good seed. A constant check of insect populations will tell him when trouble is imminent and an insecticide must be applied. If you raise these plants in your garden, you may not object to worm-eaten outer cabbage leaves or green aphids among the broccoli buds. But insect-damaged produce can hardly be put into commerce. Aside from the likelihood of consumer rejection, losses from spoilage would often be intolerable.

Insect pests of livestock and poultry can cause losses through disease transmission, reduction in appetite and feeding time, and often through debilitation by the loss of blood. Insecticides, often needed to maintain a high level of productivity, may be administered as sprays, dusts, dips, single spot or "pour-on" applications, or in feed.

Horn fly of cattle is an example of a debilitating insect that prevents animals from grazing as much as they should for full production. This common summer pest was controlled in one group of about 500 range cattle at the University of Nebraska's North Platte Station[1] through the use of dust bags, while a similar group received no control. Flies numbered less than 20/cow during the 6-month trial on the treated group, and over 500/cow on the untreated lot. The 257 steer calves from the treated group averaged 12.92 lb per calf more at weaning time than the 278 steer calves produced by the untreated cows.

In a further study at the same station,[1] 40 yearling heifers selected for uniformity were put in four screened pens at a rate of 10 per pen, and 100 horn flies per animal were introduced into each of two pens, while the other two were kept fly-free. After 100 days, the fly-free calves averaged 43 lb more and had 11% better feed efficiency than the fly-infested calves.

Weeds

Weeds have been defined as plants that are out of place. Anyone who has grown even a small vegetable garden has learned that food plants will not thrive in competition with others that grow from seed or vegetative organs that were in the soil at planting time. These may sometimes be useful plants in themselves, but they are out of place. Lamb's-quarters, for example, has edible shoots similar to spinach, but if many lamb's-quarters seedlings emerge among your row of snapbeans and are not removed, production of beans will be pitifully low. Volunteer corn from seed lost in harvesting the year before can be a serious weed in soybean fields. Most unwanted plants in crop fields have little economic or nutritional value under any circumstances, but they do have a serious impact on crop productivity if not controlled.

Since agriculture began nearly 10,000 years ago, weeds, including grass sod growing where a crop is to be planted have been destroyed by various means of stirring the soil. The plows and disks you see operating on today's farms are modern counterparts to the sticks used by early agriculturalists. The inevitable weeds that come up with the crop have traditionally been removed by pulling or stirring the soil between rows and, in modern times, by interrow cultivation.

A new era in weed control has dawned in recent decades with the discovery of chemicals highly toxic to many weeds but safe on desirable crops. If you have treated your lawn with a selective herbicide to control dandelions or other weeds, you have had firsthand experience with one of these remarkable selective materials.

The cereal grains — wheat, barley and oats — are ordinarily planted in narrow drill rows about 8 in. apart, which does not permit interrow tillage for weed control purposes. For many thousands of years these crops suffered great losses in yield because of weed competition. During the last 30 years, 2,4-D and other selective herbicides have been widely used on these crops in many parts of the world. At present there are in the world more than 200 million acres of cereals treated each year with selective weed control chemicals producing an average increase in yield of at least 5 bushels/acre. Thus the world benefits by one billion bushels or more that could not otherwise be realized. In terms of wheat, at 65 1-lb loaves of bread per bushel, this gain means the equivalent of more than 65 billion loaves, about 15 for each of the world's more than 4 billion people.

Many crops including corn, sorghum, soybean, cotton, sugar beets, sugarcane, and potatoes are grown in rows, and tillage between rows has long been practiced. No matter how carefully interrow cultivation is carried out, many weeds growing close to the crop plants remain. Aside from hand hoeing and weeding, which is not practical on the massive scale on which farming must be conducted to feed the world, there was until very recent times no way to handle these unwanted plants that so seriously reduced yields and impeded harvesting. Now that we have selective herbicides for most important crops, chemicals can be applied over the row immediately after planting to keep the weeds from coming up (preemergence herbicides), or may be sprayed after emergence to kill weeds without hurting the crop, as we do with the cereal grains (postemergence products). Some compounds are effective and safe to the crop when worked into the soil before planting (preplant incorporation).

Tremendous areas of land not topographically or climatically suited to crop production are used for grazing ruminant animals, primarily cattle and sheep. These livestock species are able to utilize roughages in their nutrition and thus contribute meat, wool, and dairy products that do not compete for crop land. Even when meat animals are "finished" with grain during the latter third of their growth period, or when dairy production is boosted with supplemental feed concentrates, the crop land used per unit of human food produced is modest because of the large utilization of forage. Grazing land and ruminant animals are truly man's benefactors if properly managed.

But pastures and ranges often become infested with nonnutritious, nonpalatable, or even poisonous vegetation; thus, production of livestock is far below the potential. Cutting these unwanted plants, which are often woody in nature, is like going to the barbershop; they grow right back, and benefits in terms of increased forage production are very temporary. Selective herbicides that will kill or greatly reduce the competitive effect of unwanted woody or herbaceous vegetation are now in wide use on grazing lands in North and South America, Australia, New Zealand, and parts of Africa. They result in vast increases in forage production and corresponding increases in the animal products man utilizes which are indirectly derived from forage.

An example of the depressing effect woody vegetation can have on forage production may be seen from data from the Gualaca Experiment Station in Panama,[2] in a zone of annual rainfall of 229 cm. The production of grass and nongrass vegetation in a woody brush-infested pasture of Jaragua grass, an important tropical forage, was measured after treatment with a mixture of picloram herbicide at 0.672 kg plus 2,4-D at 2.688 kg/ha. Cattle were withheld and clippings were made 460 days after application; results can be found in Table 2. Note the shift from brush to grass in the treated areas, with total vegetation remaining essentially constant.

Of all available approaches to improving protein supplies around the world, none offers a greater potential than the improvement of pastures and ranges for ruminant animals. Along with fertilization, liming where needed, reseeding, and wise grazing practices, the use of herbicides can thus contribute significantly to better nutrition.

Nematodes

These tiny roundworms that live parasitically on plant roots are far more detrimental to full crop productivity than was formerly realized. Among the many plant parasitic species, the best known and probably the most damaging is the root-knot nematode, which causes the formation of root galls and inhibits full underground plant development. Throughout the tropics and subtropics, root knot is a prevalent disease of a wide range of food crops including beans, tomatoes, potatoes, cabbage, and many

TABLE 2
RESULT OF TREATMENT WITH PICLORAM PLUS 2,4-D

Treatment	Jaragua grass (ton/acre)[a]	Other grasses (ton/acre)	Live brush (ton/acre)	Total vegetation (ton/acre)
None	1.80	0.28	12.65	14.73
Picloram + 2,4-D	13.55	0.29	0.50	14.34

[a] One ton per acre equals 2.72 metric tons per hectare.

other vegetables as well as fruits. Few crops are entirely free from some parasitic nematode species and, in addition to the plants mentioned, one or more attack most crops including corn, cotton, rice, pineapple, sugar beets, beans, carrots, soybeans, lettuce, onions, sweet potatoes, strawberries, citrus, grapes and peaches. Yield losses vary from modest to almost complete, depending on the nematode population and various environmental factors. Crop rotations are helpful in keeping populations at a low level, and soil drying or prolonged freezing also tends to minimize the severity of nematode damage through population reduction.

In the tropics and subtropics where crops or weeds susceptible to nematodes are growing on the land continuously, control by strictly cultural methods is most difficult. High-value crops, requiring expensive inputs of labor, seed, fertilizer, and tractor power, can lose money for the grower if he allows nematode damage to reduce yield appreciably. Reduction of nematode populations before planting or, in some instances, control on the roots of established plants through the use of nematicidal chemicals applied in irrigation water, has become quite common in recent years. Without nematicides, many of our favorite fruits and vegetables would be more expensive, might often be unavailable, and in certain areas, major crops, including sugar beets and soybeans, would be unprofitable.

Several volatile liquid chemicals which vaporize after injection into the soil have been found to be useful. With most crops they are applied preplant, but in the case of bananas and other fruits, they may be applied in irrigation water. More recently, nematicidal compounds which are not fumigants have been discovered. Applied as granules to the soil before or at the time of planting, they successfully reduce populations so the young plant can get off to a good start.

A characteristic of nematicides when used at practical levels, is that they do not eradicate the pest, but merely reduce its numbers. As the crop develops, so will more nematodes, but if the young plant has been protected from an overwhelming population of root parasites, a profitable net return can be obtained. Nematicides often also serve as insecticides reducing the population of wireworms and other insect species that inhibit soil and attack newly planted seed or the underground parts of the plants we wish to grow.

Many examples of the beneficial impact of nematicides on food costs and abundance can be cited. For example, practically all pineapple is treated with a nematicide. Costs of this crop are so high that no grower can afford the fertilizer and land preparation and the extensive labor for planting unless he obtains a very good yield. With rotation alone as a control method and without nematicides, pineapple production around the world would be unprofitable at present returns. If this favorite fruit was still grown with the inevitable low yield caused by various species of nematodes, costs would be so high that only the rich could afford it. Nematode control is one of the factors that has made pineapple a common processed fruit on our supermarket shelves and, in many areas, an economical fresh fruit as well.

Soybeans, now grown on more than 50 million acres in the U.S., are increasingly attacked by the cyst nematode and in some areas by other types. Considerable progress has been made in breeding soybeans for resistance to nematodes but when populations of this parasite are especially high help is still needed from a nematicide. Recent research by R. A. Kinloch[3] of the University of Florida showed that the soybean variety "Bragg" which is resistant to root knot was still increased in yield one third by nematicides when grown on heavily infested land. In these tests "Hood", a susceptible variety, produced next to nothing without a nematicide. Kinloch's data follow:

	Yield in bushels per acre	
Nematicide	Hood (susceptible)	Bragg (resistant)
None (untreated control)	3.1	24.6
A	25.1	38.0
B	20.4	32.6
C	17.4	38.9

A look at sugar beet production in relation to the prevalence of the nematode, *Heterodera schachtii*, indicates that, where land is available for long rotations, the population of this soil pest does not build up to highly damaging proportions. In the extensive beet-growing areas of Europe and eastern North America, rotations of 7 years are often needed to keep the pest in check. However, in many productive intermountain and coastal sugar beet-growing areas of the western U.S., there simply is not enough land to permit control by rotation alone. Dichloropropene soil fumigant has made it possible to economically produce large acreages of beets on land that would otherwise have to be turned over to some other crop. Without fumigation, yields on infested land would not exceed 10 tons per acre while with fumigation, 25 tons or more are common.

Others

Mites are among the more serious pests of apples, pears, and citrus. Certain field crops including cotton are also sometimes attacked. These tiny spider-like organisms debilitate the plant by sucking juices from the underside of leaves and sometimes lower quality by feeding on the fruit. Other species of mites attack the skin of livestock and poultry, causing mange and similar problems. Plant-feeding mite populations are often kept from reaching damaging proportions by their natural enemies, and with pest control programs that favor predators, miticide applications may not be necessary. In many situations, however, parasitic mite populations reach the point where the crop is in jeopardy and miticides must be employed to reduce the population. Outbreaks in livestock and poultry must be controlled with appropriate chemicals to avoid serious losses.

Bacteria are the cause of many plant diseases such as leaf spot disease of beans and fire blight of apples and pears, which causes the death of whole branches. Some synthetic organic chemicals are employed, but antibiotics produced by culturing specific fungi are also very useful. Like many fungus diseases of foliage, bacterial plant infections are generally associated with a humid climate and frequent rainfall. Successful control involves sanitation plus application of a bactericide when weather conditions indicate a need. There are many bacterial diseases of livestock and poultry occasionally controlled by immunization but often by use of the appropriate veterinary drug of synthetic or biological origin.

Rodents have long been among man's most threatening enemies, destroying food and harboring insects that transmit disease. It is estimated that rodents still consume 15% or more of all the grain produced in Asia, an amount that would require land the equivalent of the entire state of Kansas to produce. Protecting food against the ravages of rats and mice requires sanitation and the construction of proper storages, but rodenticides to help keep populations in check are also very useful. Much damage from rats, particularly to sugarcane and rice, is also experienced in the field. Without the use of rodenticides as one phase of a control program, populations can reach staggering proportions and cause tremendous losses of crops badly needed for human food.

Virus infections are among the more serious types of plant diseases, and must often be controlled by maintaining virus-free planting stock under special conditions so the disease will not be transmitted from one generation to another through seed or vegetative reproductive organs. Plant viruses are often transmitted by insects, particularly aphids, and in many instances aphicidal chemicals provide virus control. Animal viruses, like bacterial infections, are controlled by immunization or veterinary drugs. Proper handling and housing practices are important factors in animal disease control.

Terrestrial snails and slugs, both members of the group of organisms known as mollusks, are serious pests of gardens and sometimes field crops. Gardeners almost everywhere are troubled by these pests, and the common bait containing the chemical metaldehyde has been helpful in their control for many years.

Poultry meat was a luxury 40 years ago, often costing more than beef or pork, while today it is a common and often economical item in our diet. Tremendous advances in the efficiency of poultry production have made this change possible. Improved breeding and better nutrition are important factors, but a significant factor in lower costs has been the control of coccidiosis, an intestinal parasite, through continuous medication in the feed. This disease caused significant losses, even in the days of the farm flock, but the major reason for giving chickens a lot of space was to keep coccidiosis infection from becoming too great. Confinement rearing at lower costs would have been impossible before the development of effective, parasite-controlling chemicals, that are safe on the poultry and in meat if traces should be present.

Every species of livestock and poultry and every type of companion animal suffers from one or another internal parasite if steps are not taken for their control. Fortunately, the chemical and pharmaceutical industries in cooperation with the veterinary profession have provided us with effective controls for a wide range of organisms including roundworms, flat worms, filarial worms, bots, and other internal parasites.

No discussion of the world's serious pests would be complete without mention of birds, which can do so much damage to certain crops including fruits, rice and grain sorghum. The Quella bird in Africa sometimes destroys as much as half the sorghum crop so important to human survival in that part of the world. No effective repellents have been discovered and few chemical approaches to control have been used.

Mammals other than rodents also take their toll, but here too chemicals have had limited utility in keeping populations in check. Chemical control programs for rabbits have supplemented biological controls in Australia and New Zealand where this animal once reached such staggering populations that even pasture grass was consumed.

Pesticide Safety

Only those chemicals that have been judged in wide-scale testing to give effective pest control with safety to the host crop or livestock species are granted permits to be marketed. Furthermore, before being approved by regulatory agencies, safety to nontarget organisms in the environment must be established. Precautions required for safety in application and subsequent contact with treated crops and livestock must be clearly prescribed.

Of primary concern in the broad safety investigation now required by most countries before a new pesticide may be placed in commerce, is the level of residue in food and the safety (or hazard) of this residue if it does exist. When considering the safety of pesticide residues in food, several basic concepts must be kept in focus. Almost any substance can be hazardous if consumed in too great a quantity. Common salt, essential to the diet, is toxic if taken in too large amounts. Vitamin A, also important in the human diet, has been found to induce birth defects in laboratory animals when administered in massive doses.

Conversely, it is probable that nothing is toxic if exposure through ingestion or other routes is low enough. Toxicological investigations of potential new pesticides using laboratory animals are conducted through a range of doses administered in the feed over a long period. Based on data on growth and reproduction, and on the pathological investigation of tissues, a no-adverse-effect level is established. Using these data as a guide and providing for a wide margin of safety, allowable maximum daily intake levels are established. These form the basis for decision by regulatory agencies as to how much of a residue will be acceptable.

Only those proposed uses for a crop or livestock protection chemical that are found to result in a residue at or below this safe level are approved and published on the label. Thus the label is a legal document. It not only advises the user on timing, dosages and species on which it may be employed, but at the same time defines the only legal uses to which the product may be put.

Label specifications are arrived at after serious consideration of data by the scientists who conduct the safety tests, and regulatory officials who review them. Deviation from label directions and precautions is, in many countries, a violation of the law. Compliance assures the best chance of effective and profitable use with a wide margin of safety to all.

There has been particular concern for possible residues in food of those compounds that have been found to induce tumors in laboratory animals when they are incorporated in the diet over a long period. Some people believe that these carcinogenic compounds may not have a threshold below which there is no chance of an effect on an occasional individual. They hold to this view even though those experimental dosages, inducing a statistically significant increase in tumors in mice or other laboratory animals, were highly exaggerated. They consequently believe that no tolerance level should be established; that none whatsoever should be allowed.

Many toxicologists, on the other hand, hold to the threshold concept; they believe that there is a point below which there is no effect. Neither view can be proven correct. There is no way to statistically establish the chances of a rare occurrence, such as one in a million, without conducting experiments too vast to contemplate.

For two decades there has been a statutory bar in the U.S. to approval and commercialization of any substance that may be present in food, regardless of how miniscule the amounts, if it has been shown to be a carcinogen at any dosage in dietary tests with laboratory animals. A paragraph in the U.S. Food and Drug Law which excludes suspected carcinogens from being eligible for tolerances in food is known as the Delaney Clause.

Some crop and livestock protection chemicals have been removed from the market because when refined analytical techniques showed fantastically low amounts present, often in the parts per billion range in certain agricultural products, while at high doses, a statistically significant increase in mouse tumors occurred. Fortunately, there have been alternate pesticides available that have gone a long way toward assuring us of a continuing abundant food supply. Many toxicologists believe that the basis for demanding the banning of any useful flavoring or preservative or any crop or livestock protection chemical could probably be discovered if they work hard enough at developing a more sensitive analytical method, and conduct enough tests for carcinogenicity with varying strains of laboratory animals. If this is correct, an extreme no-risk policy could eventually present us with the greatest hazard of all, a shortage of food through the banning of one after another of the very crop and livestock protection chemicals that now help assure abundance.

As has already been stated, the broad scope of safety tests now required prior to a decision on registration of a product include many environmental considerations. Thus potential adverse effects are avoided; however, environmental benefits are seldom fully recognized.[4] If crops and livestock were not protected with chemicals, vastly greater acreages would be needed and these would often involve erodible land ill-adapted to crops. Greater acreage means more energy required for agriculture. Fertilizer requirements for a crop damaged by a pest are fully as great as for a highly-productive crop. Inadequately protected livestock and poultry are a drain on resources.

Brush-infested pastures are more subject to erosion than those composed of a thick sod. Recent trends toward reduced tillage made possible by modern herbicides makes energy savings possible and often result in less soil erosion with the concomitant silting of lakes and streams. Herbicides also reduce the need for energy-requiring tillage of cropland and at the same time decrease the chances of erosion and undesirable soil compaction.

REFERENCES

1. **Campbell, J. B.,** Effect of horn fly control on cows as expressed by increased weaning weights of calves, *J. Econ. Entomol.,* 69, 711—712, 1976.
2. **Barrons, K. C.,** Some ecological benefits of woody plant control with herbicides, *Science,* 165, 465—468, 1969.
3. **Kinloch, R. A.,** Response of soybean cultivars grown in root-knot infested soil treated with Fumizone 86 and other nematicides, *Down-to-Earth,* 31(2), 10-13, 1975.
4. **Barrons, K. C.,** Environmental benefits of intensive crop production, *Agric. Sci. Rev.,* 9(2), 33—39, 1971.

Stress

EFFECTS OF DISEASE ON ANIMAL PRODUCTIVITY

M. J. Burridge

INTRODUCTION

The world population will increase from nearly four billion in 1974 to a projected figure of seven billion by the end of this century.[1-3] In the meantime, world food production is lagging behind human requirements by a greater margin each year, particularly in the economically developing countries,in which the population growth rate is the greatest.[4] It is apparent, therefore, that there must be a marked improvement in animal and plant productivity if the critical shortage of food in many regions is to be overcome.

The role of animals in the production of food for human consumption has been stressed by many authors.[1-3,5-9] Animal proteins are of higher nutritional quality than are plant proteins, with animal products such as eggs, meat, and milk providing all the essential amino acids, along with some valuable minerals and vitamins, in a single source of protein food.[1] As sources of animal protein, poultry and swine have the advantages of maturing and multiplying rapidly. Additionally, poultry production is recognized as the most efficient and economical means of providing a rapid increase in high-quality animal protein for human consumption.[6] On the other hand, ruminants (cattle, sheep, goats, water buffalo, and camels) have the ability to convert pasture and forage crops that are unsuitable as human food into highly nutritious meat and milk.

Most arguments against the utilization of animals in the production of human food have centered around the belief that animals compete with man for plant foods. Such generalizations tend to overlook a number of important facts,[8] among which are the following:

1. Much of the earth's energy is stored in forms unsuitable for direct consumption by man.
2. Ruminants are capable of converting many plant and waste materials into high-quality foods.
3. The majority of the world's grazing lands are unsuitable for cultivation.
4. Large populations of domestic animals already exist in some of the same areas as malnourished populations, as in parts of Africa.
5. Some ruminants serve as draft animals for transportation and cultivation of crops.
6. Some domestic animals play an important role in certain social and tribal customs.
7. The people of many cultures show a strong preference for various types of animal foods.

Regarding point 3 above, it is pertinent to note that permanent grassland exceeds cropland on all continents except Europe, with the area of grassland greater than that of cropland by a factor of ten in Oceania and by a factor of four in Africa and South America (Table 1). Most of these grasslands would have little agricultural value unless they were used for ruminant production.

One of the important constraints on increased production of food for human consumption in all parts of the world is animal disease. The continuing losses from animal

Table 1
LAND USAGE BY REGIONS OF THE WORLD, 1974[10]

Region	Land area (millions of hectares)					
	Total area	Permanent meadows and pastures (grassland)	Arable land and land under permanent crops (cropland)	Forests and woodlands	Other areas	Ratio of grassland to cropland
Africa	3,031	793	218	644	1,377	3.6:1
North and Central America	2,246	326	289	730	902	1.1:1
South America	1,783	445	101	928	309	4.4:1
Asia	2,753	550	477	597	1,130	1.2:1
Europe	487	87	143	149	108	0.6:1
Oceania	851	468	47	86	250	10.0:1
U.S.S.R.	2,240	375	233	920	712	1.6:1
World	13,392[a]	3044	1,507[a]	4,053[a]	4,788	2.0:1

[a] Individual areas given to nearest million hectares. Therefore, rounding errors may occur in totals of individual areas.

disease constitute an intolerable waste of agricultural resources in a hungry world. This wastage results from death of animals, reduced productive efficiency, interference with reproductive function, and condemnation of animal products at slaughter. Additionally, certain diseases have a pronounced effect on the establishment and development of animal industries in some regions, and they can also have an inhibitory effect on international trade in animals and animal products

It has been estimated that about one quarter of the world-wide food production from animals is lost due to disease.[11] The enormity of disease losses can be appreciated from the fact that more than 50 million cattle and water buffaloes and 100 million sheep and goats die each year from disease.[3] Animal morbidity losses due to disease are of similar magnitude. Reduction of this wastage through disease control measures would produce great benefits. For example, with every 10% reduction in disease losses, an average daily increase of at least 0.6 g of animal protein would be generated for every person in the world.[12]

The scope of this contribution is broad, and it is therefore possible only to outline the major effects of disease on animal productivity and present specific examples drawn from a review of the literature. In addition, approaches to the control of animal diseases will be discussed in the light of current knowledge of veterinary epidemiology and economics.

EFFECTS OF ANIMAL DISEASES

Effect on Development of Animal Industries

The major epidemic diseases of food-producing animals include African swine fever, contagious bovine pleuropneumonia, East Coast fever, foot-and-mouth disease, Newcastle disease, rinderpest, and trypanosomiasis. These diseases limit and in some instances even preclude the development of viable animal industries wherever they occur. Today, they exert their most devastating effects primarily in Africa, Asia, and Latin America.[12]

Approximately 10 million km^2 of Africa south of the Sahara has been rendered unsuitable for livestock production by trypanosomiasis, a hemoprotozoan disease transmitted by tsetse flies (*Glossina* spp.).[13] It has been demonstrated repeatedly that, in the presence of this disease, pastoral pursuits are practically impossible. Consequently, vast areas of Africa, capable of supporting some 125 million cattle, cannot be utilized for livestock production, resulting in a potential loss estimated at $5 billion.[14] Trypanosomiasis, therefore, has a disastrous effect on the development of ani mal industries in a continent already desperately short of protein for human consumption.

Rinderpest (cattle plague) has had more influence on the world's food supply than has any other animal disease.[15] It has been a scourge of many regions for centuries, with periodic epidemic waves inflicting catastrophic losses on cattle and water buffalo populations. More than 200 million cattle died from rinderpest in Europe between 1710 and 1769.[12] The great rinderpest epidemic that swept Africa during the last decade of the 19th century has been considered one of the major natural disasters of recorded history.[16] It killed tens of millions of livestock and game animals, including 80 to 90% of the cattle, African buffalo, giraffes, and antelopes.[12,17] In South Africa alone, the losses amounted to 2.5 million cattle.[17] Apart from these direct losses to livestock productivity, rinderpest has had a profound effect upon rice production in parts of Asia. Cultivation of the paddy fields of China and Burma was badly disrupted during the 1940s by heavy mortality among water buffalo and cattle, respectively.[18] Burma at that time was the world's greatest exporter of rice. Rinderpest, together with the ravages of World War II, caused a complete loss of its annual surplus of three million tons of rice, ruining its economy and threatening famine to neighboring Bengal. More recently, an outbreak of rinderpest in Guinea required up to 5 years' calf production to replace the loss, whereas eradication of the disease from Sierra Leone has resulted in a fourfold increase in cattle production.[19]

African swine fever is potentially the most devastating of all porcine diseases. It usually takes the form of a highly contagious, peracute disease in domestic swine, with a mortality rate approaching 100%. It has the capability of destroying entire swine industries unless adequate control and eradication measures are taken. There are no effective prophylactic methods currently available for this viral disease. African swine fever caused little world-wide concern until it escaped from Africa to Portugal in 1957.[20] The subsequent spread to Spain resulted in the death of 1.5 million swine between 1959 and 1974, with direct losses estimated at $600 million.[21] In 1967, the disease struck Italy, and rapid dissemination of the virus was arrested only after more than 1.25 million swine had been slaughtered.[22] African swine fever reached the Western Hemisphere in 1971, when it spread to Cuba. Eradication of the disease from that country was accomplished only after the destruction of more than 500,000 swine.[23]

East Coast fever is a highly pathogenic tick-borne disease of cattle caused by the protozoan parasite *Theileria parva.* It killed 900,000 cattle in the Transkei region of South Africa between 1910 and 1914.[24] Today, East Coast fever is restricted to eastern and central Africa, where it is a major constraint to improved cattle production.[25] Improved breeds of cattle can only be raised in *T. parva*-endemic areas when intensive and expensive acaricide programs are continuously applied.

Virulent forms of Newcastle disease can destroy entire poultry populations, and flourishing poultry industries can be established only when the disease is adequately controlled. Contagious bovine pleuropneumonia was one of the major plagues of cattle in the past, and today it still kills tens of thousands of animals annually in Africa and Asia.[12] Foot-and-mouth disease is an extremely contagious disease of all cloven-footed animals. Although it does not produce a high mortality rate, it does cause very serious economic losses in a number of ways. The greatest losses occur as a result of severe impairment of productivity, expense of eradication, and interference with international movement of livestock and livestock products.

The major epidemic diseases must be adequately controlled before significant progress can be made toward the development of animal industries in a given area. The U.S. affords a good example. Development of its cattle industry in the South, swine industry, and intensive poultry industries was possible only after successful control of bovine piroplasmosis, hog cholera, and fowl plague and Newcastle disease, respectively.

Most of the major epidemic diseases are now limited to the economically developing nations. Nevertheless, some continue to pose serious potential threats to all economically developed countries. Foot-and-mouth disease and Newcastle disease have periodically produced disastrous epidemics in Europe and North America. Such outbreaks often result from the improperly controlled movement of live animals.[23]

Some economically developing nations have the potential to expand their animal industries through export of animals and animal products. However, all too often this potential is not realized because of disease. The U.S. in 1971 and the countries of the European Economic Community in 1972, for example, directed that domestic ruminants and swine cannot be imported from any country in which foot-and-mouth disease or rinderpest exists.[26] The latter countries additionally forbid the importation of meat from animals showing evidence of tuberculosis or cysticercosis. It is evident, therefore, that disease is also a serious constraint on the expansion of international trade in animals and animal products.

Effect on Meat Production

All diseases that cause mortality have an obvious effect on meat production. However, the less spectacular effects of some diseases, such as those that lead to retardation of growth rate and to condemnation of meat or viscera at slaughter, also produce massive economic losses throughout the world that can be even more costly than those due to mortality. Specific diseases and their resulting economic losses to meat production have been summarized by the Food and Agriculture Organization of the United Nations (FAO).[14]

Reduction in Growth Rate

Many internal parasites produce clinical or subclinical infections that reduce animal performance and result in weight loss or retarded growth of their hosts. Subclinical infections are insidious and can cause considerable losses in animal productivity without the producer being aware that a disease problem exists. G. I. nematodes commonly produce a reduction in the weight gain rate of cattle.[27-33] The major internal parasites (excluding arthropods) affecting growth rate in food-producing animals are listed in Table 2. These parasites produce their detrimental effects in a variety of ways. Reductions in weight gain can result from: (1) gross pathological changes to organs (e.g., destruction of intestinal mucosa by *Eimeria* spp. and extensive damage to bile ducts and hepatic tissue by *Fasciola* spp.), (2) anemia due to active blood sucking (e.g., *Bunostomum* and *Haemonchus* spp.), (3) migration of larvae (e.g., *Stephanurus dentatus*), (4) loss of appetite (e.g., *Cooperia, Ostertagia* and *Trichostrongylus* spp.), and (5) reduction of digestive efficiency (e.g., *T. axei*).[37,44,49,51,56,57,59,61]

A major cause of reduced weight gain, especially in beef cattle, is arthropod parasitism. Tick infestations depress growth rates of cattle.[32,62-67] Loss of appetite is responsible for the majority of the reduction in weight gain seen in cattle heavily infested with the tick *Boophilus microplus*.[65] Heavy infestations of lice also can produce pronounced anemia and weight loss in cattle.[64,68] Scabies mites cause intense pruritus in cattle, interfering with feeding and depressing growth rates.[64,69]

Table 2
PROTOZOAN AND HELMINTH INFECTIONS THAT RETARD THE RATE OF GROWTH OF FOOD-PRODUCING ANIMALS

Internal parasites	Species affected	Parts of body parasitized	Ref.
Protozoa			
Eimeria spp.	Cattle and sheep	Small and large intestine	34—37
	Poultry	Alimentary tract	38—40
Nematodes			
Ascaris suum	Swine	Small intestine[a]	41—43
Bunostomum spp.	Cattle and sheep	Small intestine	44
Cooperia spp.	Cattle and sheep	Small intestine	45—49
Haemonchus spp.	Cattle and sheep	Abomasum	50—52
Metastrongylus spp.	Swine	Lung	53
Oesophagostomum spp.	Cattle and sheep	Cecum and colon	47, 50, 54
Ostertagia spp.	Cattle and sheep	Abomasum	48, 49, 55
Stephanurus dentatus	Swine	Kidney and perirenal tissues[a]	56, 57
Strongyloides ransomi	Swine	Small intestine	42
Trichostrongylus spp.	Cattle and sheep	Abomasum and small intestine	49, 50, 58, 59
Trematodes			
Fasciola spp.	Cattle and sheep	Liver	60, 61

[a] Liver damaged by migrating larvae.

Insect pests have a marked effect on the growth rate of animals. Biting flies cause irritation and annoyance, often interrupting normal feeding patterns to such an extent that rates of weight gain are severely reduced. The biting flies that have the most pronounced effect on beef production are horn flies (*Haematobia irritans*)[64,70-72] stable flies (*Stomoxys calcitrans*),[64,70] horse flies (*Tabanus* spp.),[64,72] deer flies (*Chrysops* spp.),[64] mosquitoes,[64,73,74] and black flies (*Simulium* spp.).[75] The nonbiting face fly (*Musca autumnalis*) is also a serious pest of cattle. Its habit of clustering around the eyes, mouth, and nostrils is extremely annoying to animals, preventing normal grazing and resulting in a depressed rate of weight gain.[64] The larvae of some flies cause massive losses to beef production through myiasis (i.e., the invasion of organs and tissues of animals by larvae of dipterous insects). Most notable are cattle grubs (larvae of warble flies, *Hypoderma* spp.) and larvae of the screwworm fly (*Cochliomyia hominivorax*), which cause extensive injuries to infected animals.[64,75-77]

Respiratory infections can have profound effects on the growth rate of animals. Mycoplasmal pneumonia of pigs (previously called enzootic pneumonia and virus pneumonia of pigs) is a chronic debilitating condition that is probably the most economically important of all swine diseases.[19,78] It reduces the efficiency of food utilization by swine and seriously depresses their growth rate.[19,79-86] Experimentally, it has been shown that mycoplasmal pneumonia reduces the food-conversion efficiency of pigs by 22% and growth rate by 16%; the effects of the disease in the field are thought to be at least of this magnitude.[81] Another respiratory infection having an inhibitory effect on the growth rate of swine is atrophic rhinitis.[87,88] Respiratory diseases also markedly affect the performance of beef cattle and broiler chickens during their growing periods.[89-91]

Infectious bovine keratoconjunctivitis (pinkeye of cattle) is a condition that has an important effect on beef production. The pain, photophobia, and impaired vision associated with pinkeye cause a reduction in food intake and a depression in weight gain.[89,92-94]

Reduction in the growth rate of food-producing animals results in serious losses in potential meat production and in increased costs incurred during the extra feeding period required to bring affected animals to a satisfactory market weight. The economic impact of this effect of disease on animal productivity will be discussed in greater detail later.

Condemnation of Meat and Viscera at Slaughter

Large quantities of meat and viscera are rejected at slaughter as unfit for human consumption, constituting a great wastage of animal protein. The major cause of this wastage is disease. Unfortunately, there are few published reports on condemnation losses from specific diseases.

One of the best-documented disease losses at meat inspection is that due to liver fluke infection (fascioliasis). Bovine and ovine livers worth many millions of dollars are rejected every year in many regions because of damage caused by these trematode parasites.[14,29,60,64,95-97]

Some parasitic diseases are responsible for substantial losses of meat primarily because of their importance to public health. Bovine cysticercosis is an example. Muscles of cattle harboring cysticerci are condemned in order to prevent infection of man with the beef tapeworm *Taenia saginata.* This bovine disease has long been a problem in the large beef feedlots of California.[98] In 1953, the financial loss from meat infected with *T. saginata* cysticerci in California was reported to amount to $35 million.[99] This figure appears somewhat excessive, since an estimate of the average annual loss to all animal industries in the U.S. from all carcass condemnations during the 1950s was only $32.1 million.[100]

Other parasitic larvae also cause important losses at meat inspection. The larval stages of the large roundworms (*Ascaris suum*) and the kidney worms (*Stephanurus dentatus*) of swine produce extensive hepatic lesions during their migratory phase, resulting in the condemnation of livers worth millions of dollars annually.[64] Cattle grubs damage muscular tissue during their migration, necessitating trimming and causing a loss of affected parts of the carcass, frequently including the best steak cuts.[64,101,102] In certain regions such as Australasia and South America, a major cause of liver condemnations is hydatidosis (infection of sheep, cattle, goats, and swine with the larval hydatid cysts of the cestode *Echinococcus granulosus*).[14,103-105] Another cestode infection, ovine cystocercosis (infection of sheep with the larval stage of *T. ovis*), is a problem to the Australian mutton industry. During the first half of 1968, one eighth of all mutton exports from Australia were rejected due to infection with cysticerci of *T. ovis.*[105]

Major economic losses from bovine tuberculosis result from the rejection of infected carcasses. Meat worth approximately $150 million was condemned annually in the U.S. as a result of this disease before the tuberculosis eradication program was initiated in 1917.[106] More recent losses from bovine tuberculosis at slaughter have been documented by the Food and Agriculture Organization.[14]

A condemnation rate of 3.5% at poultry meat inspection has been reported for the U.S.[107] Important causes of this loss are infectious bronchitis, mycoplasmosis, and neoplastic diseases (Marek's disease and lymphoid leukosis).[91] In Canada, leukosis accounted for 36.5% of all birds condemned during the fiscal year 1968—1969.[6] Neoplastic conditions are also a cause of condemnation losses in other food-producing species, although to a much lesser extent than in poultry.[108]

Effect on Milk Production

Bovine mastitis continues to be one of the most important and most costly diseases confronting dairy industries throughout the world. The massive economic losses from mastitis include those due to reduced milk yield, decreased milk quality, discarded milk, increased herd replacement and labor costs, and the expense of therapy, control, and prevention.

Mastitis decreases milk production of cattle by 5 to 25% in most instances, although reductions in milk yield of as high as 83.9% have been reported.[99,109-127] Cow's milk is a highly nutritious food, containing proteins, carbohydrates, fats, minerals, and vitamins. Mastitis reduces the quality of milk by adversely affecting its composition; both the fat and solids-not-fat content of milk are lowered.[109,111,115,117,119,120,122,124,128-131] Synthesis of two of the important constituents of the solids-not-fat component, protein casein and carbohydrate lactose, is suppressed by mastitis.[111,117,118,124,128,130,132]

The detrimental effects of mastitis on the productivity of dairy cattle are a major cause of wastage in dairy herds.[95,117,121,127,133-139] The quantity and quality of milk can be affected to such an extent that infected cattle are often culled from herds before they have attained maximum production. This reduction in the lactating life of cattle creates serious economic losses not only through the drop in potential milk production but also from the increased costs incurred in purchasing or raising herd replacements.

Diseases other than mastitis that affect the udder produce appreciable losses to dairy industries. An example is vesicular stomatitis. Cattle infected with this viral disease often cannot be milked because of painful teat lesions. However, the major losses to milk production from vesicular stomatitis are a result of the slaughter of cattle with severe udder damage and from the reduced productivity of recovered animals.[140]

Diseases that cause abortion have a profound effect on milk production. It has been estimated that bovine abortions reduce milk yield by 17.3 kg for each day by which the gestation period is shortened.[96] A major cause of bovine abortions is brucellosis (*Brucella abortus* infection). Losses in milk production during the lactation following *B. abortus* abortion vary from 10 to 45%.[14,110,141-144] Similar losses occur in the fat content of milk.[143] In general, the earlier the abortion occurs during the gestation period, the greater is the reduction in quantity and fat quality of the milk produced during the subsequent lactation.[143] Even in the absence of abortion, *B. abortus* infection can decrease milk yield by as much as 21%.[110]

Parasitic diseases have an important influence on milk production. G. I. nematodes reduce the productivity of dairy cattle.[145-147] Fascioliasis can depress milk yields by as much as 20%.[29,60,95,148] Arthropods, as well as helminth parasites, cause substantial losses to dairy industries. In 1934, while researchers were attempting to determine the loss due to bovine piroplasmosis in the U.S., it was found that milk production was reduced by an average of 42.4% in cattle heavily infested with ticks.[149] More recently, it has been estimated that cattle ticks are responsible for a loss of 48% in milk production in Mexico.[67] Other arthropod parasites depressing milk yields include biting flies, face flies, lice, and cattle grubs.[64,150-153] Losses to the U.S. dairy industry due to arthropod parasitism amount to hundreds of millions of dollars/year.[64] The effects of insect pests can be truly dramatic; for example, attacks by the black fly *Simulium venustum* on dairy cattle in Canada have caused reductions of 50% in milk production.[75]

Foot-and-mouth disease has a major effect on the productivity of dairy cattle.[14,154-156] During the acute stages of the disease, milk yield can drop by 80 to 100%. Additionally, milk production is seriously impaired throughout the prolonged convalescent period. Water buffaloes are similarly affected, and there can be a general reduction of 30% in their milk yield after complete recovery from the infection.[157]

Other bovine diseases that cause losses in milk production include anaplasmosis, infectious bovine rhinotracheitis (primarily due to abortions), infectious footrot, pinkeye, tuberculosis, respiratory infections, and metabolic diseases (especially ketosis).[14,64,83,89,158-162]

Effect on Egg Production

Diseases that produce a drop in egg production are responsible for major losses to layer industries. They include protozoan infections (coccidiosis), bacterial infections (pullorum disease, paratyphoid, fowl cholera, infectious coryza, and chlamydiosis), viral infections (infectious bronchitis, laryngotracheitis, Newcastle disease, avian influenza, Marek's disease, and lymphoid leukosis), and diseases of undetermined etiology (avian monocytosis).[40,91,163-172] With some diseases such as Newcastle disease, birds may cease to lay completely. Other diseases (e.g., Marek's disease) have important indirect effects on egg production by causing heavy mortality in chickens as they come into lay.[173] These indirect effects are of considerable economic significance to the layer industry because the costly expenditure on rearing birds is only partially offset by income from egg production.

Losses to layer industries also arise from diseases that lower egg quality, such as infectious bronchitis and Newcastle disease.[91,168,170] The shells of affected eggs are often thin, rough, and misshapen, and their internal contents may be of an inferior standard.

Virulent forms of Newcastle disease periodically produce major epidemics in many areas, often causing serious losses to layer industries. The velogenic viscerotropic Newcastle disease epidemic that occurred in southern California between 1971 and 1973 affected mainly layer flocks.[174] The high mortality rate on infected premises and the measures introduced to eradicate the disease severely disrupted egg production. Eradication measures included depopulation of all infected and exposed flocks and stringent restrictions on the movement of birds and poultry products.

Effect on Production of Hides, Wool, and Mohair

Cattle grubs cause serious damage to bovine hides.[64,75,158,175] These dipterous larvae injure the most valuable portion of the hide when they emerge along the back after their migration through the body. In the U.S., hides with a few grub holes sell for reduced prices, whereas those with many holes are fit only for glue manufacture.[64] Ectoparasites are also of concern to the leather industry. The follicular mite *Demodex bovis* causes demodectic mange and the production of small holes in bovine skin, decreasing its market value.[176] Scabies mites give rise to intense pruritus in cattle, which can result in self-inflicted damage to hides.[64] Heavy cattle tick infestations leave scars that can depreciate the market value of hides by as much as 40%.[67]

Losses in wool production result from both internal and external parasitism.[14] Nodular worms (*Oesophagostomum columbianum*) and liver flukes can cause a marked impairment of wool growth and quality.[50,60] The effects of ectoparasites such as ticks, mites, lice, and keds can reduce the amount and quality of wool produced by infested sheep.[64] The louse *Bovicola ovis* is very irritating to sheep, and heavily infested animals can lose large areas of wool through biting and scratching.[177]

Internal parasites and ectoparasites (lice and mites) cause major losses in mohair production.[14,64] Lice (*Linognathus stenopsis* and *Bovicola* spp.) are of particular concern because heavily infested goats rub off considerable amounts of mohair.[177]

Effect on Animal Reproduction

One of the most serious impediments to efficient livestock production is poor reproductive performance due to infertility, abortion, and embryonic and neonatal death. The economic consequences of reproductive failure can be staggering. It was reported in 1953 that the cattle industries of the U.S. lost $824 million annually from impaired fertility.[99] Current data indicate that approximately 20% of the 71 million cows bred in the U.S. each year fail to reproduce, resulting in a loss of 14.2 million calves valued at $760 million and an annual cost of $1.8 billion to maintain barren cows.[89] Infertility and abortion are major causes of wastage in dairy herds, with economically unproductive animals culled at considerable loss to dairy industries.[133-139] There are many other causes of reduced reproductive performance, including conditions of an anatomical, genetic, immunological, nutritional, physiological, and toxicological nature.

The most important diseases causing abortion in cattle include aspergillosis, brucellosis, epizootic viral abortion, infectious bovine rhinotracheitis, leptospirosis, listeriosis, trichomoniasis, and vibriosis.[178] Brucellosis (*Brucella abortus* infection) has a profound effect on bovine productivity. The reduced milk production of infected and aborting cows is the major loss to the dairy industry, whereas decreased calving rates and interference with breeding programs are of greatest importance to the beef industry. Additional losses in productivity result from the common sequel of infertility that increases the period between lactations and between calvings. Other infectious causes of bovine infertility include vibriosis and trichomoniasis.[178] Vibriosis has been reported to be responsible for about 40% of infertility in cattle in the U.S.[14] Further losses to the potential calf crop occur as a result of neonatal diseases. It is estimated that about 10% of calves born annually in the U.S. die from diarrheic diseases, resulting in an annual loss of approximately $400 million.[89]

The diseases causing abortion in sheep include brucellosis (*B. melitensis* and *B. ovis* infections), enzootic virus abortion, leptospirosis, listeriosis, salmonellosis (*Salmonella abortus ovis, S. dublin,* and *S. typhimurium* infections), toxoplasmosis, and vibriosis.[179,180] *B. melitensis* infection is also a major cause of abortion in goats. *B. ovis* infection has an effect on the fertility of both rams and ewes. It produces epididymitis in rams, resulting in reduced fertility, shortened breeding life, and lowered lambing rates among ewes.[181] Ram epididymitis is assuming increasing importance; it causes infertility losses of more than $2 million annually in California.[182] Recent studies indicate that fascioliasis might have an adverse effect on ewe fertility.[183,184]

Bacterial diseases, especially brucellosis (*B. suis* infection) and leptospirosis, are the most frequent infectious causes of abortion in swine.[185] Infected sows that do not abort often give birth to weak piglets that exhibit a high neonatal mortality rate. Viral diseases generally cause embryonic and fetal death, with stillbirths common at farrowing. However, the more pathogenic viruses such as hog cholera, pseudorabies, and influenza can give rise to abortions. All of these diseases have important effects on swine productivity because they reduce the number of pigs weaned per litter.

Some diseases can seriously impair fertility and hatchability of eggs in the poultry industry. Pullorum disease and paratyphoid infections, for instance, can cause a decrease in the proportion of fertile eggs and a reduction in their hatchability.[163,164]

ECONOMIC IMPACT OF ANIMAL DISEASES

Study of the economic impact of disease on animal production is still an embryonic discipline utilizing input from agricultural economics, animal science, and veterinary medicine. As a result, there are few published reports on the economic aspects of either animal diseases or disease control and eradication programs at a national or regional level.

The economic losses from animal disease are not known precisely for any country. Estimation of losses is complicated by a number of factors. The most notable problems are (1) the inadequate reporting of all diseases in some countries and of certain diseases in all countries and (2) the lack of standardized nomenclature, particularly regarding diagnosis and the classification of losses. The FAO has suggested that losses be classified into the following categories:[14]

1. Direct losses suffered by owners and resulting from the direct physical effects of disease; these may be subdivided into visible losses (e.g., mortality, abortion, condemnation at meat inspection, damaged hides), invisible losses (e.g., impaired productivity, infertility), and immediate consequences (e.g., loss of production following death of animals, herd replacement costs).
2. Consequential losses suffered by the community as a result of animal disease; these may be subdivided into visible consequences (e.g., effects of zoonotic diseases, spoilage of dairy products due to mastitis) and invisible consequences (e.g., loss of foreign markets).

The direct losses from animal disease are well appreciated, and their monetary value is relatively easy to assess. Consequential losses are often more difficult to estimate, can be very high, and frequently result in the most costly impact of a disease. For example, the total compensation paid for slaughter of infected animals and contacts during the 1952 foot-and-mouth disease epidemic in Canada was $1 million, whereas the resultant closure of foreign markets to Canadian products was responsible for consequential losses of $724 million.[186] The indirect consequences of animal disease can have even farther-reaching effects. The very presence of some diseases can deny vast areas of land to animal production. The prime example of such a situation is trypanosomiasis, which prevents development of livestock production in the 10 million km^2 of Africa infested by the tsetse fly vectors. The potential capital value of livestock lost through trypanosomiasis is estimated at $5 billion.[14]

Many of the published data on economic losses from disease are presented simply as monetary figures. These values, however large, seldom achieve the desired impact and understanding unless they indicate the degree of importance of the losses to animal productivity. This can be done conveniently by expressing economic losses as a proportion of the total value of annual animal production.

The total economic impact of animal disease consists of the actual loss plus the cost of control, prevention, and eradication measures. For clarity of presentation, these two components of economic losses will be discussed separately.*

Economic Losses Caused by Animal Diseases

The most comprehensive international data on economic losses from animal disease were published by the FAO in 1963.[14] The data from this and other publications are summarized in Table 3, and they demonstrate the magnitude of the problem created by animal diseases in many areas of the world. Parasitic diseases are probably the most economically important group of diseases world-wide, producing global losses estimated at $250 billion/year.[97]

In the U.S., the majority of dramatic animal diseases have been successfully controlled or eradicated. Estimates of the major economic losses from animal diseases in that country have been published recently, showing that, at the present time, the most important disease problems are primarily those of a less spectacular nature, such as parasitism and bovine mastitis.[89,91,189-191] Economic data from these publications are summarized in Table 4.

The extent of the economic impact of arthropods on livestock and poultry production is seldom fully appreciated. Arthropods cause massive losses of about $3 billion annually to the animal industries of the U.S.[189] The relative importance of different arthropod parasites in that country is shown in Table 5. Recent estimates of losses

* All economic values are presented in U.S. dollars; where literature cited has given values in other currencies, they have been converted to U.S. dollars using foreign exchange rates in operation at that time and utilizing data supplied by the Board of Governors of the Federal Reserve System, Washington, D.C.

Table 3
ESTIMATED ECONOMIC LOSSES FROM ALL ANIMAL DISEASES BY COUNTRY

Country	Year(s)	Animal species	Annual loss from animal disease: Thousands of U.S. dollars	Annual loss from animal disease: Proportion of total value of annual production of species cited (%)	Ref.
Canada	1966	All	225,190	11.9	187
		Cattle	138,660	11.4	187
		Poultry	32,930	9.8	187
		Sheep	1,600	11.9	187
		Swine	52,000	15.8	187
Colombia	1958	Cattle	122,000	27.1	14
Cyprus	1960	All	1,540	15.0	14
Ecuador	1960	All	13,200	12.9	14
France	1960	All	650,000	15.1	14
Iran	1960	All	158,000	28.7	14
Ireland	1954—1955	All	78,500	19.8	14
		Cattle	49,660	19.2	14
		Poultry	4,900	8.7	14
		Sheep	9,940	33.1	14
		Swine	14,000	27.5	14
Italy	1960	All	400,000	19.0	14
Malawi	1960	All except poultry	800	16.8	14
Mexico	1960	All	280,000	37.3	14
Peru	1959—1960	All	40,300	36.8	14
		Cattle	20,900	35.9	14
		Goats	1,600	37.2	14
		Llamas and other aucheniae	1,200	20.5	14
		Poultry	1,000	14.0	14
		Sheep	12,100	80.8	14
		Swine	3,500	18.4	14
Tanzania	1959	All	3,500	6.8	14
Uganda	1960	All	14,000	31.1	14
U.K.	1959—1960	All	451,400	15.7	14
		All except poultry	333,860	15.0	14
		Poultry	117,540	18.0	14
U.S.	1954	All	2,409,841	13.9	188
		Cattle	1,101,723	14.4	188
		Goats	1,986	7.5	188
		Poultry	375,204	7.5	188
		Sheep	84,708	21.0	188
		Swine	819,440	23.6	188
Uruguay	1959	Cattle	47,150	31.4	14

caused by cattle tick infestations (primarily of the tick *Boophilus microplus*) in other countries emphasize the economic significance of these ectoparasites. Annual losses from cattle ticks were \$62 million in Australia, \$286.5 million in Mexico, and \$88 million in Argentina.[66,192] In addition to their direct effects on animal productivity, many arthropods are of great importance as vectors of disease.

One of the most economically disruptive diseases is foot-and-mouth disease. Endemic infection is a constant source of high losses to productivity. It has been estimated

Table 4
ESTIMATES OF MAJOR ECONOMIC LOSSES FROM ANIMAL DISEASES IN THE U.S., 1973 to 1975

Species	Disease(s)	Annual loss from animal diseases: Millions of U.S. dollars	Annual loss from animal diseases: Proportion of total income from appropriate animal industry (%)	Ref.
Cattle	Arthropod parasitism	2495	8.1	189
	Mastitis	368	4.6[a]	89
	Respiratory diseases	500	1.6	89
	Internal parasitism[b]	482	1.6	89
	Neonatal enteric diseases	400	1.3	89
Swine	Respiratory diseases	400	5.2	190
	Helminth parasitism	255	3.3	190
	Neonatal enteric diseases	108	1.4	190
	Arthropod parasitism	100	1.3	189
	Mastitis-metritis-agalactia	100	1.3	190
Sheep	Helminth parasitism	98	19.4	191
	Arthropod parasitism[c]	43	8.5	189
	Respiratory diseases	20	4.0	191
	Bluetongue	7	1.4	191
Poultry	Mycoplasmosis	250	3.6	91
	Internal parasitism[d]	233	3.4	91
	Stress-related diseases	225	3.3	91
	Salmonellosis	197	2.9	91
	Newcastle disease	154	2.2	91
	Infectious bronchitis	150	2.2	91
	Arthropod parasitism	100	1.4	189
	Neoplastic diseases[e]	83	1.2	91

[a] Proportion of total income from dairy industry only.
[b] Includes nematodiasis, coccidiosis, and anaplasmosis.
[c] Relates to sheep and goats.
[d] Predominantly coccidiosis.
[e] Marek's disease and lymphoid leukosis.

that the 1968 losses from endemic foot-and-mouth disease were approximately $4.7 million in Argentina, $11.6 million in Venezuela, and $89.8 million in Brazil.[155,156,193] Foot-and-mouth disease is an ever-present threat to the livestock industries of countries free from the disease, primarily because of the ease and rapidity with which the virus spreads and the high morbidity rates produced in all susceptible species. As a result, these countries place severe restrictions on trade in animals and animal products with infected countries, adding substantially to the consequential losses from this disease. Nevertheless, costly epidemics do occur from time to time. The serious European epidemic between 1951 and 1952 produced direct losses of $400 million.[154] The 1965 outbreak in Turkey caused losses estimated at $43 million.[194] Some authorities believe that if foot-and-mouth disease were to be introduced into the U.S., the result would be a 25% reduction in livestock production costing $8.5 billion in direct losses and up to ten times that amount in consequential losses.[22]

Some zoonotic diseases have an important economic effect on animal production. Annual losses from brucellosis were estimated to be $155 million in Argentina alone.[106] Bat-transmitted rabies causes immense losses to cattle production in Latin America,

Table 5
ESTIMATED ECONOMIC IMPACT OF ARTHROPODS ON ANIMAL INDUSTRIES IN THE U.S., 1973 to 1975[189]

Arthropods	Annual losses plus control costs by animal industry (millions of U.S. dollars)				
	Beef	Dairy	Swine	Sheep and goats	Poultry
Stable fly (*Stomoxys calcitrans*)	735	59	?[a]	?	?
Ticks	400	40	0	17[b]	?
Horn fly (*Haematobia irritans*)	300	59	0	?	0
Cattle grubs (*Hypoderma* spp.)	300	30	0	0	0
Lice	100	30	40	8	30
Face fly (*Musca autumnalis*)	70	70	5	0	5
Mites	70	10	30	7	30
House fly (*M. domestica*)	30	30	25	0	25
Mosquitoes	40	10	?	?	3
Biting gnats (*Culicoides* and *Leptoconops* spp.)	25	5	?	?	4
Black flies (*Simulium* spp.)	25	5	?	?	3
Screwworm (*Cochliomyia hominivorax*)	25	2	0	1	0
Horse flies (*Tabanus* spp.) and deer flies (*Chrysops* spp.)	20	5	?	?	?
Nose bot (*Oestrus ovis*)	0	0	0	10	0
Total	2140	355	100	43	100

[a] Loss unknown.
[b] Includes losses from sheep ked (*Melophagus ovinus*).

amounting to as much as $350 million/year.[195] The economic impact of bat-transmitted rabies is due not only to mortality but also to the loss of blood in cattle bitten by the vampire bat *Desmodus rotundus*.[196]

Economic losses from poultry diseases have been reviewed recently.[6] Newcastle disease continues to be a major economic problem to poultry industries throughout the world[197] because virulent forms of the disease periodically produce serious epidemics. The consequential losses from these outbreaks can be of great significance; for example, the most costly consequence of the 1970-1971 epidemic in the Netherlands was the import ban placed on Dutch table eggs by many countries.[197]

Cost of Eradication and Control of Animal Diseases

Morris has pointed out that inclusion of the cost of disease control in the classification of losses from animal diseases implies that disease control is a negative activity, thus leading to a neglect of the subject of control when methods of increasing animal productivity are considered.[198] Furthermore, such an all-inclusive description of losses can lead to the assumption that complete control of a disease will yield returns equal to all losses previously incurred. Obviously, this cannot be true because control will not be achieved at zero cost. For these reasons, the cost of disease control and eradication will be discussed separately so that the economic benefits from these activities can be clearly appreciated.

The cost of the regional eradication of selected diseases is shown in Table 6. These costs are relatively small in comparison with the massive economic losses from animal disease. A major economic benefit resulting from disease eradication is the freedom to export animals and animal products to other countries. Other economic advantages can be appreciated from consideration of the following data. The net benefit (after recouping all costs) from the eradication of hog cholera in the U.K. was assessed to be $90 million by 1975.[19] The eradication of velogenic viscerotropic Newcastle disease from southern California cost $56 million, whereas a control program to contain the introduced infection would have resulted in estimated losses to the poultry industry of up to $800 million during the first year with an expected annual increase of 10 to 15% in production costs.[201] Screwworm eradication rid the southeastern U.S. of an insect pest that inflicted annual losses estimated at $20 million.[200,202,203] The subsequent savings to the livestock producers of that region have been some $140 million from a program that cost only $10.25 million in eradication and research expenses.[75] *Boophilus* ticks caused annual losses of $40 million to the cattle industry of the U.S. before the national eradication program began in 1906.[189] Today, losses from cattle ticks and the tick-borne disease babesiosis would amount to an estimated $1 billion/year if that eradication program had not been successful.[189]

Some eradication programs are influenced by factors other than those of an economic nature. The initial motivation for eradication of zoonotic diseases such as brucellosis and tuberculosis was partially, if not primarily, to improve human health. Nevertheless, these programs have achieved considerable economic benefits for livestock industries. The ongoing brucellosis eradication program in the U.S. has reduced annual losses to cattle production from $100 million in 1950 to about $12 million today.[204] The 40-year cost of the bovine tuberculosis eradication program in the U.S. has been $326 million, as compared with an estimated total saving of $6 billion as a result of the program.[205]

There is a dearth of literature on the cost-benefit evaluation of alternative control policies for animal diseases. One of the few studies published considered the control of foot-and-mouth disease in the U.K. following the 1967-1968 epidemic that cost $22 million in direct eradication costs plus $111 million in consequential losses.[199] The traditional slaughter policy (eradication program) was compared with a proposed vaccination policy (control program). Although it was shown that both policies would yield huge net benefits, the eradication program was found to be less costly to the community and was therefore the approach of choice for foot-and-mouth disease in the U.K.

For many diseases in most countries, eradication is neither scientifically realistic nor economically feasible at the present level of technical knowledge. Consequently, the best course of action is to institute control programs on either a national or regional basis. Control of infectious diseases is aimed at reducing the number of cases and the opportunities for transmission to a level at which the infection no longer exists as a major economic or public health problem. Disease control has the important disadvantage that it requires a continuing effort until such a time that technical advances make eradication possible.

There are few published data on the cost of national disease control programs. The economic benefits of the foot-and-mouth disease control campaigns in Argentina and Venezuela are shown in Table 7. The data indicate the importance of foot-and-mouth disease control in reducing the disastrous effects of endemic infection on animal productivity. The reduction of losses from coccidiosis in chickens through the use of feed-additive drugs results in annual savings of about $38 million for the poultry industry of the U.S.[206]

Disease control and preventive medicine programs have received inadequate recognition as methods of reducing the costs of production and increasing animal productivity. The economic principles relating to the development of these programs have been outlined.[198,207-209] Most of the published reports on planned approaches to preventive veterinary medicine relate to dairy cattle, and they demonstrate favorable benefits from such herd health programs.[210-213]

Table 6
COST OF REGIONAL ERADICATION OF SELECTED DISEASES

Disease	Region	Date(s)	Eradication cost (U.S. dollars)	Ref.
Contagious bovine pleuropneumonia	U.S.	1887—1892	1,502,100	12
East Coast fever	South Africa	1905—1954	139,000,000	24
Foot-and-mouth disease	Canada	1952	1,000,000	186
	France	1952	126,000,000	83
	Mexico[a]	1946—1954	134,571,653	12
	U.K.	1952	7,000,000	18, 83
		1967—1968	22,000,000	199
	West Germany	1952	112,000,000	83
Hog cholera	U.K.	Undated	30,000,000	19
Newcastle disease (exotic)	U.K.	1962	25,000,000	197
	California	1971—1973	56,000,000	91
Screwworms	Southeastern U.S.	1958—1959	10,000,000	12,75,200
Vesicular exanthema	U.S.	1953—56	11,158,737	12

[a] Joint Mexico-U.S. program.

Table 7
ECONOMIC BENEFITS FROM FOOT-AND-MOUTH DISEASE CONTROL IN ARGENTINA AND VENEZUELA

Country	Year(s)	Estimated annual losses (U.S. dollars): With control program	Estimated annual losses (U.S. dollars): Without control program	Estimated annual cost of control program (U.S. dollars)	Estimates of annual savings due to control program (U.S. dollars)	Ref.
Argentina	1968	4,701,451	78,337,417	13,893,406	59,742,560	155
Venezuela	1951—1960	896,000	12,675,000	1,824,000	9,955,000	156

APPROACHES TO ANIMAL DISEASE CONTROL

Among the more serious research problems facing agricultural scientists today are methods of providing adequate supplies of animal food to an ever-increasing human population. Efforts to increase the world production of animal protein must involve improvement in the productivity of livestock and poultry through intensified research activity in disease control, nutrition, and genetics. In the absence of effective disease control, an expanded population of unproductive animals is created that cannot fulfill its genetic potential in the utilization of feed for growth and reproduction.

Epidemic disease control is the highest priority requirement for the veterinary services of the economically developing world. The epidemiology of many of the epidemic diseases is relatively simple. In most instances, the etiologic agents are single species or a few related species of pathogenic organisms which are fairly stable genetically, and their range of reservoir hosts (i.e., the hosts upon which the infectious agent actually depends for survival) is narrow.[8] In addition, diagnostic tests that can be applied to screen affected animal populations are available for the majority of these infections.

Most epidemic diseases, therefore, lend themselves to proven methods of control that involve identification and treatment of cases and carriers, removal of reservoirs of infection, quarantine and sanitary measures, and mass immunization programs.[214] Some of these diseases have not been successfully controlled in developing countries because of inadequate veterinary services, political instability, lack of local support, and insufficient financial and technological assistance.

Adequate methods of control are presently unavailable for some epidemic diseases in which the epidemiology is both more complex and poorly understood. Examples include trypanosomiasis, East Coast fever, and African swine fever. All cause great losses to livestock productivity, particularly in Africa. Recently, the International Laboratory for Research on Animal Diseases was established in East Africa to develop improved methods for control of the two hemoprotozoan infections.[21] No such intensification of African swine fever research is apparent.

Most epidemic diseases have been successfully controlled in the economically developed countries. This has allowed development of intensive systems of animal husbandry utilizing genetically improved breeds capable of high levels of production. Profit margins in these operations tend to be so narrow that subclinical endemic infections such as mastitis and GI parasitism assume major significance. Disease control is of paramount importance in these intensive systems if animal production is to be maintained at profitable levels. However, rational control measures can be developed only from a clear understanding of the underlying disease processes. Many endemic diseases are epidemiologically complex, with multiple factors influencing the prevalence and incidence of infection in a given herd or flock. Moreover, the epidemiological pattern of a disease can vary markedly between farms. Consequently, the unit of concern for epidemiological study is the whole farm or enterprise rather than the individual animal.

Development of the computer has added an invaluable dimension to the epidemiological study of complex disease processes. With this technology, powerful analytical methods such as multiple regression, factor analysis, and discriminant analysis have been applied to epidemiological data to investigate the relationships between the numerous variables that influence the patterns of many diseases. The value of these statistical procedures in epidemiological research has been demonstrated in studies on bovine brucellosis, calf diarrhea, dairy calf mortality, echinococcosis, and ovine cysticercosis.[215-221] However, these procedures have the important limitation of not interpreting causal relationships. In contrast, another analytical method, path analysis, does approach the problem of causal interpretation through the application of multiple regression procedures to a linear model that represents the causal processes assumed to operate among the variables in nature. A recent study has indicated that path analysis, by permitting interaction between epidemiological theory and statistical analysis, is a valuable additional tool to epidemiologists.[222] The identification of important causal pathways in complex biological systems is not the only use of path analysis. This technique also provides a methodology whereby the consequences of realistic manipulation of variables can be visualized, forming in the context of preventive medicine a rational basis for designing disease control programs.

The importance of carrying out detailed epidemiological studies prior to the inception of large-scale disease control programs can be seen from the New Zealand experience with the control of taeniid cestodes. The hydatid disease control program in that country produced a steady decline in the prevalence of *Echinococcus granulosus* in dogs but a concurrent and dramatic increase in the prevalence of *Taenia ovis*.[221] Due to the economic threat posed to the New Zealand export market through the condemnation of lamb and mutton infected with *T. ovis* cysticerci, a specific *T. ovis* control program had to be introduced. That action added a new dimension to taeniid control by involving urban pet dogs, diluting the resources of the hydatid control authorities, and changing the emphasis of the original program. This example demonstrates the hazards of interference with stable biological systems without sufficient understanding of the complex interrelationships between parasites, hosts, and environment.

The results of epidemiological studies often indicate that a number of control strategies are available for a given disease problem. In these situations, economic analysis is required to determine the optimum control strategy after it has been established that the disease is indeed a problem to animal productivity. The economic principles involved in such an analysis have been outlined.[198] It is necessary to demonstrate in any anticipated disease control program that the effects of control measures will result in increased profits for producers. This is essential if the farming community is to be induced to invest in disease control activities. At the national level, the agencies financing animal health activities are increasingly demanding cost-benefit analyses to justify their approval of disease control or eradication programs. These analyses involve not only comparison of the potential benefits of control or eradication against no action but also involve evaluation of alternative control strategies.[199] Such estimates require a clear understanding of the epidemiology and economic impact of the disease under consideration.

One of the most promising current approaches to animal disease control is the utilization of genetic resistance to certain diseases. Considerable evidence exists to indicate that genetic factors play an important part in the susceptibility and resistance to many diseases.[223,224] Specific genes that directly affect resistance to disease have been found in both experimental and domestic animals.[224,225] Studies in West Africa have shown that the N'dama breed of cattle possesses a high tolerance to trypanosomiasis,[226,227] and it has been suggested that this immunity to trypanosomiasis might have a genetic basis.[228] There is an urgent need to intensify research on the genetic mechanisms involved in disease resistance and to explore their practical application to the control of the major disease problems of food-producing animals.

The necessity of a multidisciplinary approach to the control of animal diseases can be seen from the case of bovine trypanosomiasis in Africa. As a result of successful control of rinderpest and contagious bovine pleuropneumonia, trypanosomiasis is now the major natural means of restraining the progressive overgrazing of the arid marginal areas in tropical Africa.[229] Therefore, research aimed at developing practical trypanosomiasis control methods must be accompanied by corresponding improvement in pastures and forages, water resources, and husbandry practices. In the absence of the latter research activities, successful control of this disease would allow the bovine population to rapidly increase beyond the carrying capacity of the land, with all of the attendant dangers to the environment.

It is apparent from the foregoing text that our knowledge of the effects of disease on animal productivity is lacking in many instances, and there is presently a relative paucity of funds allocated to such research. For example, funds for research on bovine mastitis in the U.S. amount to only 0.01% of the cash income from dairy products.[230,231] There is a real need for an intensification of research activity aimed at defining those diseases and disease complexes that have economically important effects on animal productivity and at developing practical means for their control. Standardized quantitative approaches to the epidemiological and economic assessment of disease and disease control must be evolved in terms lending themselves to comparative interpretaion. Such research objectives will be realized best through coordinated multidisciplinary effort involving input from veterinarians, agricultural economists, and animal scientists.

REFERENCES

1. **Pimentel, D., Dritschilo, W., Krummel, J., and Kutzman, J.,** Energy and land constraints in food protein production, *Science,* 190, 754—761, 1975.
2. **Hodgson, H. J.,** Forages, ruminant livestock, and food, *BioScience,* 26, 625-630, 1976.
3. **Byerly, T. C.,** Ruminant livestock research and development, *Science,* 195, 450-456, 1977.
4. **Maurer, F. D.,** Livestock, a world food resource threatened by disease, *J. Am. Vet. Med. Assoc.,* 166, 920-923, 1975.
5. **Byerly, T. C.,** The role of livestock in food production, *J. Anim. Sci.,* 25, 552-566, 1966.
6. **Cockrill, W. R.,** Economic loss from poultry disease—world aspects, in *Poultry Disease and World Economy,* Gordon, R. F. and Freeman, B. M., Eds., British Poultry Science, Edinburgh, 1971, 3-24.
7. **Hodgson, R. E.,** Place of animals in world agriculture, *J. Dairy Sci.,* 54, 442-447, 1971.
8. **Schwabe, C. W. and Ruppanner, R.,** Animal diseases as contributors to human hunger: problems of control, *World Rev. Nutr. Diet.,* 15, 185-224, 1972.
9. **Wedin, W. F., Hodgson, H. J., and Jacobson, N. L.,** Utilizing plant and animal resources in producing human food, *J. Anim. Sci.,* 41, 667-686, 1975.
10. Production Yearbook 1975, Vol. 29, Food and Agriculture Organization of the United Nations, Rome, 1976.
11. **Cunningham, I. J.,** Veterinary science and man's food, *Aust. J. Sci.,* 28, 194-200, 1965.
12. **Pritchard, W. R.,** Increasing protein foods through improving animal health, *Proc. Natl. Acad. Sci. U.S.A.,* 56, 360—369, 1966.
13. **du Toit, R. M.,** The eradication of the tsetse fly (*Glossina pallidipes*) from Zululand, Union of South Africa, *Adv. Vet. Sci.,* 5, 227-240, 1959.
14. **Anon.,** The economic losses caused by animal diseases, in FAO/WHO/OIE Animal Health Yearbook, 1962, Food and Agriculture Organization of the United Nations, Rome, 1963, 284-313.
15. **Maurer, F. D.,** Rinderpest, *J. Am. Vet. Med. Assoc.,* 141, 713-716, 1962.
16. **Branagan, D. and Hammond, J. A.,** Rinderpest in Tanganyika: a review, *Bull. Epizoot. Dis. Afr.,* 13, 225-246, 1965.
17. **Mack, R.,** The great African cattle plague epidemic of the 1890s, *Trop. Anim. Health Prod.,* 2, 210-219, 1970.
18. **Short, G. V.,** Veterinary science and the world's food, *Outlook Agric.,* 3, 39-50, 1960.
19. **Goodwin, R. F. W.,** The cost effectiveness of animal disease control, *Span,* 16, 63-64, 1973.
20. **De Tray, D. E.,** African swine fever, *Adv. Vet. Sci.,* 8, 299-333, 1963.
21. **Pritchard, W. R.,** Animal disease constraints to world food production, *Theriogenology,* 6, 305-312, 1976.
22. Control of Foreign Animal Diseases, National Research Program Publication No. 20460, U.S. Department of Agriculture, Agricultural Research Service, Washington, D.C., 1976.
23. **Ellis, P. R.,** The movement of live animals, *World Anim. Rev.,* 16, 6-12, 1975.
24. **Neitz, W. O.,** Tick-borne diseases as a hazard in the rearing of calves in Africa, *Off. Int. Epizoot. Bull.,* 62, 607-625, 1964.
25. East African Livestock Survey, Food and Agriculture Organization of the United Nations, Rome, 1967.
26. **Kafel, S.,** Exporting animals and meat from developing countries, *World Anim. Rev.,* 14, 15—19, 1975.
27. **Goldberg, A.,** Relation of feeding level to gastrointestinal nematode parasitism in cattle, *J. Parasitol.,* 51, 948-953, 1965.
28. **Durie, P. H. and Elek, P.,** The reaction of calves to helminth infection under natural grazing conditions, *Aust. J. Agric. Res.,* 17, 91-103, 1966.
29. **Honer, M. R.,** Economics of parasitic disease, *J. Parasitol.,* 56 (4), 427-428, 1970.
30. **Cornwell, R. L., Jones, R. M., and Pott, J. M.,** Bovine parasitic gastroenteritis: growth responses following routine anthelmintic treatment of sub-clinical infections in grazing animals, *Vet. Rec.,* 89, 352-359, 1971.
31. **Keith, R. K.,** Prolonged effect of previous helminth infection on cattle, *Aust. Vet. J.,* 48, 427, 1972.
32. **Turner, H. G. and Short, A. J.,** Effects of field infestations of gastrointestinal helminths and of the cattle tick (*Boophilus microplus*) on growth of three breeds of cattle, *Aust. J. Agric. Res.,* 23, 177-193, 1972.
33. **Williams, J. C. and Knox, J. W.,** Effect of nematode parasite infection on the performance of stocker cattle at high stocking rates on coastal bermudagrass pastures, *Am. J. Vet. Res.,* 37, 453-464, 1976.
34. **Salisbury, R. M., Muir, J., and Stirling, J.,** Coccidiosis as a probable cause of unthriftiness and deaths in lambs, *N. Z. Vet. J.,* 1, 72-77, 1953.

35. **Shumard, R. F.,** Ovine coccidiosis — incidence, possible endotoxin, and treatment, *J. Am. Vet. Med. Assoc.,* 131, 559-561, 1957.
36. **Fitzgerald, P. R. and Mansfield, M. E.,** Effects of bovine coccidiosis on certain blood components, feed consumption, and body weight changes of calves, *Am. J. Vet. Res.,* 33, 1391—1397, 1972.
37. **Blood, D. C. and Henderson, J. A.,** *Veterinary Medicine,* 4th ed., Williams & Wilkins, Baltimore, 1974, 585-588.
38. **Long, P. L.,** The pathogenic effects of *Eimeria praecox* and *E. acervulina* in the chicken, *Parasitology,* 58, 691-700, 1968.
39. **Soulsby, E. J. L.,** *Helminths, Arthropods & Protozoa of Domesticated Animals (Mönnig),* 6th ed., Baillière, Tindall & Cassell, London, 1968, 644-669.
40. **Reid, W. M.,** Coccidiosis, in *Diseases of Poultry,* 6th ed., Hofstad, M. S., Calnek, B. W., Helmboldt, C. F., Reid, W. M., and Yoder, H. W., Eds., Iowa State University Press, Ames, 1972, 944-989.
41. **Spindler, L. A.,** The effect of experimental infections with ascarids on the growth of pigs, *Proc. Helminthol. Soc. Wash.,* 14, 58-63, 1947.
42. **Spindler, L. A.,** Effect of parasites on the growth of pigs, *Vet. Med.,* 46, 421-427, 1951.
43. **Soulsby, E. J. L.,** *Helminths, Arthropods & Protozoa of Domesticated Animals (Mönnig),* 6th ed., Baillière, Tindall & Cassell, London, 1968, 152-157.
44. **Blood, D. C. and Henderson, J. A.,** *Veterinary Medicine,* 4th ed., Williams & Wilkins, Baltimore, 1974, 633-635.
45. **Alicata, J. E. and Lynd, F. T.,** Growth rate and other signs of infection in calves experimentally infected with *Cooperia punctata, Am. J. Vet. Res.,* 22, 704-707, 1961.
46. **Herlich, H.,** The effects of the intestinal worms, *Cooperia pectinata* and *Cooperia oncophora,* on experimentally infected calves, *Am. J. Vet. Res.,* 26, 1032-1036, 1965.
47. **Keith, R. K.,** The effect of repeated anthelmintic treatment on body weight gains of calves, *Aust. Vet. J.,* 44, 326—328, 1968.
48. **Smith, H. J. and Calder, F. W.,** The development, clinical signs and economic losses of gastrointestinal parasitism in feeder cattle on irrigated and non-irrigated dikeland and upland pastures, *Can. J. Comp. Med.,* 36, 380-388, 1972.
49. **Blood, D. C. and Henderson, J. A.,** *Veterinary Medicine,* 4th ed., Williams & Wilkins, Baltimore, 1974, 635-642.
50. **Gordon, H. McL.,** Some aspects of parasitic gastro-enteritis of sheep, *Aust. Vet. J.,* 26, 14-28, 1950.
51. **Blood, D. C. and Henderson, J. A.,** *Veterinary Medicine,* 4th ed., Williams & Wilkins, Baltimore, 1974, 642-645.
52. **Allonby, E. W. and Urquhart, G. M.,** The epidemiology and pathogenic significance of haemonchosis in a Merino flock in East Africa, *Vet. Parasitol.,* 1, 129-143, 1975.
53. **Soulsby, E. J. L.,** *Helminths, Arthropods & Protozoa of Domesticated Animals (Mönnig),* 6th ed., Baillière, Tindall & Cassell, London, 1968, 255-258.
54. **Andrews, J. S. and Maldonado, J. F.,** Some clinical aspects of experimental esophagostomiasis in cattle, *Am. J. Vet. Res.,* 4, 211-225, 1943.
55. **Soulsby, E. J. L.,** *Helminths, Arthropods & Protozoa of Domesticated Animals (Mönnig),* 6th ed., Baillière, Tindall & Cassell, London, 1968, 227-230.
56. **Soulsby, E. J. L.,** *Helminths, Arthropods and Protozoa of Domesticated Animals (Mönnig),* 6th ed., Baillière, Tindall & Cassell, London, 1968, 200-203.
57. **Blood, D. C. and Henderson, J. A.,** *Veterinary Medicine,* 4th ed., Williams & Wilkins, Baltimore, 1974, 631-633.
58. **Stewart, W. L. and Crofton, H. D.,** Parasitic gastritis in cattle, *Vet. Rec.,* 53, 619—621, 1941.
59. **Spedding, C. R. W.,** Effect of a sub-clinical worm-burden on the digestive efficiency of sheep, *J. Comp. Pathol. Ther.,* 64, 5-14, 1954.
60. **Taylor, S. M.,** The cost of liver fluke in Northern Ireland, *Agric. North. Ireland,* 49, 264-268, 1974.
61. **Blood, D. C. and Henderson, J. A.,** *Veterinary Medicine,* 4th ed., Williams & Wilkins, Baltimore, 1974, 602-609.
62. **Francis, J.,** The effect of ticks on the growth-rate of cattle, *Proc. Aust. Soc. Anim. Prod.,* 3, 130-132, 1960.
63. **Little, D. A.,** The effect of cattle tick infestation of the growth rate of cattle, *Aust. Vet. J.,* 39, 6-10, 1963.
64. **Anon.,** Livestock and poultry losses, in Losses in Agriculture, Agriculture Handbook No. 291, U.S. Department of Agriculture, Agricultural Research Service, Washington, D.C., 1965, 72-84.
65. **Seebeck, R. M., Springell, P. H., and O'Kelly, J. C.,** Alterations in host metabolism by the specific and anorectic effects of the cattle tick (*Boophilus microplus*). I. Food intake and body weight growth, *Aust. J. Biol. Sci.,* 24, 373-380, 1971.

66. **Springell, P. H.**, The cattle tick in relation to animal production in Australia, *World Anim. Rev.*, 10, 19-23, 1974.
67. **Castillo Lavie, R.**, The national tick eradication campaign in Mexico, in PAHO Scientific Publication No. 316, Pan American Health Organization, Washington, D.C., 1976, 106-111.
68. **Collins, R. C. and Dewhirst, L. W.**, Some effects of the sucking louse, *Haematopinus eurysternus*, on cattle on unsupplemented range, *J. Am. Vet. Med. Assoc.*, 146, 129-132, 1965.
69. **Tobin, W. C.**, Cattle scabies can be costly, *J. Am. Vet. Med. Assoc.*, 141, 845—847, 1962.
70. **Cheng, T.-H.**, The effect of biting fly control on weight gain in beef cattle, *J. Econ. Entomol.*, 51, 275—278, 1958.
71. **Duren, E. and O'Keeffe, L. E.**, Horn fly control with dust bags: effect on weight gains, *Anim. Nutr. Health*, 27 (8), 3—4, 1972.
72. **Roberts, R. H. and Pund, W. A.**, Control of biting flies on beef steers: effect on performance in pasture and feedlot, *J. Econ. Entomol.*, 67, 232—234, 1974.
73. **Steelman, C. D., White, T. W., and Schilling, P. E.**, Effects of mosquitoes on the average daily gain of feedlot steers in southern Louisiana, *J. Econ. Entomol.*, 65, 462—466, 1972.
74. **Steelman, C. D., White, T. W., and Schilling, P. E.**, Effects of mosquitoes on the average daily gain of Hereford and Brahman breed steers in southern Louisiana, *J. Econ. Entomol.*, 66, 1081—1083, 1973.
75. **Steelman, C. D.**, Effects of external and internal arthropod parasites on domestic livestock production, *Annu. Rev. Entomol.*, 21, 155—178, 1976.
76. **Collins, R. C. and Dewhirst, L. W.**, The cattle grub problem in Arizona. II. Phenology of common cattle grub infestations and their effects on weight gains of preweaning calves, *J. Econ. Entomol.*, 64, 1467—1471, 1971.
77. **Campbell, J. B., Woods, W., Hagen, A. F., and Howe, E. C.**, Cattle grub insecticide efficacy and effects on weight-gain performance on feeder calves in Nebraska, *J. Econ. Entomol.*, 66, 429—432, 1973.
78. **Switzer, W. P. and Ross, R. F.**, Mycoplasmal diseases, in *Diseases of Swine*, 4th ed., Dunne, H. W. and Leman, A. D., Eds., Iowa State University Press, Ames, 1975, 741—764.
79. **Betts, A. O.**, Respiratory diseases of pigs. V. Some clinical and epidemiological aspects of virus pneumonia of pigs, *Vet. Rec.*, 64, 283—288, 1952.
80. **Betts, A. O. and Beveridge, W. I. B.**, Virus pneumonia of pigs: the effect of the disease upon growth and efficiency of food utilization, *Vet. Res.*, 65, 515—520, 1953.
81. **Betts, A. O., Whittlestone, P., Beveridge, W. I. B., Taylor, J. H., and Campbell, R. C.**, Virus pneumonia in pigs: further investigations on the effect of the disease upon the growth-rate and efficiency of food utilization, *Vet. Rec.*, 67, 661—665, 1955.
82. **Young, G. A., Caldwell, J. D., and Underdahl, N. R.**, Relationship of atrophic rhinitis and virus pig pneumonia to growth rate in swine, *J. Am. Vet. Med. Assoc.*, 134, 231—233, 1959.
83. **Beveridge, W. I. B.**, Economics of animal health, *Vet. Rec.*, 72, 810—815, 1960.
84. **Goodwin, R. F. W.**, The economic effect of enzootic pneumonia in a large herd of pigs, *Br. Vet. J.*, 119, 298—306, 1963.
85. **Goodwin, R. F. W.**, The economics of enzootic pneumonia, *Vet. Rec.*, 89, 77—81, 1971.
86. **Braude, R. and Plonka, S.**, Effect of enzootic pneumonia on the performance of growing pigs, *Vet. Rec.*, 96, 359—360, 1975.
87. **Kristjansson, F. K. and Gwatkin, R.**, The effect of infectious atrophic rhinitis on weight for age in swine, *Can. J. Agric. Sci.*, 35, 139—142, 1955.
88. **Shuman, R. D. and Earl, F. L.**, Atrophic rhinitis. VII. A study of the economic effect in a swine herd, *J. Am. Vet. Med. Assoc.*, 129, 220—224, 1956.
89. Control of Cattle Diseases, National Research Program Publication No. 20420, U.S. Department of Agriculture, Agricultural Research Service, Washington, D.C., 1976.
90. **Hemsley, L. A. and Durrant, R. J.**, The effect of respiratory disease, age of litter and disinfection practices on the performance of young chickens, *Br. Vet. J.*, 120, 567—575, 1964.
91. Control of Poultry Diseases, National Research Program Publication No. 20450, U.S. Department of Agriculture, Agricultural Research Service, Washington, D.C., 1976.
92. **Scott, G. C.**, The use of cortisone in the treatment of infectious keratoconjunctivitis (pink-eye) in cattle, *J. Am. Vet. Med. Assoc.*, 130, 257—259, 1957.
93. **Thrift, F. A. and Overfield, J. R.**, Impact of pinkeye (infectious bovine kerato-conjunctivitis) on weaning and postweaning performance of Hereford calves, *J. Anim. Sci.*, 38, 1179—1184, 1974.
94. **Killinger, A. H., Valentine, D., Mansfield, M. E., Ricketts, G. E., Cmarik, G. F., Neumann, A. H., and Norton, H. W.**, Economic impact of infectious bovine keratoconjunctivitis in beef calves, *Vet. Med. Small Anim. Clin.*, 72, 618—620, 1977.
95. **Harnett, P.**, The significance of veterinary science in the national economy, *Ir. Vet. J.*, 10, 130—142, 1956.

96. **Leech, F. B.**, Food losses through animal diseases, *Proc. Nutr. Soc.*, 20, 20—24, 1961.
97. **Gibson, T. E.**, The cost of animal parasites, *Span*, 7, 99—102, 1964.
98. **Schultz, M. G., Hermos, J. A., and Steele, J. H.**, Epidemiology of beef tapeworm infection in the United States, *Public Health Rep.*, 85, 169—176, 1970.
99. **Meyer, K. F.**, Animal diseases and human welfare, *Adv. Vet. Sci.*, 1, 1—48, 1953.
100. **Anon.**, Marketing and processing losses, in Losses in Agriculture, Agriculture Handbook No. 291, U.S. Department of Agriculture, Agricultural Research Service, Washington, D.C., 1965, 85—94.
101. **Lassahn, P. L.**, Grubs eat into cattle profits, *Iowa Farm Sci.*, 23, 284—286, 1968.
102. **Rich, G. B.**, The economics of systemic insecticide treatment for reduction of slaughter trim loss caused by cattle grubs, *Hypoderma* spp., *Can. J. Anim. Sci.*, 50, 301—310, 1970.
103. **Anon.**, The present hydatid situation in New Zealand and the urgent need for a new approach, *N.Z. Med. J.*, 56, 138—139, 1957.
104. **Trejos, A. and Williams, J. F.**, The problem of hydatidosis in the Americas, in PAHO Scientific Publication No. 196, Pan American Health Organization, Washington, D.C., 1970, 122—126.
105. **Arundel, J. H.**, A review of cysticercoses of sheep and cattle in Australia, *Aust. Vet. J.*, 48, 140—155, 1972.
106. **Szyfres, B.**, Zoonoses, public health, and livestock development in Latin America, in PAHO Scientific Publication No. 196, Pan American Health Organization, Washington, D.C., 1970, 99—103.
107. **Gordon, R. F.**, The economic effect of ill health, *Vet. Rec.*, 89, 496—500, 1971.
108. **Steiner, P. E. and Bengston, J. S.**, Research and economic aspects of tumors in food-producing animals, *Cancer*, 4, 1113—1124, 1951.
109. **Shaw, A. O. and Beam, A. L.**, The effect of mastitis upon milk production, *J. Dairy Sci.*, 18, 353—357, 1935.
110. **Minett, F. C. and Martin, W. J.**, Influence of mastitis and of *Brucella abortus* infection upon the milk yield of cows. *J. Dairy Res.*, 7, 122—144, 1936.
111. **McDowall, F. H.**, Studies on the detection of mastitis in New Zealand dairy herds. V. Composition of milk from quarters reacting to the bromthymol blue test for mastitis, *N.Z. J. Sci. Technol. Sect. A*, 27, 258—269, 1945.
112. **Crossman, J. V., Dodd, F. H., Lee, J. M., and Neave, F. K.**, The effect of bacterial infection on the milk yield of the individual quarters of the cow's udder, *J. Dairy Res.*, 17, 128—158, 1950.
113. **McLeod, D. H. and Wilson, S. M.**, Milk yield in relation to infection with *Streptocuccus agalactiae*, *J. Dairy Res.*, 18, 235—239, 1951.
114. **Watts, P. S.**, Mastitis in Ayrshire from 1938 to 1950, *Vet. Rec.*, 63, 32—39, 1951.
115. **O'Donovan, J., Dodd, F. H., and Neave, F. K.**, The effect of udder infections on the lactation yield of milk and milk solids, *J. Dairy Res.*, 27, 115—120, 1960.
116. **Hale, H. H., Plastridge, W. N., and Williams, L. F.**, The effect of *Streptococcus agalactiae* infection on milk yield, *Cornell Vet.*, 46, 201—206, 1956.
117. **Landrey, J. S. A.**, The effect of mastitis on herd milk production and composition, *J. S. Afr. Vet. Med. Assoc.*, 36, 515—519, 1965.
118. **Wheelock, J. V., Rook, J. A. F., Neave, F. K., and Dodd, F. H.**, The effect of bacterial infections of the udder on the yield and composition of cow's milk, *J. Dairy Res.*, 33, 199—215, 1966
119. **King, J. O. L.**, The effect of mastitis on the yield and composition of heifers' milk, *Vet. Rec.*, 80, 139—141, 1967.
120. **Philpot, W. N.**, Influence of subclinical mastitis on milk production and milk composition, *J. Dairy Sci.*, 50, 978, 1967.
121. **Dobbins, C. N.**, Mastitis losses, *Mod. Vet. Pract.*, 50(9), 38—41, 1969.
122. **King, J. O. L.**, The effects of different bacterial infections causing mastitis on the yield and quality of cow's milk, *Br. Vet. J.*, 125, 57—62, 1969.
123. **Roberts, S. J., Meek, A. M., Natzke, R. P., Guthrie, R. S., Field, L. E., Merrill, W. G., Schmidt, G. H., and Everett, R. W.**, Concepts and recent developments in mastitis control, *J. Am. Vet. Med. Assoc.*, 155, 157—166, 1969.
124. **Janzen, J. J.**, Economic losses resulting from mastitis. A review, *J. Dairy Sci.*, 53, 1151—1161, 1970.
125. **Marx, G. D.**, Quarter milking machine and post-milking teat dip to study factors involved in mastitis, *J. Dairy Sci.*, 54, 797, 1971.
126. **Natzke, R. P., Everett, R. W., Guthrie, R. S., Keown, J. F., Meek, A. M., Merrill, W. G., Roberts, S. J., and Schmidt, G. H.**, Mastitis control program: effect on milk production, *J. Dairy Sci.*, 55, 1256—1260, 1972.
127. **Dobbins, C. N.**, Mastitis losses, *J. Am. Vet. Med. Assoc.*, 170, 1129—1132, 1977.
128. **Rowland, S. J.**, The protein distribution in normal and abnormal milk, *J. Dairy Res.*, 9, 47—57, 1938.
129. **Rowland, S. J. and Zein-El-Dine, M.**, The effect of subclinical mastitis on the solids-not-fat content of milk, *J. Dairy Res.*, 9, 182—184, 1938.

130. **Vanlandingham, A. H., Weakley, C. E., Moore, E. N., and Henderson, H. O.,** Mastitis. I. The relationship of the development of mastitis to changes in the chlorine, lactose and casein number of milk, *J. Dairy Sci.*, 24, 383—398, 1941.
131. **Rathore, A. K.,** The influence of age and mastitis on the solids-not-fat content of milk in cattle, *Br. Vet. J.*, 126, xvi—xvii, 1970.
132. **Schalm, O. W.,** Pathologic changes in the milk and udder of cows with mastitis, *J. Am. Vet. Med. Assoc.*, 170, 1137—1140, 1977.
133. **Pegg, S. E. and Rice, E. B.,** A survey of herd wastage and other factors on Queensland dairy farms, *Queensl. Agric. J.*, 69, 346—350, 1949.
134. **Asdell, S. A.,** Variations in amount of culling from D.H.I.A. herds, *J. Dairy Sci.*, 34, 529—535, 1951.
135. **Withers, F. W.,** Wastage and disease incidence in dairy herds, *Vet. Rec.*, 67, 605—612, 1955.
136. **Clark, C. H.,** A survey of dairy herd wastage in Queensland, *Queensl. Agric. J.*, 83, 653—658, 1957.
137. **O'Bleness, G. V. and Van Vleck, L. D.,** Reasons for disposal of dairy cows from New York herds, *J. Dairy Sci.*, 45, 1087—1093, 1962.
138. **McClure, T. J. and Dowell, A. E.,** Survey of dairy herds in the Moss Vale district of New South Wales. I. Disease wastage, *Aust. Vet. J.*, 44, 536—542, 1968.
139. **Amiel, D. K. and Moodie, E. W.,** Dairy herd wastage in south eastern Queensland, *Aust. Vet. J.*, 49, 69—73, 1973.
140. **Ellis, E. M. and Kendall, H. E.,** The public health and economic effects of vesicular stomatitis in a herd of dairy cattle, *J. Am. Vet. Med. Assoc.*, 144, 377—380, 1964.
141. **Simms, B. T. and Miller, F. W.,** Practical results of attempts to control abortion disease, *J. Am. Vet. Med. Assoc.*, 68, 455—458, 1925-1926.
142. **Fritz, B. S. and Barnes, M. F.,** Bang disease control work in fourteen state institution herds, *J. Am. Vet. Med. Assoc.*, 76, 490—504, 1930.
143. **Rich, L. H.,** Economic factors of abortion in cattle, *Cornell Vet.*, 21, 15—24, 1931.
144. **Huddleson, I. F.,** The relation of brucellosis to human welfare, *Ann. N.Y. Acad. Sci.*, 48, 415—428, 1947.
145. **Todd, A. C., Myers, G. H., Bliss, D., and Cox, D. D.,** Milk production in Wisconsin dairy cattle after anthelmintic treatment, *Vet. Med. Small Anim. Clin.*, 67, 1233—1236, 1972.
146. **Bliss, D. and Todd, A. C.,** Milk production by Wisconsin dairy cattle after deworming with Baymix, *Vet. Med. Small Anim. Clin.*, 68, 1034—1038, 1973.
147. **Bliss, D. H. and Todd, A. C.,** Milk production by Wisconsin dairy cattle after deworming with thiabendazole, *Vet Med. Small Anim. Clin.*, 69, 638—640, 1974.
148. **Ross, J. G.,** The economics of *Fasciola hepatica* infections in cattle, *Br. Vet. J.*, 126, xiii—xv, 1970.
149. **Schwabe, C. W.,** *Veterinary Medicine and Human Health,* 2nd ed., Williams ™ Wilkins, Baltimore, 1969, 465.
150. **Freeborn, S. B., Regan, W. M., and Folger, A. H.,** The relation of flies and fly sprays to milk production, *J. Econ. Entomol.*, 18, 779—790, 1925.
151. **Granett, P. and Hansens, E. J.,** The effect of biting fly control on milk production, *J. Econ. Entomol.*, 49, 465—467, 1956.
152. **Granett, P. and Hansens, E. J.,** Further observations on the effect of biting fly control on milk production on cattle, *J. Econ. Entomol.*, 50, 332—336, 1957.
153. **Anderson, J. R. and Voskuil, G. H.,** A reduction in milk production caused by the feeding of blackflies (Diptera: Simuliidae) on dairy cattle in California, with notes on the feeding activity on other animals, *Mosq. News*, 23, 126—131, 1963.
154. **Henderson, W. M.,** Foot-and-mouth disease and related vesicular diseases, *Adv. Vet. Sci.*, 6, 19—77, 1960.
155. **Borsella, J.,** Foot-and-mouth disease campaign in Argentina: results, benefits, and projections, in PAHO Scientific Publication No. 196, Pan American Health Organization, Washington, D.C., 1970, 58—65.
156. **Delgado, M. V.,** Foot-and-mouth disease campaign in Venezuela: results, benefits, and prospects, in PAHO Scientific Publication No. 196, Pan American Health Organization, Washington, D.C., 1970, 69—75.
157. **Kassem, M. H. and Soliman, K. N.,** Diseases of the buffalo, in *The International Encyclopedia of Veterinary Medicine,* Dalling, T., Ed., Green, Edinburgh, 1966, 527—533.
158. **Harnett, P.,** The significance of veterinary science in the national economy, *Ir. Vet. J.*, 10, 164—172, 1956.
159. **Pierson, R. E. and Vair, C. A.,** The economic loss associated with infectious bovine rhinotracheitis in a dairy herd, *J. Am. Vet. Med. Assoc.*, 147, 350—352, 1965.
160. **Weaver, A. D.,** Solar penetration in cattle: its complications and economic loss in one herd, *Vet. Rec.*, 89, 288—296, 1971.

161. **Foley, R. C., Bath, D. L., Dickinson, F. N., and Tucker, H. A.,** *Dairy Cattle: Principles, Practices, Problems, Profits,* Lea & Febiger, Philadelphia, 1972, 486—487.
162. **McCallon, B. R.,** Anaplasmosis, *J. Dairy Sci.,* 59, 1171—1174, 1976.
163. **Snoeyenbos, G. H.,** Pullorum disease, in *Diseases of Poultry,* 6th ed., Hofstad, M. S., Calnek, B. W., Helmboldt, C. F., Reid, W. M., and Yoder, H. W., Eds., Iowa State University Press, Ames, 1972, 83—114.
164. **Williams, J. E.,** Paratyphoid infections, in *Diseases of Poultry,* 6th ed., Hofstad, M. S., Calnek, B. W., Helmboldt, C. F., Reid, W. M., and Yoder, H. W., Eds., Iowa State University Press, Ames, 1972, 135—202.
165. **Heddleston, K. L.,** Avian pasteurellosis, in *Diseases of Poultry,* 6th ed., Hofstad, M. S., Calnek, B. W., Helmboldt, C. F., Reid, W. M., and Yoder, H. W., Eds., Iowa State University Press, Ames, 1972, 219—251.
166. **Yamamoto, R.,** Infectious coryza, in *Diseases of Poultry,* 6th ed., Hofstad, M. S., Calnek, B. W., Helmboldt, C. F., Reid, W. M., and Yoder, H. W., Eds., Iowa State University Press, Ames, 1972, 272—281.
167. **Page, L. A.,** Chlamydiosis (ornithosis), in *Diseases of Poultry,* 6th ed., Hofstad, M. S., Calnek, B. W., Helmboldt, C. F., Reid, W. M., and Yoder, H. W., Eds., Iowa State University Press, Ames, 1972, 414—447.
168. **Hofstad, M. S.,** Avian infectious bronchitis, in *Diseases of Poultry,* 6th ed., Hofstad, M. S., Calnek, B. W., Helmboldt, C. F., Reid, W. M., and Yoder, H. W., Eds., Iowa State University Press, Ames, 1972, 586—606.
169. **Hanson, L. E.,** Laryngotracheitis, in *Diseases of Poultry,* 6th ed., Hofstad, M. S., Calnek, B. W., Helmboldt, C. F., Reid, W. M., and Yoder, H. W., Eds., Iowa State University Press, Ames, 1972, 607—618.
170. **Hanson, R. P.,** Newcastle disease, in *Diseases of Poultry,* 6th ed., Hofstad, M. S., Calnek, B. W., Hemboldt, C. F., Reid, W. M., and Yoder, H. W., Eds., Iowa State University Press, Ames, 1972, 619—656.
171. **Easterday, B. C. and Tumova, B.,** Avian influenza, in *Diseases of Poultry,* 6th ed., Hofstad, M. S., Calnek, B. W., Helmboldt, C. F., Reid, W. M., and Yoder, H. W., Eds., Iowa State University Press, Ames, 1972, 670—700.
172. **du Bose, R. T.,** Avian monocytosis, in *Diseases of Poultry,* 6th ed., Hofstad, M. S., Calnek, B. W., Helmboldt, C. F., Reid, W. M., and Yoder, H. W., Eds., Iowa State University Press, Ames, 1972, 781—784.
173. **Coles, R.,** The economic significance of the incidence of mortality in fowl, *Br. Vet. J.,* 111, 235—252, 1955.
174. **Burridge, M. J., Riemann, H. P., Utterback, W. W., and Sharman, E. C.,** The Newcastle disease epidemic in southern California, 1971—1973: descriptive epidemiology and effects of vaccination on the eradication program, in U.S. Animal Health Assoc., 1975 Proc., Vol. 79, U.S. Animal Health Association, 1976, 324—333.
175. **James, M. T. and Harwood, R. F.,** *Herm's Medical Entomology,* 6th ed., Macmillan, New York, 1969, 289—292.
176. **Blood, D. C. and Henderson, J. A.,** *Veterinary Medicine,* 4th ed., Williams & Wilkins, Baltimore, 1974, 676—677.
177. **Medley, J. G. and Drummond, R. O.,** Tests with insecticides for control of lice on goats and sheep, *J. Econ. Entomol.,* 56, 658—660, 1963.
178. **Blood, D. C. and Henderson, J. A.,** *Veterinary Medicine,* 4th ed., Williams & Wilkins, Baltimore, 1974, 378—379.
179. **Blood, D. C. and Henderson, J. A.,** *Veterinary Medicine,* 4th ed., Williams & Wilkins, Baltimore, 1974, 384.
180. **Jensen, R.,** *Diseases of Sheep,* Lea & Febiger, Philadelphia, 1974, 39—72.
181. **Jensen, R.,** *Diseases of Sheep,* Lea & Febiger, Philadelphia, 1974, 8—13.
182. **Crenshaw, G. L., Schultz, G., Bills, C. J., Cameron, H. S., and Timm, O.,** Ram epididymitis in California, *Calif. Vet.,* 17(6), 42—44, 1963.
183. **Hope Cawdery, M. J.,** The effects of regime therapy in fascioliasis. I. The effects of therapy on the prevalence of fascioliasis and on fertility in ewes maintained in one paddock over a period of four years, *Ir. Vet. J.,* 26, 118—127, 1972.
184. **Hope Cawdery, M. J.,** The effects of fascioliasis on ewe fertility, *Br. Vet. J.,* 132, 568—575, 1976.
185. **Dunne, H. W.,** Abortion, stillbirth, fetal death, and infectious infertility, in *Diseases of Swine,* 4th ed., Dunne, H. W. and Leman, A. D., Eds., Iowa State University Press, Ames, 1975, 918—952.
186. **Wells, K. F.,** Foot-and-mouth disease: eradication and preventive measures in Canada, in PAHO Scientific Publication No. 196, Pan American Health Organization, Washington, D.C., 1970, 76—81.

187. **Nadeau, J. D.**, Importance du controle des maladies animales dans l'efficacite des productions, *Can. Vet. J.*, 7, 142—147, 1966.
188. **Boughton, D. C.**, Effective control of internal parasites, *Adv. Vet. Sci.*, 2, 380—410, 1955.
189. Control of Insects Affecting Livestock, National Research Program Publication No. 20480, U.S. Department of Agriculture, Agricultural Research Service, Washington, D.C., 1976.
190. Control of Swine Diseases, National Research Program publication no. 20430, U.S. Department of Agriculture, Agricultural Research Service, Washington, D.C., 1976.
191. Control of Sheep and Other Animal Diseases, National Research Program Publication No. 20440, U.S. Department of Agriculture, Agricultural Research Service, 1976.
192. **Lombardo, R. A.**, Socioeconomic importance of the tick problem in the Americas, in PAHO Scientific Publication No. 316, Pan American Health Organization, Washington, D.C., 1976, 79—89.
193. **Freire de Faria, J.**, Foot-and-mouth disease campaign in Brazil: results and benefits, in PAHO Scientific Publication No. 196, Pan American Health Organization, Washington, D.C., 1970, 66—68.
194. **Nazlioglu, M.**, Economic losses caused by foot-and-mouth disease in Turkey and sanitary measures taken, *Off. Int. Epizoot. Bull.*, 68, 533—540, 1967.
195. **Malaga Alba, A. and Acha, P. N.**, The status of rabies in the Americas, in PAHO Scientific Publication No. 196, Pan American Health Organization, Washington, D.C., 1970, 112—121.
196. **Kverno, N. B. and Mitchell, G. C.**, Vampire bats and their effect on cattle production in Latin America, *World Anim. Rev.*, 17, 1—7, 1976.
197. **Lancaster, J. E.**, A history of Newcastle disease with comments on its economic effects, *World's Poult. Sci. J.*, 32, 167—175, 1976.
198. **Morris, R. S.**, Assessing the economic value of veterinary services to primary industries, *Aust. Vet. J.*, 45, 295—300, 1969.
199. **Power, A. P. and Harris, S. A.**, A cost-benefit evaluation of alternative control policies for foot-and-mouth disease in Great Britain, *J. Agric. Econ.*, 24, 573—600, 1973.
200. **Baumhover, A. H.**, Eradication of the screwworm fly, *JAMA*, 196, 150—158, 1966.
201. **Sharman, E. C. and Walker, J. W.**, Regulatory aspects of velogenic viscerotropic Newcastle disease, *J. Am. Vet. Med. Assoc.*, 163, 1089—1093, 1973.
202. **Braumhover, A. H.**, Florida screwworm control program, *Vet. Med.*, 53, 216—219, 1958.
203. **Diamant, G.**, Screwworm eradication in southeastern United States, *Am. J. Public Health*, 53, 22—26, 1963.
204. **Becton, P.**, Brucellosis status report, *J. Dairy Sci.*, 59, 1163—1165, 1976.
205. **Schwabe, C. W.**, *Veterinary Medicine and Human Health*, 2nd ed., Williams & Wilkins, Baltimore, 1969, 464.
206. **Reid, W. M. and Kowalski, L.**, Economics of coccidiosis in poultry production, *J. Parasitol.*, 56 (4), 279—280, 1970.
207. **Morris, R. S. and Blood, D. C.**, The economic basis of planned veterinary services to individual farms, *Aust. Vet. J.*, 45, 337—341, 1969.
208. **Bens, R. J.**, The economics of preventive medicine and swine production, *Can. Vet. J.*, 12, 186—189, 1971.
209. **Morris, R. S.**, Economic aspects of disease control programmes for dairy cattle, *Aust. Vet. J.*, 47, 358—363, 1971.
210. **Herschler, R. C., Miracle, C., Crowl, B., Dunlap, T., and Judy, J. W.**, The economic impact of a fertility control and herd management program on a dairy farm, *J. Am. Vet. Med. Assoc.*, 145, 672—676, 1964.
211. **Roberts, S. J. and DeCamp, C. E.**, Study of a planned preventive health program for dairy herds, *Vet. Med. Small Anim. Clin.*, 60, 771—777, 1965.
212. **Morrow, D. A.**, Analysis of herd performance and economic results of preventive dairy herd health programs — part I, *Vet. Med. Small Anim. Clin.*, 61, 474—483, 1966.
213. **Barfoot, L. W., Cote, J. F., Stone, J. B., and Wright, P. A.**, An economic appraisal of a preventative medicine program for dairy herd health management, *Can. Vet. J.*, 12, 2—10, 1971.
214. **Derbyshire, J. B.**, Microbial diseases and animal productivity, *Symp. Soc. Gen. Microbiol.*, 21, 125—147, 1971.
215. **Kellar, J., Marra, R., and Martin, W.**, Brucellosis in Ontario: a case control study, *Can. J. Comp. Med.*, 40, 119—128, 1976.
216. **Franti, C. E., Wiggins, A. D., Lopez-Nieto, E., and Crenshaw, G.**, Factor analysis: a statistical tool useful in epizootiological research, with an example from a study of diarrhea in dairy calves, *Am. J. Vet. Res.*, 35, 649—655, 1974.
217. **Martin, S. W., Schwabe, C. W., and Franti, C. E.**, Dairy calf mortality rate: influence of meteorologic factors on calf mortality rate in Tulare County, California, *Am. J. Vet. Res.*, 36, 1105—1109, 1975.

218. **Martin, S. W. Schwabe, C. W., and Franti, C. E.,** Dairy calf mortality rate: influence of management and housing factors on calf mortality rate in Tulare County, California, *Am. J. Vet. Res.,* 36, 1111—1114, 1975.
219. **Martin, S. W., Schwabe, C. W., and Franti, C. E.,** Dairy calf mortality rate: the association of daily meteorological factors and calf mortality, *Can. J. Comp. Med.,* 39, 377—388, 1975.
220. **Burridge, M. J. and Schwabe, C. W.,** Epidemiological analysis of factors influencing rate of progress in *Echinococcus granulosus* control in New Zealand, *J. Hyg.,* 78, 151—163, 1977.
221. **Burridge, M. J. and Schwabe, C. W.,** An epidemiological analysis of factors influencing the increase in *Taenia ovis* prevalence during the New Zealand *Echinococcus granulosus* control program, *Aust. Vet. J.,* 53, 374—379, 1977.
222. **Burridge, M. J., Schwabe, C. W., and Pullum, T. W.,** Path analysis: application in an epidemiological study of echinococcosis in New Zealand, *J. Hyg.,* 78, 135—149, 1977.
223. **Plant, J. and Glynn, A. A.,** Natural resistance to *Salmonella* infection, delayed hypersensitivity and Ir genes in different strains of mice, *Nature* (London), 248, 345—347, 1974.
224. **Spooner, R. L., Bradley, J. S., and Young, G. B.,** Genetics and disease in domestic animals with particular reference to dairy cattle, *Vet. Rec.,* 97, 125—130, 1975.
225. **Bradley, J. S.,** Genetic aspects of disease in cattle, *Proc. Roy. Soc. Med.,* 69, 6, 1976.
226. **Chandler, R. L.,** Comparative tolerance of West African N'dama cattle to trypanosomiasis, *Ann. Trop. Med. Parasitol.,* 46, 127—134, 1952.
227. **Chandler, R. L.,** Studies on the tolerance of N'dama cattle to trypanosomiasis, *J. Comp. Pathol. Ther.,* 68, 253—260, 1958.
228. **Roberts, C. J. and Gray, A. R.,** Studies on trypanosome-resistant cattle. II. The effect of trypanosomiasis on N'dama, Muturu and Zebu cattle, *Trop. Anim. Health Prod.,* 5, 220—233, 1973.
229. **Ormerod, W. E.,** Ecological effect of control of African trypanosomiasis, *Science,* 191, 815—821, 1976.
230. **Pilchard, E. I.,** Economic importance of mastitis research in the United States, *Agric. Sci. Rev. Coop. State Res. Serv. U.S. Dep. Agric.,* 10 (2), 30—35, 1972.
231. **Anon.,** Justifications for veterinary animal health research, *Am. J. Vet. Res.,* 35, 875—887, 1974.

MICROBIAL DISEASE AND ANIMAL PRODUCTIVITY

J. B. Derbyshire

INTRODUCTION

Microbial infections of farm livestock may be either beneficial or detrimental to the host animal. Some components of the alimentary microflora fall into the former category and may play a major role in nutrition, particularly of the ruminant. [1] This contribution, however, will discuss only disease-producing microbes. Microbial disease has been broadly defined as any infection with bacteria, viruses, or protozoa that decreases the productive capacity of an animal.[2] In the present context, we are concerned with domesticated farm livestock maintained for food production, although infections of draft animals that have an essential role in agriculture will not be excluded.

The definition of animal productivity also requires some clarification, particularly as distinct from animal production. At the level of the individual animal, productivity is best measured in terms of efficiency of feed conversion, but from the point of view of the livestock producer, productivity includes a high return on the capital and labor costs of his operation. At the national level, additional factors include the efficient utilization of national resources and the economic benefits to be gained from increased exports or savings on imports. It is important to recognize that under certain circumstances, an increase in animal production, which may result from the application of effective disease-control measures, may not necessarily result in increased productivity. If the disease-control procedures are not accompanied by improved breeding and diets, the result may merely be an expanding population of unproductive animals. On occasion, failure of the industry to compensate for increased numbers when a disease is successfully controlled may so depress the market value of the product in the short-term as to render the procedure unproductive, in spite of the benefits at the level of the individual animal.

Unfortunately, there is a relative lack of statistics on both the productivity losses due to microbial disease[3] and the benefits that accrue from successful control of disease. International organizations such as the Food and Agriculture Organization (FAO) and L'Office Internationale des Epizooties (OIE) have directed their attention towards the major epidemics of farm livestock such as foot-and-mouth disease, rinderpest, bluetongue, and Newcastle disease. The World Health Organization (WHO) shows special concern for zoonoses, such as rabies, that pose a direct threat to the human population. The development of disease surveillance, particularly with reference to the major epidemics, was discussed recently by Steele.[4] Certain less clearly characterized diseases, such as neonatal enteric infections and infections of the respiratory tract, that are emerging under conditions of intensive animal husbandry, are poorly monitored. The need for improved monitoring of these diseases was stressed by several contributors to a recent symposium.[5] In a number of diseases in this category, environmental factors, in addition to microbial infection, play an essential part in the etiology. Certain of these diseases commonly occur in a subclinical form and may cause serious losses without ever showing clinical signs. Thus, while the scope of this contribution is broad, relatively little solid data is available. This report will briefly review the ways in which microbial diseases can contribute to reduced animal productivity and discuss the value of control measures. Specific examples will be cited from the literature whenever information is available. A more general discussion of the effects of disease on animal production in relation to human nutrition can be found in a review by Schwabe and Ruppanner.[6]

PRODUCTIVITY LOSSES DUE TO MICROBIAL DISEASES

The kinds of productivity losses associated with microbial disease include mortality, production losses, and indirect or consequential losses. Although death is the most obvious and dramatic effect of the introduction of a microbial disease into a susceptible population, mortality is frequently of less significance than production and consequential losses, examples of which are discussed below. However, in certain of the major epidemics, such as rinderpest in cattle[7] and Newcastle disease in poultry,[8] mortality may approach 100%; infections of neonatal animals, such as transmissible gastroenteritis in swine, [9] are frequently characterized by high mortality.

Production losses due to microbial disease represent a major burden on the livestock industry in all parts of the world. Those associated with major viral epidemics are best recognized, and their control is well advanced in many countries. Foot-and-mouth disease[10] is a classic example of a debilitating infection involving major losses in meat and milk production. Eichhorn[11] estimated that this disease could cost a country as much as 25% of its annual production. In 1952, foot-and-mouth disease cost Germany, France, and Britain $245 million in compensation to farmers;[12] the 1971—1972 epidemic in Italy cost $11 million.[13] At the level of the individual producer, losses due to epidemic disease can be equally dramatic. Ellis and Kendall[14] studied the economic effects of an outbreak of vesicular stomatitis in a dairy herd in Alabama in 1964. The total loss, including animals culled for slaughter and decreased milk production, was estimated at $40,000.

Endemic bacterial infections such as bovine brucellosis and those associated with mastitis in cattle can cause major production losses in dairy cattle, mainly in lost milk production. In brucellosis, milk is lost because the cows fail to lactate normally after abortion; in acute mastitis (caused by streptococcal or staphylococcal infection of the udder), there may be a total cessation of lactation. In chronic mastitis, milk-yield reductions of at least 10% are common. Mastitis has been estimated to cost at least $50 per cow annually in lost milk production, which in Canada means a national loss of $100 million/ year.[15] In 1960, the average annual loss due to bovine mastitis in France was put at the same figure,[13] which included the cost of replacing incurable cows and losses in the manufacture of dairy products as well as the direct loss of milk. The milk loss from brucellosis in Great Britain was estimated in 1961 at 0.5% of that country's total milk production.[16]

Infections of the respiratory tract of farm livestock are another significant cause of production losses. In beef cattle, losses due to infectious bovine rhinotracheitis were estimated at 36 pounds sterling per animal in 1979.[17] Pneumonia in housed calves and "shipping fever" in calves maintained under feedlot conditions are associated with a variety of viral and bacterial agents and lead to productivity losses. Mortality is usually relatively low in calf pneumonia, but in this condition the growth rate of the animals may be chronically depressed and the unproductive animals may have to be culled. In uncomplicated enzootic pneumonia of swine, deaths rarely occur, but again, growth and feed-conversion rates are impaired. The national economic loss from this disease in Britain was estimated at 10 million pounds sterling annually in 1961.[12] In these respiratory diseases, production losses are associated with impairment of the normal function of the lung,[18] which causes the infected animal to divert more energy than normal to respiration.

While enteric infections are frequently fatal in neonatal animals, slightly older stock usually recover; and enteric disease tends to be of a less chronic nature than respiratory disease. The damage caused to the intestinal epithelium, characterized in viral infections by atrophy of the villi of the small intestine, is relatively transient. If the animal is able to survive the dehydration associated with the diarrhea that marks the acute disease, the intestinal epithelium will normally regenerate rapidly. Thus, the check in growth rate in this type of infection is usually more transient than in respiratory infections, in which permanent tissue damage is more frequent, and the economic consequences may be correspondingly less severe.

In a recent paper, Loew[19] made some interesting calculations of the wastage of feed energy involved in febrile conditions in sick animals. Many microbial infections of livestock are accompanied by fever, often of several days duration. Loew assumed a 5 to 7% increase in energy requirement per degree Fahrenheit of fever and on this basis calculated that cattle in Canada might consume as much as 11,812 tons of grain per year to compensate for febrile reactions rather than for more productive purposes.

In economic terms, the consequential losses (particularly those associated with the major epidemics) may outweigh the direct effects of the infection at the local level. In the case of zoonoses such as rabies, the threat of human infection is a significant consequence of the disease in animals. Fatal or debilitating disease in draft animals can have far-reaching effects on agriculture. In 1960, between 200,000 and 300,000 horses and mules in Asia died from African horsesickness following the emergence of this disease from the African continent,[20] indirectly causing extremely serious crop production losses. Loss of export markets is an important consequence of the presence of contagious diseases in certain countries. In an outbreak of foot-and-mouth disease in Canada in 1951, $1 million was paid in compensation for the direct losses suffered, but greater losses accrued from the closure of foreign markets. In Ireland, an estimated $10 million was spent annually on the eradication of bovine tuberculosis in order to protect the U.K. export market, worth $110 to 140 million/year.[13] In certain situations, local production losses associated with some diseases may be regarded as relatively unimportant; the stimulus for their control relates to the export trade. Thus, rinderpest in some African countries and foot-and-mouth disease in parts of Africa and South America are of prime importance in relation to the loss of potential or actual export markets for meat from these countries.

One of the more far-reaching consequences of the presence of an infectious disease in an indigenous animal population, particularly in a developing country, is the constraint that this places on livestock development. The presence of reservoirs of infection in the wildlife population of an area, together with vectors of the infections, may preclude the development of large tracts of land for livestock production.The trypanosomiases provide an excellent example of this situation. FAO estimated in 1963[13] that the capital value lost in the tsetse fly-infested areas of Africa, in relation to their potential cattle-carrying capacity, was as much as $5 million. In less extreme situations, the presence of infection in domesticated native stock may prevent the introduction of susceptible high-grade stock to replace unproductive animals. This was recognized relatively early in South Africa, where preventive veterinary medicine has long been successfully practiced.

It is necessary to include the cost of control measures among the consequential losses associated with a disease, particularly in relation to national productivity. The application of a slaughter and quarantine policy for the control of a disease or a widespread vaccination program can be expensive measures, although if they are effective they can be regarded as an investment to prevent even greater losses in productivity.

The advent of increased trade and more rapid transportation between livestock-producing areas has increased the risk of introducing infection into fully susceptible populations that were hitherto free of the disease. A number of important diseases have emerged in this manner in relatively recent years. One of the more costly examples of this emergence relates to African swinefever, which reached Europe from Africa and in 1960 caused losses amounting to more than $11 million in Portugal and Spain.[20] This viral disease subsequently appeared in Cuba in 1971, necessitating the slaughter of 33,254 pigs, which were either infected or had come into contact with infected animals.[21] Eradication from Cuba was successful, but the disease is now believed to be endemic in parts of Spain and Portugal. Subsequent spread of the virus to Brazil and the Dominican Republic occurred in 1978.[43]

CONTROL OF MICROBIAL DISEASE IN RELATION TO PRODUCTIVITY

Somewhat different approaches are made to the control of major epidemics and endemic infections of intensively reared livestock. In the former, eradication is the ultimate aim, while in the latter, control measures are usually directed towards minimizing the effectof the infections on productivity, although attempts to establish disease-free herds have met with limited success in the livestock industry.

Major strides have been made towards the eradication of many costly animal diseases at the local and national levels. However, global eradication has been claimed for only one such infection, vesicular exanthema,[22] and the relatively recent isolation of this virus from marine mammals calls into question the validity of even this modest claim.[23] Nonetheless, the number of successes and the contributions that these have made to animal productivity are impressive. The main efforts have involved the vigorous application of quarantine and sanitary measures, including the compulsory slaughter of infected and contact stock. In some situations, widespread vaccination is an essential preliminary to the use of slaughter in order to reduce the prevalence of infection to economically manageable proportions. However, by using quarantine and sanitary measures alone, Great Britain eradicated rinderpest and contagious bovine pleuropneumonia at the end of the last century. Australia eradicated foot-and-mouth disease in 1872 and rinderpest in 1923. In Great Britain, the eradication of foot-and-mouth disease has been interspersed, sometimes with disastrous economic consequences, with repeated reintroductions of the virus from the carcasses of food animals imported from endemic areas. While eradication programs are costly, the benefits in terms of increased productivity are considerable. Through an intensive and successful vaccination campaign, rinderpest was eradicated from Burma in 1958, and the government of that country estimated that this resulted in an annual saving of $5 million. Eradication of brucellosis in Sweden eliminated an annual $7 to 10 million food loss. In the U.S., the bovine tuberculosis eradication program cost $326 million over a period of 40 years, but the resulting saving was estimated at $150 million/year.[20] In Canada, Wells[24] claimed in 1964 that the control efforts against just three diseases, bovine tuberculosis, brucellosis, and hog cholera, saved food worth $27 million, a figure that was considerably greater than the whole operating budget of the government agency involved.

Unfortunately, disease eradication is not always possible. Reid[25] listed certain general and specific requirements for disease eradication, some of which cannot always be met. The general requirements included stable government, the support of the local population, and, sometimes, financial and technological assistance. Clearly, political instability can lead to the diversion of manpower and funds from disease control, and the illegal movement of livestock and their products can render quarantine measures useless. Todd[26] described two historical examples of the spread of infectious disease of livestock in Europe as a result of smuggling, and Cockerill[27] referred to more recent problems in Latin-American countries. The need for financial and technological assistance in controlling the major epidemics is apparent from a study of the global distribution of these diseases, which tend to be more prevalent in less-developed countries.[2]

Among the specific requirements for disease eradication[25] are the identification of cases and carriers and the removal of reservoirs of infection. Although some diseases can be readily recognized in a population, others such as brucellosis and tuberculosis may require sophisticated laboratory or field procedures for their identification, and even these may leave something to be desired in terms of sensitivity and specificity. In some areas, the system of livestock husbandry, such as nomadic grazing,[28] makes effective disease control impossible. The establishment of an infection in the wildlife population makes eradication from domesticated stock unusually difficult; under these circumstances, vaccination gives greater hope of success as a control procedure than the application of a slaughter policy.

Vaccination programs have played a major role in the control of microbial diseases in farm livestock, with corresponding gains in productivity. Particular success has been achieved in Africa, initially as a result of the pioneer work carried out at the Onderstepoort Research Institute. Some of the data given by Jansen[29] on the use of vaccines in South Africa provide an impressive record of the scope of the practice and its effectiveness in terms of increased productivity. One of the earliest vaccines to be introduced was against anthrax, for which vaccination is compulsory in affected areas. Only 18 outbreaks of anthrax were recorded in 1967, compared with 1121 in 1927. Millions of doses of vaccine are produced annually against bluetongue and African horsesickness. The latter disease, which had earlier killed up to 40% of the horses in one season, has virtually disappeared from South Africa. Jansen[29] indicated that 105 million doses of vaccine directed against 27 diseases were being manufactured annually at Onderstepoort. It is clear that the costs of such an operation are considerable, although if the use of vaccines is well planned, the recovery of the costs in terms of increased productivity may be anticipated. Henderson[10] discussed several aspects of vaccination programs in relation to foot-and-mouth disease, emphasizing the need for the vaccination of a high proportion of all susceptible species, revaccination at appropriate intervals, and adequate facilities for the storage, distribution, and quality control of the vaccines. The application of some vaccines in the field may be limited by cost factors; increasingly, cost-benefit analyses[6] are sought as a basis for the financing of national vaccination programs. Felton and Ellis[30] demonstrated a 50% annual return on investment in a large scale rinderpest vaccination campaign in Nigeria in which there was a tenfold reduction in the number of outbreaks.

The endemic infections of intensively reared livestock present control problems that are somewhat different in character. Although effective control of epidemic disease is a prerequisite for intensive husbandry, which involves the rearing of genetically improved stock in large groups so as to minimize labor costs, the intensity involved has created disease problems that are more severe than under less intensive conditions. Mild or subclinical infections assume major importance because of the low-profit margins involved, and productivity can only be increased and maintained if a high standard of preventive medicine is practiced. This trend towards larger units of highly productive animals is now well developed in the poultry, dairy, beef, and swine industries.

Many of the infections that cause losses in intensively produced livestock are extremely widespread, making eradication feasible only at the local level. This involves the isolation of individual production units and the introduction of new stock only from sources of known health history. An extreme example of this concept is the use of specific pathogen-free (SPF) animals for the repopulation of herds and flocks — newborn animals are obtained free of infection by hysterectomy or hysterotomy and reared in strict isolation. This technique was pioneered for swine in the U.S.[31] and there have been fairly extravagant claims for the productivity benefits of the procedure. Although interpretation of the latter is frequently difficult, one study showed that in one SPF swine herd in Britain, the feed conversion rate was 2.8 as compared with a national average of 3.95.[32] Other workers have stressed the problems of maintenance of SPF pigs[33] and poultry.[34] Undoubtedly, the exclusion of infections that are widespread in the environment or in the general animal population is extremely difficult. Organisms can be brought into intensive units in food and bedding, by attendants, or through the air.[35] There is some evidence that airborne disease may be preventable in buildings ventilated with filtered air under positive pressure.[36]

The value of vaccines in controlling endemic infections such as bovine mastitis, coliform infections in young animals, and respiratory infections in calves is less well established than in the major epidemic diseases discussed previously. Their use in controlling endemic infections attests more to the intractable nature of the infections than to a proven prophylactic value.

In the control of bovine mastitis, considerable success has been attained with the application of sanitation measures coupled with the strategic use of antibiotics, which can minimize the spread of infection within herds. However, some infected cows are untreatable and must be culled. Notable productivity successes have been claimed in mastitis control, such as an average gain per cow of nearly 2.5 lb of butterfat in the first year of a control program in California[20] and a substantial increase in the production of higher quality milk in New York as a result of that state's mastitis program.[37] A mastitis-control scheme in Norway reduced the annual loss of milk by $2.3 million, providing a return of $32 per dollar invested in control.[13]

Finally, some reference should be made to the use of feed medication as a disease-control measure in intensive animal production. The inclusion of suitable concentrations of antibiotic or chemotherapeutic substances in the diet as a prophylactic against coccidiosis and mycoplasmosis in poultry has been both spectacularly successful and economically sound.[38] Feed medication has been widely practiced in the swine industry in the control of enteric disease due to bacterial infection in piglets, and medicated early weaning has been suggested recently as a method of obtaining piglets free from certain bacterial pathogens in the herd of origin.[39] The pharmacological basis for the routine use of antimicrobial food additives to improve general performance is less sound than the strategic use of medication against specific infections because the mechanisms involved in the former situation are poorly understood, although antibiotic growth promoters have undoubtedly contributed to productivity. However, concern over the possible transference of drug resistance from animal to human strains of enteric bacteria has cast doubts on the wisdom of the widespread use of antibiotics in this way.

Areas that require further attention in relation to the control of endemic microbial disease include more widespread epidemiological studies of the infections involved and improved disease monitoring so that economic losses may be better characterized. An exciting area is the development of computer simulation in the design, evaluation, and monitoring of animal disease control programs. Success has already been demonstrated for this technique when applied to brucellosis,[40,41] bovine mastitis,[40] and dairy calf mortality.[42]

REFERENCES

1. **Lewis, D. and Swan, H.**,The role of intestinal flora in animal nutrition, in *Microbes and Biological Productivity,* Hughes, D. E. and Rose, A. H., Eds., Cambridge University Press, Cambridge, 1971, 149—175.
2. **Derbyshire, J. B.**, Microbial disease and animal productivity, in *Microbes and Biological Productivity,* Hughes, D. E. and Rose, A. H., Eds., Cambridge University Press, Cambridge, 1971, 125—147.

3. **Blaxter, Sir Kenneth,** The limits to animal production, *Vet. Rec.,* 105, 5—9, 1979.
4. **Steele, J. H.,** The development of disease surveillance: its uses in disease control that relate to public and animal health, in *Animal Disease Monitoring,* Ingram, D. G., Mitchell, W. R., and Martin, S. W., Eds., Charles C Thomas, Springfield, Ill., 1975, 7—19.
5. **Ingram, D. G., Mitchell, W. R., and Martin, S. W., Eds.,** *Animal Disease Monitoring,* Charles C Thomas, Springfield, Ill., 1975.
6. **Schwabe, C. W. and Ruppanner, R.,** Animal diseases as contributors to human hunger. Problems of control, *World Rev. Nutr. Diet.,* 15, 185—224, 1972.
7. **Scott, G. R.,** Rinderpest, *Adv. Vet. Sci.,* 9, 113—224, 1964.
8. **Lancaster, J. E. and Alexander, D. J.,** Newcastle disease virus and spread, *Can. Dep. Agric. Monogr.* No. 11, 1975.
9. **Woode, G. N.,** Transmissible gastroenteritis of swine, *Vet. Bull. (London),* 39, 239—248, 1969.
10. **Henderson, W. M.,** Foot and mouth disease: a definition of the problem and views on its solution, *Br. Vet. J.,* 126, 115—120, 1970.
11. **Eichhorn, E. A.,** To protect our food supply, *Americas* (Washington, D.C.), 5, 3—5 and 42—43, 1953.
12. **Beveridge, W. I. B.,** Economics of animal health, *Vet. Rec.,* 72, 810—815, 1960.
13. **Anon.,** The economic losses caused by animal diseases, in *Animal Health Yearbook, 1962,* Food and Agriculture Organization, Rome, 1963.
14. **Ellis, E. M. and Kendall, H. E.,** Public health and economic effects of vesicular stomatitis in a herd of dairy cattle, *J. Am. Vet. Med. Assoc.,* 144, 377—380, 1964.
15. **Nelson, F. C. and Saucier, A.,** Dry Cow Management, Ayerst Laboratories, Montreal, 1973, 3.
16. **Leech, F. B.,** Food losses through animal diseases, *Proc. Nutr. Soc.,* 20, 20—24, 1961.
17. **Wiseman, A., Selman, I. E., Msolla, P. M., Pirie, H. M., and Allan, E., The financial burden of infectious bovine rhinotracheitis,** Vet. Rec., *105, 469, 1979.*
18. **Thomson, R. G.,** Pathology and pathogenesis of the common diseases of the respiratory tract of cattle, *Can. Vet. J.,* 15, 249—251, 1974.
19. **Loew, F. M.,** A theoretical effect of fever on feed efficiency in livestock, *Can. Vet. J.,* 15, 298—299, 1974.
20. **Schwabe, C. W.,** *Veterinary Medicine and Human Health.* 2nd ed., Williams & Wilkins, Baltimore, 1969, 461—470.
21. **Anon.,** Preliminary report on the African swine fever epizootic in Cuba. Methods of diagnosis and control, *Off. Int. Epizoot. Bull.,* 75, 415—437, 1971.
22. **Bankowski, R. A.,** Vesicular exanthema, *Adv. Vet. Sci.,* 10, 23—64, 1965.
23. **Prato, C. M., Akers, T. G., and Smith, A. W.,** Serological evidence of calicivirus transmission between marine and terrestrial mammals, *Nature (London),* 249, 255—256, 1974.
24. **Wells, K. F.,** The role of the Health of Animals Branch in zoonosis, *Can. J. Public Health,* 55, 93—99, 1964.
25. **Reid, D.,** General aspects of disease eradication, *Vet. Rec.,* 84, 626—627, 1969.
26. **Todd, F. A.,** Defense against imported animal diseases, *Adv. Vet. Sci.,* 4, 1—50, 1958.
27. **Cockerill, W. R.,** The changing status of animal quarantine, *Br. Vet. J.,* 119, 338—349, 1963.
28. **Wilde, J. K. H.,** East Coast fever, *Adv. Vet. Sci.,* 11, 207—259, 1967.
29. **Jansen, B. C.,** Past, current and future control of epizootic diseases in South Africa, *Trop. Anim. Health Prod.,* 1, 96—102, 1969.
30. **Felton, M. R. and Ellis, P. R.,** Studies on the control of rinderpest in Nigeria, Veterinary Epidemiology Unit, Department of Agriculture, University of Reading, England, 1978.
31. **Young, G. A.,** SPF swine, *Adv. Vet. Sci.,* 9, 61—112, 1964.
32. **Heard, T. W. and Jollans, J. L.,** Observations on a closed, hysterectomy-founded pig herd, *Vet. Rec.,* 81, 481—487, 1967.
33. **Goodwin, R. F. W.,** The possible role of hysterectomy and related procedures for the eradication and control of pig diseases in Britain, *Vet. Rec.,* 77, 1070—1076, 1965.
34. **Cooper, D. M.,** Poultry: principles of disease control. I. Production of specific pathogen-free stock by management-environment control, *Vet. Rec.,* 86, 388—396, 1970.
35. **Hyslop, N. St. G.,** Observations on pathogenic organisms in the airborne state, *Trop. Anim. Health Prod.,* 4, 28—40, 1972.
36. **Drury, L. N., Patterson, W. C., and Beard, C. W.,** Ventilating poultry houses with filtered air under positive pressure to prevent airborne diseases, *Poult. Sci.,* 48, 1640—1646, 1969.
37. **Fincher, M. G.,** "Crash plan" — New York State mastitis control program, *Vet. News,* 26, 9—10, 1962.
38. **Oakley, R. G.,** Poultry: principles of disease control. IV. Medication, *Vet. Rec.,* 86, 429—430, 1970.
39. **Alexander, T. J. L., Thornton, K., Boon, G., Lysons, R. J., and Gush, A. F., Medicated early weaning to obtain pigs free from pathogens endemic in the herds of origin,** Vet. Rec., *106, 114—119, 1980.*

40. **Morris, R. S. and Roe, R. T.,** The use of computer simulation in the design, evaluation and monitoring of animal disease control programs, in *Animal Disease Monitoring,* Ingram, D. G., Mitchell, W. R., and Martin, S. W., Eds., Charles C Thomas, Springfield, Ill., 1975, 80—101.
41. **Hugh-Jones, M. E.,** Brucella: a computer model of bovine brucellosis, in *Animal Disease Monitoring,* Ingram, D. G., Mitchell, W. R., and Martin, S. W., Eds., Charles C Thomas, Springfield, Ill., 1975, 102—112.
42. **Martin, S. W. and Wiggins, A. D.,** A model for the economic costs of dairy cattle mortality, *Am. J. Vet. Res.,* 34, 1027—1031, 1973.
43. Anon., African swine fever — an emerging problem, *Vet. Rec.,* 103, 129, 1978.

EFFECTS OF POLLUTION ON ANIMAL PRODUCTIVITY

Harry E. Smalley

Before we address ourselves to current pollution problems, we must first define the terms pollution and animal productivity and include or exclude certain aspects of these that would becloud the issues beyond recognition.

What is pollution? A graphic word currently in vogue to denote a highly undesirable condition. By definition, to pollute is to contaminate an environment with man-made wastes. Is this enough? We have ample evidence of whole countries, even the world, being exposed to clouds of noxious gases and dusts caused by volcanic eruptions, which contribute many times more noxious gases and dusts to the atmosphere than has man during his entire existence. Can we exclude these because they are not man-made? Could we not use the word contaminate? The definition of contaminate is "to render unfit for use by introduction of unwholesome or undesirable elements." I prefer the use of contaminate not only because it has a more precise definition, but also because it excludes the words "wastes" and "environment." Many of our contamination problems arise from elements or compounds not considered as "wastes" but merely as matter out of place.

The word environment has been used so extensively and so often incorrectly that a backlash has evolved to the point that those who use it are derided as being fanatics — "A man who is determined that the millions of tons of crude sewage that goes into Lake Erie every year should be free from DDT".[1]

To further define our terms, animal productivity is that productivity leading to utilization by man of major animal products, i.e., meat, milk, and fiber. We will only mention by-products, such as manure for fertilizer, and certain body constituents, such as hyperimmune sera or endocrine glands, for hormone production. Also excluded are wild, companion, and laboratory animals, exotic fur-bearers (e.g., mink and chinchilla), and beasts of burden (e.g., water buffalo and camel).

We are all aware that many of the toxic elements are essential to life in very low doses; many compounds increase productivity when used sparingly or in correct proportions to other elements and to the diet. Additionally, some are utilized by lower orders, with a resultant better balance of nature. We must recognize two dictums here long recognized by the toxicologists: The first is the difference between hazard and toxicity, the *possibility* of harm, and the *probability* of harm. The classic example is that of the bottle of poison on the shelf that is not in itself harmful until someone drinks it. Second is the fact that only the dose of any chemical determines its toxic effect. Ingestion of too much water can kill just as effectively as too much cyanide; the effects are the same, but the dosage makes the difference.

The harmful effects of contamination can be direct or indirect; they may be immediate or long-lasting; they may affect the animal or the consumer of the animal; or they may affect the progeny of the animal. Contamination of the atmosphere may affect the animal directly when it is breathed into the body; or, more likely, the contaminant settles upon the animal's feed and is ingested later. Indirect effects include contamination of growing plants to the extent that they become unavailable to the animal as feed. Upon introduction of the contaminants to the body, the animal may die or its metabolism may be slowed to the extent that growth or weight increase is inhibited. Those who consume the animal may be affected, while the animal itself exhibits no toxic effects; or the animal may not be obviously affected, while the offspring may die or be deformed to the extent that further reproduction is impossible.

In addition, the harmful effects of contaminants may include all gradations in between. It is of great concern that, while the animal may not be affected, chemical residues of the compound may contaminate the meat to the extent that it is rendered unfit for consumption.

Sources of contamination in the atmosphere must be necessarily linked to man, despite the earlier reference to volcanic action. Tremendous and increasing industrialization throughout the world and mismanagement of wastes and emissions have concomitantly increased the flow of contaminants into the "biggest wastebaskets in the world", — the sea and the atmosphere. However, we have recognized that even these huge depositories have limits; dilution or dispersion can no longer be considered the solution due to high concentrations over small areas. Localized contamination episodes have been recognized for many years. Hydrogen sulfide or sulfur dioxide in closed swine houses and lethal ammonia accumulations in closed poultry houses, for instance, were recognized early and were relatively easily corrected by opening a window. Larger scale regional episodes were recognized as well and had a much greater impact not only on man but also on domestic animals and regional productivity. Air inversion episodes in Donora, Pa., London, the Meuse and Ruhr valleys in Europe, and New York City received publicity because of dramatic loss of human life.

The classic instance of regional loss of productivity, which occurred in Copper Hill, Tenn., received little publicity until recent years. Effluent from extensive copper smelting operations before 1900 led to complete denudement of some 7000 acres, partial or complete denudement of an additional 17,000 acres, and measurable harm seen on a total of 70,000 acres. This episode remained of local interest only, even after Hursh's classic monograph in 1948 in which he showed that the effects of contamination were not only long-standing but affected parameters little recognized at the time.[2] The completely denuded area of 7000 acres not only lost all vegetation and ground cover, but also lost soil nutrients and even the biota, including microorganisms necessary to support life of any kind. He found that the climate itself changed: The ambient temperature rose 2° to 4°F during the summer and was from 0.6° to 2°F lower during winter; the soil temperature was 22°F higher during the summer, rainfall was lower but disasterous, and wind velocity was 5 to 15 times higher than the surrounding area. Although these effects alone were negative enough, later workers found that adjacent areas were harmed to the extent that, although foliage slowly returned, the more hardy and prolific weeds and woody plants essentially predominated. In addition, trees further away from "ground zero" were weakened and much more susceptible to diseases and invasion and attack by harmful insects. In spite of the fact that this indirect effect of contamination was localized by geography and climate and limited to forests, the fact remains that, in Copper Hill, there are approximately 70,000 acres which have been out of production since the late 1800s.

Intolerable in this enlightened age? Perhaps. But consider this: The number of ore smelters has increased by many thousands since that time. New manufacturing processes, new types of plants, and new products have increased contamination beyond the point-source effects seen in Tennessee. Fluoride emissions have been studied probably more extensively and for a longer period of time than other toxic chemicals. Fluoride emissions from aluminum works, super phosphate factories, steel works, and enamel and ceramic factories contribute up to 20 kg of fluoride gases for each ton of aluminum produced, very often in isolated parts of the world.[3] Other contaminants in the atmosphere include sulfur and ammonia gases, carbon monoxide, nitrogen oxides, ozone, particulate matter, and others, as well as combinations of these. Plant losses due to industrial emissions have been estimated at $85.6 million annually, but these figures are admittedly low.[4] Industrial emissions having a direct toxic effect upon livestock include arsenic, beryllium, cadmium, lead, manganese, mercury, molybdenum, magnesium, copper, sulfur, selenium, titanium, vanadium, zinc, and others.[3]

More contaminants are being recognized due to greater sophistication in methods of collecting and quantitating harmful levels. It must be emphasized at this point that much of the evidence accumulated is circumstantial at best, or derived from laboratory tests on laboratory animals. Many judicial proceedings have limited admission of evidence to the crucial questions: Is the contaminant present on feedstuffs? Did the animal actually eat the contaminated feed or graze? Did the contaminate actually do the damage in the animal? Did the contaminate come from the source indicted? There are so many variable conditions involved in pollution episodes that it is extremely difficult to prove an actual cause and effect.

Industrial emissions not only contribute to the contamination in the atmosphere, but also to contamination in the water. Many of the same contaminants are found in the latter and may be concentrated to a higher degree, although their introduction into the animal is still essentially by ingestion and has nearly the same effects. Inhalation of toxic particles or direct deposition on skin can cause problems, but not to the same extent that ingestion can. Therefore, the primary concern of this chapter will be to consider the effects of ingested contaminants, with minor mention of the other effects.

ARSENIC (AS)

Arsenic is an element found in high levels in coal and other ores. It has been discovered to be one of the industrial contaminants emitted from copper smelting plants. The earth's crust has been found to contain about 10 ppm As, naturally, and because it is poorly taken up by plants, As ingestion by animals has been from deposits on the surface of plants from atmospheric fallout. Levels of up to 33 kg As per kilometer^2 per year have been recorded, and plants have been found to have levels of greater than 227 mg/kg dry weight.[5] As is usually in low concentration in natural waters, probably due to fixation to iron-hydroxide. Certain localities, e.g., New Zealand, of the world are known to have high levels of As in water naturally and may even protect animals from selenium-accumulator plants.[6] A standard of 0.05 mg/ℓ As in drinking water has been set by the U.S. Public Health Service.

The toxicity of As depends upon its state of oxidation; the trivalent form is more toxic than the pentavalent; and the inorganic form is more toxic than the organic. As behaves primarily as a nonmetallic agent, but recently inorganic As was found to be converted to the organic form through methylation by intestinal flora.[7] Chronic toxicity due to ingestion of As is relatively rare due to a certain built up tolerance and a rapid urinary excretion rate; however, tissues do become saturated, and toxicity is often found to be a function of solubility (see Table 1).

Symptoms of As poisoning due to acute exposure are well known and indicate acute G.I. distress, along with inflammation of oral, nasal, and ocular mucous membranes. Staggering, thirst, emaciation, salivation, and prostration are frequently seen. Postmortem lesions are nearly pathognomonic, with an intense, rosy-red inflammation of the G.I. tract. Chronic intoxication of cattle due to ingestion is relatively rare, but not unknown; its symptoms are emaciation, rough hair coat (with some loss of hair), eczema, and occasionally muscular paralysis. Very low levels of As tend to increase appetite, accentuate the bloom and hair coat, and clear inflamed eyes.

Exposure of cattle to dermal deposits of As are known through dipping for tick infestations and spraying. Intoxication by As has been reported to one tenth the oral dose and would hardly be expected from atmospheric contamination.[12] Ocasionally, cattle show a rosy-red skin reaction following dipping and exposure to sunlight;

Table 1
LETHAL SINGLE ORAL DOSE OF INORGANIC TRIVALENT ARSENIC (g)[8]

Species	Arsenic trioxide (insoluble)	Sodium arsenite (soluble)
Horse	10—45	1—3
Cow	15—45	1—4
Sheep	3—10	0.2—0.5
Pig	0.5—1.0	0.05—0.1
Fowl	0.05—0.3	0.01—0.1

Reeve's report suspects carcinogenic activity following dermal exposure in man, but this has not been proven.[13,14]

After single doses, As is eliminated from the body rather quickly through the urine and is almost entirely excreted within 3 days, but exposed cattle should be withheld from market for 6 weeks following chronic poisoning.[11]

As poisoning has been seen in cattle, horses, and sheep grazing on pastures near smelters.[7,9-11] Milk yield has been lowered by as much as 12.5% among cattle grazing near these smelters, and butterfat has been reduced by 8%. Abortions and failure to breed have been greater in the contaminated than in the noncontaminated area.[15,16]

Ruminants may selectively graze contaminated pastures, apparently developing a taste for As.[8] Because this element is used extensively as a dessicant on cotton in the form of arsenic acid and monosodium acid methanearsanate (MSMA), levels as high as 600 ppm have been found in cotton-gin trash and cotton burrs. Therefore, producers should not use these waste products as roughage. Residues in the liver were reported as 5.5 to 60 ppm and 8.8 ppm in muscles of cattle exposed to 300 ppm MSMA for 7 days.[17]

BERYLLIUM (BE)

Beryllium is relatively abundant in coal and its pyrolysis products; with the current depletion of oil and gas fuels and increased use of coals, especially from Kentucky, stack emissions from coal-burning operations show concentrations well above acceptable levels. Additionally, liquification and gasification of coal yield not only higher concentrations of Be but much higher amounts within the atmosphere.[18]

Inhalation studies in the laboratory showed that there are serious problems when exposure is prolonged at rather high rates. Exposure for 14 days at levels of 100 mg/m^3, 51 days at 50 mg/m^3, and 100 days at 1 mg/m^3 was lethal.[19] Effects included typical pneumonitis symptoms such as labored breathing, mucosal irritation, coughing, convulsions, and death. Changes in nitrogen metabolism were seen probably due to competitive inhibition of certain metabolic enzymes. By far the most serious effects due to Be exposure were found after prolonged (6 to 9 month) exposures and included inflammatory changes leading to fibrosis and thickening of alveolar walls and, on continued exposure, to epithelial proliferation and neoplasia — cancer.[20]

CADMIUM (CD)

The exact place of the element Cadmium in the natural order of the body has not been precisely determined. Certainly Cd has been used for years in metal plating and in Cd-nickel or Cd-silver alloys. Fairly recent studies done on incineration of various synthetic plastic materials have shown that Cd is present in the fly ash of incinerated polyethylene and polyvinylchloride plastics in excess of 1%; it was found at lower levels (less than 100 ppm) in pyrolysis of polystyrene and phenolic resins. Some adhesive tapes, notably the cellulose-base (clear) tapes, release high levels (>1%) of Cd upon incineration, while lower levels (100 ppm) are found on incineration of colored embossing tapes.[21] Cd has been found in ground water contaminated by electroplating wastes at 3.2 mg/ℓ and in mine water at more than 1000 mg/ℓ.[22]

Episodes of acute toxicity due to inhalation of Cd are rare and have been done mostly in the laboratory. When rabbits, goats, and rats were exposed to Cd fumes in doses of up to 1000 min mg/m^3 (referring to minutes of exposure times fume concentration), an acute pulmonary edema developed 24 hours after exposure and led to proliferative interstitial pneumonitis; 250 min mg/m^3 dose levels led to permanent lung damage, primarily a fibrosis or scar tissue formation.[23] The sequence of pathological events appears to be lung edema leading to acute respiratory distress. If the animal recovers, there is a pneumonitis and finally pulmonary emphysema. Cd is distributed throughout the body and localized in the kidney with little excretion.

Ingestion of Cd by swine, as an anthelminthic containing 0.044% Cd anthranilate, revealed increased susceptibility in this species, with deaths approaching 50%. Necropsies showed anemia, enlarged spleen, enlarged mulberry-shaped heart, and fatty degeneration in liver and kidney.[24] Analysis of milk samples from 61 different localities showed an average content of between 0.017 and 0.030 ppm. The safe level for man has been determined to be 0.01 ppm, and the toxic level is 3 mg.[25] Lambs were found to prefer drinking water contaminated with 12 mg Cd/ℓ to noncontaminated water.[26] Certain water plants, e.g., naiad weeds, appear to concentrate Cd, contaminating the water at levels of up to 5000 ppm.[27]

Apparently, ingested or inhaled Cd is concentrated in the kidneys, and dose-related structural changes in tubular epithelium have been noted. These changes impair renal reabsorption and excretion mechanisms, resulting in loss of urinary protein, amino acids, glucose, and certain enzymes; Cd concentrations in the kidney reached a plateau at 271 ppm, and this is regarded as the critical renal level above which toxicity results.[28] Toxic manifestations due to renal impairment of tubular reabsorption and excretion include copper deficiency and anemia, iron deficiency and anemia, and zinc deficiency. Additionally, calcium metabolism is impaired, the indirect results of which are bone growth and osteomalacia.

FLUORIDES (F)

Airborne fluoride has caused more damage to domestic animals than has any other atmospheric contaminant. Voluminous reports and excellent reviews have been cited in the literature for many years.[29-37] Much work has been done concerning the researching and detailing mechanisms of toxicity, in the field and in the laboratory, but only highlights are given here.

Sources of airborne F include volcanoes, emissions from industrial plants producing phosphate fertilizers, aluminum, iron, steel, tile, enamel, and brick, and other industries. Combustion of coal and incineration of certain plastics add to the burden, as does production of fluoride itself and defluorination of rock phosphate for mineral supplements in feed. Additionally, F is found in groundwaters at toxic levels.

The great majority of F toxicosis cases occur as a result of ingestion of F deposited on vegetation rather than direct inhalation of F itself. Fluoride-contaminated vegetation can be consumed directly in pastures and grazing lands or as hay stored for relatively long periods in barns. Hay stored in the open can also become contaminated because there is little or no uptake of F by the growing plant. Fluorosis is, simply, due to airborne contaminants being deposited on feed.

As with all airborne contamination, the degree of F deposition varies directly with prevailing winds from the source, distance, rainfall, type and solubility of F, length of exposure, and efficacy of precautions and management practices at the source.

Ruminants are most affected due to their slower digestion rate, which permits longer alimentary absorption time; horses, swine, poultry, and man are not as affected because of less exposure.

Acute fluorosis in domestic animals is rare, primarily because animals refuse to eat vegetation heavily contaminated with F. In one study, however, signs of acute poisoning included staggering gait, muscular tremors, excitability, and conjunctivitis.[38]

The symptoms of fluorosis in cattle have been well defined and include dental and skeletal changes leading to lameness, stiffness, lack of appetite, muscular weakness, emaciation, and death.

Long-term ingestion of F-contaminated vegetation apparently interferes with calcium metabolism in the teeth and bones. The mottling of teeth is often the first sign of fluorosis and includes a softening of the enamel, which wears quickly to the point that the animal cannot masticate properly. Skeletal changes involve calcification of ligaments and bony outgrowths, or exostoses, chiefly on the lower leg. Exostoses are painful and interfere with normal use of the legs; they undoubtedly play a major role in lameness and in refusal of the animal to rise. It is believed that F, when present in amounts greater than 25 ppm in the forage over a short period of time, induces lameness in cattle.

Excessive dental wear leads to poor digestion of food, with consequent loss of weight, condition, appetite, rumination, and milk production, as well as lowered butterfat content of the milk.

F in serum concentrations of two to ten times that found normally in teeth and bone, i.e., 1.5 to 400 ppm in teeth and bones, respectively, has apparently proven to be indicative of fluorosis. Little deposition of F in soft tissue is encountered, although this is not unknown, and levels found in muscle tissue do not constitute a threat to the consumer. Small quantities of F may cross the placenta, but excessive levels in calves are thought to be due to milk ingestion.

Ingestion of vegetation containing F at levels of 15 ppm led to dental fluorosis and bone and joint lesions after 30 days.[39] Death occurred in animals that consumed hay containing F levels of between 0.01 to 0.1% (100 to 1000 ppm) within several weeks to 1 month.[40] The threshold value for cattle is thought to be consumption of 2 to 3 mg F per kilogram body weight per day.[41]

Since many of the F-emitting industrial plants are found in Utah, Washington, and Oregon, sheep have been studied rather extensively, but do not differ markedly from cattle. Levels of F on vegetation above 15 ppm produce dental and skeletal effects and, in addition, cause abortion in ewes. There is apparently greater movement of F across the placenta in sheep than in cattle.[42]

Growth in chicks was seriously depressed when they were fed rock phosphate containing F at a level of 3% of the diet. The 3% rock-phosphate diet depressed egg production in layers by 8%.[43]

The immune response to several bacterial diseases (including anthrax) in man, pigeons, rabbits, and other animals was lowered by the presence of F in the diet.[44]

Aluminum sulfate or aluminum chloride salts are often used in mineral blocks to partially counteract the effects of F; its retention in bones was found to be reduced by 30 to 45%.[45]

LEAD (PB)

Lead is widely distributed throughout nature, and these naturally occurring Pb salts are usually insoluble; the least soluble salt is lead sulfide (PbS), the most prevalent form. Pb is found in the earth's crust as lead sulfate ($PbSO^4$), and concentrations generally do not exceed 15 mg/g. Pb from automobile exhaust is in particulate form as lead bromochloride; from smelters it is found as elemental Pb, PbS, or $PbSO_4$.[46] Certain microorganisms have the ability to methylate the inorganic Pb to an organic form. Gasoline, lead-based paint, and the insecticide lead arsenate contain significant amounts of Pb and are sources of toxicity for both man and animals. In addition, Pb is found in discarded storage batteries, fumes from industrial concerns, Pb seams in utensils or containers, and in pottery glaze. Lead mine tailing leachate has been suspect as well. Lead poisoning is considered to be the most prevalent form of accidental poisoning in the U.S. and ingestion of lead-based paints is the method by which this poisoning occurs most frequently. Toxicity due to inhaled Pb has only been reported rarely, and there is some question of those few instances.

Cattle are the species which are usually affected by Pb poisoning. There have been numerous reports made of cattle grazing on pastures contamined by Pb emissions from factories.[5] While the form of Pb ingested is water insoluble, gastric juices render it fairly soluble, and it is readily absorbed. In contaminated areas, the Pb content of hay and silage has ranged up to 139 ppm; uncontaminated hay has background levels of up to 1.8 ppm. A value of 0.15 mg/m^3 of Pb is considered to be the maximum permissible atmospheric concentration for cattle.[5]

Dollahite and Younger have found that horses are ten times as resistant as cattle to chronic Pb poisoning, a finding that contrasts with those of earlier workers.[47] Singer has reported an increased incidence of Pb from automobile exhaust systems, contaminating pastures near busy highways and intersections.[48] Sheep are believed to be more resistant than cattle, but this may represent the greater vigilance of shepherds in keeping flocks farther from civilization.

Swine are susceptible to both inhaled and ingested Pb, but there are few instances of airborne contamination reported in the literature. Ingestion of Pb by swine has occurred in garbage-feeding operations, but such reports have been sparse recently.

Lead is absorbed and stored mainly in the liver, kidneys, and bone; it is accumulative in these tissues, and signs of poisonings are generally not seen until a blood-lead level of 0.35 to 0.45 ppm is seen.[49] Lead affects the synthesis of heme and inhibits enzyme activity in several reactions involving free sulfhydryl groups. Signs of acute Pb poisoning are nonspecific, i.e., loss of appetite, constipation, rough hair coat, salivation, delirium, and reduced milk yield. Signs of chronic Pb poisoning are emaciation, cachexia, nervous disorders, convulsions, blindness, anemia, weakness, diarrhea, incoordination, stupor, and rough hair coat. Abortions are often seen in chronic Pb poisoning, and calves have shown Pb residues in their bodies from ingestion of contaminated milk as well as from cross-placental movement.

Pb is slowly excreted in the urine after removal of contamination, with bone-lead remaining in the animal for weeks or even months. The use of calcium ethylene-diamine-tetra-acetic acid (Ca-EDTA) as a Pb chelator has been advocated with variable success. It is known that Ca itself affords some degree of protection and hastens excretion as well. Tissue levels, except for high blood levels, do not give as good a correlation with levels of ingestion, as might be expected; calves consuming 100 ppm Pb for 100 days had liver and kidney Pb residues of 2.3 and 4.7 ppm, respectively. Lead poisoning is complicated by interactions and translocations of Cu, Fe, and Zn. All these may be present in atmospheric contamination from smelters and industrial effluents.

MERCURY (HG)

Mercury poisoning in animals has been primarily due to direct contamination of feedstuffs. Hg has been used extensively as a fungicide on seeds; accidental consumption of such mercury-treated grain has accounted for most of the toxic catastrophes in livestock. It is widely distributed in the environment, and the normal concentration in the earth's crust is estimated at 50 to 80 μg/kg.[6] Hg occurs as a free metal, and mercury sulfide as fumes from certain industrial processes. Inhalation of Hg can be fatal at 1 to 2 mg/m^3. Ingestion of Hg by livestock from atmospheric pollution is rare. However, due to industrial emissions into water, Hg is mentioned as a major contaminant causing mercurialism in humans or Minamata disease. Although animals have been affected, the effects in humans who have ingested contaminated fish are so horrible and dramatic that world-wide attention has been focused upon such catastrophes.[49] Other episodes of human illness due to ingestion of Hg-contaminated pork have received extensive notice as well.

Hg accumulates in the tissues of animals, primarily in the liver and kidneys, and is quite toxic, especially in the organic form. Excretion is through the feces and is slow; thus, there is an accumulation in the liver. Metabolically, Hg interacts with sulfhydryl groups in certain enzymes and serves to block their action; nervous symptoms predominate.[50]

ENVIRONMENTAL POLLUTANTS

Pollution control has become an extremely important issue that has been recognized for years but emphasized greatly only in the last few years. Population surveys show that environmental cleanup ranks behind only inflation and unemployment as the major public concern. Reasons for this concern have been listed and include esthetics, damage to material, damage to vegetation, harm to wildlife and domestic animals, and protection of human health. With regard to the major air pollution problems identified below, the order of public concerns indicated above can be understood. The original and most important air pollutants to be identified are suspended particles, sulfur dioxide, oxides of nitrogen, carbon monoxide, ozone and peroxacetyl nitrates (PAN), hydrocarbons, noise, toxic materials, agricultural dust, and pollen. With the exception of toxic materials, and rare instances of the others, there has been little concrete evidence of damaging effects on livestock in actual field situations. As mentioned before, laboratory conditions reveal their potential toxicity, but most of the atmospheric pollutants mentioned here occur in highly industrialized, urban areas. All air pollution problems are caused by high concentrations of contaminate in rather localized areas, and this concentration is generally reduced by the time dispersal to rural areas is noted. Certainly carbon monoxide is lethal at high concentrations, but these concentrations are rarely found in farming situations. The major elemental toxic contaminants covered in this chapter have caused harm to livestock in field situations. A number of other contaminants have been reported, such as copper, iron, manganese, selenium, zinc, chromium, nickel, vanadium, molybdenum, and cobalt, but these are more than adequately covered elsewhere in this series.

Control of air pollution depends mainly upon control at the source. Through 1975, industry has spent over $6.6 billion in attempting to comply with regulations. Their efforts have been partially successful. Sulfur dioxide levels in urban areas have declined more than 50% since the 1960s; average ambient total suspended-particulate levels have declined by 26% during this same period despite an overall increase in emissions.

Similarly, water pollution is a very visible and exciting problem, especially in urban and suburban areas. This is logical because most water pollution is due to urban activities, e.g., domestic sewage, industrial wastes, and storm drain discharges. Agricultural runoff of fertilizer and agricultural chemicals are well recognized contributors to the burden of water pollution, but their amounts are much less than those due to industrial contributions. Where atmospheric contaminants can be dispersed, contaminants in water are concentrated and can be a problem in waterways, but this is not generally the case in farming and ranching areas. The major problems in water pollution have been identified as reduction of oxygen levels and thermal pollution, and except for rare "blooms" of toxic algae, they do not present a problem to livestock. Of course, it can be argued that water pollution affects us all, and so it does, but the effects are extremely hard to quantify. Another exception, more common than algae blooms, is the contamination of water supplies with nitrates from fertilizers; unfortunately, children are most susceptible to nitrate poisoning and incidences are increasing. Nitrate poisoning in animals is seen generally as a result of direct application of fertilizers to growing crops and graze.

Water pollution is not only highly visible, but the means for controlling it are visible as well. In contrast to air pollution, water pollution is primarily a community contribution, e.g., sewage; control has been funded, therefore, from public expenditures to the amount of some $3.3 billion. Water quality has been improved primarily through increased sewage treatment efforts.

Recently, several instances have shown that the problems of pollution or contamination are more widespread than was previously thought. Pentachlorobenzene (PCB) has been found to be ubiquitous in its distribution, due to its widespread use in electrical transformers and in carbon paper; its use in these situations and many others has been banned. Other halogenated compounds, notably pentabromobenzene (PBB) were distributed, in error, over large areas of the Midwest with disastrous results to the livestock industry. A highly toxic contaminant (9TCDD or dioxin) has been found in some widely used herbicides — 2, 4, 5, T, — and its use has raised a number of questions in the human population. Chemical waste disposal sites have become major concern in that migration of toxic chemicals through the soil and possibly into the water supply may prove harmful to the human population as well as the food animal population. Contamination of feed and foodstuffs by microorganisms, fungi, or mycotoxins, has been detected and is currently being investigated.

The effects of these recently exposed hazards have not been thoroughly researched or evaluated as yet. Some are very adequately covered elsewhere in this series and do not fall within the scope of this chapter. The effects of pollutants, or contaminants, on livestock have been, and can be, considerable. However, these effects must be considered in relation to all other effects. Correlations are only indicative of a problem, and evidence is often circumstantial. Efforts to clean up the environment are succeeding, at great cost, but they will ultimately benefit us all.

REFERENCES

1. **Ebling, F. J. and Heath, H. W., Eds.,** Future of man, *Symp. Inst. Biol.,* 20, 197, 1972.
2. **Hursh, C. R.,** Local climate in the copper basin of Tennessee, *U.S. Dep. Agric. Circ.,* No. 744, 1948.
3. **Allcroft, R.,** Fluorosis in farm animals. The effects of air pollution on living material, *Symp. Inst. Biol.,* 8, 95—102, 1959.
4. **Bartik, M.,** Industrial poisonings of domestic animals, *Vet. Med. (Prague),* 12, 52—53, 1962.
5. **Lillie, R. J.,** Air pollutants affecting performance of domestic animals, *U.S. Dep. Agric. Agric. Handb.* No. 380, 1972, 20.
6. **O'Hara, P. J.,** personal communication, Agric. Bur., New Zealand, 1967.
7. **Lakso, J. U. and Peoples, S. A.,** Methylation of inorganic arsenic by mammals, *J. Agric. Food Chem.,* 23, 674—676, 1975.

8. **Clarke, E. G. C. and Clark, M. L.,** *Garner's Veterinary Toxicology,* 3rd ed., Williams & Wilkins, Baltimore, 1967, 477.
9. **Bartik, M. and Havassay, I.,** Toxicosis of animals caused by arsenic exhalations from thermal power plants and metallurgical plants, *Veterinarstvi,* 13, 460—462, 1963.
10. **Phillips, P. H.,** The effects of air pollutants on farm animals, in *Air Pollution Handbook,* Section 8, Magill, P. L., Holden, F. R., Ackley, C., and Sawyer, F. G., Eds., McGraw, New York, 1956, 1—12.
11. **Strauch, D.,** Death came with industrial smoke, *Ubersicht,* 10, 217—219, 1959.
12. **Selby, L. A., Case, A. A., Dorn, C. R., and Wagstaff, D. J.,** Public health hazards associated with arsenic poisoning in cattle, *J. Am. Vet. Med. Assoc.,* 165, 1010—1014, 1974.
13. **Smalley, H. E.,** personal observation, 1968.
14. **Reeves, G. I.**The arsenical poisoning of livestock, *J. Econ. Entomol.,* 18, 83—89, 1925.
15. **Harkins, W. D. and Swain, R. E.,** The chronic arsenical poisoning of herbivorous animals, *J. Am. Chem. Soc.,* 30, 928—946, 1908.
16. **Hradil, M., Masek, J., and Hais, K.,** Experiments to evaluate the economic losses caused by the effect of industrial exhalations on the productivity of beef in the Ostravia region, *Veterinarstvi,* 14, 462—474, 1964.
17. **Dickinson, J. O.,** Toxicity of the arsenical herbicide monosodium acid metharasonate in cattle, *Am. J. Vet. Res.,* 33, 1889—1892, 1972.
18. **Luckens, M. M.,** Some aspects of the toxicology of beryllium, *Proc. 1st Int. Congr. Toxicology,* Academic Press, New York, 1977.
19. **Stokinger, H. E., Ashenburg, N. J., and DeVoldre, J.,** Acute inhalation toxicity of beryllium, *Arch. Ind. Hyg. Occup. Med.,* 1, 398—410, 1950.
20. **Vorwald, A. J. and Reeves, A. C.,** Pathologic changes induced by beryllium compounds, *Arch. Ind. Health,* 19, 190— 199, 1959.
21. **Scott, R. O.,** Problems in trace element analysis, *Trace Element Metabolism in Animals,* Mills, C. F., Ed., E. & S. Livingstone, Edinburgh, 1970, 497—504.
22. National Research Council, Nutrients and Toxic Substances in Water for Livestock and Poultry, Report of Subcommittee on Nutritional Toxic Elements in Water, National Academy of Sciences, Washington, D.C., 1974.
23. **Paterson, J. C.,** Studies on the toxicity of inhaled cadmium. III. The pathology of cadmium smoke poisoning in man and in experimental animals, *J. Ind. Hyg.,* 29, 294—301, 1941.
24. **Alber, C. L.,** Cadmium toxicity in swine, *Vet. Med. J.,* 58, 893, 1963.
25. **Murphy, G. K. and Thea, U.,** Cadmium and silver content of market milk, *J. Dairy Sci.,* 51, 610—613, 1968.
26. **Doyle, J. J. and Pfander, W. H.,** Acceptability by lambs of cadmium in feed and water, *Nutr. Rep. Int.,* 9, 273—276, 1974.
27. **Cearley, J. E. and Coleman, R. L.,** Cadmium toxicity and accumulation in southern Naiad, *Bull. Environ. Contam. Toxicol.,* 9, 100—101, 1973.
28. **Cousins, R. J., Barber, K. A., and Trout, J. R.,** Cadmium-induced anemia in growing pigs: protective effect of oral or parenteral iron, *J. Anim. Sci.,* 36, 1122—1124, 1973.
29. **Allcroft, R.,** Fluorosis in farm animals. The effects of air pollution on living material, *Symp. Inst. Biol.,* 8, 95—102, 1959.
30. **Cass, J. S.,** Fluorides: A critical review. IV. Response of livestock and poultry to absorption of inorganic fluorides, *J. Occup. Med.,* 3, 471—543, 1961.
31. **Huffman, W. T.,** Effects on livestock of air contamination caused by fluoride fumes, *U. S. Tech. Conf. Air Pollution Proc.,* McGraw-Hill, New York, 1952, 59—63.
32. **Largent, E. J.,** The effects of air-borne fluorides on livestock, Air Pollution, *U.S. Tech. Conf. Air Pollution Proc.,* McGraw-Hill, New York, 1952, 64—72.
33. **Pedini, B.,** Clinical observations of fluorosis in cattle, *Vet. Ital.,* 18, 23—26, 1967.
34. **Shupe, J. L., Miner, M. L., and Greenwood, D. A.,** Clinical and pathological aspects of fluorine toxicosis in cattle, *Ann. N.Y. Acad. Sci.,* 11, 618—637, 1964.
35. **Suttie, J. W.,** Fluorosis in livestock, *Proc. Am. Coll. Vet. Toxicol.,* 2, 64—68, 1964.
36. **Lillie, R. J.,** Air pollutants affecting the performance of domestic animals, U.S. Department Agric. Handb. No. 380, Government Printing Office, Washington, D.C., 1972, 41—61.
37. **Underwood, E. J.,** *Trace Elements in Human and Animal Nutrition,* 3rd ed., Academic Press, New York, 1971, 369—402.
38. **Botija, R. S.,** Fluorine poisoning of cattle from industrial processes, *Rev. Patron. Biol. Anim.,* 1, 183—196, 1955.
39. **Boddie, G. F.,** Fluorine alleviators: a review, *Vet. Rec.,* 67, 827—830, 1955.
40. **Cristiani, H. and Gautier, R.,** Chronic poisoning from ingestion of fluorine, *C. R. Soc. Biol.,* Paris, 92, 139—141, 1925.

41. **Klussendorf, R. C.,** Fluorosis, *N. Am. Vet.*, 35, 585—586, 1954.
42. **Liegeosis, F. and Derivaux, J.,** Several cases of chronic fluorosis in sheep, *Ann. Med. Vet.*, 100, 221—224, 1956.
43. **Halpin, J. G. and Lamb, A. R.,** The effect of ground phosphate rock fed at various levels on the growth of chicks and on egg production, *Poult. Sci.*, 11, 5—13, 1932.
44. **Fridlyand, I. G.,** The effect of industrial poisons on the immunobiological state of the organism, *Gegiena i Sanitariya*, 24, 55—61, 1959.
45. **Greenwood, D. A., Shupe, J. L., Stoddard, G. E., Binns, W., Miner, W. L., Nielson, H. M., Bateman, G. Q., and Harris, L. E.,** Fluorosis in cattle, *Utah Agric. Exp. Stn. Spec. Rep.*, 17, 1—36, 1964.
46. **Olson, K. W. and Skogerboe, R. K.,** Identification of soil lead compounds from automotive sources, *Environ. Sci. Technol.*, 9, 227, 1975.
47. **Dollahite, J. W., Younger, R. L., Crookshank, H. R., Jones, L. P., and Petersen, H. D.,** Chronic lead poisoning in horses, 1977, *Am. J. Vet. Res.*, 39(6), 96—964, 1978.
48. **Singer, R. H.,** personal communication, Central Kentucky Animal Disease Diagnostic Laboratory, Lexington, Ky., 1976.
49. **Buck, W. B., Osweiler, G. D., and Van Gelder, G. A.,** *Clinical and Diagnostic Veterinary Toxicology*, 2nd ed., Kendall Hunt, Dubuque, Ia., 1976, 319—332.
50. **Doyle, J. J., Spaulding, J. A., and Smalley, H. E.,** Low level ingestion of metallic ions in the environment, Toxic and essential trace elements in meat — a review, J. Anim. Sci., 47, 398—419, 1978.

Index

INDEX

A

B

C

D

E

F

G

H

I

M

N

O

P

Q

R

S

T

U

X

Y

Z

16 x 3 + 3